ESSENTIAL NOTES IN
GENERAL
SURGERY

Mohammed Othman Almaimani

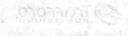

Order this book online at www.trafford.com
or email orders@trafford.com

Most Trafford titles are also available at major online book retailers.

Print information available on the last page.

ISBN: 978-1-6987-0355-8 (sc)
ISBN: 978-1-6987-0356-5 (hc)
ISBN: 978-1-6987-0354-1 (e)

Library of Congress Control Number: 2020924671

Because of the dynamic nature of the Internet, any web addresses or links contained in
this book may have changed since publication and may no longer be valid. The views
expressed in this work are solely those of the author and do not necessarily reflect the
views of the publisher, and the publisher hereby disclaims any responsibility for them.

Trafford rev. 06/24/2021

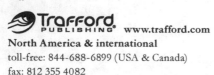

www.trafford.com
North America & international
toll-free: 844-688-6899 (USA & Canada)
fax: 812 355 4082

Contents

Section I
Basic Surgical Principles

Section II
General Surgery

Section III
Subspecialty

Preface

Essential Notes in General Surgery is a summary of years of work, after reading several text books, articles, attending the conferences, hospital daily rounds, and many review courses.

It is précis, digested, updated and provides essential knowledge that will help you pass the board exams, especially the American, Canadian, and Saudi board exams.

This book was designed to be sufficiently used by medical students, general surgery residents and senior general surgeon.

The book contains basic knowledge of the anatomy, physiology, pathology as well as history, physical examination, investigation, detailed management, operative intervention, and follow-up of each disease.

The material is divided into three main sections:
- Basic surgical principles
    Fluids, hemostasis, shock, surgical infection, trauma, wound healing, and critical care
- General surgery
    Upper GIT, Colorectal, Hepatobiliary, and Endocrine surgery
- Subspecialty
    Pediatric, Vascular, Bariatric and Thoracic surgery.

Acknowledgments

In the name of the Almighty Allah, the beneficent and most merciful. We are immeasurably thankful to Allah, whose blessings flourished our thoughts and thrived our ambitions.

To **my parents**, thank you for everything you have done in my entire life, for your love and support throughout my academic career. There is no way for me to express my utmost gratitude and thanks to you two.

I thank my wife, sweetheart, and best friend, **Shaimaa Althubaity**. Through the good and bad times, you have always been there for me.

I thank my sons, **Othman and Abdulrahman**, who endured my absence and motivates me to be the best.

I thank my brother and sisters.

Special thanks to **Mansul H. Amsud** for typing the book.

Special thanks to **Khalaf Shehab** for algorithms and figures design.

I thank the general surgery departments in Makkah City: **Al Noor** Specialist Hospital, **KFH, KAAH** and **KAMC** for their support.

Mohammed Othman Almaimani
General Surgery Senior Registrar
Pediatric Surgery Fellow

Section I

Basic Surgical Principles

Fluid and Electrolyte

Body Fluids

Total Body Water
- The total body weight contains 50%–60% water. It differs from male to female.
- Lean tissue (i.e., muscles and solid organs) has more fluid than fat and bones.
- Obese people has 10%–20% less body water than the normal population.
- An infant's total body weight is 80% water. At the end of its first year, it decreases to 65%.

Fluid Compartments
- The total body weight is 60% water, which is distributed as follows:

% Of total body weight	Volume of TBW	Male (70 kg)	Female (60kg)
Transcellualar <1%		500 mL	500 mL
Plasma 5%	Extracellular Volume	3500 mL	2500 mL
Interstitial Fluid 15%		10.500 mL	7500 mL
Intracellular Volume 40%	Intracellular Volume	28.000 mL	20.000 mL
Total		42.500 mL	30.500 mL

1

Spaces

1st Intracellular fluid (ICF)

2nd ECF (plasma, interstitial, transcellular)

3rd Always no physiologic fluid (peritoneum, pleura)

NB Transcellular fluid: it is the smallest component of extracellular fluid. These fluids are contained within <u>epithelial</u> lined spaces e.g. CSF <u>aqueous humor</u>, inner ear fluid, <u>joint fluid</u> and respiratory secretions.

Composition of Fluid Compartment

Plasma		Interstitial		ICF	
Cation	**Anion**	**Cation**	**Anion**	**Cation**	**Anion**
Na$^+$ 142	Cl 103	Na$^+$144	Cl 114	K$^+$ 150	HPO$_3$ 150
K$^+$ 4	HCO$_3$ 27	K$^+$ 4	HCO$_3$ 30	Mg^{++} 150	SO$_4$ 150
Ca$^+$ 5	Protein 16	Ca^{++} 3	Protein 1	Na$^+$ 10	Protein 40
Mg^{++} 3		Mg^{++} 2			

Osmotic Pressure

$$\text{Molal} = \frac{N}{Vol.\ in\ kg}$$

$$\text{Molar} = \frac{N}{Vol.\ in\ Liter}$$

- Number of particles per unit volume (mmol/L)
- Number of electric charges per unit volume (mEq/L)
- Number of osmotically active per unit volume (mOsmol/L)
- Equivalent = atomic weight (g)/valance
- For Na$^+$ (univalent) 1 mEq = 1 mmol
- For Mg^{++} 2 mEq = 1 mmol
- Serum osmolarity = $2\,Na^+ + \frac{Glucose}{18} + \frac{BUN}{2.8}$
  $\approx$ 290–310 mOsmol in each compartment.

Body Fluid Changes

- A healthy person consumes 2 L/day.
- 75% of oral intake is fluid, and 25% is extracted from solid food.

- Daily fluid losses are 800–1,200 mL in urine (sensible), 200–600 mL in sweating, and 250 mL in stool (sensible).
- Insensible loss is 600 mL, 75% by skin (evaporation) and 25% by lungs.
- Kidney excretes a minimum of 500–800 mL/day to clear metabolites, regardless of intake.
- Normally, the daily intake of salt is 3–5 g.
  → Balanced by kidney, it can excrete 1–500 mEq/day.

Classification

    a. Volume   b. Concentration   c. Composition

  A. **Volume**

    By osmoreceptor and baroreceptor
- Osmoreceptor: the kidney either excretes or reabsorbs through the thalamus & vasopressin.
- Baroreceptor: a specialized pressure sensor in the aortic arch and carotid sinus, responds to neural stimulus (sympathomimetic and parasympathomimetic) or hormonal renin-angiotensin-aldosterone, ANP.

  B. **Concentration**
- Total body water reflects serum Na^+ level.
- Normal range of Na^+ 135–145 mEq/L.
- **Hyponatremia**, classified as follows:
  - Hypervolemic hyponatremia
    - The most common type
      → Excess water intake or administration of IV hypotonic fluid
    - Postoperative patient → ↑ ADH → ↑ reabsorption of water by the kidneys
  - Normovolemic hyponatremia
    - Drugs such as ACE inhibitor, antipsychotic, antidepressant
  - Hypovolemic hyponatremia
    - ↓ intake, vomiting, NGT, or diarrhea

Symptoms
- Nausea, vomiting, headache, confusion, fatigue, irritability, weakness, spasm or cramps, seizures, and coma

NB:
- Pseudohyponatremia: (hyperglycemia, hyperlipidemia, hyperproteinemia) $\rightarrow$ shift of water from ICF to ECF.
  - $\rightarrow$ For every increase of 100 mg/dL in plasma glucose
  - $\rightarrow$ $\downarrow$ Na^+ by 1.6 mEq/L

- **Hypernatremia**
  - Loss of water or gain in Na^+
  - Serum osmolarity > 300 and urine Na^+ > 20 mEq/L
    - Hypervolemic hypernatremia
      - Administration of IVF with Na^+ such as normal saline, $NaHCO_3$, mineralocorticoids, congenital adrenal hyperplasia
      - Cushing syndrome
    - Normovolemic hypernatremia
      - Diabetes insipidus, diuretic use, renal disease, or from nonrenal water loss from the GI tract or skin
    - Hypovolemic hypernatremia
      - Isotonic GI fluid losses such as that caused by diarrhea
      - Hypotonic skin fluid losses such as loss due to fever or losses via tracheostomies during hyperventilation
      - Water loss caused by thyrotoxicosis
      - Use of hypertonic glucose solutions for peritoneal dialysis.
      - Urine sodium concentration is < 15 mEq/L
      - Urine osmolarity is > 400 mOsm/L

Symptoms are rare unless > 160 mEq/L.
- Confusion, muscle twitching, seizures and coma

Sodium Deficit = 0.6 × weight × (desired Na^+ − actual Na^+)

C. Composition Changes
Potassium (K^+)
- Intake is 50–100 mEq/day.
- Normal range is 3.5–5 mEq/L.
- Excretion by kidneys is 10–700 mEq/day.
- Only 2% of total K^+ is located in ECF.
- K^+ in ECF: 4.5 mEq/L × 14 L = 63 mEq.
- Minor change can have major effect on heart.

- **Hyperkalemia**
    - ↑ intake
    - Hemolysis, rhabdomyolysis, crush injury
    - Acidosis → ↑ ECF osmolality → shift K^+ to ECF
    - Spironolactone, ACE inhibitor, NSAIDs
    - ARF, CRF
    Symptoms
    CNS: weakness to paralysis
    CVS: arrhythmia, cardiac arrest
    ECG: peaked T wave, wide QRS complex, flattened P wave, and prolonged PR interval (first-degree block)

- **Hypokalemia**
    - Much common than hyperkalemia
    - ↓ intake, ↑ excretion, e.g., loss of GI section, diarrhea, enterocutaneous fistula, NGT, alkalosis
    - Potassium decreases by 0.3 mEq/L for every 0.1 increase in pH
    - ↓ Mg^{++} → decrease Mg^{++} intracellular → release of Mg^{++}-mediated inhibition of ROMK channel → ↓ K^{++} secretion from intracellular

- Symptoms related to failure of normal contraction, ileus, constipation, ↓ tendon reflex, paralysis.
- ECG: U wave, flattening T wave

K^+ deficit = (normal K^+ − measured K^+) × body weight × 0.4

Calcium (Ca⁺⁺)

- Vast majority is in the bone.
- Extracellualr Ca^{++} represents 1% of total calcium in the body.
- Normal range is 8.6–10.5 mg/dL.
- Three forms are as follows:
    - Protein bound, 40%
    - Complex to phosphate or another ions, 10%
    - Ionized, 50%
- Ionized is responsible for neuromuscular stability.
- decrease in Ca^{++} 0.8 mg/dL for every decrease of 1 g/dL in albumin.
- Acidosis ↓ Ca^{++} binding to protein → ↑ ionized Ca^{++}.
- Daily intake is 1–3 g.

- **Hypercalcemia**
    - Above 8.5–10.5 mg/dl
    - Or above ionized Ca^{++} 4.2–4.8 mg/dL
      Causes: hyperparathyroidism in outpatients and malignancy in hospitalized patients
    - Symptoms: nausea, vomiting, constipation, abdominal pain, confusions, headache, and depression
    - ECG: prolonged PR–QRS, high-voltage QRS, flattening of T wave

- **Hypocalcemia**
    - Causes: pancreatitis, necrotizing fasciitis, renal failure, small bowel fistula, hypothyroidism, toxic shock syndrome, low Mg^{++}, and tumor lysis syndrome from hyperphosphatemia
    - Transient after parathyroid adenoma excision → bone hunger

- Malignant with osteoblastic activity: lung, breast and prostatic CA.
- Symptoms: paresthesia in face, extremities, muscle cramps, carpopedal spasm, stridor, tetany.
- Chvostek sign (spasm when tapping over facial nerve)
- Trousseau sign (spasm when pressure over nerve and vein of upper limb)
- ECG: prolonged QT, inverted T wave

Phosphate

- Primary intracellular, energy production.
- Controlled tightly by renal excretion.

Hyperphosphatemia

- ↓ urine excretion, ↑ intake
- Mostly in renal failure
- Hypoparathyroidism, hyperthyroidism
- Rhabdomyolysis, tumor lysis syndrome, hemolysis, sepsis, hyperthermia, malignant hyperthermia
- Laxative: sodium phosphate
- If hyperphosphatemia prolonged → metastatic deposition of calcium-phosphorus complexes in the soft tissue.

Hypophosphatemia

- Most cases due to shift of phosphate to ICF in response to respiratory alkalosis, insulin therapy and hungry bone syndrome.
- Symptoms related to adverse effect on O_2 availability and ↓ energy.

Magnesium (Mg^{++})

- Fourth most common mineral in the body.
- Normal range 1.3 – 2.1 mEq/L
- Half in the bone and ⅓ is complex to albumin,.
- Normal daily intake is 400 mg/day.

- **Hypermagnesemia**
    - Antacids, laxative, TPN, massive trauma, thermal injury, severe acidosis
    - Symptom: neuromuscular dysfunction similar to hypercalcemia
    - ECG similar to hyperkalemia

- **Hypomagnesemia**
    - Mg^{++} depleted in critically ill
    - Kidney is responsible for Mg^{++} and Ca^{++} homeostasis
    - Prolonged IVF, TPN, not sufficient Mg^{++}
    - Alcohol abuse, amphotericin B
    - Diarrhea, primary aldosterone, acute pancreatitis
    - ECG: inversion of P wave or flattened, torsades de pointes.

Acid-Base Balance
- The important buffer intracellularly is protein, phosphate and extracellularly is bicarbonate and carbonic system.
- Compensation of acid-base derangement by respiratory system for metabolic cause and metabolic mechanism if respiratory cause (Kussmaul breathing).
- Change in ventilation in response to metabolic derangement mediated by H^+ sensitive receptor.
- Acidosis stimulates chemoreceptor to increase ventilation, and alkalosis decreases it.
- Kidney compensates respiratory abnormalities by ↑ or ↓ bicarbonate, and it is delayed compensation for 6 hrs to days.

Metabolic Acidosis
- Increase acid intake, increase generation of acid, or significant loss of HCO_3 → Kussmaul respiration, increase HCO_3 reabsorption and H^+ execration.
    - **Anion gap (AG)** $= Na^+ - (CT + HCO_3)$
    - Normally is < 12.
    - Correct AG = actual AG − (2.5 [4.5 − albumin])

- Metabolic acidosis with high AG
  - Ingestion of exogenous acid, salicylate, methanol.
  - $\uparrow$ production of acid, ketoacidosis, $\uparrow$ lactate, renal failure.
  - Common cause in surgery is lactic acidosis. Lactate is produced by hypoxic tissue.
    - $\rightarrow$ Treatment: resuscitation for adequate perfusion
  - The liver metabolizes lactate.
  - Administration of bicarbonate does not improve mortality and cellular function.
    - $\rightarrow$ Overzealous $\rightarrow$ alkalosis, curve shifts to the left
  - Interfere with $O_2 \rightarrow$ arrhythmia and increase intracellular acidosis to form carbonic acid
  - $HCO_3 + H^+ = H_2CO_3 \rightarrow CO_2 + H_2O \rightarrow$ higher $PCO_2 \rightarrow$ ventilation problem in patient already with respiratory distress.

- Metabolic acidosis with normal AG
  - Result of acid administration (HCl^-, NH_4) or from bicarbonate loss (e.g., diarrhea, fistula, ureterosigmoidostomy, or from renal losses).
    - $\rightarrow$ Carbonate loss and gain of Cl^-
      - $\rightarrow$ Proximal renal tubular acidosis from $\downarrow$ tubular reabsorption of HCO_3, while distal renal tubular acidosis from $\downarrow$ acid excretion

Metabolic Alkalosis
- Loss of acid or gain of bicarbonate.
- Associated with low K^+ because alkalosis enhances K^+ to enter the cell.
- Excess HCO_3, milk alkali syndrome, citrate in blood transfusion.
- Hyperchloremic metabolic alkalosis occurs in infant with pyloric stenosis or adult with duodenal ulcer.

- The loss in patent pylorus will be gastric, pancreatic, and biliary content.
    - → Urine HCO_3 is high, H^+ reabsorption + K^+ excretion.
    - → If hypokalemia persists → H^+ excretion → paradoxical aciduria.
- Treatment is volume repletion with isotonic saline

Respiratory Acidosis
- Retention of CO_2, hypoventilation.
- Delayed response from kidney, so correct by treating underlying cause.
- CNS: narcotic.
  Pulmonary: PE, atelectasis.
  Abdomen: abdominal compartment syndrome, distention.
- Treatment may require intubation after trial of noninvasive methods.

Respiratory Alkalosis
- Common in surgical patients because of alveolar hyperventilation caused by pain, anxiety, CNS injury.
- Drugs: salicylate, fever, gram-negative bacteria, thyrotoxicosis, hypoxemia.
- Treat the underlying cause of hyperventilation.

Fluid and Electrolyte Therapy
- Ringer's lactate is slightly hypotonic and contains 130 mEq/L of lactate, which is converted in the liver to bicarbonate after infusion (lactate more stable in storage than bicarbonate).
- Used in resuscitation in trauma.
- Normal saline: NaCl mildly hypertonic, contains 154 mEq/L of Na^+ and 154 mEq/L of Cl^-.
  Disadvantage → chloride load in kidney → hyperchloremic metabolic acidosis.
- Used to correct hyponatremia and replace GI losses.
- 5% dextrose (hypotonic) contains dextrose 50 g/L.
    - → 170 kcal/L to prvent catabolism + ½ NS to maintain osmolarity and prevent lysis of RBCs and.

Alternative Resuscitation Fluid
- Hypertonic saline is 3%, 5% to correct severe hyponatremia.
- 7.5% used in closed-head injury → ↑ perfusion, ↓ ICP, ↓ edema.
- Colloid (volume expander): high molecular weight, not used in severe hemorrhagic shock → enters the interstitial space and worsens the edema.
- Types: (1) albumin, (2) dextran, (3) hetastarch, (4) gelatin

1. Albumin
   - 5%, 25%
   - Induce allergic reaction and renal impairment
2. Dextran
   - Glucose produced by bacteria in sucrose media
   - 40,000–70,000 medium weights
   - Used to lower blood viscosity + normal saline → maintain IV volume
3. Starch (hetastarch)
   - Molecular weight is 1000 - 3000,000
   - 6% solution
   - Cause hemostatic derangement, ¯ vWF and factor VIII → renal dysfunction
   - Hextend, a modified form
4. Gelatin: Bovine collagen

Correction of Electrolyte Abnormality
Hypernatremia
- Treatment of water deficit.
- D5% or D5 in ¼ NS or enteral water.
  Water deficit = % body water × weight (kg) × $\frac{serum\,Na - 140}{140}$
- No more than 1 mEq/hr or 12 mEq /day → rapid correction → cerebellar edema, demyelination and herniation.

Hyponatremia
- Treatment with free water restriction.
- If severe, administer Na^+Cl^-.
- In normal patients, they usually become symptomatic if Na^+ is less than 120 mEq/L.
- Sodium deficit = 0.6 × weight (kg) × (desired Na^+- actual Na^+)

11

- Use 3% NS but no more than 1 mEq/hr until it reaches 130 mEq/L and maximum 12 mEq/L/day.

Hyperkalemia
- Stop exogenous K^+.
- Kayexalate 15–30 g in 20–100 mL of 20% sorbitol.
- Shift K^+ to intracellular with glucose + insulin and bicarbonate infusion.
  → Nebulizer albuterol (10–20 mg)
- When ECG changes, Ca^{++} gluconate or Ca^{++} chloride (5–10 mL 10% solution) over 10 min.
- If high K^+ persists → dialysis.

Hypokalemia
- Potassium deficit = (K^+ lower normal − K^+ measured) × body weight (kg) × 0.4.
- Oral KCl syrup if mild or asymptomatic.
- If symptomatic, correct K^+ deficit first then administer maintenance therapy.
- KCl 10 mEq diluted in 100 mL normal saline with no monitoring → can be up to 40 mEq/hr but through large veins, diluted in 200–400 mL normal saline, slowly over 2–4 hrs.

Hypercalcemia
- Treatment indicated if Ca^{++} is > 12 mg/dL.
- NS infusion to treat volume deficit + diuretic if severe hypercalcemia.

Hypocalcemia
- Asymptomatic → oral Ca^{++} carbonate 600–1,200 mg PO.
- Symptomatic → IV 10 mg Ca^{++} gluconate with concentration 10% over 10 min to achieve 7–9 mg/dL.
- If associated Mg, K^+ deficiency should be corrected.

Hyperphosphatemia
- Phosphate binder such as sucralfate or aluminum-containing antacid.
- Ca^{++} acetate tablet can be used.
- Dialysis if failed.

Hypophosphatemia

- If phosphate is 1–2.5 mg/dL,
    - → tolerating enteral nutrition → Neutra-Phos 2 packets Q6H.
    - → parenteral $KPHO_4$ (0.15 mmol/kg) IV over 6 hrs for 1 dose.
- If phosphate is < 1 mg/dL, IV $KPHO_4$ or $NapHO_4$ 0.25 mmol/kg over 6 hrs for 1 dose.

Hypermagnesemia

- Eliminate exogenous cause and correct acidosis.
- If acute symptom, Ca^{++} chloride 5–10 mL IV STAT.

Hypomagnesemia

- If asymptomatic, oral administration.
- If level 1–1.8 mEq/L, magnesium sulfate 0.5 mEq/kg in 250 cc NS IV over 24 hrs × 3 days.
- If < 1 mEq/L, magnesium sulfate 1 mEq/kg in 250 cc NS over 24 hrs × 1 day, then 0.5 mEq/kg in 250 cc NS IV over 24 hrs × 2 days.
- If severe, 1–2 g of magnesium sulfate IV over 15 min with monitoring.

Fluid Therapy
Preoperative

- IV fluid calculation:

    | First 10 kg | 100 mL/kg/day |
    | Second 10 kg | 50 mL/kg/day |
    | For every 1 kg | 20 mL/kg/day |

- Other formulas:
    - 4 mL/kg/hr for first 10 kg
    - 2 mL/kg/hr for second 10 kg
    - 1 mL/kg/hr for every kilogram
- Mostly D5 ½ NS 125 cc/hr + KCl^- 20 mEq/L.
- Consider volume deficit (GI and third space losses).
- Maintain UOP at 0.5–1 mL/kg/h.
- If hypernatremia, unsafe to give D5 alone; it should be accompanied with ¼ NS or RL.

13

Intraoperative

- During induction → compensatory mechanism lost → ↓ BP.
- Consider blood loss in major abdominal surgery.
- During major abdominal surgery, the water loss is 500–1,000 mL/hr.
- No colloid administration.
- Best is RL; in the past, it was NS (salt intolerance).

Postoperative

- Any deficit during preoperative or intraoperative therapy should be corrected with isotonic saline.
- Usually RL or NS for the first 24 hrs then change to D5% ½ NS + K^+.
- Should Replace deficit and all losses: NGT, drain, UOP + insensible losses.

Special Consideration Postoperative

- Don't exceed actual need.
- Early sign of volume overload is weight gain.
- Postoperative weight loss should be 0.23 kg.
- Symptoms of volume deficit: tachycardia, orthostasis, oliguria, and hemoconcentration.

Electrolyte Abnormalities in Specific Patients

Secretion on Inappropriate Antidiuretic Hormone (SIADH)

- After head injury or CNS surgery.
- Also associated with administered morphine, NSAIDs, oxytocin.
- Pulmonary and endocrine disease: hypothyroidism, glucocorticoid deficiency.
- Malignant: small cell CA (lung), pancreatic CA.
- Patient has euvolemic hyponatremia with elevation of urine Na^+.
- Furosemide to induced free water loss along with fluid restriction.

Diabetes Insipidus (DI)

- Disorder of ADH stimulation.
- Diluted urine with hypernatremia.
- Seen in closed-head injury, pituitary surgery.

- There is nephrogenic DI + low K^+ associated with contrast dye and use of aminoglycosides and amphotericin B.
- Diagnosis by high urine osmolarity in response to water deprivation.
- In mild cases free water replacement is adequate therapy.
- If severe → vasopressin 5 units SC Q6–8H.

Cerebral Salt Wasting
- Diagnosis of exclusion.
- Hyponatremia occurs with secondary events, which can be differentiated from SIADH.

Refeeding Syndrome
- Rapid excessive feeding in malnourished patient.
- Shifting metabolism from fat to carbohydrate → ↑ insulin release → ↑ cellular uptake of electrolyte Mg, K, Ca, phosphate, as well as glucose (hypoglycemia).
- Symptoms: arrhythmia, confusion, respiratory failure, death.
- Correct electrolyte and volume deficit.
- Add thiamine before feeding.
- To prevent: ↑ fat administration and ↓ carbohydrate with slowely progression.

Acute Renal Failure
- Azotemia → correct volume deficit.
- Acute renal tubular necrosis → fluid restriction.
- Correct high K^+.
- Hyponatremia is a result of breakdown of protein, fat, carb.
- Low Ca^{++}, high Mg^{++}, high phosphate.
- Measure ionized Ca^{++} as patient usually experiences hypoalbuminemia.
- Bicarbonate can benefit, but dialysis is a must.

Cancer Patients
- Hyponatremia by caused by diuretics, salt-wasting nephropathy, cisplatin.
- Cerebral salt wasting, SIADH.
- Hyponatremia also occurs with poor oral intake.
- Hypokalemia from diarrhea, chemotherapy and atrophy of villi
- Hypocalcemia: thyroid surgery, bone hunger, high phosphate.

-   Hypomagnesemia: cisplatin, hypophosphatemia, hyperparathyroidism
    → Low phosphate reabsorption, oncogenic osteomalacia, multiple myeloma
-   The tumor lysis syndrome occurs when tumor cells release their contents into the bloodstream, either spontaneously or in response to therapy, leading to the characteristic findings of hyperuricemia, hyperkalemia, hyperphosphatemia, and hypocalcemia.

Hemostasis

Biology of Hemostasis
1. Vasoconstriction
2. Platelet plug formation
3. Fibrous formation
4. Fibrinolysis

Vasoconstriction (VC)
- VC is an initial response, more evident in medium and large vessels, depending on smooth muscle.
- Subsequent link to platelet formation.
- TXA_2 is produced at the site of injury via release of arachidonic acid from the platelet membrane, a potent VC of smooth muscle + endothelin and serotonin (from injured vessel) released during platelet aggregation.
- Bradykinin and fibrinopeptide is involved in coagulation + VC.
- The extent of VC correlates with the degree of vessel injury.

Platelet Function
- Anucleate fragment from megakaryocyte.
- Count: 150,000–450,000.
- Up to 30% sequestrated in spleen, and average life span is 7–10 days.
- Platelet aggregation → thrombus formation.
- Injury to intimal layer (vWF) → exposes subendothelial collagen that allows platelet adhesion.
- vWF binds to glycoprotein (GP) I/IX/V on platelet membrane.
- Up to this point → primary hemostasis.
- Platelet aggregation is reversible.
- Arachidonic acid, which is released from the platelet membrane, is converted by cyclooxygenase to prostaglandins PGG_2; PGH_2 converted to TXA_2 which is a potent VC, ↑ platelet aggregation.
- Arachidonic acid may shutter and convert.
- Platelet cyclooxygenase inhibited by aspirin (irreversible) and NSAIDs (reversible), but not affected by COX-2 inhibitor.
- Second wave of platelet aggregation → fibrinogen required.
- Cofactor acting as bridge for GP IIb, IIIa in activated platelet.

- If platelet plug formed (irreversible).
- Thrombospondin: stabilized fibrinogen binding to activated platelet.
- Platelet factor 4 and α-thrombomodulin are secluded during this reaction.
- PF4 is a potent heparin antagonist.
- Second wave of platelet aggregation is inhibited by aspirin and NSAIDs and nitric oxide (NO).
- Alteration of phospholipid in platelet membrane (PF3) allows Ca^{++} and clotting factor bind platelet membrane.

Coagulation

- Hemostasis is a combination of interaction between platelet + endothelin + coagulation factor.
- Coagulation 2 pathways converting to common pathway.
- Intrinsic factors are XII → XI → IX → (VIII), then common pathway X → (V) → II → I.
- Extrinsic factors are tissue factors (III) → VII, then common pathway X → (V) → II → I.
- PTT measures: I, II, V, VIII, IX, X, XI, XII.
- PT (INR)measures: I, II, VII, X.
- Vitamin K and warfarin affect factor II, VII IX, X.
- Factor X + Va + Ca^{++} + phospholipid (prothrombin complex) convert prothrombin → thrombin → fibrinogen → fibrin.
- Last step, thrombin activates fibrinolysis inhibitor (TAFI), which stabilizes the colt.
- Balanced mechanism to prevent propagation of clot beyond site of injury.
    1. Feedback inhibition to deactivate cascade → activated protein C → inhibit factors V and VIII.
    2. Tissue plasminogen activator (tPA) is released from endothelin following injury → fibrinolysis.
- Tissue factor pathway inhibitor (TFPI) → block tissue factor and VIIa (7) complex.
- Antithrombin III inhibits tissue factor, VIIa.
- Activated protein C system with cofactor protein S inhibit factors V and VIII to form TF-7a.
- Factor V Leiden, resistant to cleavage by activated protein C.
- Plasmin degrades clot.

- Other major plasminogen activator is uPA (urokinase plasminogen activator).

Fibrinolysis
- Plasminogen → plasmin → degrade fibrous mesh → production of circulating fragment (fibrous degradation product or FDP) cleaned by liver, kidney.
- Clot lysis FDP → E-nodules, D-dimer.
- D-dimer is a marker for thrombolysis (fibrinolysis).

Coagulation Factor Deficiency
Four most common are the following:
1. Hemophilia A factor VIII
2. Hemophilia B (Christmas disease) factor IX
3. vWF disease
4. Factor XI deficiency

- Hemophilia A (VIII), Hemophilia B (IX)
  - Inherited sex-linked recessive disorder.
  - Severity depends on factor level in the blood:

    | < 1% | severe disease |
    | 1%–5% | moderate disease |
    | 5%–30% | mild disease |

  - Symptoms: hemarthrosis, ICH, GI hemorrhage.
  - Patient with moderate disease is less likely to bleed spontaneously but ↑ the risk with trauma or surgery.
  - Mild, no spontaneous bleeding, only minor bleeding after trauma or surgery.
  - Platelet function is normal, i.e., plug formation and aggregation.
  - For hemophilia A and B, give factors VIII and IX.
  - Consider factor VII if not received previously.
  - Activity level should be:

    | 30%–40% | in mild hemorrhage |
    | 50% | in severe bleeding |
    | 80%–100% | in life-threatening bleeding |

- von Willebrand's Disease (vWD)

- Most common congenital bleeding disorder.
- is characterized by a quantitative or qualitative defect in vWF
- vWF is a glycoprotein responsible carrying factor VIII and platelet adhesion.
- Symptoms: easy bruising, mucosal bleeding, menorrhagia in female.
  - Types:
Type I	partial quantitative
Type II	qualitative
Type III	total deficiency

  - Therapy:
Type I	responds to DDAVP
Type II	may respond to DDAVP
Type III	unresponsive and require vWF

- Factor XI Deficiency
  - Referred as hemophiliac.
  - Spontaneous bleeding is rare, but trauma or surgery can produce bleeding.
  - Treatment: FFP.
  - Each 1 mL of FFP contains 1 unit of factor XI.
  - Antifibrinolytic may be useful in menorrhagia.
  - Factor VII recommended in patient with factor XI antibody.

- Deficiency in Factors II, V, X
  - Bleeding is treated with FFP.
  - Half-life of factor II is 72 hrs, 25% needed to achieve hemostasis.

- Factor VII
  - Bleeding varies and does not always correlate with factor VII level.
  - Bleeding is uncommon unless < 3%.
  - Treatment: FFP or recombinant factor VII, half-life of 2 hrs.

- Factor XIII
    - Associated with liver failure, IBD, myeloid, leukemia.
    - Clot and coagulation is normal but with early fibrinolysis.
    - Treatment: FFP, cryoprecipitate, factor XIII.

Platelet Function Defect

- Either abnormal surface protein or platelet granules or enzyme defect.
- The major surface of protein abnormality is thrombasthenia (Glanzmann's disease) or Bernard-Soulier syndrome.
- Glanzmann's disease → lack or dysfunctional IIb/ IIIa → Tx is platelet transfusion.
- Bernard-Soulier syndrome defect in GP Ib/IX/V receptor, vWF necessary for platelet adhesion.
- Most common intrinsic platelet defect is storage pool disease, i.e., loss of dense granule.
- Treatment: DDAVP, if severe platelet transfusion.

Acquired Hemostatic Defect
Platelet Abnormalities

- Failure of production: bone marrow disorder; leukemia, vitamin B12 deficiency, folate deficiency, chemotherapy, radiotherapy
- Decrease survival with ITP, HITT, DIC, TTP
- Sequestration, portal HTN, lymphoma, Gaucher disease
- Massive transfusion, antiplatelet, liver disease

- **Quantitative**
    - Idiopathic thrombocytopenic purpura (ITP): impaired platelet production and T cell destructs the platelets.
    - Heparin-induced thrombocytopenia and thrombosis (HITT):
        - drug induces immunity against PF4 after exposure to heparin → thrombocytopenia + IV thrombosis.
        - Platelet ↓ 5–7 days after heparin administration.
        - Increase suspicions if platelet is < 100,000 or drops 50% of initial platelet count.

- Can occur with LMWH as well.
- Occurs in 17% with unfractionated 8% with LMWH.
- Diagnosis: serology or ELISA.
- Treatment: stop heparin or LMWH and start thrombin inhibitor (argatroban) for renal insufficiency and lepirudin, danaparoid with normal renal function.
  - Hemolytic uremic syndrome (HUS) → secondary to infectious E. coli or shigella associated with renal failure, HIV, SLE → plasmapheresis.
  - One unit platelet 5.5×10^{10} = increase 10,000.

- **Qualitative**
  - Aspirin, clopidogrel (Plavix), irreversible antiplatelet.
  - General recommendation to stop 5–7 days before elective procedure. If emergent operation → platelet transfusion.
  - Uremia → dialysis or DDAVP (desmopressin)

Acquired Hypofibrinogenemia
Disseminated Intravascular Coagulopathy (DIC)
  - Systemic activation of coagulation pathway → excessive thrombin generation and formation of microthrombi → depletion of platelet and coagulation factor → resultant classic picture of diffuse bleeding.
  - Fibrin thrombi developing in the microcirculation may cause microvascular ischemia and subsequent end-organ failure if severe.
  - Predisposing factor: severe hemorrhage, embolization of material from brain, bone marrow, amniotic fluid, severe pancreatitis, liver dysfunction, malignancy, snakebite, large aneurysm.
  - Diagnosis: low platelet, low fibrinogen level.
  - Treatment: FFP, cryoprecipitate, platelet, fibrinogen.
  - Heparin is not helpful.

Primary Fibrinolysis
- Acquired hypofibrinogen.
- Risk factor, prostate surgery when urokinase release during surgery.
- Treatment: antifibrinolytic, Ɛ-aminocaproic acid, or tranexamic acid that inhibits activation.

Myeloproliferative Diseases
- Polycythemia → spontaneous thrombosis, polycythemia vera, neoplasm.
- Treatment: low dose of aspirin, phlebotomy.

Coagulopathy with Liver Disease
- Liver synthesized many coagulation factors.
- Factors I, II, III, V, VII, VIII, IX, X, XI, XII, XIII, protein C, S, plasminogen are synthesized in the liver except factors VIII and vWF, which are synthesized in liver sinusoidal endothelial cells.
- IL-11: cytokines stimulate proliferation of hematopoietic stem cells and megakaryocytes → good for cancer patients as well as cirrhotic patients.
- Treatment of coagulation caused by liver disease is usually with FFP.
- If fibrinogen is < 200 mg/dL → cryoprecipitate, rich in factor VIII.

Coagulopathy in Trauma
- Acidosis, hypothermia, and dilution of coagulation factor are the components of the triad of death.
- Patient arrived with coagulopathy → ↑ mortality in the first 24 hrs.
- Tranexamic acid ↓ mortality.

Acquired Coagulation Inhibitor
- Most common antiphospholipid syndrome → lupus anticoagulant and anticardiolipin antibody.
- Arterial or venous thrombosis.
- Antiphospholipid antibody common with rheumatoid arthritis, Sjogren's syndrome.

Anticoagulation and Bleeding
- Spontaneous bleeding can happen with any anticoagulant.
- Heparin, LMWH, warfarin, factor Xa inhibitor, direct thrombin inhibitor.
- The most reliable is LMWH.
- Warfarin for long term treatment: DVT, PE, heart disease, MI.
    → ↓ effect of warfarin: OCP, barbiturate, estrogen, steroid
    → ↑ effect of warfarin: anabolic steroid, L-thyroxine, glucagon, cephalosporin
- Reversal, in emergency situation: FFP, vitamin K (it takes at least 6 hrs)
Life-threatening: prothrombin complex, FFP, factor VII, cryoprecipitate with vitamin K.
    → New generation: dabigatran, rivaroxaban, but no detectable level, no reversal → only dialysis, may be reversed by prothrombin complex.
    → If not urgent, stop 36–48 hrs when aPTT less than 1.3 times or INR 1.5, reversal not necessary.
- Patient on anticoagulant → stop heparin. If emergent surgery → protamine sulfate (can produce allergy).
- Vitamin K for biliary obstruction, malabsorption.
- Vitamin K is ineffective in hepatic failure.
- If patient for surgery and he is on warfarin → need (bridging) therapy, i.e., stop warfarin and start IV heparin.
    → Heparin should be held 4–6 hrs preoperative and restart 12–24 hrs postoperative along with warfarin.

Cardiopulmonary Bypass (CPB)
- Patient underwent CPB.
- contact with circuit tubing and membranes results in abnormal platelet and clotting factor activation, as well as activation of inflammatory cascades, that ultimately result in excessive fibrinolysis and a combination of both quantitative and qualitative platelet defect.
- Empiric FFP, cryoprecipitate used for bleeding.
- TEG gives better assay for coagulation.
- Platelet given when patient bleeds postoperative.
- Desmopressin stimulates factor VIII.

Local Hemostasis
- Mechanical Procedure
    - Oldest method: direct digital pressure.
    - Tourniquet if limb is bleeding.
    - Liver packing, Pringle maneuver if liver is bleeding.
    - Small vein → ligation.
    - Large vein → transfixation.
- Thermal Agent
    - Denaturation of protein that results in coagulation.
    - 20–100 mA.
- Topical
    - Absorbable, biologic, synthetic agent.
    - Absorbable: gelatin foam (Gelfoam), oxidized cellulose (surgicel), microfibrillar collagen (Avitene).
        - → Gelfoam: physical matrix for clotting initiation.
        - → Avitene: platelet adherence.
    - Biologic: Floseal, Vitagel.
    - Caution should be undertaken: thrombotic enter circulation → thrombosis.

Transfusion
Replacement Therapy
- 15% is −ve Rh.
- Administer Rh +ve for Rh −ve if not available, accepted unless female is in childbearing age.
- In emergent situation, −ve to all people but not more than 4 units → hemolysis.
- Crossmatch RBCs of donor and recipient.
- If antibody is present → avoid use.
- Crossmatch if administering dextran.
- Autologous transfusion (patient's own blood), 40 days before OR, but Hb > 11 and hematocrit > 34%; last donation should be 3 days before surgery.
- Another modality cell saver machine (in trauma or long surgery).

Banked Whole Blood
- Rarely done.
- Shelf life is 42 days.

- During storage, ↓ ADP, 2, 3 DPG, alter oxygen dissociation curve

  → acidic, ↑ lactate, ↑ K^+, ↑ ammonia.
- Recent evidence has demonstrated that the age of red cells may play a significant role in the incidence of inflammatory response and MOF.

Platelet

- Transfusion for thrombocytopenia.
- Shelf life is 120 hrs.
- One unit contains 50 mL.
- Therapeutic platelet level is 50,000–100,000.
- If the patient previously received platelet transfusion → HLA matching.

Fresh Frozen Plasma (FFP)

- Usual source of vitamin K dependent factor and is only source of factor V.
- Stored up to 5 days.

Tranexamic Acid (TXA)

- Antifibrinolytic agent.
- ↓ bleeding especially in CABG.
- ↓ risk of death due to ↓ hemorrhage by 21%.
- S/E: nausea, vomiting, blurred vision, DVT, PE, PV thrombosis.
- In urinary bleeding → TXA → ureter obstruction from thrombosis.
- Contraindicated in aneurysm, SAH.
- TXA: inhibit plasmin and plasminogen.
- TXA is ten times potent than aminocaproic acid.
- Not effective on platelet.
- Half-life is 2 hrs.
- No adjustment needed.

Indication for Replacement of Blood Products

- ↑ O_2-carrying capacity.
- Treatment of anemia → if Hb 10 and hematocrit is < 30%

→ RCT study compares Hb > 10 vs. Hb 7–9 → no difference in mortality.
- Volume replacement → blood loss up to 20% → crystalloid. If more, give blood (RBCs, platelet, FFP).

New Concept in Resuscitation
- New concept damage control resuscitation.
  → ½ death before reaching hospital and all nonpreventable.
  → Truncal trauma → shock → ↑ death.
- Defined as administer ≥ 4–6 units within 4–6 hrs.

Damage Control Resuscitation (DCR)
- Composed of permissive hypotension, decreased crystalloid administration, and immediate release and administer PRBCs, platelet, FFP.
- Rate is 1:1:1.

Complication of Transfusion
- Related to blood-induced pro-inflammatory response.
- 10%, less than 0.5% is serious.
- Transfusion-related acute lung injury (TRALI), 16%–20%.
- ABO hemolytic transfusion reaction, 12%–15%.
- Bacterial contamination, 11%–18%.

Nonhemolytic Reaction
- Febrile nonhemolytic reaction, ↑ temperature > 1°C, associated with transfusion (1% of transfusion).
- Cytokines of donated blood to recipient antibody.
- Decreased due to ↓ leukocyte in blood product.
- Treatment: paracetamol.
- Bacterial contamination is rare, −ve gram stain capable of growing at 4°C.
  → Mostly from platelet stored at 20°C.
  → FFP in container with water both repeated.
  → Death and sepsis, 25%.
  → Symptoms: chills, tachycardia, hypotension, abdominal pain, diarrhea.
  → Treatment: stop transfusion, blood culture.

$\rightarrow$ Adrenergic blocking agent and use leukocyte filter.

Allergic Reactions
- 1% with all transfusions.
- Usually mild rash, urticaria, and flushing, rarely anaphylactic shock.
- Caused by antibody of donor to recipient antigen.
- Affects all blood product, but platelet and FFP are common.
- Treatment: antihistamine; if shock $\rightarrow$ epinephrine and steroid.

Respiratory Complication
- Transfusion associated with circulatory overload (TACO).
    - $\rightarrow$ Rapid infusion of blood, plasma expander, crystalloid.
    - $\rightarrow$ Increase heart disease.
        - CVP should be monitored.
        - Overload, high CVP, dyspnea, cough, basal lung rales.
        - Treatment: diuresis, $\downarrow$ blood administer rate.

- Transfusion-related acute lung injury (TRALI)
    - Noncardiogenic pulmonary edema.
    - Occurs with transfusion of any blood product.
    - Symptoms: as TACO and hypoxemia + fever, rigor, bilateral lung infiltrate on CXR.
    - Within 1–2 hrs after transfusion and before 6 hrs.
    - $\downarrow$ TRALI with $\downarrow$ transfusion of plasma due to $\downarrow$ HLA class II antibody + HNA antibody.
    - Treatment: D/C transfusion, ventilation support.

Hemolytic Reaction
- Acute and delayed

    - Acute ABO incompatibility = 6% fatal, caused by laboratory technical error
        - $\rightarrow$ IV destruction of RBCs $\rightarrow$ anemia, hemoglobinuria
        - $\rightarrow$ Activation of coagulation cascade $\rightarrow$ acute renal failure from tubular necrosis

- Delayed 2–10 days
  - Extravascular hemolysis, mild anemia, and high bilirubin (indirect)
    - → Occurs in population with low antibody titer at time of transfusion
    - → Reaction to non-ABO antigen → IgG by RES
    - → Facial flushing, back and chest pain, fever, respiratory distress, hypotension, pulse in awake patient
    - → In anesthetized patient → diffuse bleeding + hypotension
  - Diagnosis: laboratory—hemoglobinuria and serology for incompatibility of donor and recipient of blood
  - +ve Coombs test
  - Delayed hemolytic transfusion fever, recurrent anemia, jaundice, low haptoglobin
  - Treatment: hydrate and stop transfusion, send blood for retest from both samples
  - Delayed reaction has no special treatment

Transmission of the Disease
- Malaria, Chagas disease, brucellosis disease, syphilis (rare).
  - → Malaria's incubation period is 8–100 days.
- Symptoms: shaking chills and spiking fever.
- CMV: infectious mononucleosis.
- HIV, HCV decreased by screening.
  - → Risk is 1:1,000,000.
- HBV residual risk is 1:100,000.
- HAV is rare.
- West Nile virus.
- Creutzfeldt-Jakob disease (CJD) can also be transmitted.

Tests for Hemostasis and Blood Coagulation
- Bleeding time, clotting time, PTT, PT and INR, TEG.
- Platelet > 1,000,000, ↑ thrombotic complications.
- If major surgery, need to be > 50,000.
  - → With minor intervention, > 30,000.

Spontaneous hemorrhage occurs when < 20,000.

- Platelet transfusion if < 100,000 in ophthalmology and neurosurgery procedures.

- The PT test measures the function of factors I, II, V, VII, and X.

- Factor VII is part of the extrinsic pathway, and the remaining are part of the common pathway.

- PT is to detect vitamin K deficiency and warfarin therapy.

- $INR = \dfrac{measured\ PT}{normal\ PT}$

- PTT measures factors I, II, V, and (VIII, IX, X, XII [intrinsic pathway]).

- Heparin action is measured by PTT.

- Bleeding time for platelet action, Ivy test, if prolonged, either platelet or vWF dysfunction.

- TEG is the only test measuring all dynamic steps of clot formation till clot lysis.

    → Also can identify thromboembolic complication after injury and postoperative

    → Can predict the need for lifesaving intervention and 24-hr mortality

    → Useful to guide administration of TXA to injured patients with hyperfibrinolysis.

Systemic Response to Injury

Overview: Injury Associated with Systemic Inflammatory Response
- Minor host insults: localized inflammatory response that is transient and most often beneficial.
- Major host insults: leads to amplified reaction, resulting in systemic inflammation, remote organ damage, and multiple organ failures.
- SIRS should meet two of the following:
  - Temperature > 38°C or < 36°C
  - Heart rate 90 beats/min
  - Respiratory rate > 30 breaths/min or arterial CO_2 < 32 mmHg
  - WBCS > 12,000 or < 4,000
- Sepsis: SIRS + documented or suspected source of infection; in addition, other possible manifestations include elevations of procalcitonin, c-reactive protein, hyperglycemia in those without diabetes, altered mental status.
- Severe sepsis: sepsis + evidence of organ dysfunction.
  - Arterial hypoxemia (PaO_2/FiO_2 < 300)
  - Acute oliguria (urine output < 0.5 mg/dL)
  - Increase in creatinine > 0.5 (INR > 1.5, PTT > 60 s, platelets < 100,000)
  - Hepatic dysfunction (elevated bilirubin)
  - Paralytic ileus
  - Decreased capillary refill or skin mottling
- Septic shock sepsis with hypotension refractory to fluid resuscitation, needs pressor.

Detection of Cellular Injury
- Mediated by members of damage-associated molecular pattern family. Systemic inflammatory responses that limit damage and restore homeostasis:
  1. Acute pro-inflammatory response: innate immune system recognizes ligands.
  2. Anti-inflammatory response: modulate pro-inflammatory phase and return homeostasis.

Alarmins or Damage-Associated Molecular Patterns (DAMPs)
- With pathogen-associated molecular patterns (PAMPs), interact with specific cell receptors on cell surface and intracellular.
- It includes HMGB1, formyl peptides (mitochondrial DNA), S100 protein, biglycan.

High-Mobility Group Protein B1 (HMGB1 protein)
- It is the best characterized DAMP.
- It was first described as a constitutively expressed nonhistone chromosomal protein that participated in a variety of nuclear events, including DNA repair and transcription.
- It has been shown to signal via the toll-like receptors (TLR2, TLR4, TLR9).
- HMGB1 is actively secreted from immunocompetent cells stimulated by PAMPs (e.g., endotoxin) or by inflammatory cytokines (e.g., tumor necrosis factor and interleukin-1).
- It has the ability of HMGB1 to influence its activity, including cytokine production.
- It is rapidly released into circulation within 30 min following trauma.

Pro-Inflammatory Biologic Responses from HMGB1 Signaling
1. Release cytokines and chemokines from macrophages, monocytes, and dendritic cells
2. Neutrophil activation and chemotaxis
3. Altered epithelial barrier function
4. Increased procoagulant by platelets
5. Mitochondrial DAMPs

DAMPs—Ligands for Pattern Recognition Receptors (PRR)
Four distinct classes of PRR:
1. Toll-like receptors (TLRS)
2. Calcium-dependent (C-type) lectin receptors (CLRS)
3. Retinoic acid-inducible gene (RIG)-I–like receptors (RLRs)
4. Nucleotide-binding domain (NDB), leucine-rich repeat (LRR)–containing receptors

CNS Regulation of Inflammation in Response to Injury
-   DAMPs and inflammatory molecules convey stimulatory signals to CNS via multiple routes.
-   Inflammatory stimuli interact with receptors on brain to generate pro-inflammatory mediators (cytokines, chemokines, adhesion molecules, proteins of complement system, and immune receptors).
-   Inflammation can also signal the brain via afferent fibers (vagus nerve).

Neuroendocrine Response to Injury
-   **Hypothalamic-Pituitary-Adrenal (HPA) Axis**
    -   Results in the release of glucocorticoid hormones and the sympathetic nervous system, which results in release of the catecholamines, epinephrine, and norepinephrine
    -   Corticotropin-releasing hormone (CRH) → acts on anterior pituitary to stimulate ACTH secretion → acts on zona fasciculata to synthesize and secrete glucocorticoids

-   **Growth Hormone**
    -   Promotes protein synthesis and insulin resistance, enhances mobilization of fat stores
    -   Enhances immunocyte phagocytosis by increased lysosomal superoxide production

-   **Insulin-like Growth Factor (IGF)-1**
    -   Anabolic growth factor that improves metabolic rate, gut mucosal function, and protein loss after traumatic injury

-   **Ghrelin**
    -   Natural ligand for GH
    -   Appetite stimulant secreted by stomach
    -   Promotes GI secretion and glucose homeostasis, lipid metabolism, and immune function

-   **Catecholamines**
    -   Fight-or-flight response
    -   Effects: ↑ HR, myocardial contractility, conduction velocity, and BP

- Redirects blood flow to skeletal muscle
- ↑ cellular metabolism, mobilization of glucose from liver via glycogenolysis, gluconeogenesis, lipolysis, and ketogenesis

- **Aldosterone**
  - Mineralocorticoid released by zona glomerulosa
  - Interferes with insulin-signaling pathways and reduces expression of insulin-sensitizing factors, adiponectin, and peroxisome proliferator–activated receptor

- **Insulin**
  - Hormone secreted by pancreas
  - Mediates overall host anabolic state through hepatic glycogenesis and glycolysis, peripheral glucose uptake, lipogenesis, and protein synthesis

Cellular Stress Responses
1. Reactive oxygen species (ROS) and oxidative stress response
2. Heat shock proteins (HSP)
3. Unfolded protein response
4. Autophagy
5. Apoptosis
6. Necroptosis

Mediators of Inflammation
1. **Cytokines**
   - Mediate invading organism and promote wound healing

2. **Eicosanoids**
   Omega-6 polyunsaturated metabolites: arachidonic acid
   - Prostaglandins, thromboxane, leukotrienes
   - Anti-inflammatory
   - Inflammatory mediators

3. **Plasma Contact System**
   A. Complement
      - Eliminates immune complexes and damaged cells

- Mobilizes hematopoietic stem cells and lipid metabolism
- Classical pathway, lectin pathway, and alternative pathway

B. Kallikrein-Kinin System
- Group of proteins that contribute to inflammation, blood pressure control, coagulation, and pain responses

4. **Serotonin**
- Monoamine neurotransmitter (5-hydroxytryptamine)
- Potent vasoconstrictor and modulates cardiac inotropy
- Released by platelets

5. **Histamine**
- Short-acting endogenous amine
- Rapidly released or stored in neurons, skin, gastric mucosa, mast cells, basophils, and platelets
- Increased with hemorrhagic shock, trauma, thermal injury, and sepsis

Tumor Necrosis Factor
- TNF was thought to be produced primarily by macrophages, but it is produced also by a broad variety of cell types, including lymphoid cells, mast cells, endothelial cells, cardiac myocytes, adipose tissue, fibroblasts, and neurons.
    - Large amounts of TNF are released in response to lipopolysaccharide, other bacterial products, and interleukin-1 (IL-1).
    - In the skin, mast cells appear to be the predominant source of preformed TNF, which can be released upon inflammatory stimulus.
    - It has a number of actions on various organ systems, generally together with IL-1 and IL-6.
- On the hypothalamus:
    - o Stimulation of the hypothalamic-pituitary-adrenal axis by stimulating the release of CRH
    - o Suppressing appetite
    - o Fever

- On the liver: stimulates the acute phase response, leading to an increase in C-reactive protein and a number of other mediators. It also induces insulin resistance by promoting serine phosphorylation of insulin receptor substrate-1 (IRS-1), which impairs insulin signaling.
- It is a potent chemoattractant for neutrophils and promotes the expression of adhesion molecules on endothelial cells, helping neutrophils migrate.
- On macrophages: stimulates phagocytosis and production of IL-1 oxidants and the inflammatory lipid prostaglandin E_2 (PGE_2)
- On other tissues: increases insulin resistance. TNF phosphorylates insulin receptor serine residues, blocking signal transduction.
- On metabolism and food intake: regulates bitter taste perception.

Lymphocytes and T Cell Immunity
- The expression of genes associated with the adaptive immune response is rapidly altered following severe blunt trauma.
- Significant injury is associated with adaptive immune suppression that is characterized by altered cell-mediated immunity, specifically the balance between the major populations of T cells.
- T lymphocytes are functionally divided into subsets, which principally include Th1 and Th2 cells, as well as Th17 and inducible Treg cells.

Eosinophils
- Immunocytes whose primary functions are antihelminthic.
- Are found mostly in tissues such as the lung and gastrointestinal tract, which may suggest a role in immune surveillance.
- Can be activated by IL-3, IL-5, GM-CSF, and platelet-activating factor. Eosinophil activation can lead to subsequent release of toxic mediators, including ROSS, histamine, and peroxidase.

Mast Cells
- Important in the primary response to injury because they are located in tissues.
- TNF release from mast cells has been found to be crucial for neutrophil recruitment and pathogen clearance.

- It is known to play an important role in the anaphylactic response to allergens.
- On activation from stimuli including allergen binding, infection, and trauma, mast cells produce histamine, cytokines, eicosanoids, proteases, and chemokines, which leads to vasodilatation, capillary leakage, and immunocyte recruitment.

Monocyte/Macrophages

- Monocytes are mononuclear phagocytes that circulate in the bloodstream and can differentiate into macrophages, osteoclasts on migrating into tissues.
- Macrophages are the main effector cells of the immune response to infection and injury, primarily through mechanisms that include phagocytosis of microbial pathogens, release of inflammatory mediators, and clearance of apoptotic cells.

Neutrophils

- Neutrophils are among the first responders to sites of infection and injury and, as such, are potent mediators of acute inflammation.
- Chemotactic mediators from a site of injury induce neutrophil adherence to the vascular endothelium and promote eventual cell migration into the injured tissue.
- Neutrophils are circulating immunocytes with short half-lives (4–10 hrs).
- However, inflammatory signals may promote the longevity of neutrophils in target tissues, which can contribute to their potential detrimental effects and bystander injury.
- Once primed and activated by inflammatory stimuli, including TNF, IL-1, and microbial pathogens, neutrophils are able to enlist a variety of killing mechanisms to manage invading pathogens.

Vascular Endothelium

- Under physiologic conditions, vascular endothelium has overall anticoagulant properties mediated via the production and cell surface expression of heparin sulfate, dermatan sulfate, tissue factor pathway inhibitor, protein S, thrombomodulin, plasminogen, and tissue plasminogen activator.

Nitric Oxide
- Nitric oxide (NO) was initially known as endothelium-derived relaxing factor due to its effect on vascular smooth muscle.
- Normal vascular smooth muscle cell relaxation is maintained by a constant output of NO that is regulated in the endothelium by both flow- and receptor-mediated events.
- NO can also reduce microthrombosis by reducing platelet adhesion and aggregation.

Prostacyclin
- Prostacyclin is a potent vasodilator that also inhibits platelet aggregation. In the pulmonary system, PGI_2 reduces pulmonary blood pressure and bronchial hyperresponsiveness.

Metabolism after Injury
Lipid Metabolism
- Lipid—nonprotein and noncarbohydrate fuel sources that minimize protein catabolism in the injured patient
- Triglycerides—predominant energy source (50%–80%) during critical illness and after injury and responsible for fat mobilization, lipid absorption, lipolysis, and fatty acid oxidation

Carbohydrate Metabolism
- Primarily refers to the utilization of glucose
- Minimizes muscle wasting—primary goal for maintenance glucose administration in surgical patients

Protein and Amino Acid Metabolism
- Average protein intake in healthy young adults is 80–120 g/d.
- Every 6 g of protein → 1 g of nitrogen.
- Degradation of 1 g of protein → 4 kcal of energy.
- Protein catabolism after injury provides substrates for gluconeogenesis.
- Amino acid cannot be considered a long-term fuel reserve.

Nutrition in Surgical Patients

Goals

- Prevent or reverse the catabolic effects of disease or injury
- Ultimate validation of nutritional support
- Improvement in clinical outcome restoration of function
- Estimating energy requirements

Nutritional Assessment

Caloric need is approximately 20–25 calories/kg/day.

Calories:

Fat	9 calories/g
Protein	4 calories/g
Oral carb	4 calories/g
Dextrose	3.4 calories/g

Nutritional Requirements for Average Healthy Adult Male

- 20% protein calories (1 g protein/kg/day, 20% should be essential amino acids)
- 30% fat calories—important for essential fatty acids
- 50% carbohydrate calories.
- Trauma, surgery, or sepsis stress can increase caloric requirement to 20%–40%.
- Pregnancy increases kilocalorie requirement to 300 kcal/day.
- Lactation increases kilocalorie requirement to 500 kcal/day.
- Protein requirement also increases with above.
- Burns:
    - Calories: 25 kcal/kg/day + (30 kcal/day × % burn)
    - Protein: 1–1.5 g/kg/day + (3 g × % burn)
- Most of the energy expenditures is used for heat production.
- Fever increases basal metabolic rate (10% for each degree above 38.0°C).
- If overweight and trying to calculate caloric need, use this equation:
- Weight = ([actual weight − ideal body weight] × 0.25) + IBW
- Harris-Benedict equation calculates basal energy expenditure based on weight, height, age, and gender.
- Central line TPN—glucose based.

- Maximum glucose administration is 3 g/kg/hr.
- Peripheral parenteral nutrition (PPN)—fat-based short-chain fatty acids (e.g., butyric acid), fuel for colonocytes.
- Glutamine—fuel for small bowel enterocytes and common amino acid in bloodstream and tissue.

Respiratory Quotient (RQ)

- Ratio of CO_2 produced to O_2 consumed is a measurement of energy expenditure.
- RQ > 1 → lipogenesis (overfeeding).
  Tx: ↓ carbohydrates and caloric intake.
- High carbohydrate intake can lead to CO_2 buildup and ventilator problems.
- RQ < 0.7 = ketosis and fat oxidation (starving).
  Tx: ↑ carbohydrates and caloric intake.
  Pure fat utilization − RQ = 0.7.
  Pure protein utilization − RQ = 0.8.
  Pure carbohydrate utilization − RQ = 1.0.

Refeeding Syndrome

- Occurs when feeding after prolonged starvation/malnutrition
- Results in ↑ glucose, ↑ insulin → shifting of glucose and insulin with concomitant electrolyte into intracellular → ↓ K, Mg, and PO_4
- Causes cardiac dysfunction, profound weakness, encephalopathy
- Tx: gradual feeding, gradual carbohydrate administration, electrolyte replacement

Overfeeding

- Results from overestimation of caloric needs
- May contribute to clinical deterioration via increased oxygen consumption
- Increased CO_2 production
- Prolonged need for ventilatory support fatty liver
- Suppression of leukocyte function hyperglycemia
- Increased risk of infection.

Enteral Nutrition

Rationale for Enteral Nutrition
- Lower cost of enteral feeding
- Associated risks of the intravenous route
- Reduced intestinal atrophy
- Reduced infectious complications and acute-phase protein production

Types of Enteral Formulas
1. Immune nutrients
2. Low-residue isotonic formulas
3. Isotonic formulas with fiber
4. Immune-enhancing formulas
5. Calorie-dense formulas
6. High-protein formulas
7. Elemental formulas
8. Renal failure formulas
9. Pulmonary failure formulas
10. Hepatic failure formulas

Access for Enteral Nutritional Support
- Nasogastric or enteric tubes
- Percutaneous endoscopic gastrostomy
- Jejunostomy and direct endoscopic jejunostomy
- Surgical gastrostomy and jejunostomy

Parenteral Nutrition
- Continuous infusion of a hyperosmolar solution containing carbohydrates, proteins, fat, and other necessary nutrition through an indwelling catheter inserted into the superior vena cava.

Rationale for Parenteral Nutrition
- Malnutrition.
- Sepsis.
- Surgical/traumatic injury.
- In patients for whom use of feeding is not possible, intravenous nutrition may be used to supplement inadequate oral intake.

Types

- Total parenteral nutrition requires access to a large-diameter vein to deliver the entire nutritional requirements of the individual.
- Peripheral parenteral nutrition allows administration via peripheral veins for short period. Considered if central routes are not available and supplemental nutritional support is required.

TPN Preparation Guideline

- Basically, TPN contains the following:
  - o Macroelement (dextrose, amino acid, fatty acid)
  - o Microelement (minerals and vitamins)
  - o Additive (insulin, heparin, etc.)
- TPN requires water (30–40 mL/kg/day).
- Energy required is 30–35 kcal/kg/day, depending on energy expenditure.
- Amino acids required is 1.0–2.0 g/kg/day, depending on the degree of catabolism.
- Essential fatty acids, vitamins, and minerals.
- Children who need TPN may have different fluid requirements and need more energy (up to 120 kcal/kg/day) and amino acids (up to 2.5 or 3.5 g/kg/day).
- Basic TPN solutions are prepared using sterile techniques, usually in liter batches according to standard formulas.
- Normally, 2 L/day of the standard solution is needed.
- Solutions may be modified based on laboratory results, underlying disorders, hypermetabolism, or other factors.
- Most calories are supplied as carbohydrate.
- Typically, about 4–5 mg/kg/min of dextrose is given.
- Standard solutions contain up to about 25% dextrose.
- 3% to 5% crystalline amino acids.
- 20%–30% of total calories are usually supplied as lipids.
- Minerals such as Na^+, Ca^{++}, Cu^{++}, chromium, Cl^-, Mg^{++}, phosphorus, K^+, zinc.
- Vitamins such as K, E, D, A, C, B1-12, folic acid, cobalamin, thiamin.

Initiation of Parenteral Nutrition
- Urine/capillary blood glucose level is checked every 6 hrs.
- At least 1 day—serum glucose concentration.
- K^+ essential to achieve positive nitrogen balance and replace depleted intracellular stores.

Wound Healing

Definition

- *Wounding* disrupts tissue integrity, leading to division of blood vessels and direct exposure of extracellular matrix to platelets.

Phases of Wound Healing

a. Hemostasis and inflammation
b. Proliferation
c. Maturation and remodeling

- **Inflammatory phase (1–10 days)**
    - Exposure of subendothelial collagen to platelets results in platelet aggregation, degranulation, and activation of the coagulation cascade, VC for a while then VD by prostacyclin (PGI_2).
    - Platelet α-granules release a number of wound-active substances, such as PDGF, TGF-β, PAF, fibronectin, and serotonin.
    - PMNs are the first infiltrating cells to enter the wound site, peaking at 24–48 hrs.
    - Increased vascular permeability, phagocytosis, local prostaglandin release, and the presence of chemotactic substances such as complement factors IL-1, TNF-α, TGF-β, platelet factor IV.
    - The second inflammatory cell is macrophages, which are recognized as being essential to successful healing, derived from circulating monocytes; macrophages achieve significant numbers in the wound by 48–96 hrs postinjury and remain present until wound healing is complete.
    - Macrophages, like neutrophils, participate in wound debridement via phagocytosis and contribute to microbial stasis via oxygen radical and nitric oxide synthesis.
    - T lymphocytes comprise another population of inflammatory/immune cells that routinely invades the wound, peak at about 1 week postinjury, and truly bridge the transition from the inflammatory to the proliferative phase of healing.

44

- **The proliferative phase (5 days to 3 weeks)**
  - is the second phase of wound healing and roughly spans days 4 through 12.
  - It is during this that fibroblasts and endothelial cells are the last cell populations to infiltrate the healing wound, and the strongest chemotactic factor for fibroblasts is PDGF.
  - Fibroblasts isolated from wounds synthesize more collagen.
  - Lactate, which accumulates in significant amounts in the wound environment over time (~10 mmol), is a potent regulator of collagen synthesis.
  - Endothelial cells also proliferate extensively during this phase of healing. These cells participate in the formation of new capillaries (angiogenesis).
  - Collagen, the most abundant protein in the body, plays a critical role in the successful completion of adult wound healing.

- **The maturation and remodeling phase (3 weeks to 1 year)**
  - begins during the fibroblastic phase and is characterized by a reorganization of previously synthesized collagen.
  - Epithelialization occurs while tissue integrity and strength are being reestablished; the external barrier must also be restored. This process is characterized primarily by proliferation and migration of epithelial cells adjacent to the wound. The process begins within 1 day of injury and is seen as the thickening of the epidermis at the wound edge.
  - Reepithelialization is complete in less than 48 hrs in the case of approximated incised wounds but may take substantially longer in the case of larger wounds.
  - Wound contraction—all wounds undergo some degree of contraction. For wounds that do not have surgically approximated edges, the area of the wound will be decreased by this action (healing by secondary intention).
  - The myofibroblast has been postulated as being the major cell responsible for contraction, and it differs from

the normal fibroblast in that it possesses a cytoskeletal structure.

- Typically, this cell contains α-smooth muscle actin.

Collagen Types

o Type I collagen is the major component of extracellular matrix in skin; it's the most common type in the body + the primary collagen in wound healing.

o Type II is mostly in cartilage.

o Type III is found in granulation tissue, blood vessels, fetal skin.

o Type IV is found in basement membrane, eye, lens.

Heritable Diseases of Connective Tissue

Ehlers-Danlos Syndrome (EDS)

- Ehlers-Danlos syndrome is a group of ten disorders that present as a defect in collagen formation.

- Autosomal recessive form characterized by tenascin-X deficiency. The defect is a quantitative loss of protein.

- Alpha chains of collagen type V, causing it to be either quantitatively or structurally defective.

- Finding includes thin, friable skin with prominent veins, easy bruising, poor wound healing, atrophic scar formation, recurrent hernias, and hyperextensible joints.

- Gastrointestinal problems include bleeding, hiatal hernia, intestinal diverticula, and rectal prolapse.

- Small blood vessels are fragile, making suturing difficult during surgery.

- Large vessels may develop aneurysms, varicosities, or arteriovenous fistulas or may spontaneously rupture.

Marfan Syndrome

- Patients with Marfan syndrome have tall stature, arachnodactyly, lax ligaments, myopia, scoliosis, pectus excavatum, and aneurysm of the ascending aorta.

- Patients who suffer from this syndrome also are prone to hernias.

- Surgical repair of a dissecting aneurysm is difficult as the soft connective tissue fails to hold sutures.

- Skin may be hyperextensible but shows no delay in wound healing.
- The genetic defect associated with Marfan syndrome is a mutation in the FBN1 gene.

Osteogenesis Imperfecta (OI)

- Patients with osteogenesis imperfecta have brittle bones, osteopenia, low muscle mass, hernias, and ligament and joint laxity.
- This is a result of a mutation in type I collagen.
- Patients experience dermal thinning and increased bruisability.
- Scarring is normal, and the skin is not hyperextensible.
- Surgery can be successful but difficult in these patients as the bones fracture easily under minimal stress.

Epidermolysis Bullosa (EB)

- Epidermolysis bullosa is classified into four major subtypes: EB simplex, junctional EB, dystrophic EB, and Kindler syndrome. The first three are determined by location in various skin layers; the last can present as multiple blisters.
- The disease manifestations include impairment in tissue adhesion within the epidermis, basement membrane, or dermis, resulting in tissue separation and blistering with minimal trauma.
- Characteristic features of EB are blistering and ulceration.
- The recessively inherited dystrophic type is characterized by defects in the COL7A1 gene, encoding type 7 collagen, important for connecting the epidermis to the dermis.

Essentials for Wound Healing

- Moist environment (avoid desiccation).
- Oxygen delivery—optimize fluids, no smoking, pain control, arterial revascularization, supplemental oxygen.
- Want transcutaneous oxygen measurement (TCOM) > 25 mmHg.
- Avoid edema—leg elevation.
- Remove necrotic tissue.

Impediments to Wound Healing

- Bacteria > 105/cm^2—↓ oxygen content, collagen lysis, prolonged inflammation.
- Devitalized tissue and foreign bodies—retards granulation tissue formation and wound healing.
- Cytotoxic drugs—5FU, methotrexate, cyclosporine, FK-506 can impair wound healing in the first 14 days after injury.
- Diabetes—can contribute to poor wound healing by impeding the early-phase inflammation response (hyperglycemia causes poor leukocyte chemotaxis).
- Albumin < 3.0—risk factor for poor wound healing.
- Steroids—prevent wound healing by inhibiting macrophages, PMNs, and collagen synthesis by fibroblasts; ↓ wound tensile strength as well.
- Vitamin A (25,000 IU)—counteracts effects of steroids on wound healing.
- Wound ischemia (hypoxia)—can be caused by fibrosis, pressure (sacral decubitus ulcer, pressure sores), poor arterial inflow (atherosclerosis), poor venous outflow (venous stasis), smoking, radiation, edema, vasculitis.

Healing in specific tissues

Gastrointestinal tract

- Healing of full-thickness wounds begins with a surgical or mechanical reapposition of the bowel ends, which is most often the initial step in the repair process.
- Failure of healing results in dehiscence, leaks, and fistulas, which carry significant morbidity and mortality.
- excessive healing can be just as troublesome, resulting in stricture formation and stenosis of the lumen.
- The gross anatomic features of the GI tract are remarkably constant throughout most of its length.
- The submucosa is the layer that imparts the greatest tensile strength and greatest suture-holding capacity, a characteristic that should be kept in mind during surgical repair of the GI tract.
- Serosal healing is essential for quickly achieving a watertight seal from the luminal side of the bowel.

- The importance of the serosa is underscored by the significantly higher rates of anastomotic failure observed clinically in the bowel that are extraperitoneal and lack serosa (i.e., the esophagus and rectum).

Bone
- The initial stage of hematoma formation consists of an accumulation of blood at the fracture site.
- The next stage accomplishes the liquefaction and deg- radation of nonviable products at the fracture site.
- The normal bone adjacent to the injury site can then undergo revascularization.
- This is similar to granulation tissue in soft tissue.
- In the next stage (soft callus stage).
- The next phase (hard callus stage) consists of mineralization of the soft callus and conversion to bone. This may take up to 2 to 3 months.
- This stage is followed by the remodeling phase, in which the excessive callus is reabsorbed and the marrow cavity is recanalized.

Cartilage
- Unlike bone, cartilage is very avascular and depends on diffusion for transmittal of nutrients.
- The healing response of cartilage depends on the depth of injury.

Tendon
- Tendon and ligament healing progresses in a similar fashion as in other areas of the body (i.e., through hematoma formation, organization, laying down of reparative tissue, and scar formation).
- Matrix is characterized by accumulation of type I and III collagen along with increased water and glycosaminoglycan content.

Nerve
- There are three types of nerve inju- ries: neurapraxia (focal demyelination), axonotmesis (interrup- tion of axonal continuity but preservation of schwann cell basal lamina), and neurotmesis (complete transection).

- The nerve ends progress through three crucial steps:
  o survival of axonal cell bodies.
  o regeneration of axons that grow across the transected nerve to reach the distal stump.
  o migration and connection of the regenerating nerve ends to the appropriate nerve ends or organ targets.
- Schwann cells help in remyelinating the regenerating axons.
- Proximal budding leads to sprouting axon that migrate at 1mm/day to connect distal end.

Classification of wounds

Wound class	example	Expected infection rate
Clean I	Hernia, breast	1%–2%
Clean contaminated IIa	Cholecystitis Gi (not colon)	2%–9%
Clean contaminated IIb	Colon	4%–12%
Contaminated III	Penetrating injury	3%–13%
Dirty IV	Perforation diverticulitis necrotizing fasciitis	3%–13%

- Wound closure
  I, II primarily
  III, IV primarily closure achieved in 25%–50%
- If infected wound, i.e., class III, IV, left to heal in secondary intention with bid dressing → VAC is helpful.

Chronic wounds

- The majority of wounds that have not healed in 3 months are considered chronic.
- Unresponsiveness to normal regulatory signals also has been implicated as a predictive factor of chronic wounds.
- Fibroblasts from chronic wounds also have been found to have decreased proliferative potential.
- Malignant transformation of chronic ulcers can occur in any long-standing wound (marjolin's ulcer).

Excess healing

Keloids
- autosomal dominant, dark-skinned.
- Collagen goes beyond original wound.
- Tx: intralesional steroid injection, silicone, pressure garments, xrt.

Hypertrophic scar
- dark-skinned, flexor surfaces of upper torso.
- Collagen stays within confines of original scar.
- Often occurs in burns or wounds that take a long time to heal.
- Tx: steroid injection, silicone, pressure garment.

Treatment of wounds

Local care
- Irrigation to visualize all areas of the wound and remove foreign material is best accomplished with normal saline (with- out additives). High-pressure wound irrigation is more effective in achieving complete débridement of foreign material and non-viable tissues.
- Iodine, povidone-iodine, hydrogen peroxide, and organically based antibacterial preparations have all been shown to impair wound healing due to injury to wound neutrophils and macrophages, and thus should not be used.

Antibiotics
- Antibiotics should be used only when there is an obvious wound infection.
- Signs of infection to look for include erythema, cellulitis, swelling, and purulent discharge.
- Indiscriminate use of antibiotics should be avoided to prevent emergence of multidrug-resistant bacteria.

Dressings
- The type of dressing to be used depends on the amount of wound drainage.
    o A nondraining wound drainage of less than 1 to 2 ml/d
    o Moderately draining wounds (3–5 ml/d)
    o Heavily draining wounds (>5 ml/d)

- Absorbent dressings.
- Nonadherent dressings (petroleum jelly, or water-soluble jelly) for use as nonadherent coverage.
- Occlusive and semiocclusive dressings.
- Hydrophilic and hydrophobic dressings.
- Hydrocolloid and hydrogel dressings.
- Hydrogel is a cross-linked polymer that has high water content → allow a high rate of evaporation without compromising wound hydration → useful in burn wound treatment.
- Alginates.
- Absorbable materials, include collagen, gelatin, oxidized cellulose.
- Medicated dressings include benzoyl peroxide, zinc oxide, neomycin, and bacitracin-zinc.
- Mechanical devices The vacuum-assisted closure (VAC) system, assists in wound closure by applying localized negative pressure to the surface and margins of the wound, very effective in removing exudates from the wound.

Burn

- A burn severity grading system was developed to help providers distinguish between types of burn.
- Minor burn—the total burn surface area (TBSA) must be less than 10% in adults and less than 5% in children.
- Moderate burns—the TBSA burn in adults is 10%–20% and 5%–10% in children.
- Major burns—TBSA is greater than 20% in adults and greater than 10% in children.
- The American Burn Association (ABA) has published the classification system.
  - *Superficial.* or epidermal burns involve only the epidermal layer of skin. They do not blister but are painful, dry, red, and blanched with pressure. This process is seen with sunburns.
  - *Partial-thickness.* burns involve the epidermis and portions of the dermis. They are either superficial or deep.
    - Superficial partial-thickness—these burns characteristically form blisters. They are painful, red, and weeping and blanched with pressure.
    - Deep partial-thickness—these burns extend into the deeper dermis.
  - *Full-thickness.* These burns extend through and destroy all layers of the dermis and often injure the underlying subcutaneous tissue.
  - *Extension to deep tissues.* Fourth-degree burns are deep and potentially life-threatening injuries that extend through the skin into underlying soft tissue and can involve muscle and/or bone.

Methods of Estimation
- Lund-Browder—this chart is the most accurate method for estimating TBSA for both adults and children.
- Rule of nines (for adult assessment):
  - The head represents 9% TBSA.
  - Each arm represents 9% TBSA.
  - Each leg represents 18% TBSA.

- The anterior and posterior trunk each represent 18% TBSA.
- Genitalia represent 1% TBSA.
  o Palm method—small burns can be approximated by using the surface area of the patient's palm; entire palmar surface including fingers represent 1 percent in children and adults.

Admission Criteria

- Second- and third-degree burns > 10% BSA in patients aged < 10 or > 50 years
- Second- and third-degree burns > 20% BSA in all other patients
- Second- and third-degree burns to significant portions of hands, face, feet, genitalia, perineum, or skin overlying major joints
- Third-degree burns > 5% in any age-group
- Electrical and chemical burns
- Concomitant inhalational injury, mechanical traumas, preexisting medical conditions
- Injuries in patients with special social, emotional, or long-term rehabilitation needs
- Suspected child abuse or neglect

Burn Assessment

- Parkland formula, use for burns ≥ 20%—give 4 cc/kg × % burn in first 24 hrs.
- Give ½ the volume in the first 8 hrs.
- Use lactated ringer (LR) in first 24 hrs.
- Urine output best measure of resuscitation: 0.5–1.0 cc/kg/hr in adults, 2–4 cc/kg/hr in children < 6 months.
- Caloric need: 25 kcal/kg/day + (30 kcal × % burn).
- Protein need: 1 g/kg/day + (3 g × % burn).

Types of Grafts

- Autograft (split-thickness or full-thickness)
- Homograft (allografts, cadaveric skin)
- Xenografts (porcine)—not as good as homograft, last 2 weeks, do not vascularize
- Dermal substitutes—not as good as homograft or xenografts
- Meshed grafts—used for back, flank, trunk, arms, and legs

Wound Care
- No role for prophylactic IV antibiotics
- Pseudomonas is the most common organism in burn wound infection, followed by staph, E. coli, and Enterobacter, which are more common in burns > 30% BSA.
- Topical agents have decreased incidence of burn wound bacterial infections.
- Flamazine (silver sulfadiazine)—an antibacterial cream, S/E neutropenia.
- Silver nitrate—can cause electrolyte imbalances (hyponatremia, hypochloremia, hypocalcemia, and hypokalemia), discoloration.
- MEBO cream—use on daily basis.

Complications after Burns
- Seizures: usually iatrogenic and related to Na^+.
- Curling's ulcer: gastric ulcer that occurs with burns.
- Marjolin ulcer: highly malignant squamous cell CA that arises in chronic nonhealing burn wounds or unstable scars.
- Hypertrophic scar.

Surgical Infections

Pathogenesis of Infection
   Host Defenses
- Barrier: epithelial mucosa in GI, respiratory, urogenital.
- Most of the extensive physical barrier is the skin.
- Disease of skin (eczema, dermatitis) associated with overgrowth of skin commensal organism.
- In respiratory system:
  - → Upper: mucus → cleared by cough
  - → Lower: phagocytosis by alveolar macrophage
  - → GI: killing bacteria by high acidity but only small colony of 100–1,000 CFU/mL bacteria that is not destroyed by stomach juice
  - → Small bowel: 10^5–10^8 CFU/mL
  - → In distal colon: 10^{11}–10^{12} CFU/g bacteroides, small amount of E. coli, enterococcus, *Candida albicans*, *Enterococcus faecalis*.
- Microflora prevent invasion of enteric pathogens such as salmonella, shigella, vibrio.
- Once microbe enters the body, e.g., pleural, peritoneal (sterile body compartment), host defense → limit or eliminate these pathogens.
- Lactoferrin or transferrin sequesters microbial growth.
- Also, fibrinogen traps long numbers of microbes.
- In the peritoneal cavity, unique host defense mechanism
  - → Include diaphragmatic breathing mechanism
  - → Thoracic lymphatic channel + omentum → gatekeeper
  - → Microphage + complement
- Foreign organism → recognize microbial PAMPs and DAMPs, TLR.
  - → Macrophage cytokines upregulated → TNF-α, IL-1, IL-6, IL-8, and IFN-α → microbial opsonization.
- Several possible outcomes:
  1. Eradication
  2. Containment
  3. Locoregional infection (cellulitis soft tissue infection)

4. Systemic infection (bacteria)
- Sign of inflammation: (rubor, calor, dolor, tumor, function laesa) + systemic manifestation fever, high WBC, tachycardia, or tachypnea (SIRS).
- Sepsis = SIRS + infection.
- Severe sepsis = sepsis + new onset of organ failure.
- Septic shock = high ventilation, oliguria, not responding to fluid resuscitation or require vasopressor.

Criteria of SIRS
- General
  Temperature < 36 or > 38.3
  HR > 90, tachypnea
- Altered mental status
  Edema (generalized), high RBS with no DM
- Inflammatory variables
  WBCs < 4,000 or > 12,000, high CRP
- Hemodynamic variable
  MAP < 70
- Organ dysfunction
  Hypoxia, high creatinine, ileus, thrombocytopenia, high bilirubin
- Tissue perfusion
  High lactate
  Low CRT (capillary refill test)
- Septic shock, MR 30%–66%

Bacteria
- Stain: blue for +ve, red for −ve
- Cocci or bacilli
- Single or group (diplococcic, cluster, chain)
- Gram +ve SSI, nosocomial infection UTI

Fungi
- Special stain KOH, Indian ink
- Growth is 25°C–37°C

Virus
- EBV, CMV, HSV, hepatitis B, C

Prevention and Treatment of Surgical Infection
General Principles
- Exogenous (surgeon, OR environment) and endogenous (patient)

Source Control
- Drain all purulent material, debride all infected and devitalized tissue, and remove debris of all foreign bodies.
- Wall off purulent fluid collection (abscess), either percutaneous or open drainage.
- Soft tissue infection: radical debridement.

Appropriate Use of Antimicrobial
- Prophylaxis is limited to the time prior to and during procedure (skin incision).
    - Only single dose, but if prolonged → additional dose.
    - No evidence to give postoperative antibiotics → discouraged → costly and increase resistance.

- Empiric
    - Given when the risk of surgical infection is increased (rupture appendicitis) or when inadequate bowel preparation, i.e., high contamination.
    - Critically ill with severe sepsis or septic shock.
    - Should be limited to 3–5 days and should stop ASAP if C/S is −ve.

- Therapy of established infection
    - UTI, pneumonia with SIRS + C/S
    - Perforated or gangrenous appendix → IV antibiotic for 3–5 days or longer, e.g., ciprofloxacin, metronidazole.
    - For monoclonal infection:

UTI	3–5 days
Pneumonia	7–10 days
Bacteremia	7–14 days
Osteomyelitis endocarditis	6–12 weeks

- Minimum inhibitory concentration (MIC) is the lowest concentration of chemical (drugs), which prevents visible growth of bacteria.
- Oral agent should achieve high serum level, e.g., fluoroquinolones.
- Penetrating GI without contamination 12–24 hrs
  Perforated or gangrenous appendicitis 3–5 days
  Peritoneal spillage (perforated viscus) 5–7 days
  Extensive spillage (feculent peritonitis) 7–14 days
- You can stop antibiotic if WBC is not high, no fever, no PMN on peripheral smear.
  → If persistently high → complete and search for another source.
- Penicillin allergy is 0.7%–10% → cross-reactivity is 5%–7% with cephalosporins, 1% carbapenem.
  → Should do intradermal testing, as it decreases 16% of vancomycin use in patient reported to have penicillin allergy.

Antibiotics Types
- Penicillin: cell wall inhibitor
  Penicillin G, piperacillin

- Penicillin / beta-lactamase inhibitor: inhibit cell wall / beta-lactamase inhibitor
  (Ampicillin − sulbactam), (ticarcillin − clavulanate [augmentin]) (piperacillin/tazobactam [tazocin])

- Cephalosporin: cell wall inhibitor
  1st, 2nd, 3rd, 4th generation

- Carbapenem: cell wall inhibitor
  Imipenem, meropenem

- Aminoglycosides: alteration of cell membrane / inhibit ribosomes
  Gentamycin, amikacin

- Fluoroquinolones: DNA synthesis inhibitor
  Ciprofloxacin, levofloxacin

- Glycopeptides: cell wall synthesis inhibitor
  Vancomycin, lizolid, clindamycin, rifampicin, Metronidazole.

- Macrolides: protein synthesis inhibitor (ribosomes)
  Erythromycin, azithromycin

- Tetracycline: protein synthesis inhibitor (ribosomes)
  Doxycycline, tigecycline

Infections in Surgical Patients
Surgical Site Infection (SSI)
- Infection to skin or deeper
- Development related to three factors:
    1. Degree of contamination during surgery
    2. Duration of surgery
    3. Host factors, e.g., DM, obesity, malnourishment
- Risk factors
    o Patient factor
        - Old age, low immunity, obesity, DM, chronic inflammation, malnutrition, smoking, RF, peripheral vascular disease, anemia, history of radiation, chronic skin disease, recent OR
    o Local factor
        - Open vs. laparoscopy, poor skin preparation, contaminated instrument, inadequate antibiotic, prolonged procedure, hypothermia, hypoxia, blood transfusions
    o Microbial factor
        - Prolonged hospitalization, toxin secretion, resistance

Intra-Abdominal Infection
- Primary microbial peritonitis
  - When normally sterile peritoneum invaded by infection via hematogenous dissemination:
    - → More common in patients with ascites, CRF with PD catheter
    - → Monomicrobial, no surgical intervention
    - → Diagnosis based on risk factor as noted previously
    - → Diffuse abdominal tenderness (not localized), no pneumoperitoneum
  - If paracentesis → WBCs/mL = 100.
  - Treatment: antibiotic for 14–21 days + removal of catheter, e.g., VP shunt.

- Secondary microbial peritonitis
  - Perforation or severe infection in intra-abdominal organ

- Tertiary (persistent) peritonitis → from leak after OR
  - Abscess → diagnosis by CT and usually treated by interventional radiology
  - Surgery for multiple abscesses, adjacent to vital organ
    - → Catheter for drainage → leave in situ till output is 10–20 mL/day
    - → Antibiotic for 3–7 days

Organ with Specific Infection
- Liver abscess, rare → 80% pyogenic, 20% amoebic, fungal
  - Pyogenic → due to neglected appendicitis or diverticulitis.
    But nowadays, manipulation of biliary tract becomes most common cause, 50%.
    - → Organism: E. coli, K. pneumoniae, and bacilli such as enterococcus, pseudomonas, anaerobic bacteria
  - Large → percutaneous drainage with IV antibiotic
  - Fungal: candida

- Splenic abscess, rare
    → Recurrent hepatic and splenic may need operative intervention (unroofing, marsupialization, splenectomy).

- Secondary pancreatic infection (infective pancreatic necrosis or pancreatic abscess)
    - 10–15 days with severe pancreatitis
        → Previously: debridement
        → Currently: staging CT, no prophylactic IV antibiotic, ICU, enteral feeding, N-J to decreased translocation of bacteria
        → Should be suspected if high WBC, high SIRS, and MOF
        → CT-guided aspiration for C/S if +ve culture or gas pocket in pancreatic CT scan
    - Open necrosectomy → ↑ mortality and morbidity
        → Endoscopic mortality (5%–30%) laparoscopic (6% mortality)
    - If failed endoscopic or laparoscopic → VARD vs. open necrosectomy mortality → 40% vs. 69%.

Infection of Skin and SC Tissue
- Classified to surgical and nonsurgical infection.
- Superficial skin infections: cellulitis, erysipelas, and lymphangitis → IV antibiotic alone.
- Furuncle = boil → only I&D, but antibiotic may be considered if cellulitis, suspected MRSA, or infection is persisting after treatment.
- Severe infections: gas gangrene, necrotizing soft tissue infection (necrotizing fasciitis).
    → Patient at risk: ↓ immunity, DM.
    → Invasion through fascial plane (destroy blood supply of fascia).
    → Sepsis or septic shock.
    → Extremities, perineum, trunk, and torso are most commonly affected in that order.
    → History: pain out of proportion.
    → Nausea, vomiting, fever, and mental status changes.

→ Late sign: skin erythema, blistering (hemorrhagic bullae), turbid semipurulent discharge (dishwater pus), skin crepitus.

→ Radiology → some → use x-ray or CT to diagnose air in fascial plane.

- 50% polymicrobial.
- IV antibiotic vancomycin, carbapenem, penicillin G → clostrial.
- Debridement for devitalized tissue, tissue C/S, and swab from discharge.

Postoperative Nosocomial Infection

- UTI > 10^4 CFU/mL microbes in symptomatic or > 10^5 CFU/mL microbes in asymptomatic
    - → Antibiotic for 3–5 days
    - → Risk of Foley catheter → should disconnect ASAP
- Prolonged ventilation → VAP
    - → Purulent sputum, high WBC, fever, CXR
- Indwelling catheter:
    - o 25% colonized, 5% bacteria
    - o PICC is better than CVP → tunnel
    - o Most common organism: Staph. epidermidis, 50%–60%
    - o Antibiotic for 14–21 days
    - o No routine antibiotic to prevent this event

Five Ws Mnemonic for Postoperative Fever
- Wind (atelectasis), postoperative day 1–2
- Water (UTI), postoperative day 3–5
- Wound (SSI), postoperative day 5–7
- Walking (DVT), postoperative day 5–7
- Wonder drugs, transfusion

Blood-Borne Pathogen
- Hep. B needlestick risk is 3%
- Hep. C needlestick risk is 1.8%.
- HIV needlestick is 0.3%.

Tetanus Vaccine

Type of wound	Patient not immunized or partially immunized	Patient completely immunized Time since last booster dose	
		5- 10 years	> 10 years
Minor – clean	Begin or complete vaccination: tetanus toxoid 1 dose of 0.5 ml	None	Tetanus toxoid 1 dose of 0.5 ml
Minor – Clean or tetanus prone	In one am: Human tetanus immunoglobulin 250 l. U In other arm: tetanus toxoid 1 dose of 0.5 ml	Tetanus toxoid: 1 dose of 0.5 ml	In one arm: Human tetanus immunoglobulin 250 IU In other arm: tetanus toxoid: 1 dose of 0.5 ml
Tetanus prone: delayed or incomplete debridement	In one arm: Human tetanus immunoglobulin 500 IU In other arm: tetanus toxoid: 1 dose of 0.5 ml Antibiotic therapy	Tetanus toxoid: 1 dose of 0.5 ml Antibiotic therapy	In one am: Human tetanus immunoglobulin 500 IU In other arm: tetanus toxoid: 1 dose of 0.5 ml Antibiotic therapy

Shock

Overview
- Failure to meet metabolic need of the cell
- Inadequate tissue hypoperfusion, marked by ↓ delivery of O_2 and metabolic needs, ↓ removal of waste products

Pathophysiology of Shock
- Tissue hypoperfusion + cellular injury → imbalance of supply and demand leads to neuroendocrine and inflammatory process.
- It differs according to type.
- Regulation of many organs to maintain perfusion to cerebral and coronary circulation includes the following:
  - → Stretch receptor and baroreceptor
  - → Chemoreceptor
  - → Cerebral ischemia response
  - → Release of endogenous VC
  - → Shift of fluid to intravascular space
  - → Renal reabsorption (salt and water)
- In hemorrhagic shock, the body compensates primarily by neuroendocrine (compensated phase) then decompensates by microcirculatory dysfunction, parenchymal tissue damage, inflammatory cells activation (perpetuate hypoperfusion).
- Ischemia and reperfusion → exacerbate the initial result.
- This affects at cellular level if untreated → MOF and vicious cycle.
- Persistent hypoperfusion → irreversible phase.

Types
- Cardiogenic
- Hypovolemic (hemorrhagic)
- Distributive (septic, neurogenic [spinal])
- Obstructive (tension pneumothorax, PE)

Neuroendocrine and Organ-Specific Responses to Hemorrhage
- The goal is to maintain perfusion to the brain and heart.
- Peripheral VC + inhibit fluid secretion.

- Autonomic control of peripheral vascular tone and cardiac contractility.

Afferent Signals
- CNS: expand plasma volume, maintain peripheral perfusion and O_2 delivery.
    - The initial inciting event usually is loss of circulating blood volume.
        - → Other stimuli: pain, hypoxemia, hypercarbia acidosis, infection, change in temperature, hypoglycemia
    - Sensation of injured tissue transmitted through spinothalamic tract → activation of hypothalamic pituitary − adrenal axis + ANS → direct sympathetic stimulation of adrenal medulla to release catecholamines.

- Baroreceptors: initiate adaptive response to shock; it's sensitive to change in both chamber pressure and wall stretch (in the atrium).
    - Activated when slight drop of BP.
    - Receptor in aortic arch and carotid bodies respond to alteration of stretch in arterial wall if ↓ in intravascular pressure.

- Chemoreceptor in aorta and carotid body are sensitive to O_2 tension.
    - → Stimulation → VD of coronary artery, ↓ HR and VC of splanchnic and skeletal circulation.

Efferent Signals
- CVS
    - Change in CVS result of neuroendocrine response and autonomic nervous system (ANS)
    - Hemorrhage → ↓ VR → ↓ COP → ↑ HR and contractility + VC
    - Stimulation of sympathetic fiber, which innervate the heart → activation of β_1 + VD of coronary (adrenergic receptor)

- Sympathetic of peripheral vessels α receptor $\rightarrow$ VC $\rightarrow$ $\uparrow$ SVR
- increase sympathetic output $\rightarrow$ catecholamines (peak within 24–48 hrs) + hepatic glycogenolysis and gluconeogenesis to increase glucose
- Increase of muscle glycogenolysis $\rightarrow$ decrease insulin, $\uparrow$ glucagon

- Hormonal response
  - Stress $\rightarrow$ ANS activation + activation of hypothalamic pituitary adrenal axis $\rightarrow$ ACTH.
    - $\rightarrow$ Cortisol $\rightarrow$ gluconeogenesis, insulin resistance
    - $\rightarrow$ Proteolysis, lipolysis $\rightarrow$ hepatic gluconeogenesis
    - $\rightarrow$ No $-$ve feedback
  - Renin-angiotensin system:
    - $\rightarrow$ $\downarrow$ renal artery perfusion
    - $\rightarrow$ β-adrenergic stimulation
    - $\rightarrow$ $\uparrow$ Na^+ reabsorption in renal tubule $\rightarrow$ release of renin from juxtaglomerular cells in kidney
    - $\rightarrow$ Angiotensinogen (liver) $\rightarrow$ angiotensin I $\frac{ACE}{lung}$ $\rightarrow$ angiotensin II.
    - $\rightarrow$ Angiotensin I has no function, while angiotensin II is a potent VC of splanchnic and peripheral vessels (can cause intestinal ischemia)
    - $\rightarrow$ Stimulant ACTH + ADH
    - $\rightarrow$ Aldosterone (mineralocorticoid), Na^+ reabsorption
    - $\rightarrow$ K^+ + H^+ exchange with Na^+
  - In septic shock, endotoxin stimulates ADH independent to blood pressure or osmotic or IV volume.
  - ADH = vasopressin.
  - Pro-inflammatory cytokines $\rightarrow$ stimulate ADH.

Circulatory Homeostasis
Preload
- A vast majority of blood in venous system.
- VR = end diastolic wall tension.

- If low blood flow in arteriole → contraction of venous.
- Sympathetic has minor effect on smooth muscle but dramatic effect on splanchnic blood volume (normally 20%).
- Acute response ↑ venous tone, ↑SVR, ↑ intrathoracic pressure.

Ventricular Contraction
- Frank-Starling law.

Afterload
- Force that resists myocardial work during contraction.
- Arterial pressure is the major component (EF).
- Blood viscosity has high vascular resistance.
- COP = SV × HR.

Microcirculation
- Integral role in cellular perfusion.
- Innervated by sympathetic.
- Capillary leak → ↓ ECV → ↓ energy → no K^+/Na^+ pump.
    → capillary occlusion (no reflow)

Metabolic Effect
- Cellular metabolism based on ATP.
- Majority of ATP through aerobic metabolism and oxidation phosphorylation in the mitochondria.
    → Depends on O_2
    → If low → ↓ oxidation phosphorylation → ↓ ATP
    → Only 2 mol of ATP from 1 mol of glucose (compare to complete oxidation 1 mol glucose = 38 ATP)
- Hypoxic condition → pyruvate → lactate (anaerobic metabolism) leading to an intracellular metabolic acidosis.
- Epinephrine and norepinephrine → increase liver glycogenolysis, glycogenolysis, skeletal muscle breakdown, lipolysis and glucagon, ↓ insulin resistance.

Cellular Hypoperfusion
- Hypoxia → O_2 + nitrogen radicals → ↑ VEGF, ↑ cytokines, ↑ NO.

Immune and Inflammatory Response

- Increase in response to trauma, infection, ischemia, toxic, and autoimmune.
- Failure to activation escalation or suppression of inflammatory response → SIRS → MOF.
- Both innate and adaptive immunity work.
- Activation of leukocyte, neuron, mast cell.

Cytokines and Chemokines

- TNF-α: first cytokines released, peak in 90 min and return to baseline within 4 hrs, can be released by bacteria and endotoxin.
  - → No correlate (level) in mortality.
  - → ↑ in trauma but less than in septic shock.
  - → VD and activate other cytokines.
  - → During stress → ↑ protein breaks down and cachexia.
  - → Monocyte, macrophage, T cells is potent pro-inflammatory.

- IL-1
  - Same with TNF-α.
  - Half-life is 6 min.
  - Produces fever in response to injury by activation of prostaglandin in post hypothalamus and causes anorexia by activation of satiety center.
  - ↑ ACTH, steroid and b endorphin.
  - TNF-α + IL-1 = stimulate IL-2, IL-4, IL-6, IL-8, macrophage, and interferon.

- IL-2
  - Produced by activated T cells.
  - Some investigation → ↑ IL-2 → increase injury → increase shock.
  - Increase initially and decrease later → progression of shock.

- IL-6
  - Increases in response to hemorrhagic shock.
    - → Contributes in lung, liver, gut injury.
    - → May play role in alveolar damage and ARDS.
    - → IL-6 and IL-1 are mediators in acute liver injury.
    - → ↑ activity of CRP, fibrinogen, haptoglobin.

- IL-10
  - Anti-inflammatory: immunosuppression.
  - ↑ after shock and trauma, increase infection.
  - Secreted by T cells.
  - ↓ cytokines production.

Complement
- Activated by injury, shock.
- C3a − C5a + C4a increase vascular permeability; ↑ smooth muscle contraction, ↑ histamine → release TNF-α, IL-1.
- Development of ARDS, MODs correlate with activation of component.

Neutrophil
- First cell to recruit to the site of injury (PMNs).

Inflammatory Mediators of Shock

Pro-Inflammatory	Anti-Inflammatory
TNF-α	IL-4
IL-1	IL-10
IL-2	IL-13
IL-6	Prostaglandin E_2
IL-8	TGF-β
Interferon	IL-15
PAF	

Forms of Shock

Hypovolemic/Hemorrhagic

- Acute blood loss → decrease baroreceptor stimulation from stretch receptor → decrease inhibition of VC in brain stem → increase chemoreceptor stimulation of VMC and ↓COP from atrial stretch receptor → increase VC in periphery and peripheral arterial resistance.
- Hypovolemia → increase epinephrine and norepinephrine, activation of renin-angiotensin system and increase vasopressin.
- VC is prominent while lack of sympathetic effect on cerebral and coronary vessel.

- Diagnosis
  - Search for the cause of hypotension.
  - Symptom: agitation, cool and clammy extremities, tachycardia, weak or absent peripheral pulse, and hypotension.
  - Usually loss of > 25%–30% of blood volume.
  - Young will maintain BP, sometimes suddenly collapse.
  - Elderly may be on anticoagulant or β-blocker.
    - → Atherosclerotic → decrease cardiac compliance → inability to increase HR, also acidosis → cardiac muscle inhibition.
  - Classification of hemorrhage:

	I	II	III	IV
Blood loss (mL)	< 750	750–1,500	1.5–2	> 2 L
Blood loss (%)	< 15%	15%–30%	30%–40%	> 40%
HR	< 100	> 100	> 120	> 140
BP	N	Orthostatic	Hypo	Hypo
CNS	N	Anxious	Confused	Obtunded

  - If < 110 mmHg SBP, it's hypotension.
  - Some authors and studies said ↑ HR is not a reliable sign.
  - Serum lactate and base deficit to estimate bleeding and shock.
  - Lactate is an indirect marker for tissue hypoperfusion.

- Several studies show initial and serial lactate levels are reliable predictors for mortality.
- Also, base deficit marker for tissue hypoperfusion
  → Base deficit:

Mild	3–5 mmol/L
Moderate	6–9 mmol/L
Severe	> 10 mmol/L

  → Correlate with needs of transfusion and MOF and death
- Hematocrit (Hct) may not rapidly reflect the total volume of blood loss.
- If no decrease in Hct, it won't rule out in ongoing bleeding.
- Substantial blood loss in prehospital must be documented.
- Each pleural cavity can accommodate 2–3 L.

- Treatment
  - Control of hemorrhage is an essential compound of resuscitation.
  - If patient has abdominal bleeding requiring laparotomy, there's an increase probability of death with ↑ length of stay in ER to 1% for each 3 min.
  - Damage control to keep SBP 80–90 (permissive hypotension) to prevent rebleeding from clotted vessel.
  - If you aggressively resuscitate with high BP in uncontrolled bleeding → ↑ bleeding and mortality.
  - PRC study: delayed resuscitation vs. standard resuscitation in patient with hypotension and penetrating torso injury → results in decrease mortality and morbidity in delayed resuscitation.
  - Any uncontrolled bleeding with attempt to achieve normal BP → increase mortality.
  - Avoid hemodilution by early transfusion of RBCs.
  - Ratio: 1:1:1
  - Current recommendation for stable ICU patient is to keep Hb 7–9.
  - Early use of tranexamic acid decreases rebleeding and decreases mortality.
  - TEG (thromboelastography) for coagulopathy and fibrinolysis.

- Minimize heat loss (prevent hypothermia).
- Triad of death: acidosis, hypotension, hypothermia.

Traumatic Shock

- Systemic response after trauma → combining effect of soft tissue injury, long bone fracture, blood loss.
- Development of MOF, ARDS.
- Ischemia → ischemia reperfusion → pro-inflammatory activation → release of DAMP (damage-associated molecular pattern) like ribonucleic acid.
- Treatment: control of hemorrhage, resuscitation, O_2 debt, debridement.

Septic Shock (Vasodilatory Shock)

- Normally VC occurs with hemorrhage.
- Vasodilatory shock is a result of dysfunction of endothelin and vasculature secondary to activation of inflammatory mediator and cells or as response to prolonged and severe hypoperfusion.
- Failure of vascular smooth muscle to constrict appropriately.
- Peripheral VD → hypotension and resistance to vasopressin
    → Catecholamines, renin-angiotensin system activated; other causes of vasodilatory shock are composing hypoxic lactic acidosis and irreversible hemorrhagic shock.
- Mortality rate from severe sepsis is 30%–50%.
- Each 1-hr delay in diagnosis and management (antibiotics) increases mortality rate by 6.7%.
- Immune and endothelial cells → soluble mediators that enhance macrophage and neutrophil → ↑ procoagulant, ↑ microvascular blood flow → symptom of sepsis.
    → such as ↑ COP, peripheral VD, fever, leukocytosis, hyperglycemia, and tachycardia.
- Nitric oxide in vessel wall predisposes VD.

- • Treatment
    - Airway and ventilation may need intubation.
    - Resuscitation should be 30 mL/kg for the first 4–6 hrs.
    - Avoid starch, colloid fluids.

- Empiric antibiotic (−ve, +ve, anaerobes), but long-term empiric antibiotic avoided → pseudomembranous colitis (C. diff).
- Vasopressin (norepinephrine) is the first option pressor, then epinephrine in case of arterial resistance.
- ↑ COP.
- Dobutamine for patient with cardiac dysfunction.
- Use of surviving sepsis campaign bundles:
  - To be completed within 3 hrs
    1. Measure lactate level.
    2. Blood C/S.
    3. Broad-spectrum IV antibiotic.
    4. IVF 30 mL/kg for low HTN or lactate ≥ 4 mmol/L.
  - To be completed within 6 hrs
    1. Vasopressor MAP ≥ 65.
    2. If persistent hypotension → measure CVP and $SCVO_2$.
    3. Remeasure lactate if first one is high.
- These measurements are important to decrease mortality and morbidity.
- Hyperglycemia and insulin resistance → intensive insulin therapy reduces septicemia by 46% + antibiotic and ventilation.
- ↓ tidal volume → ↓ ARDS.
- Use steroid (corticosteroids and fludrocortisone) if adrenal insufficiency is suspected in form of persistant hypotension despite of IVF and vasopressor.
  → consider hydrocortisone, 200 mg daily × 7 days.
- Antitoxin antibody, anticytokine antibody should be obtained.

Cardiogenic Shock
- Circulatory pump failure → hypoxia
- Criteria: SBP < 90 at least for 30 min
  Low cardiac index < 2.2 L/min
  PAWP > 15 mmHg
- Mortality rate is 50%–80%.

-   Extensive acute MI is the most common cause, and the other is related to heart function.
-   Degree of coronary flow after perfusion correlates with hospital mortality:
    a. 33% with complete perfusion
    b. 50% with incomplete perfusion
    c. 80% with no perfusion
-   Cardiogenic shock → ↓40% of left ventricle (damage).
-   ↓ COP with good preload → ↑ sympathetic stimulation,
-   ↑ HR, ↑ catecholamines → heart failure.

• Diagnosis
-   Low COP, hypotension.
-   Exclude other cause of hypotension such as sepsis, PE.
-   Dysrhythmia.

• Treatment
-   A, B, C → ↓ work of breathing.
-   Adequate O_2.
-   Avoid fluid overload → pulmonary edema.
-   Common electrolyte, low K^+, low Mg^+ should be corrected.
-   Anti-arrhythmic drugs.
-   Morphine for pain.
-   Dobutamine → stimulate cardiac β_1 → ↑ COP but lower dose produce VD to periphral vascular bed and lower SBP through effect on β_2.
-   Dopamine in low dose stimulates β_1 → VC, β_2 → VD.
-   Dopamine is preferable over dobutamine in cardiac dysfunction with hypotension.
-   Epinephrine stimulates both α, β → ↑ peripheral VC → impair cardiac performance.
-   Catecholamines, ↑ coronary perfusion, ↓ O_2 demand.
-   pH, base deficit, and lactate should be measured.
-   Some require intra-aortic balloon pump.
-   Thrombolytics decreases mortality.
-   b-blocker to lower HR and low O_2 consumption.
-   ACE inhibitor to ↓ VC.
        → PCI treatment of choice.

Obstructive Shock
- Tension pneumothorax.
- Cardiac tamponade.
- PE.
- IVC obstruction, DVT, neoplasm.
- High intrathoracic pressure (high PEEP).
- 200 mL can produce cardiac tamponade.

- Diagnosis and Treatment
    - Beck's triad: hypotension, muffled heart sound, and distended neck veins.
    - Echo for cardiac tamponade → pericardiocentesis.
    - Treatment according to the cause, i.e., chest tube for tension pneumothorax.
    - Diagnostic pericardial window is the most direct method in OR by median sternotomy or left anterior thoracotomy or bilateral anterior thoracotomy (clamshell).

Neurogenic Shock
- Decrease tissue perfusion due to loss of vasomotor tone on peripheral vascular bed → ↓ VR → ↓ COP.
- Cause: spinal trauma, spinal neoplasm, spinal epidural anesthesia.

- Diagnosis
    - Bradycardia, hypotension, cardiac dysrhythmia, low COP, and low PVR.
    - Absence of reflexive tachycardia due to disruption of sympathetic discharge.
    - Paralysis.

- Treatment
    - A-B-C.
    - Vasoconstrictor.
    - Exclude other cause of hypotension.
    - Pure α-agonist phenylephrine.

Hemodynamic responses to different types of shock

types of shock	Cardiac index	SVR	Venous capacitance	CVP / PCWP	SVO2
Hypovolemic	↓	↑	↓	↓	↓
Septic	↑↑	↓	↑	↓↑	↓↑
Cardiogenic	↓↓	↑↑	Little effect	↑	↓
Neurogenic	↑	↓	Little effect	↓	↓

End Point in Resuscitation
- Resuscitation is completed when O_2 debt is repaired, acidosis is corrected, and aerobic metabolism is resorted.
- In trauma, ↑ lactate and ↓ mixed venous O_2.
- If lactate is high and not normalized within 12 hrs in spite normal HR, BP, and UOP and its > 3 times the normal individual with normal lactate → mortality is fourfold.
- End point in resuscitation can be divided into systemic or global parameter, tissue specific parameter and cellular parameter
- Global end point include: vital signs, lactate, base deficit, COP, O_2 delivery and consumption

Assessment of End Point Resuscitation
- The ability to repay O_2 debt increases mortality and morbidity.
    - → Known by HR, BP, UOP, and CVP, PAOP is a poor indicator, but lactate and base deficit show correlation with O_2 debt.

- Lactate
    - Generated by conversion of pyruvate to lactate dehydrogenase in absence of O_2.
    - Metabolized by kidney and liver, 30% and 50%, respectively.

- Admission lactate, highest lactate, normal ≥ important prognostic indicator for survival.
- Base deficit and volume of blood transfusion required in first 24 hrs of resuscitation is a better indicator of mortality than lactate alone.

- **Base Deficit**
  - Is the amount of base in mmol that is required to titrate 1 L of blood to return pH 7.4 with the sample fully saturated with O_2 at 37°C and P pressure of CO_2 40.
  - Usually measured by ABG.
  - This indicates metabolic acidosis.
  - A positive number is called base excess and indicates metabolic alkalosis.
  - Base deficit > 15 mmol/L → mortality, 70%

    | Mild | 3–5 mmol/L |
    | Moderate | 6–14 mmol/L |
    | Severe | 15 mmol/L |

  - Trauma admitted with a base deficit greater than 15 mmol/L requires twice the volume of fluid and six times blood transfusion in the first 24 hrs.
  - High base deficit correlates with ARDS.
  - Factors comprising the utility of base deficit: administration of bicarbonate, hypothermia, hypocapnia, heparin, ethanol, ketoacidosis.

- **Gastric Tonometry**
  - Lactate and base deficit indicate global tissue acidosis (systemic) rather than tissue specific.
  - Many authors suggest tissue-specific end-point are more predictive of outcome and adequate tissue resuscitation in trauma.

Trauma

Initial Evaluation of Injured Patient
ATLS Protocol
    Primary Survey
       - ABCDE

        Airway and C-Spine
- Airway is the priority.
- C-spine is protected by hard neck collar.
- Generally, if the patient is conscious, no tachypnea, normal voice → no airway intervention except the following:
    - Penetrating neck injury with expanding hematoma
    - Chemical or thermal injuries to mouth, nares (nostril), pharynx
    - Extensive SC air in the neck
    - Complex maxillofacial injury
    - Airway bleeding
- In comatose patients, hypopharynx falls backward → obstruction → chin lift or jaw thrust maneuver.
- Rapid sequence intubation → if failed ETT → surgical airway → cricothyroidotomy vertical (longitudinal) skin inicision, SC dissection→ incise the membrane → horizontal (transverse) incision then tube size 6.0 introduced.
- Contraindicated in low age-groups < 11 years → subglottic stenosis → tracheostomy is better.
- Tracheostomy in patient with laryngeal separation in OR.
- Clothesline injury, distal trachea clamp to prevent retraction.

        Breathing and Ventilation
- All O_2 supply and pulse oximetry
- Life-threatening: Tension pneumothorax
                          Open pneumothorax
                          Flail chest with underlying contusion
                          Massive air leak

- Tension pneumothorax
    → Needle decompression in second intercostal space (recently in fifth intercostal space, just anterior to midaxillary line)
- Open (sucking wound)
    → Occlusive dressing that tape in three sides
- Flail chest need generous analgesia with O_2 supplement
- Massive air leak; injury to major tracheobronchial tree
    Type I—with 2 cm of carina (no pneumothorax)
    Type II—distal injury (pneumothorax)

Circulation and Hemorrhage
- Hypotension when SBP < 90.
- Assumed hemorrhage till proven otherwise.
- If IV access is difficult → all medications via intraosseous infusion but should be removed ASAP → osteomyelitis.
- Blood drawn for CBC, chemistry, ABG, crossmatching, and coagulation.
- Venous cutdown: Cordis introducer catheter (saphenous), 1 cm anterior and 1 cm superior of medial malleolus, 14 gauge introduced.
- CVP: femoral for thoracic trauma, subclavian or jugular for abdominal trauma.
- External control of hemorrhage (manual) with gauze 4 × 4 and glare hand → OR.
- Covering with excess gauze → unrecognized bleeding.
- Blind clamping avoided.
- If extremities → tourniquet → warm ischemia.
- Scalp → diffuse → clips or deep continuous prolene suture.
- Life-threatening:
    - Massive hemothorax > 1,500 mL
    - Cardiac tamponade
    - Massive hemoperitoneum
    - Unstable pelvic fracture
- FAST, eFAST.
- Cardiac tamponade: acute > 100 cc.
    → Beck's triad (Δ) hypotension, muffled heart sound, and distended neck veins. diagnosis by US or FAST.

Pericardiocentesis 15–20 mL, 80% success rate.
- Resuscitation thoracotomy (RT)
   → Is associated with the highest survival rate after isolated cardiac injury, 35%.
   → For all penetrating wounds, survival rate is 15%.
   → Conversely, patient outcome is poor when RT is done for blunt trauma, with 2% survival among patients in shock and < 1% survival among those with no vital signs.

- • Indication:
   - Patient with penetrating trauma to torso arrested < 15 min of hospital arrival.
   - Patient with blunt trauma arrested < 10 min of hospital arrival.
   - Patient with penetrating neck trauma arrested < 5 min of hospital arrival.
   - Air embolism.
   - Cardiac tamponade.
- • Contraindication: if prolonged presentation, i.e., arrested for a long time.
   Steps:
   - Generous left thoracotomy → longitudinal pericardiotomy.
   - Identify phrenic nerve.
      → Cross-clamp aorta to improve cerebral and coronary blood flow.
- Tranexamic acid decreases number of transfusions, ↑ SR → thrombotic complication if given > 3 hrs.

Disability
- GCS

15–13	Mild
12–9	Moderate
≤ 8	Severe

- Neurological shock, hypotension, bradycardia, paralysis, low rectal tone, or priapism

Glascow coma scale

Eye	Spontaneous 4	To voice 3	Pain 2	None 1		
Verbal	Oriented 5	Confused 4	Inappropriate ward 3	Incomprehensive word 2	None 1	
Motor	Obey command 6	Localize the pain 5	Pain Withdrawn 4	Abnormal flexion 3	Abnormal extension 2	None 1

Exposure

- Cover to prevent hypothermia and to proceed to adjuncts such ECG, NGT, Foley catheter, log roll and DRE,

  e-FAST and secondary survey

Shock Classification and Initial Fluid Resuscitation

- Classic signs and symptoms of shock are tachycardia, hypotension, tachypnea, altered mental status, diaphoresis, and pallor.
- In general, the quantity of acute blood loss correlates with physiologic abnormalities.
- The goal of fluid resuscitation is to reestablish tissue perfusion.
- Fluid resuscitation begins with 2 Liters (adult) or 20 mL/kg (child) IV bolus of isotonic crystalloid, typically Ringer's lactate.
- For persistent hypotension (SBP < 90 mmHg in an adult), the current trend is to activate a massive transfusion protocol (MTP) in which red blood cells (RBC) and fresh frozen plasma (FFP) are administered early.
- Peripheral perfusion (warm fingers and toes with normal capillary refill) is presumed to have adequate overall perfusion → UOP 0.5–1 mL/kg for adult and 2 mL/kg in pediatric indicate stability.
- Tachycardia is the earliest sign of hemorrhage, bradycardia can occur with severe blood loss, myocardial inhibition from severe acidosis or patient on β-blocker.

Persistent Hypotension

- Ongoing hemodynamic instability.
- Consider hemorrhage, cardiogenic, neurogenic, septic shocks
  → FAST

- → CVP → patient with distended neck vein CVP > 15 → cardiogenic shock
  - → Patient with flat neck vein CVP < 5 → hypovolemic shock
- Persist arterial base deficit > 8 → organ cellular shock.
- Near IR spectroscopy → noninvasive of O_2 to tissue.
- Neurogenic (spinal) → bradycardia or normal pulse + hypotension + unable to move the legs if conscious; no rectal tone.
- Differential diagnosis of cardiogenic shock:
  1. Tension pneumothorax
  2. Pericardial tamponade
  3. Blunt cardiac injury
  4. MI
  5. Air embolism
- ⅓ of blunt trauma to chest → has cardiac injury.
- Patient with dysrhythmia → ECG monitoring and anti-arrhythmia.
- ECG is first and adequate toll to r/o cardiac injury.
- Normal ECG + troponin at admission and after 8 hrs to rule out cardiac injury.
- Echo for valvular or septal injury, and most common finding is right ventricular dyskinesia.
- If cardiogenic shock persists → intra-aortic balloon pump.
  If MI → lytic therapy or angioplasty.
- Air embolism can be in blunt and penetrating trauma from bronchial venous fistula.
- Should be on Trendelenburg position to trap air at apex of left ventricle, to force air exit from coronary arteries; if failed → aspiration from right coronary.
- Once circulation is restored → keep on Trendelenburg and clamp pulmonary hilum till injury is repaired (Satinsky).
- During evaluation of the cause of hypotension, give blood type O^+ and O^- for female in childbearing age + plasma 2:1.
- Gunshot → AXR.
- If penetrating weapon, don't remove.

- If in neck → CT to see arterial injury.
- Five potential causes of bleeding: scalp, chest, abdomen, pelvis, and extremities.
- Blood loss

Each	Rib fracture	100–200 cc
	Tibial fracture	300–500 cc
	Femur fracture	800–1,000 cc
	Pelvic fracture	> 2,000 cc

- Concept of hypotensive resuscitation (permissive hypotension), i.e., sealing of clot disrupted at SBP > 90, as in aortic dissection.
- On the other hand, traumatic brain injury (TBI) is prevented by maintaining SBP > 100.

Secondary Survey
- AMPLE (history)
- Then physical examination from head to toe.
  With special attention to axilla, perineum, back.
  DRE: tone, blood, perforation, overriding prostate and vaginal examination.
- Adjunct: CVP monitoring, ECG, Foley catheter, NGT, radiography, urinalysis, base deficit, and repeat FAST.
- NGT to all intubated patient.
- If maxillofacial or basilar skull fracture → OGT.
- If hematoma or sign of urethral injury, deferred till urology examination → if can't → suprapubic catheter.
- Pan CT scan.

Mechanism of Injury
- Most affected organs by blunt injury—liver, spleen, kidney.
- Penetrating small bowel, liver, colon.
- Severe mechanism, pedestrian, MVC if exceeding 20 mph, falls from height of 20 ft.
- Front impaction → trauma to chest and upper abdomen, hit steering column.
- Side C-spine, thoracic, diaphragm.
- Ejected from vehicle → any.
- Penetrating stab, gunshot, shotgun.

→ Gunshot: high and low velocity
→ Shotgun: close (like high velocity) range < 20 ft, long range

Regional Assessment and Special Diagnostic Test

- Head
  - Scalp, eye, nose, mouth, ears, facial bone.
  - Lateral canthotomy is needed to relief periorbital pressure.
  - Basilar skull fracture—raccoon sign, battle sign.
  - Epidural (Extra-dural) hematoma between skull and dura → middle meningeal artery.
  - Subdural between dura and cortex → venous bleeding.
  - Due to associated brain parenchymal injury, with subdural, its worse prognosis.
  - SAH → vasospasm → ↓ cerebral blood flow.
  - Diffuse axonal injury (DAI)—high-speed deceleration injury from shear effect → blurring of gray and white matter.
  - MRI is the accurate test.
  - Stroke syndrome → CT angiography for carotid and vertebral arteries.

- Neck
  - Ligamentous injury not visible by x-ray or CT but by MRI.
  - Spinal cord injuries can vary in severity; complete injuries cause either quadriplegia or paraplegia, depending on the level of injury.
  - Central cord syndrome → hyperextension.
  - Anterior cord syndrome → ↓ motor function and pain.
  - Brown-Sequard syndrome → transected one-half of spinal cord → loss of ipsilateral motor and proprioception.
  - Look for SC emphysema, hoarseness, palpable fracture.

- Neck zones:
  - ○ Zone I—sternal notch till cricoid cartilage.
  - ○ Zone II—from carotid cartilage and angle of mandible.
  - ○ Zone III—above angle of mandible till nose.
- Penetrating neck injury in unstable pateint → OR.
- Stable with specific symptoms or signs that should be identified include dysphagia, hoarseness, hematoma, venous bleeding, minor hemoptysis, and subcutaneous emphysema; should undergo diagnostic imaging before operation if they remain hemodynamically stable.
- Less than 15% with penetrating neck injury require exploration.
- Zone III can be managed by selective angioembolization.

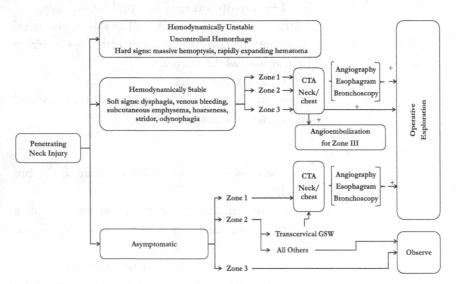

- Chest
  - Persistent pneumothorax after chest tube → fiber-optic bronchoscopy to exclude tracheobronchial injury or foreign body.
  - Persistent hemothorax not drained by two chest tube → caked hemothorax → thrombolytics therapy or VATS, if failed → thoracotomy.

- Wide mediastinum → great vessels injury.
  - Left-side hematoma → descending aorta.
  - Right-side hematoma → innominate artery.
- Other CXR findings suggested aortic tear:
  1. Wide mediastinum
  2. Abnormal aortic contour
  3. Tracheal shift
  4. NGT shift
  5. Left apical cap
  6. Depression of left bronchus
  7. Obliteration of aortopulmonary window
  8. Left pulmonary hilar hematoma
- 7% with aortic dissection have normal CXR.
- 95% of injuries is distal to left subclavian artery at ligamentum arteriosum.
- 2.5% in ascending or aortic arch or at the level of the diaphragm.
- Needs two views of CXR, pericardial US, CVP.
- Bronchoscopy for persistent air leak.
- Esophagoscopy can miss injury → water-soluble contrast esophagram followed by barium (for contrast extravasation).
- If suspected subclavian artery injury → brachial–brachial index should be measured.
- CT angiography for vascular injury.

- Abdomen
  - Diagnostic black box.
  - Differs in either blunt or penetrating.
  - Gunshot penetrates peritoneum → laparotomy, except if in RUQ and stable patient.
  - Anterior abdominal wall stab → exploration under local anesthesia to see if fascia is violated or not.
    - → If not → discharge the patient home.
    - → If yes, 50% require serial abdominal examination and further image or operative intervention (laparotomy).

- If the stab wound is tangential in stable patient → CT to exclude peritoneal penetration.
- Laparoscopic exploration is another option.
- Diaphragmatic injury—laparoscopy (diagnostic and therapeutic).
- DPL or DPA → ↓ use nowadays.
- Patients with free intra-abdominal fluid without solid organ injury are closely monitored for evolving signs of peritonitis.
- If the patients have a significant closed-head injury or cannot be serially examined → DPL should be performed to exclude bowel injury:
  - Infraumbilical approach is used.
  - After placement of the catheter, a 10 mL syringe is connected and the abdominal contents aspirated (termed as diagnostic peritoneal aspiration).
  - The aspirate is considered to show positive findings if > 10 mL of blood is aspirated.
  - If < 10 mL is withdrawn, a liter of normal saline is instilled (lavage).
  - The effluent is withdrawn via siphoning and sent to the laboratory for RBC, WBC, amylase, bilirubin, and alkaline phosphatase levels.
  - Criteria for "positive" finding on diagnostic peritoneal lavage:

Red blood cell count	> 100,000/mL
White blood cell count	> 500/mL
Amylase level	> 19 IU/L
Alkaline phosphatase level	> 2 IU/L
Bilirubin level	> 0.01 mg/dL

- FAST 100% sensitive if > 250 mL.
- If FAST +ve → stable → CT.
  - → unstable → OR.

- Guideline for nonoperative management:
  - → Stable, no blush, minimal amount of intraperitoneal hemorrhage, no peritonitis, no pseudoaneurysm.
  - → 24 hrs serial abdominal examination.
  - → But delay recovery and ↑ stay.
- CT is part of nonoperative management.
- Bowel injury—thickening of bowel wall + streaking in mesentery, free fluid without solid organ injury, free air.
- Location is important → anterior → ↑ risk of injury followed by UQ (thoracoabdominal); the flanks have the least risk of organ injury.
- In gunshot injuries, 90% has +ve finding → blast effect.
- Complication of laparotomy—iatrogenic injury, ileus, evisceration, small bowel adhesion and obstruction, infection, incisional hernia, death (8%–41%).

- Pelvis
  - Complex fracture → major hemorrhage.
  - X-ray shows gross abnormal deformity, but CT is necessary.
  - Organs in danger are bladder, rectum, or vagina.
  - CT cystogram if urinalysis is +ve.
  - Urethral injury—blood at meatus, scrotal or perineal hematoma, high-riding prostate on DRE.
    - → Urethrogram before Foley catheter.
  - Injury to major vessels is uncommon, but thrombosis may occur.
    - → CT angiography.

- Extremities
  - Hard signs: pulsate hemorrhage, absent pulse, acute ischemia.
  - Soft signs: hematoma + (A-A index) < 0.9, thrill, or bruit.

- Bone fracture and knee dislocation should align before vascular examination.
- Most common approach to evaluate vascular injury is to measure SBP using Doppler and compare to opposite side (A-A index).
  If injury > 10% → CT angiography is indicated.
- Pseudoaneurysm if bleeding → compartment syndrome and may lose the limb.

General Principle of Management
Transfusion Practice
- Severe injury with life-threatening hemorrhage will develop an acute coagulopathy of trauma (ACOT).
- Protein C and fibrinolysis are major complements.
- Occurs in 5% of injured patient and 20% with massive transfusion.
- Manifestation of coagulopathy:
  → INR > 1.5, PTT > 1.5, platelet > 50,000, fibrinogen > 100 mg/dL
    → Guidelines replaced all this by TEG and ROTEM.
- Optimal ratio is 1:2 blood—plasma in massive transfusion (10 units of RBCs in 6 hrs) → crossmatching in 45 min → O+ group is transfused, if female better to transfuse O⁻ if available.
- TEG—clot capacity and fibrinolysis within 10 min.

Prophylactic Measures
- Antibiotic to all patients before OR.
- Extended postoperative antibiotic only for contaminated open fracture.
- Tetanus prophylaxis.
- LMWH initiated as soon as bleeding is controlled → anti-Xa and antiplatelet in high-risk patient, obese, with multiple pelvic fractures, with spinal cord injury.
- Thermal protection, can become hypothermic on 34°C.

Operative Approach and Exposure

Cervical Exposure

- Two finger breadth above sternal notch. For bilateral exploration, it can be extend accordingly.
- Unilateral—incision from mastoid till clavicle along anterior border of sternomastoid.
- Facial vein marks carotid bifurcation → ligate it to expose internal carotid.

- Exposure of distal carotid artery in zone III is difficult but can be by:
    1. Division of ansa cervicalis to expose hypoglossal nerve.
    2. Transect posterior portion of digastric muscle.
    3. Mandibular subluxation.
    4. Resection of parotid gland, be careful (facial nerve).

Thoracic Incision

- o Anterolateral thoracotomy (emergency exploration)
    - → Can be extended across sternum (clamshell).
    - → Internal mammary artery is ligated.
    - → Access to heart, lung, esophagus, hilum of lung, descending aorta.
    - → Can be extended to left supraclavicular incision (trap door).
    - → Access left subclavian artery (if intrathoracic) after resuscitation thoracotomy; if out thoracic outlet → medial sternotomy.
- o Median sternotomy for stab wounds in the heart.
- o Median sternotomy with cervical extension → for proximal subclavian, innominate, proximal carotid arteries.
    - → Take care for phrenic and vagus nerves (RLN).
- o Posterolateral incision:
    - → Right posterolateral thoracotomy, exposure of trachea or main bronchus (near carina).
    - → Left posterolateral thoracotomy if descending aorta and thoracic esophageal injury.

Emergent Abdominal Exploration
- Drape—from chin to knees to posterior axillary line, arms are out.
- For adult, longitudinal midline incision.
- For pediatrics < 6 years, transverse incision.
- Incision with scalpel and ignoring bleeding from incision.
- Evacuate fluid using pad.
- Palpate spleen and liver for injury.
- Inspect infracolic mesentery (zone I) for vascular injury and upper lateral (zone II), and the pelvis (zone III).
  If bleeding → digital pressure or clamp aorta at diaphragm level.
- If severe bleeding from the liver, clamp hepatic pedicle (Pringle maneuver).
- If splenic injury → clamp splenic artery after mobilization and medial rotation to expose lateral peritoneum.
- For abdominal vascular injury either supracolic injury or infracolic
  → Supracolic for aorta, celiac, SMA, left renal artery → best approach by left medial visceral rotation (Cattell maneuver)
- SMA injury (Fullen zone I, II, III, IV):

  I   Posterior to pancreas (left medial visceral rotation)

  II   From pancreatic edge till middle colic (lesser sac) and pancreatic body may be divided

  III, IV   Directly through mesentery
- Venous bleeding behind pancreas → i.e., junction of SMV + splenic vein → divide neck of pancreas.
- IVC: right medial visceral rotation (Mattox maneuver)
- The iliac bifurcation is anterior to IVC (Satinsky clamp).
- Venous injuries are not controlled with aortic clamping, tamponade with a folded pads.
  → If hemostasis is not adequate to expose the vessel proximal and distal to the injury, sponge sticks can be strategically placed.
  → Alternatively, complete pelvic vascular isolation may be required to control hemorrhage for adequate visualization, the right iliac artery may require

division to exposed venous injuries in this area, and the artery must be repaired after the venous injury is treated.

- Injury to iliac vessels: proximal control at infrarenal aorta to avoid splanchnic and renal ischemia.
- Hematoma should be unroofed to see associated bowel injury.
- Anterior and posterior stomach should be inspected.
- Duodenal injury → Kocher maneuver.
- During exploration of the lesser sac → visualization and palpation of pancreas.
- In patients with multisystem trauma → gastrostomy or jejunostomy tube feeding could be introduced.
- In closure, use warm saline wash and close fascia with running heavy suture.
- Necrotizing fasciitis, wound dehiscence, evisceration after laparotomy are not uncommon complications.
    - → If edematous bowel → temporary closure.
    - → When diuresis occurs → close definitely.

Damage Control Surgery (DCS)

- In case of instability, hypothermia, metabolic acidosis, coagulopathy.
- DCS: limit operative time → control bleeding and spillage → restore physiology then definitive treatment.
- Aortic injury must be repaired with PTFE.
- Venous bleeding is treated by ligation, except IVC, popliteal vein.
- Extensive injury to kidney and spleen is treated with excision.
- Hepatic injury → perihepatic packing.
- Translobar gunshot controlled by balloon catheter tamponade, deeper by Foley catheter.
- Thoracic: wedge resection using stapler in bleeding peripheral pulmonary injuries; in penetrating injuries, pulmonary tractotomy is used to divide the parenchyma. Individual vessels and bronchi are then ligated using a 3-0 (PDS) and the tract left open.
- Cardiac injury by running 3-0 nonabsorbable or skin stapler.

→ Pledgeted repair performed in thin right ventricle.
- Hallow viscus → GIA stapler, no stromas.
- Pancreatic injury: packed, drained, and looked later on.
- Urological injuries needs catheter diversion and temporary abdominal closure by towel clip to decrease abdominal compartment.
- Two Jackson-Pratt drains.
- Return to OR within 24 hrs.

Vascular Repair Technique
- Direct digital pressure.
- Sharp dissection around vessels.
- Fogarty catheter, proximally and distally.
- Heparin saline of 50 mL units/mL injection, proximally and distally.
- Shunt or saphenous vein interposition reconstruction.
- Repair for aorta, carotid, innominate, brachial, SMA, proper hepatic, renal, iliac, femoral, and popliteal arteries.
- Ligation of these named vessels usually tolerate the ligation of right hepatic, left hepatic, and celiac arteries.
- In lower limb, the artery with distal runoff should be salvaged.
- Injury with pseudoaneurysm, intimal dissection or small intimal flap in upper limb and lower limb → nonoperative management.
- Follow up image after 1–2 weeks.
- Venous repair for SVC, renal vein, Portal vein, but PV can be ligated in some circumstances.
    - → SMV repaired optimally but can be ligated, and 80% will survive.
    - → Lateral vein ligation adjacent to IVC as there is collateral.
- Arterial defect 1–2 cm → ligate small branch to elongate it.
    - → If it cannot be → parachute technique.
    - → If it cannot be reapproximated → interposition graft.
    - → If < 6 mm → saphenous interposition.
    - → If larger → PTFE is better than Dacron, lower rate of infection.

→ If there's contamination → control it then irrigate the abdominal cavity, repair the vessel, cover with peritoneum or omentum, then repair bowel.

- Internal carotid injury: carotid transposition is an effective approach for treating injuries of the proximal internal carotid artery.
    → Ligate external branch and anastomosis to internal carotid.
    → Iliac A. can be done in the same fashion.
- Small injury with no loss of tissue → lateral suture repair.
- If graft thrombosed 1–2 weeks → collateral.

Definitive Management of Specific Injury
Head Injury
- GCS ≤ 8 → measure ICP by intraventricular catheter.
- ICP = 10 is upper limit of normal pressure, and you should start the following measurement if ICP is above 20.
    - OR intervention to remove space occupying lesion.
    E.g., hematoma is + clot volume
    + amount of midline shift
    + location of clot
    + GCS
    + ICP
    → If midline shift > 5 mm → OR.
    - Diffuse brain edema → high ICP → decompression craniotomy.
    - Skull fracture → either open or depressed.
    - Penetrating skull injury → OR.
    - Epidural (extradural) hematoma → lucid interval and ipsilateral dilated pupil (third Cranial nerve) with contralateral hemiparesis.
    - Subdural can be delayed.
- After OR → ICU → avoid hypotension, hypoxia, and hypo- or hypernatremia that causes secondary brain insult.
- CPP = MAP − ICP.
- CPP increased by MAP or ↓ ICP.
- PCO_2 should be normal, 35–40 mmHg (if ↑ → VD)
- Intracranial HTN treated by cerebral VC by hyperventilation

- Moderate hypothermia improves outcome at least 48 hrs (32°C–33°C).
- With hematoma → prophylactic anticonvulsant → phenytoin after injury for 7 days.

Maxillofacial Injury
- Three regions:
    Upper face: frontal sinus and brain
    Midface: nose, orbit, zygomaticomaxillary
    Lower face: mandible
- If bleeding, Foley catheter or packing.
- Open fracture → need antibiotic.
- Examine the vision, smell, taste.

Cervical Injury
Spine
- Treating patient with cervical injury depends on the stability of the spine, the presence of subluxation, the extent of angulation, and the level of neurologic deficit.
- Immobilization is achieved by spinal orthosis.
- Surgical fusion typically is performed in patients with neurologic deficit, those with angulation of > 11 degrees or translation of > 3.5 mm and those who remain unstable after halo placement.
- Historically → cortisone for spinal trauma.
    → Small benefit within 24 hrs.
    → Current guideline → no longer.
- The time of surgery is debated.
    → Urgent decompression of bilateral locked facets in patients with incomplete tetraplegia or with neurologic deterioration.

Vascular
- Blunt or penetrating.
- Carotid → end to end anastomosis, can use graft interposition.
    → All injury should be repaired.
    → Temporary shunt.
- IJV: lateral venorrhaphy.

- Vertebral artery is difficult to repair (foramen transversarium).
- Blunt injury → risk of dissection, thrombosis.
- Anticoagulant if no contraindications (ICH)
    → Heparin (15 mg/kg/hr) → PTT (40–50 s) or antiplatelet aspirin (325 mg) or clopidogrel (75 mg) for 6 months.
    → Carotid stent for grade III is controversial, but if aggravated edema → stent.

Aerodigestive

- Fractured larynx, trachea → SC emphysema.
- Thyroid cartilage fracture, vocal cord tear, cricoid fracture → after debridement of trachea end to end, interrupted absorbable suture (PDS).
    → Vascularized tissue between trachea and esophagus.
    → Drain (suction).

Chest Injury

- Blunt and penetrating → mostly hemothorax or pneumothorax.
- 85% treated with chest tube.
- Indication of thoracotomy:
    o Initial tube thoracotomy (hemothorax) > 1,500 mL or > 200 mL/hr for 3 hrs
    o Caked hemothorax despite of two chest tubes
    o Selected descending torn aorta
    o Great vessels injury
    o Pericardial tamponade
    o Cardiac herniation
    o Massive air leak
    o Tracheal or main bronchial injury
    o Esophageal perforation
    o Air embolism

Great Vessels

- 90% is penetrating injury but blunt trauma to innominate, subclavian; descending aorta can cause pseudoaneurysm or rupture.

- Ascending and transverse aorta can be repaired with lateral aortography.
    → If posterior → interposition graft repair with cardiopulmonary bypass.
- Innominate artery → repair using exclusion technique.
    → No bypass (cardiopulmonary).
    → Bypass from proximal aorta to distal innominate using PTFE then oversewn.
- Subclavian: lateral aortography or PTFE, end-to-end anastomosis not advocated if there's significant loss.
- Descending aorta: urgent intervention.

NB OR intervention: intracranial, intra-abdominal hemorrhage, or unstable pelvic fracture takes precedence.
- To prevent aortic rupture → β antagonist esmolol
- target SBP < 100 mmHg (permissive hypotension) and HR < 100/min.
- Endovascular stenting is mainstay, but open operative reconstruction is warranted in selected patients.

Heart
- Penetrating or blunt injuries.
- Hemorrhage control by Satinsky clamp to atria and digital pressure to occlude wound.
    → Foley catheter → temporary control using skin stapler.
    → Definitive repair running nonabsorbable suture polypropylene 3-0 or interrupted pledgeted 2-0 polypropylene.
- Pledgeted is used more in atrium (thin).
- Injury adjacent to coronary artery → repaired by horizontal mattress because running suture → coronary occlusion.
- Gunshot → after repair → bioGel.
- Echo can diagnose injury.
- Valvular damage requires cardiopulmonary bypass.
- Patient with blunt cardiac injury → tachycardia and cardiac tamponade.

Trachea-Bronchi and Lung Parenchyma
- 1% of trauma patient sustained to tracheobronchial injury.
- Only few of them requires surgical intervention.
- Blunt injury is most common and occurs 2–5 cm from carina.
- Massive air leak → emergent exploration.
    → Similar to tracheal injury 3-0 PDS, end to end
        → vascularized tissue; pleura, pericardium, intercostal muscle imposed over the repair.
- Peripheral bronchial injury → endoscopy, bronchoscopy → fabric glue to seal it.
- Peripheral laceration of lung → wedge resection.
- If central → tractotomy and ligation of vessels and bronchioles to prevent air embolism.
- If proximal vascular injury → formal lobectomy, because pneumonectomy is usually fatal (right heart decompensation).

- Post-trauma:
    - Pseudocyst (pneumatocele)
        → If with fever, high WBCs → CT → antibiotic + CT guide drainage.
    - Empyema, CT-guided drainage, if failed → VATS if multiple locations.

Esophagus
- Often occurs with tracheobronchial injury.
- End-to-end anastomosis after debridement.
- If cervical injury with trachea or bronchial injury → interposition of vascularized tissue.
- Perforation at GE junction → Nissen fundoplication or segmental resection and gastric pull-up.
- If large destruction injury or delay presentation with sepsis, esophageal exclusion with wide drainage → diverting loop esophagostomy + gastrostomy tube.

Chest Wall
- Rib fracture is treated nonoperatively with chest tube if indicated.
    → For pain, rib block by bupivacaine → thoracic epidural catheter for multiple fractures.
- Persistent hemorrhage from intercostal artery → thoracotomy with direct ligation or angioembolization.
- Scapula and sternum rarely need operative intervention; if significant displacement → sternal plating.
- Clavicle is treated nonoperatively if dislocation occurred, can injure subclavian vessels.

Diaphragmatic injury
- Incidence is 0.8%–8%, penetrating more than blunt.
- More in the left side than the right, 2.3:1.
- Liver protects right hemidiaphragm.

Anatomy
- Origin: lower ribs, lumbar, sternum and inserted in central tendon.
- Foramen at

8th T	Esophagus, vagus nerve
10th T	IVC
12th T	Aorta, thoracic duct, azygos vein

- Artery: phrenic artery from aorta + intercostal artery.
- Venous drainage: IVC
- Nerves: Motor   Phrenic nerve
        Sensory Central–phrenic nerves
                Peripheral–intercostal nerves

Diagnosis
- Chest: dyspnea respiratory distress, chest pain, shallow breathing, ↓ breath sound on affected area, can hear bowel sounds.
- FAST can be diagnostic.
- CXR can miss 20%–50%.
- Contrast study can be performed.
- CT: sensitivity and specificity, 71%–100%.

- MRI for chronic cases.

Grade

I	Contusion
II	Laceration $\leq$ 2 cm
III	Laceration 2–10 cm
IV	Laceration > 10 cm loss tissue $\leq$ 25 m²
V	Laceration > 25 cm² tissue loss

- Usually Penetrating injury grade I, II
  Blunt injury III–V

Treatment
- If spillage in chest → irrigation.
- Zero or one nonabsorbable, continue locking or interrupted sutures to approximate the defect.
- Laparoscopy can be performed but with risk of tension pneumothorax.
- If detachment → reattach.
- If large defect → synthetic mesh; if infection → biological mesh.
  Alternative: omentum, fascia lata, latissimus dorsi, intercostal muscle flaps.
- Chronic hernia better approached by thoracotomy or thoracoscopy.

Abdominal Injury
Liver and Biliary Injuries

Liver Injury Grade	Subcapsular Hematoma	Laceration
I	< 10%	< 1 cm
II	10%–50%	1–3 cm
III	> 50%	> 3 cm
IV	25%–75% of hepatic lobe	
V	> 75% of hepatic lobe	
VI	Hepatic pedicle avulsion	

- The liver is the most common organ injured related to blunt trauma.
- The liver's large size makes it the most susceptible to blunt trauma, and it is frequently involved in upper torso penetrating wounds.
- Patient with grade II or more → admit to surgical ICU.
- Usually nonoperative management, less than 20% require OR.
- Success rate of non operative is 80%–90%.
- Transfer to nonmonitor bed after 24 hrs with grades I and II; with high grade, monitor 2–3 days more.
- Bed rest is controversial, but for grades III and higher → can be ambulant after 2 days.
- Failure of non operative management according to grade:

  I, II   Failure rate is 3%–7.5%.
  IV, V   Failure rate is 14%–23%.
- Contraindication of non operative management → unstable patient, high injury grade, large hemoperitoneum, contrast extravasation, pseudoaneurysm.
- Angiography, ERCP can ↑ success rate.
- Indication of angiography to control hepatic hemorrhage:
  → Transfusion 4 units in 6 hrs or 6 units in 24 hrs with stable patient.
- Laparotomy → perihepatic packing with extensive hemorrhage.
- Packing between liver and diaphragm up to 10–15 pads.
- Usually, packing for left lobe is not effective as no abdominal wall muscle as well as thoracic cage for compression.
- Clamp protocol triad → Pringle maneuver occlusion, 15 min and 5 min off → if still bleeding, this is from IVC (hepatic vein) → better to place stent by interventional radiologist.
- Can ligate right or left hepatic arteries, but ligation of right hepatic artery mandates cholecystectomy.
- If destructive injury → shunt → reversed saphenous vein graft (RSVG).

- If avulsion in superior border of pancreas or retropancreatic → transect pancreas.
- If still bleeding →
  1. Direct repair of IVC
  2. Temporary shunt
  3. Venovenous bypass
  4. Hepatectomy
- Minor laceration → manual compression.
- Typical hemostatic technique includes the following:
  o Electrocautery (100 watts)
  o Organ beam coagulation
  o Microcrystalline collagen
  o Fibrin glue
  o BioGlue
- Suture liver parenchyma by chromic round blunt needle → running suture for small laceration while interrupted, pledgeted horizontal mattress suture for deep injuries.
  → Finger fracture to identify bleeding vessel followed by clip or suture.
- Gallbladder, if injured → cholecystectomy.
- Extrahepatic biliary ducts associated with vascular injury because proximity from IVC, portal v.
  → Small laceration with no devitalized tissue → T tube and lateral suture using 6-0 monofilament absorbable suture.
  → If significant tissue loss → Roux-en-Y choledochojejunostomy.
  → Single-layer 5-0 absorbable monofilament →· to decrease tension, jejunum suture to porta hepatis → can intubate the duct for external drainage then attempt a repair when patient is recovered or stent via ERCP.
  → Can ligate the duct if the other lobes are functioning.
- After packing → ICU → second look to remove pack after 24 hrs (earlier if ongoing bleeding) and exploration, i.e., low Hb, accumulation of blood, blood from drain.
- Angioembolization is another option if still bleeding.

- If prolonged Pringle maneuver → LFT will elevate like ligation of hepatic artery → hepatic necrosis.
- Liver fever → 5 days after injury.
- Complications: biloma, arterial pseudoaneurysm, biliary fistula.
- Biloma—loculated collection of bile may infect → treatment like abscess → if small → reabsorption → biliary ascites if major duct disrupted → exploration, irrigation, and subhepatic drain.
- Primary repair of intrahepatic duct is unlikely to be successful.
   - → If pseudoaneurysm → rupture to ducts → hemobilia → RUQ pain + UGIB and jaundice.
   - → If rupture to PV → portal HTN → hepatic angioembolization.
- Bilio venous fistula → ERCP + sphincterotomy.
- If diaphragmatic defect → bronchobiliary → OR closure or ERCP + sphincterotomy → will close spontaneously.
- DVT prophylaxis (anticoagulant) → hold use till Hb is stable and patient is recovering.

Splenic injury

Splenic Injury Grade	Subcapsular Hematoma	Laceration
I	< 10%	< 1 cm
II	10%–50%	1–3 cm
III	> 50%	> 3 cm
IV	> 25% Devascularization	Hilar
V	Shattered spleen Complete devascularization	

- Non operative management (NOM):
   - o Serial Hb at 6–8 hrs.
   - o Period of bed rest = grade + 1 (days).
   - o Early initiation of VTE within 48 hrs does not affect failure rate of NOM.
- 60% failure rate on first day and 1% delay failure after discharge.

- Unlike liver, which rebleeds within 48 hrs, spleen can up to weeks.
- Overall success rate is 80%–90%
- Success rate with grade:

Grade	Percentage (%)
I	90%–95%
II	70%
III	50%
IV	16.9%
V	1.3%

- Failure of non operative management → splenectomy.
- Angioembolization is controversial.
- Splenectomy considered when: instability, hilar injury, grade > II in patient with coagulopathy or multiple injuries, contrast extravasation, requires many blood transfusion within 12 hrs.
- Autotransplant in young immunocompromised → no drain.
- Options: splenectomy, partial splenectomy, splenorrhaphy.
- Partial splenectomy for injury in superior or inferior pole, also horizontal mattress suture with gentle compression → as in liver → electrocautery, organ beam.
- Postoperative bleeding → mostly slipped suture.
- Postsplenectomy → high WBCs, high platelet, but if > 15 WBCs and platelet / WBCs ration > 20 → underlying infection → mostly subphrenic collection → percutaneous drainage.
- High morbidity if unrecognized pancreatic tail injury or gastric perforation.
- To prevent OPSI → vaccine at fourteenth day.

Stomach, Small Bowel injuries

- Gastric oversewn with running single-layer suture or stapler.
  - → If single layer → full-thickness bite to ensure hemostasis.
  - → Missed injury usually in the posterior wall.

- To check → digital occlusion of pylorus, methylene blue injection through NGT or air.
- Partial or distal gastrectomy if destructive injury with Billroth reconstruction.
- If damage nerve of latarjet or vagus nerve → drainage procedure.
- Small bowel → transverse running 3-0 PDS if less than ⅓ of circumference.

    → If destructive → segmental resection and anastomosis → end-to-end continuous suture 3-0 polypropylene.

- Mesenteric injury → may mandate resection.
- Following GI surgery → paralytic ileus → return of bowel function is indicated by decrease output of NGT.
- Early total enteral nutrition (TEN) in trauma patient:
    o Patient with non operative management if solid organ ≥ II → NPO at least 48 hrs.
    o If patient opens his bowel → start feeding.
    o TEN fascial closure.

Duodenal and Pancreatic injuries
Duodenum

- Hematoma, perforation, or combined with pancreatic injury.
- Majority of hematoma → non operative with NGT and TPN.

    → If suspected associated perforation suggested by clinical deterioration, retroperitoneal free air or contrast extravasation → exploration.

    → Mark drop in NGT output → resolution of hematoma within 2 weeks and some within 3–4 weeks, and repeat image to confirm.

    → If patient shows no clinical or radiological improvement within 3 weeks → operative intervention is warranted.

- Small perforation or laceration → primary repair using single-layer suture of 3-0 monofilament.

    → Wound should be closed in direction result in largest residual lumen.

- Extensive injury (consider pyloric exclusion) will open spontaneously 3–4 months + gastrojejunostomy.
  o First part (proximal to duct of Santorini) → debridement and end-to-end anastomosis.
  o Second part, i.e., tethered head of pancreas → no more than 1 cm can be mobilized away from pancreas → patch with vascularized jejunal graft.
  o Distal to ampulla of Vater and proximal to SMA and SMV → Roux-en-Y duodenojejunostomy.
  o Third, fourth duodenal injury behind SM vessels → resection & duodenojejunostomy.

Pancreas

- To identify the pancreatic injury:
  1. Squeeze gallbladder
  2. Cholangiography
  3. By palpation
- No Whipple procedure (no trauma Whipple) ↑ mortality > 80%.
- So if no clear ductal injury → drain.
- If extensive, i.e., avulsion of papilla of Vater from duodenum or if destruction to entire secondary part of duodenal → pancreaticoduodenectomy may be considered.
- If in the distal pancreas → stable patient → distal pancreatectomy and preserve spleen or Roux-en-Y pancreaticojejunostomy or pancreaticogastrostomy.
  → If patient is unstable → distal pancreatotectomy and splenectomy.
- Regardless, definitive treatment → ligation or stapler TA of proximal duct.
- Pyloric exclusion if complex duodenal injury → gastrotomy in greater curvature and pylorus is grasped with Babcock and oversewn with zero polypropylene + gastrojejunostomy. Vagotomy is not necessary for marginal ulcer. This is temporary for 3–4 weeks. The most durable technique is TA stapler.
- If drain placed → keep it till tolerated orally.

- Pancreatic fistula at day 5 will appear in patient with output > 30 mL/day and the drainage contain amylase triple than normal.
- If injury to head of pancreas:
  → Distal pancreatectomy (rare)
  → Central pancreatectomy with preserve CBD and mobilization of pancreatic body and Roux-en-Y pancreaticojejunostomy
  → Pancreaticoduodenectomy in complex injury
- Pancreatic fistula in 20%.
- Pancreatic pseudocyst in patient managed non operatively → ERCP.
- If late cyst → manage as pancreatitis with pseudocyst.
- Abscess → percutaneous drainage.

Colon and Rectum
Three methods:
1. Primary repair
2. End colostomy
3. Primary repair + diverting ileostomy
- Primary repair is either lateral suture repair or resection anastomosis.
- All suture is running single layer.
- Colonic injury with spillage but intact mesentery → primary anastomosis.
- If devastating colon injury → damage control, i.e., temporary colostomy or colocolostomy with diverting ileostomy.
- Rectal = colon → loop ileostomy or loop colostomy.
  → If extensive injury → Hartmann's procedure → remove affected rectum and stapler the distal end + end colostomy.
  → Some place drain (Penrose) along Waldeyer's fascia via perineal incision.
- Complication: intra-abdominal abscess and fistula → 10%, 1%–3% respectively.
- Necrosis, obstruction, prolapse stenosis of stoma, 5%.
- If rectal injury adjacent to bone → osteomyelitis → bone Bx → antibiotic and debridement.

Abdominal and Pelvic Vasculature
- All vessels are liable for penetration injury.
- Blunt → renal artery, aorta (abdomen).
- Repair with lateral suture 4-0 polypropylene or PTFE patch or end-to-end and PTFE interposition.
- To avoid fistula, cover suture line with omentum.
- SMA is rarely involved, but if Pruitt-Inahara shunt can prevent bowel necrosis and definitive end-to-end interposition RSVG.

  → if associated with pancreatic injury → tunneling from distal aorta behind duodenum to distal SMA.
- SMV → digital compression then venorrhaphy → but ligation is life-threatening → temporary abdominal closure then second look.
- Following aortic interposition grafting, SBP should not exceed 120 mmHg for 72 hrs if interposition graft was used.
- Gunshot to pelvis → injury of iliac vessels → temporary shunt can help.
- If IVC ligation → lower limb edema → wrap elastic bandage from toe to hip and elevate limb 45–60 degrees.
- For SMV thrombosis, either ligation or graft or venorrhaphy → bowel edema → fluid resuscitation (aggressive) and measure IAP frequently.
- After repair → long-term antiplatelet is not routine.

Genitourinary Tract
Kidney
- Usually non operative if grades I–IV, and 50% of grade V is managed non operatively.
  - → Irrigate urinary bladder to dispel blood clot.
  - → Persist hematuria → embolization.
  - → Urinoma → percutaneous drainage.
- Indication for angioembolization:
  1. Persistent bleeding from renal artery.
  2. Unstable with grade III–V.
  3. Pseudoaneurysm or AVF.
  4. Persistent gross hematuria.

    5. Rapid drop in hematocrit requiring 2 units PRBCs.
- Indication for renal exploration:
  1. Persist life threat from renal injury.
  2. Renal pedicle avulsion (V).
  3. Exploring pulsate hematoma, either repair or nephrectomy.
- Arterial injury → graft.
- If destructive parenchymal or irreparable vascular injury → nephrectomy, and you have to palpate another kidney as it might be absent 0.1%.
- Operative intervention → destructive kidney injury + hypotension.
- Success rate of renal artery repair is 0%, but attempt is reasonable if < 5 hrs.
      → As with traction of artery → intimal rupture → thrombosis.
      → If left in place, may induce HTN and abscess.
- Collecting system closes separately.
- Renal vein avulsed from IVC → hypotension requires intervention.
- During laparotomy → if expanding or pulsatile hematoma, it should be explored.

Ureter
- If injury is suspected, IV methylene blue or indigo carmine is injected.
- Injuries are repaired with 5-0 absorbable suture and mobilization of kidney.
- Distal injury → reimplant to urinary bladder with psoas flap and DJ stent.
- Damage control can ligate it bilaterally → bilateral nephrostomy.
- Urinary bladder injury can be intra- or extraperitoneal.
      → Intraperitoneal → single-layer 3-0 absorbable monofilament can be laparoscopic, then Foley catheter for 2 weeks to decompress the bladder.
      → Extraperitoneal → Foley catheter for 2 weeks.

- Urethral injury can be treated with bridging Foley catheter with or without suture repair.

Female Reproductive Tract
- Occasionally, vaginal wall from bony pelvis → repair is not mandatory.
- If bleeding from genital tract → use hemostatic agent.
- Repair of fallopian tube is uncommon but attempt unjustified as suboptimal repair → high risk of tubal pregnancy.
  - → Transection and proximal ligation and distal salpingectomy are more prudent.

Pelvic Fracture and Hemorrhage Control
- Options: stabilization, fixation, and peritoneal packing with or without angioembolization.
- If unstable patient → Immediate stabilization by sheet should be done before radiology confirmation.
- 85% of bleeding is due to pelvic fracture → venous bleeding or bony bleeding → anterior external fixation.
- Pelvic packing with 6 laparotomy pads; 4 in children are placed by suprapubic incision → in paravesical space.
- But most cases are managed with blood transfusion.
- Angioembolization is for patient who is admitted to SICU and require > 4 units PRBCs after packing by 12 hrs.
- Packing is removed after 48 hrs → repacking if ongoing oozing.
- To decrease infection → diverting sigmoid colostomy.
- Debridement if needed + irrigation and wound left open to heal by secondary intervention with VAC.

Extremity Vascular Injury, Fracture, and Compartment Syndrome
- Immediate stabilization of fracture.
- Open fracture → Betadine gauze + antibiotic.
- Fixation is either internal or external.
- Vascular injury → either alone or with bone fracture → OR.
  - → Common combined injury → bone fixed first with temporary shunt then definitive vascular repair.

- o Clavicle and first rib fracture → subclavian artery.
  - o Dislocation humerus → axillary artery.
  - o Supracondylar fracture → brachial artery.
  - o Femur fracture → femoral artery.
  - o Knee dislocation → popliteal artery.
- → Angiography facilitates rapid intervention.
- Occlusion of artery → fixation of bone → repair artery.
- If the nerve transected along with the artery and bone → amputation.
- Subclavian or axillary artery injury → 6 mm PTFE or RSVG → because associated injury to brachial plexus → need neurological examination.
- Operative approach for brachial artery → medial upper extremity longitudinal incision → proximal control S-shaped extension through antecubital fossa → excision of injured vessel, end-to-end interposition of RSVG graft.
- Upper limb fasciotomy is rarely required unless patient is suffering from neurological diminish.
- For SFA injury → external fixation followed by end-to-end RSVG → be careful from compartment.

Compartment Syndrome
- ↑ pressure inside close space.

Causes
- Arterial hemorrhage in the compartment
- Venous ligation
- Thrombosis of veins
- Crushed injury
- Reperfusion injury

Symptoms
- Pain with active and passive motion
- Paresthesia
- Numbness
- Progress to paralysis
- Loss of pulse (late sign)
  → Fasciotomy if gradient is < 35 mm

Gradient = DBP − compartment pressure

Ischemic period of 6 hrs → 2 incisions

Treatment
- Anterior and lateral compartment → lateral incision (avoid peroneal nerve)
- Posterior → medial just 1 cm from tibial shaft

Surgical Intensive Care Management
Postinjury Resuscitation
- Optimizing tissue perfusion.
- Ensuring normothermia.
- Restoring coagulopathy.
- The first 24 hrs, Hb > 10; after 24 hrs, better Hb ≈ 7 to adverse effect of inflammatory effect from stored RBCs.
- Daily expose wound for dressing and debridement.
- Keep MAP ≥ 60.

Abdominal Compartment Syndrome
- Primary: intra-abdominal HTN due to intra-abdominal injury.
- Secondary: splanchnic reperfusion after massive resuscitation.
- Source of high intra-abdominal pressure (IAP): gut edema, ascites, bleeding packs.
- Diagnosis: by physical examination and measuring intraperitoneal pressure → by UB catheter → 50 cc of normal saline injected and drainage tube clamped (three-way) then water manometer measures.
- IPP = MAP − IAP.

Grade	mmHg	cm H_2O
I	10–15	13–20
II	16–25	21–35
II	26–35	36–47
IV	> 35	> 48

113

- Condition of unreliable test: rupture UB, extend compression from pelvic packing, neurogenic bladder, adhesive disease.
- No therapeutic intervention till pressure > 35 mmHg.
- Mortality rate affected by time of decompression: if presumptive, 60%; if delayed, 70%.
- Decompressive laparotomy can be in ICU or OR.
- If primary, better by percutaneous drainage.
- UB is measured every 4 hrs.
- Patient with open abdominal wound lose between 500–2,500 mL/day.
- Controversial to use albumin-rich fluid.
- Avoid open abdomen as it increases the need of fluid.
- Closure of the abdomen using the following methods:
  o Re operation → reapproximation of fascia by mesh (biological or prosthetic).
  o Cover bowel by split-thickness graft, removed after 9–12 months then definitive repair of hernia by component separation → high morbidity.
  o VAC revolution of fascial closure, change in OR Q48H.
      → Success rate is 95%.
      → Complication: intra-abdominal abscess, fistula, bowel perforation.

Special Population
Pregnant Patient
- During pregnancy, 7% of pregnant women are injured.
- 11% of fetal deaths are because of mother's death.
- 70% from MVC fall down.
- 30% are from domestic violence.
- Pregnancy: Increase HR, 10–15 b/pm
                Decrease BP, low SVR
  → Pregnancy loss of 35% of blood before sign of shock.
  → ↑ tidal volume (TV), ↓ FRC → ↓ CO_2 → respiratory alkalosis.
- DPL → supraumbilical.

- Lower Esophageal sphincter → ↓ tone, heart burn, ↑ aspiration risk.
- High LFT, alkaline phosphatase, progesterone, ↑ biliary stasis → Gallstones, this may not affect trauma but becomes important in a prolonged ICU stay.
- Albumin decreases to 3.
- Renal flow increases by 30% → ↓ urea and creatinine, also compress ureter → hydronephrosis.
- Anemia and Hb < 11.
- ↑ WBCs, ↑ hypercoagulability, and ↓ fibrinolytic.
- O_2 supply always as usually pregnant ↑ O_2 consumption and demand.
- Need to monitor fetal heart sound, CTG.
- If > 160, hypoxia, hypotension.
- If < 120, fetal distress.
- PV bleeding is an early sign of cervical dilation, abruptio placenta, placenta previa.
- Amniotic fluid rupture → prolapse of umbilical cord → must have OB-GYN evaluation.
- Fundal height in twentieth GA at umbilicus and fortieth GA at costal margin.
- Use FAST + fetal movement.
- Radiation is harmful in preimplantation, organogenesis in 3–16 weeks but after 16 weeks → accepted dose < 5 radiation.
    CXR, 0.07 in radiation.
    CT chest, < 1 radiation.
    CT abdomen, 3.5 radiation.
    → Better to protect the mother's belly by shield.
- Indication of emergent C/S:
    1. Serial maternal shock
    2. Uterine injury

Geriatric Patient
- > 65 of age, loss of SC fat → hypothermia.
- Should be recognized if patient is taking β-blocker.
- Head injury is more severe.
- Easily fractured: osteoporosis.

115

- Age is not the best predictor of outcome but the presence of preexisting conditions.
- Injury severity score is probably the best overall predictor of patient outcome in the elderly.

Pediatric Patient
- 1:4 children is injured /year.
- Female: Male = 1:2.
- All age-groups: infant and toddler and children.
  - → Children, bicycle
  - → Adolescent, MVA
- Tongue is larger than oropharynx, compromise the airway.
- Larynx is funnel in shape.
- Intubation by straight laryngoscopy, not the curve.
- Atropine before rapid sequence intubation to prevent bradycardia.
- O_2 supplement as O_2 consumption double in adult.
- If airway is not secured → surgical airway.
  - → If ≥ 11 → cricothyrotomy.
  - → If less → tracheostomy to prevent subglottic stenosis.
- IVF 2–3 boluses, 20 mg/kg.
- CT head → monitor CPP to prevent secondary insult from hypoxia, hypovolemia.
- In adult chest trauma, 70% of them are with rib fracture; in pediatric, 40% are with rib fracture (cartilaginous).
- Indication of thoracotomy is initially 80 mL/kg or, if it persists, 1–2 mL/kg/hr.
- If trauma (bicycle) at epigastric → duodenal or pancreatic injury.
- Seat belt syndrome: bowel perforation, spine, diaphragm rupture, aortic dissection.
- In solid organ injury, non operative is the standard of care.
- If deterioration, instability or requires transfusion > 40 mL/kg → surgery.
- In non operative, success rate is 95%.

Section II

General Surgery

Abdominal Wall, Omentum, Mesentery, and Retroperitoneum

Anatomy of abdominal wall
- Originates from mesoderm.
- Rectus abdominis
    Origin: fifth, sixth, seventh ribs, and xiphoid (superiorly)
    Insertion: pubic bone
    Lateral border: linea semilunaris
    Three tendinous intersection: xiphoid, umbilicus, and halfway between them
- External oblique
    Runs inferior and medially, origin from seventh, eighth costal cartilage
- Internal oblique
    Arises from lateral inguinal ligament, iliac crest runs superior and medially
    Inferiorly continues as cremaster muscle
- Transversus abdominis
    Deepest, runs transversely from sixth ribs, lumbosacral fascia, iliac crest laterally to lateral border of rectus abdominis
- Arcuate line
    Lies roughly at level of anterior superior iliac spine (ASIS)
    → Above arcuate line, internal oblique muscle fuses to anterior and posterior rectus sheath.
    → Below arcuate line, internal oblique and transversus muscles all beneath the rectus sheath.
- Blood supply: superior and inferior epigastric arteries
    → Superior arises from internal thoracic artery (internal mammary).
    → Inferior arises from external iliac artery.
- LNs: major nodal basin
- Nerve supply: motor—T6–T12
    Sensory (skin) T4-L1, at (umbilicus T10)

Physiology

- ↑ IAP, abdominal wall contracts when diaphragm relaxes → expiration.
- If diaphragm contracts while abdominal wall contracts → Valsalva maneuver.

Abdominal Wall Incisions

- Longitudinal midline (vertical)
  Horizontal (transverse)
  Subcostal (Kosher) right or left, chevron incision
  Paramedian, gridiron, Lanz, Pfannenstiel incisions

Congenital Abnormalities

- Abdominal wall develops within first week of gestational age.
- Large central defect passes the vitelline duct, which connects midgut by yolk sac.
- On sixth week, abdominal content grows too large and midgut herniate → undergoes 90 degrees counterclockwise rotation.
- At the end of twelfth week → returns to abdominal wall and rotate 180 degrees i.e. total rotation 270 degrees, if there is defect in abdominal wall closure → omphalocele or gastroschisis.
  - → Omphalocele viscera protrudes through open umbilical ring and covered by sac.
  - → Gastroschisis viscera protrudes through defect lateral to umbilicus and no sac.
- During third trimester → vitelline duct regresses → persistent duct → Meckel's diverticulum and complete failure → vitelline duct fistula.
- If persist duct remnant → cyst, may cause volvulus.
- Urachus: fibromuscular extension, developed where urinary bladder descends.

Acquired Abnormalities

- o Rectus Abdominis Diastasis
  - ▪ Can be congenital or acquired, obesity, pregnancy → identify by physical examination, US or CT scan.

o Rectus Sheath Hematoma
- History of trauma, cough, sneezing, sudden movement (Ballet)
- Occurs spontaneously in elderly on anticoagulant.
- Painful swelling ↑ with contraction.
- Fothergill sign: palpable abdominal mass that remains unchanged with contraction of rectus muscle.
- Diagnosis: CBC, chemistry, coagulation.
- US, CT.
- Treatment:
    - Small—OPD.
    - Large or bilateral—hospitalization for resuscitation.
    - Angioembolization—if large hematoma, free bleeding or clinical deterioration.
    - Surgical intervention—if failed angioembolization → evacuation of hematoma + ligation of the vessels.

o Desmoid Tumor
- Fibrous neoplasm originating from musculoaponeurotic structures.
- No metastasis potential.
- Common in female.
- Sporadic or familial (FAP).
- In non-FAP, postpartum in surgical scar.
- Needs radical resection and immediate reconstructions.
- If it involves margin, the recurrence is 80%
- Medical: cisplatin → induce remission, 50%.
- Prognosis with FAP is poor → 5 years, survival rate is 50%.
- Imatinib can benefit.
- Radiotherapy can be given as adjuvant or palliative therapy.

o Other Abdominal Wall Tumors
- Various: lipoma, neurofibroma.
- Surgery is not always mandatory, but excision is recommended for symptomatic or enlarged mass.
- Sarcoma is rare.
- CT, MRI for diagnosis.
- If suspected sarcoma → CNBx.
- May need reconstruction flap or by synthetic mesh.

Omentum
- Greater and lesser omentum are fibrous, fatty aprons.
- Developed in fourth week.
- Spleen develops between two layers of omentum.
- Greater omentum lies between anterior abdominal wall and hollow viscera and extended to pelvis.
- Lesser omentum—hepatoduodenal, hepatogastric.
- Blood supply is right to left gastroepiploic and venous parallel to arteries.

Physiology
- Omentum tends to wall off the area of infection (abdominal policeman).
- Some studies showed intrinsic hemostatic characteristic → tissue factor in omentum → activation of coagulation at the site of inflammation, ischemia and infection.

Omental Infarction
- Interruption of the blood supply to omentum is a rare cause of acute abdomen.
- Secondary to torsion of omentum around its vascular pedicle.
- Diagnosis: CT or US.
  Localize inflammatory mass of fat density.
- May need laparoscopic exploration.

Omental Cyst
- Results from peritoneal inclusion or degeneration of lymphatic structure.
- Less common than mesenteric cyst.
- Usually asymptomatic, but there could be mass or pain.
- CT, US → cystic lesion.
- Treatment: resection by laparoscopy.

Omental Neoplasm
- Primary tumor is rare.
- Benign neoplasm such as lipoma, myxoma, and desmoid.
- Like GIST, c-KIT is diagnostic.

- Metastasis to omentum is common, ovarian tumor is the highest, GIT, melanoma, uterus, kidney tumor is also common.

Mesentery
Surgical Anatomy

- Mesenteric tissue originate from dorsal attachment of foregut, midgut, hindgut of posterior abdominal wall.
- During fetal development → after herniated midgut and rotation to 90 degrees → return intraperitoneum to complete rotation 270 degrees → duodenum and lateral colon fixed its retroperitoneum.

Sclerosing Mesenteritis

- Or retractile mesenteritis.
- Fibrosis to mesentery.
- High in 50s age-group.
- Discrete nonneoplastic mass.
- Symptoms: pain, mass, intestinal obstruction → rare.
- CT: could be incidental.
  - → Fat ring sign.
  - → Exploration → Bx is diagnostic and rules out neoplasm.
  - → Resection if possible.
- PET-CT to rule out neoplasm.
- Most cases are self-limited.
- Aggressive surgical resection is not recommended.
- Medical treatment: steroid, colchicine, tamoxifen.

Mesenteric Cyst

- Theory: degeneration of lymphatics.
- Asymptomatic, acute, or chronic mass.
- Acute from rupture or torsion or hemorrhage.
- Can be symptomatic, such as nausea, vomiting, and anorexia.
- Physical examination: mass, mobile (Tillaux sign) shifting from left to right and vice versa.
- CT, US, MRI.
  - → Unilocular, without solid component.
  - → Multiple or multilocular, less common.

- Difficult to distinguish from cystic stromal tumor.
- If symptomatic → complete excision.
- Cyst unroofing or marsupialization is not recommended because of high risk to recur.
- If attached to bowel → segmental bowel resection + cyst.

Mesenteric Tumor
- Primary tumor is rare.
- Benign neoplasm such as lipoma, cystic lymphangioma, desmoid tumor.
- Malignant like liposarcoma, lipoblastoma, histiocytoma → wide resection of the mass and sometimes includes bowel.

Retroperitoneum
Anatomy
- Bounded superiorly by diaphragm, posteriorly by spinal column and iliopsoas muscle, inferiorly by levator ani, and anteriorly by peritoneum reflection.

Retroperitoneal Infection
- Causes: retrocecal appendicitis, contained perforation of duodenal ulcer, iatrogenic EGD perforation, pancreatitis.
- Symptoms: pain, fever, and pain in the back, pelvis, and thigh.
- Erythema in flank or periumbilical.
- CT is diagnostic: collection.
- Treatment:
  o Treat underlying condition.
  o IV antibiotic.
  o Image-guided drainage or operative intervention if complex or multiple.
- Mortality rate is 25%.
- Rarely → necrotizing fasciitis of retroperitoneum.

Retroperitoneum Fibrosis
- Idiopathic (Ormond disease) or secondary reaction.
- Men: women = 2:1.
- Linked to autoimmune disease such as SLE, DMI, myasthenia gravis,.

- T cells, macrophage, plasma cell invasion.
    → Fibrosis of IVC aorta and start to renal artery.
- Associated secondary to AAA, TB, actinomycosis, pancreatitis, and malignancy of pancreas, stomach, Hodgkin lymphoma.
- Medication association: β-blocker, hydralazine, α-methyldopa.
    → If stopped, fibrosis will regress.
- Symptom depends on involved organ.
- HTN, lower limb edema.
- Laboratory: ↑ urea, creatinine, and ESR.
- Diagnosis: US, IVP, CT, MRI.
- Biopsy to rule out malignancy.
- Steroid with or without surgery: ureterolysis, stent if significant hydronephrosis.
- Medical: cyclosporine, tamoxifen.
- 5 years, SR is 90%–100%.

Skin and Subcutaneous Tissue

Anatomy and Histology
- Skin represent 15% of total body weight and the largest organ in the body.
- Layers of skin:
  o Epidermis and appendages (ectoderm)
  o Dermis (mesoderm)
  o Hypodermis (mesoderm)

Epidermis
- Stratified epithelium.
- 90%–95% derived from keratinocytes.
- From deep to superficial:
  1. Stratum basale.
  2. Stratum spinosum.
  3. Stratum granulosum.
  4. Stratum corneum—divides to deep compact stratum compactum and superficial loose stratum disjunction.
     In palmoplantar area, an additional layer is stratum lucidum.
- 30 days to shed.
- Thickness: 50 mm on eyelid to 1 mm in sole.

Components
- Keratinocyte
- Langerhans cells
- Melanocyte (1 melanoma: 4–10 kertinocyte)
- Merkel cells
- Lymphocyte
- Toker cells
- Epithelial appendage: specialized cells located in dermis and hypodermis and connected to epidermis.
  → Function: lubrication, sensation, contractility, heat loss.
- Sweat glands
  1. Eccrine sweat gland (main)

2. Apocrine sweat gland, pilosebaceous follicles
3. Artichial gland

Dermis

- Compressible, elastic connective tissue, supports and protects epidermis, dermal appendages, neurovascular plexus.
- Synthetic and degradation of protein.
- Thickness depends on the location.
- Dermal papilla ↑ surfaces between epidermis and dermis.
- Contains fibroblast, dendrocytes, mast cells, veins, nerves.
- In distal extremities → tactile corpuscle.
  - Dermal fiber
    - 90% of collagen is I, III.
    - Type IV in dermal-epidermal junction.
    - Elastic fiber → for retractile properties.
  - Cells
    - Fibroblast is the most found in dermis.
    - Myofibroblast.
    - Dermal dendrocyte → immunological function.
  - Cutaneous vasculature
    - Epithelium is a nonvascular tissue.
    - Cutaneous vessels come from perforator.
    - Deep plexus in the dermal-hypodermal junction → supply nutrient to sweat glands and hair follicle.
    - Cutaneous enervation.

Hypodermis

- I.e., SC tissue.
- Thermoregulation.
- Storage of energy.
- Main cells: adipocyte.

Inflammatory Condition
Hidradenitis Suppurativa

- Chronic inflammatory disease, painful SC nodules.
- Multiple abscesses and internetwork sinus tract.
- Foul-smelling exudate.

- Atrophic and hypertrophic scars, ulceration, and infection.
- Diagnosed clinically.
- Affected site: axilla, inguinal, perianal, mammary, and inframammary (milk line distribution).
- Risk factors: follicular occlusion, poor hygiene, smoking, alcohol, and bacterial infection.
- Treatment:

  Early: Topical or systemic IV antibiotics
  Antiandrogen
  Ablating hair follicles
  Radiation therapy
  RFA
  CO_2 laser ablation
  Biologic (Humira)

  For refractory cases (wide locl excision [WLE] + skin graft)
- Recurrence is 50% in inguinal and perianal region.
- Options: primary wound closure, grafting, healing by secondary intention or locoregional flap.

Pyoderma Gangrenosum

- Noninfectious neutrophilic dermatosis.
- Commonly associated with IBD, rheumatoid arthritis, hematologic malignancy.
- Sterile pustule → ulceration.
- Lower extremities are the most common sites.
- Others: upper airway, eye, genitalia, lung, spleen.
- Secondary infection is common.
- More in female aged 30 and 60 years old.
- Lesion border is purplish with erythematous edge.
- Five lesion types:
  - I.   Ulcerative
  - II.   peristomal
  - III. Pustular
  - IV.   Bullous
  - V.   Vegetative
- Treatment:
  - o Treat the underlying disease, i.e., CD.
  - o Systemic steroid.
  - o Calcineurin inhibitor (T cell inhibitor).

- o   Others: sulfa drug, cyclophosphamide → infliximab, TNF-α inhibitor.
- o   Ulcer → topical antimicrobial.
- o   Wound care and debridement.

Toxic Epidermal Necrolysis (TEN) and Stevens-Johnson Syndrome (SJS)

- Autoimmune reaction to stimuli such as drugs → defect in epidermal-dermal junction.
- Follow prodromal period of URTI.
- Eruption from face to neck to extremities.
- Nikolsky sign, lateral pressure → epidermal detachment.
- Process progresses 7–10 days.
- Re-epithelization for over 1–3 weeks.
- ↑ risk with immunosuppressants.
- Historically considered erythema multiforme.
- TEN involves > 30% of total body surface area → between 10%–30%, consider Stevens-Johnson syndrome.
- Prognosis is related to extension of primary or secondary disease and associated ICU morbidity.
- Also affect mouth, esophagus, small bowel, colon → slough mucosa
  → GI bleeding and malabsorption.
- Drugs that induce TEN, SJS:
  - o   Anticonvulsant, sulfonamide, allopurinol
  - o   NSAID, nevirapine, same antibiotic

Treatment:
- o   Stop offending drug.
- o   Supportive care (pain, IVF, enteral feeding).
- o   Wound care.
- o   Wound cover by temporary biologic dressing.
- o   Wood's lamp exam Q1H to look for corneal sloughing.
- o   Steroid, increase sepsis, delay wound healing, prolonged admission.
- o   IVIG to inhibit fast mediated cells apoptosis, improve SR.

o Plasmapheresis, to decrease the load of drug, cytokines, and anti-TNF-α.

Radiation-Induced Injury
- Environmental, industrial, occupational and medical.
- Keratinocyte, stem cell hair follicles, and melanocyte are radiosensitive.
- Damage → burst of free radicals → irreversible break → inflammation.
- Within weeks, erythema, edema, alopecia → repair → hyperpigmentation.
- Chronic changes result from thrombosis, necrosis of capillary → this includes → thinning, ↓ vascularity, telangiectasia, ulceration fibrosis.
- Treatment:
    o Moisture.
    o Surgical excision of damaged tissue.
- Environment-induced injury such as UV radiation.
- UV reaches the earth 700–4,500 nm, and the ozone filters it.
    UV A has low energy, 95% more penetration.
    UV B has high energy, 5% less penetration.
- 70% absorbed by stratum corneum.
- Radiation effect starts by erythema and pigmentation.
- UV A is less effective in tanning.
- Long-term UV pigmentation → irregular pigmentation and hyperpigmentation, melasma → actinic lentigines (sunspot).
- Loss of collagen and impaired collagen, I:III ratio.

Trauma-Induced Injury
Mechanical Injury
- Penetration, blunt, shear force.
- Clean laceration → irrigation +/− debridement and primary closure within 6 hrs, but no evidence regarding time of closure.
- Contaminated wound—healing by secondary intention or delayed primary closure (tertiary).
- Tangential abrasion like burn in care.
- Superficial partial-thickness wound, left to heal spontaneously with topical antimicrobial.

- Deep wound may require split-thickness graft.
- Degloved skin—temporary dressing then closure.

Bite Wound
- 4.5 million injuries/year.
- Bacteria of normal mouth flora is infective.
- Dogs: pasteurella species.
- Human bite: staph, strep, peptococcus, bacteroides → antibiotic gram +ve and anaerobic.
   → Penicillin + clavulanic acid and clindamycin, as well as irrigation.

Caustic Injury
- 2.4%–10.7% is chemical injury.
- 30% of death in burn is because of chemical injuries.
- Acid induces superficial injury due to scar formation and coagulative necrosis.
- Basic fluid: liquefactive necrosis → deeper injury.
- Treatment for both: irrigation of distilled water or saline for 30 mintues for acids and 2 hrs of alkaline with topical emollient and analgesia.
- If second-degree deep injury → debridement, silvadene, petroleum gauze.
- Injuries with hydrogen fluoride (conditioner and petroleum) → administration of intra-arterial Ca^{++} gluconate, relieves pain and preserves artery from necrosis and repletes Ca^{++} resorption.
- Ca^{++} carbonate cream to detoxify fluoride ions.
- Chemotherapy (doxorubicin) direct toxicity → cell death → cell lysis and no healing.
- IV cannula site present with erythema, blistering, and pain, especially in hand and feet because fragile vein, poor perfused tissue (specially Ca^{++} administration and K^+).
   → Treatment is limb elevation, saline infusion to dilute. This is effective in early phase of extravasation.
   → Cold and warm compresses should be avoided.
   → Surgery (debridement) if devitalized tissue.

Thermal Injury
- Depth depends on time (duration) and temperature.
- Zone of coagulation, zone of stasis, zone of marginal perfusion.
- Hypothermia (frostbite) → microvascular thrombosis → rewarming 40°C–42°C, analgesic, aspirin, antimicrobial.

Pressure Injury
- If the pressure exceeds 30 mmHg (microcirculation) → ischemia.
- Area of bony prominence is more liable to ischemia.
- Ischium, 28%; trochanter, 19%; sacrum, 17%; head, 9%.
- In ischial region, pressure is 300 mmHg; sacrum, 150 mmHg.
- Muscle is more susceptible to ischemia than skin.
- Stages of pressure sore:
    - I   Nonblanching erythema (intact skin)
    - II   Partial-thickness (epidermis or dermis)
    - III   Full-thickness down but not including fascia
    - IV   Full-thickness with destruction of muscle bone, tendon
- Treatment of pressure sore:
    - o Pressure relief (air mattress)
    - o Nutritional supplement
    - o Wound care
    - o Surgery: incision and drainage, debridement, removal of bone ostectomy + musculocutaneous or fasciocutaneous flap.
- Stage 2 and 3 are left to heal in secondary intention.
- VAC: remove interstitials fluid, lower bacterial load, increase vascularity and granulation tissue formation.

Bacterial Infection and Skin SC
- Complicated and uncomplicated
- Staph, 44%; enterococcus, 9%; β-hemolytic strep, 4%; coagulation −ve staph, 3%; pseudomonas, 11%; E. coli, 7.2%; enterobacter, 5%; klebsiella, 4%

Uncomplicated Skin Infection

- Limited to epidermis or its appendages and < 75 cm^2 → impetigo, cellulites, erysipelas, folliculitis, furuncle, simple abscess.
- Folliculitis is the infection of hair follicles and may progress to furuncle or carbuncle.
- Minor → topical ointment.
- Furuncle and carbuncle → incision and drainage or excision.
- Uncomplicated cellulitis β-hemolytic strep → cephalexin; if not responding in 48–72 hrs and there is fever, chills, expanding erythema, or MRSA → clindamycin, linezolid, or a combination of tetracycline and β-lactam, vancomycin.
- Purulent cellulitis but not complicated → MRSA cover.

Complicated Skin Infection

- Deep tissue infection (below dermis), extensive cellulitis, necrotizing fasciitis, and myonecrosis.
- History of trauma, DM, cirrhosis, neutropenia, bite, IV or drug abuse.
- Physical examination: crepitus, fluctuant, purpura, bullae, lymphangitis, and SIRS.
- CT and MRI diagnose deep infarction but should not delay debridement.

  - Necrotizing Fasciitis (Necrotizing soft tissue infection)
    - Skin manifestation + SIRS.
    - Lower limb, genitalia, perineum, Fournier's gangrene, and abdominal wall are the common sites.
    - Necrotizing fasciitis involves SC and the fascia overly the muscle, ↓ blood supply.
    - If the muscle involved → Necrotizing myositis.
    - Necrotizing fasciitis: dull, gray avascular, murky dishwater with hemorrhagic bullae
    - Three types of necrotizing fasciitis:
      - Type I (most common)—polymicrobial gram +ve, −ve, anaerobic (bacteroides, C. perfringens, septicum), occurs in trunks

and perineum, can result from intestinal perforation.

- o Type II (less common)—monomicrobial, strep, staph (MRSA, 40%), associated with toxic shock, occurs in trunk and extremity with history of trauma.
- o Type III—rare but fulminant from V. vulnificus or trauma to skin in sea diver.
- Laboratory: ↑ WBCs, ↓ $Ca^{++,}$ ↑ lactate, ↑ CPK, ↑ creatinine coagulopathy and acidosis, ↑ CRP.
- Laboratory risk indicator for necrotizing fasciitis (LRINEC) score includes CRP, WBCs, Hb, plasma Na^+, creatinine, glucose.
- Treatment:
  - ICU, resuscitation
  - Broad spectrum IV antibiotic
  - Debridement
  - Second look in 24–48 hrs.
  - Topical cream, good nutrition.
  - IVIG.
  - Mortality rate is 25%–40%.

- **Actinomycosis**
  - Should be considered in acute, subacute, chronic cutaneous, swelling in head and neck.
  - Acute pyogenic infection in paramandibular and maxillary region.
  - Can spread to scalp, orbit, ear.
  - Oral spread, pharynx, trachea, salivary.
  - Mimic to chronic osteomyelitis.
  - Treatment: penicillin + debridement.

Viral Infection

Human papilloma virus (HPV)

- DNA, 100 types.
- Cutaneous or mucosal involvement.
- HPV 1, 2, 4 → wart.
- HPV 5, 8 → dysplasia, malignant transformation → epidermodysplasia.

- HPV 6, 11 → low malignant transformation.
- HPV 16, 18 → high malignant transformation.
- Regression is immunity mediated.
- Clinical picture: hyperkeratosis, papillomatosis.
- Plantar wart HPV 1, 4 (keratin plug and black dots) from thrombosed capillary.
- Condyloma acumination (anogenital).
- Sexually transmitted 6, 11 (90%) of genital wart.
- Epidermodysplasia, 30%–50% → malignant.
- Treatment:

  Salicylic acid, silver nitrate

  Cryotherapy

  H_2 antagonist, zinc sulfate

Cutaneous Manifestation in HIV

- Associated with morbilliform rash.
- Kaposi's sarcoma.
- Early stage: recurrent varicella zoster, hyperkeratosis, warts, seborrheic dermatitis.
- Late stage: Herpes simplex and CMV, mycobacterium and candidiasis, impetigo and folliculitis.
- Kaposi's sarcoma, 5%.
- Basal cell carcinoma.

Benign Tumor

Hemangioma

- Benign proliferation of endothelial cells that surround blood-filled cavity.
- If large → heart failure because it takes from COP (hyperdynamic circulation).
- Prednisolone, b-blocker, interferon alpha can regress tumor.
- Embolization or surgery if medical treatment failed.
- Port wine: stain of trigeminal nerve distribution.

Nevi

- Overgrowth of melanocyte in epidermal-dermal junction.
- Congenital nevi, 1% of neonate.
- 5% to develop as malignant melanoma.
- Treatment: excision.

Cystic Lesion
- Three types of cutaneous cyst:
  1. Epidermal (sebaceous)
  2. Dermoid
  3. Trichilemmal
- Epidermal cyst: most common, mature epidermis complete with granular layer.
- Trichilemmal cyst: second most common, in female scalp with lack of granular layer and outer layer in sheath of hair follicle.
- Dermoid cyst is congenital between forehead to nose tip. Contains squamous epithelial in eccrine glands and pilosebaceous unit developing bone, tooth, nerve. Eyebrow is the most common site. Asymptomatic but can be inflamed or infected.

Keratosis
Actinic Keratosis
- Abnormal proliferation of intraepidermal keratinocytes.
- Premalignant lesion.
- 10 years → transformation to SCC, 6.1%.
- 60% of SCC originates from this lesion.

Seborrheic Keratosis
- Premalignant, light brown, velvetlike texture appear in sun-exposed skin.
- Transformed to SCC, rarely metastasized
- Treatment: excision.

Soft Tissue Tumor
- o Acrochordons hyperplastic cells of epidermis attached to fibrous connective tissue (fibroma).
  - Appears in trunk, eyelid, axilla as pedunculated mass; BCC can be found in this lesion (rare).
  - Excision.
- o Lipoma: most common SC neoplasm, no malignancy, excision if symptomatic.

Neural Tumor
- Arises from nerve sheath.
  - o Neurofibroma, nontender.
- Associated with café au lait spots and Lisch nodules in NF1 (Recklinghausen's disease).
  - o Neurilemmoma from Schwann cell → resection.

Malignant Tumor
Basal Cell Carcinoma
- Arises from basal layer of nonkeratinocytes.
- 75% of all skin CA. (most common)
- Risk of UV B more than UV A, others: immunosuppressants HIV, TPx, chemical exposure, radiation.
- Local invasion rather than metastasis.
- 30% in nose, bleeding, itching, ulceration.
- 60% (most common form) is nodular, raised, pearly pink papules, and occasionally depressed tumor center and raised border (rodent ulcer) → sun exposure and present in those aged above 60s → difficult to differentiate from nodular melanoma.
- Histopathological types nodule, 50%; superficial, 15%; and infiltration.
- Treatment: Mohs microsurgery, excision, cautery.
- Recurrent, 1%.
- Need 4 mm–free margin with extension to SC.
  - **NB**
  - R0 −ve margin
  - R1 microscopic +ve margin on tumor (ink)
  - R2 +ve margin
- If patient is poor candidate for surgery patient → radiotherapy.
- Radiation for questionable resection margin or microscopically +ve.
- Annual follow-up, full-body examination.
- 66% of recurrence developed in first 3 years.

Squamous Cell Carcinoma
- Second most common skin CA.
- Risk factor is UV exposure, chemical and physical agent, HPV 16 and 18, smoking, chronic nonhealing wound, burn scar, chronic dermatosis in darker-skinned population.
- Xeroderma pigmentosum, epidermolysis bullosa, albinism.
- SCC has in situ (Brown disease, erythroplasia of Queyrat in penis).
- In situ is well-demarcated papules.
- Invasive slightly pink- or skin-colored raised plaques.
- Bleeding is uncommon related to trauma; pain is rare.
- Most of in situ grow slowly and do not progress to malignancy, except Brown, erythroplasia of Queyrat in penis.
- Invasive disease if located in mucocutaneous junction → metastasis is 30%, while if in skin arising from sun exposure, cell is likely to spread and has better prognosis.
- Perineural involvement → high recurrence and LNs metastasis has poorer survival.
- Other feature indicates aggressive disease → poorly differentiated; thickness more than 4 mm; adenoid, adenosquamous, and desmoplastic subtype.
- Treatment: cautery, ablation, cryotherapy, drug therapy (imiquimod), surgical excision, Mohs microsurgery, and radiation.
    - → Cautery and ablation → high recurrence.
    - → Surgical excision is the treatment of choice.
        - o For < 2 cm → WLE with 4 mm margin for low grade and 6 mm in high grade.
        - o For lesion > 2 cm involve of SC → Mohs microsurgery → low recurrence.
        - o If poor surgical candidate → radiation → also as adjacent in lip CA (microscopic +ve margin).
    - → LNs if palpable → resection and/or radiation.
    - → Isolated LNs involvement → follow up.
    - Follow-up surveillance:
        - o 1–3 months in first year
        - o 2–4 months in second year
        - o 4–6 months in third year
        - o 6–12 months for rest of life

Melanoma

Background

- Incidence is high.
- Arises from melanocytes-epidermal junction but also originates from mucosal surface, oropharynx, nasopharynx, eye, proximal esophagus, anorectum, female genitalia.
- Risk factor: solar UV radiation; they report more than 10 tanning beds ↑ risk by twofold.
- Dysplastic nevi has 10% life risk.
- Dysplastic nevi syndrome (B-K mole), autosomal dominant, 100% lifetime risk to develop melanoma.
- Congenital nevi has 5%–8% to develop melanoma.
- 5%–10%, p14 ARF, HMD2, p53 tumor suppressor genes, and MEK-ERK oncogene.

Pathology and Clinical Picture

- Subtype: lentigo maligna, acral lentigious, mucosal, nodular, polypoid, desmoplastic, superficial spreading.
- Common anywhere, except hands and feet.
- Nodular, 15%–30%.
- Acral lentigious, 29%–72% of dark skin.
- Melanoma manifests as ABCDE: asymmetry, irregular border, color variation, diameter > 6 mm, elevation
  → others like pigmented, enlarged, ulcerated, or bleeding.
  → Lesion: pink-purple papule.

Diagnosis and Staging

- History and physical examination of entire skin, LNs.
- Tumor marker: S100.
- Suspension lesion → excisional biopsy with 1–2 mm margin.
- If large or cosmetically or anatomically challenging, incisional biopsy includes punch biopsy site.
- Should include full-thickness and small section of normal tissue to aid pathologist.
- If suspicious LNs → FNA.
- According to AJCC → stage I and II are localized diseases.
- Stage III is regional, and stage IV is metastatic disease.
- Tumor thickness, ulceration, mitotic rate are most important prognostic indications for survival.

- If SLNBx contains melanoma along with above indicator → poor prognosis.
- With clinically +ve LNs and above indicator → stage IV
- ↑ LDH → worse prognosis.
- No CXR or CT unless +ve regional LNs.
  E.g., T4b especially in Lower limb → PET-CT or CT pelvis.
- If clinically palpable LNs → CT CAP, whole body.
- SLNBx is standard staging for clinically −ve LNs → first draining LNs.
  - → Preoperative lymphoscintigraphy with intradermal injection of technetium or intraoperative injection of 1 mL of methylene blue.
- Complication: skin necrosis at the site of injection, anaphylactic shock, lymphedema, SSI, seroma, hematoma.

Surgical Management of Primary Tumor and LNs
- Appropriate excision margin based on tumor depth.
- −ve margin of 0.5–1 cm is sufficient.
- Many studies (Swedish, English) showed that < 2 mm thickness of melanoma → margin of 2 cm vs. 5 cm showed no difference in SR or recurrence.
- Tumor thickness   < 1 mm   requires 1 cm margin
                     1–2 mm   requires 1–2 cm
                     2–4 mm   requires 2 cm
                     > 4 mm   requires 2 cm
- For fascial and scalp large lesion → advancement flap.
- SLNBx for LNs metastasis in < 1 mm is < 5%.
  - → NCCN guideline: > 0.75 mm thickness, > 1 mitosis/mm, ulcerated.
- 5 years SR is better when lymphadenectomy is done at the time of SLNBx vs. delayed until patient developed clinical finding.
- Individual with face, anterior scalp, and ear, primary → also +ve LNs → superficial parotidectomy + MRND.
- Patient with +ve SLNBx in inguinal, femoral node should undergo an inguinofemoral lymphadenectomy that includes removal of Cloquet's node.
- If Cloquet's node is +ve → ilio-obturator lymphadenectomy.

Surgery for Regional and Distant Metastasis

- If patient is not amenable to complete excision → isolated limb perfusion (ILP) and isolated limb infusion (ILI), administer high dose of chemotherapy (melphalan).
- ILI provides 31% response, while hyperthermic IPL → 63%.
- Most common sites of metastasis are liver, brain, GI tract, distant skin, and SC.
- Brain, GI, skin → surgical resection or gamma knife radiation.
- Liver metastases are better dealt without surgical resection unless they arise from an occult primary.
- Radiotherapy for symptomatic bony or brain metastases provides palliation in diffuse disease.

Adjuvant and Palliative Therapies

- Thick melanoma > 4 cm with LNs → by interferon (high dose).
- Many studies showed efficacy of interferon in metastatic disease.
- BRAF inhibitor, anti PDI, high dose of IL-2.

Special Circumstances

- Pregnant outcome = nonpregnant.
- SLNBx in pregnant is safe, but blue dye is contraindicated.
- General anesthesia should be avoided in first trimester, but local anesthesia can be used.
- Unknown primary, 2%, i.e., present with LNs +ve, 5%.
- NB: melanoma could regress in response to immunity.
- Ocular melanoma is the most common noncutaneous disease.
- Treatment: photocoagulation, partial resection, radio enucleation, ocular melanoma exclusively metastasized to liver, not LNs.
- Patient with mucocutaneous melanoma has worse prognosis, 5 years, 10% in oral cavity, nasopharyngeal, anus, rectum, vulva.
- Treatment: excision, −ve margin, radical excision, e.g., APR should be avoided because role of surgery in locoregional control is not curative.
- Generally, LNs dissection benefit is not clear.

Merkel Cell Carcinoma

- Rare, aggressive NET.
- In white men at 70s.
- UV radiation, PUVA, immunosuppressants.
- ⅓ of cases in the face.
- Rapid-growing flesh-colored papule or plaque.
- Regional LNs, 30%.
- Systemic metastasis is 50% to liver, lung, bone, and brain (LLBB).
- No standard diagnostic image: CT CAP, octreotide scan.
- Treatment: WLE + SLNBx
    - If +ve LNS → completion lymphadenectomy and/or radiation.
    - If −ve LNs → observation or radiation.
- WLE with wide margin and down to fascia margin of 1–3 cm.
- Mohs microsurgery may play role to ensure −ve margin.
- Chemotherapy used, but no data.
- Recurrence is common, 47% (80% within 2 years, 96% within 5 years).
- 70% LNs metastasis after 2 years of diagnosis.
- 5 years, SR is 40%–60%.

Kaposi's Sarcoma

- Proliferation and inflammation of endothelial-derived spindle cell lesion.
- Five major forms:
    - Mediterranean
    - African endemic
    - HIV −ve
    - AIDS associated
    - Immunosuppressants associated
- All driven by human herpes virus (HHV).
- Age-group of 50s.
- Affects the skin, but can be anywhere.
- Multifocal, rubbery blue nodules.
- Treatment of Kaposi + AIDS → antiviral → dramatic response, cryotherapy, radiation.
- Biopsy is important to diagnose.
- High local recurrence → systemic rather than local.

Dermatofibrosarcoma Protuberans

- Rare.
- Low grade sarcoma in 30s.
- Low risk of distant metastasis.
- Spreads fingerlike extension.
- Depth is the most important prognostic factor.
- Head, neck, upper and lower limbs.
- Treatment: WLE, 3 cm margin down to fascia or Mohs microsurgery.
- No LN dissection.
- Radiation and biologic (imatinib) in advanced disease.
- Local recurrence is 50%–75% within 3 years → resection.

Malignant Fibrous Histiocytoma (Undifferentiated Pleomorphic Sarcoma and Myxofibrosarcoma)

- Uncommon, cutaneous, spindle cell soft tissue sarcoma occurs in upper and lower limbs, head, neck.
- Solitary, soft to firm, skin-colored nodules.
- Surgical resection + adjuvant radiation.
- Recurrence in post gross resection is 30%–35%.
- 50% present with metastasis.

Angiosarcoma

- Uncommon, aggressive, arises from vascular endothelial cells.
- Four variants, all with poor prognosis.
- Occurs in older than 40s.
- Red patch in head or scalp with satellite lesion and distant metastasis.
- Medial survival of 18–28 months.
- Lymphedema-associated angiosarcoma (Stewart-Treves) on extremities and medial arm, all axillary LNs, nonpitting edema.
- Radiation-induced angiosarcoma occurs 4–25 years.
- Postradiation for acne and malignancy (breast).
- WLE.
- High recurrence.
- Adjuvant radiation.
- Case of extremity → amputation.
- For metastatic disease → palliative chemoradiation.

Extramammary Paget Disease
- Rare adenocarcinoma of apocrine gland occurs in perianal and axilla.
- Erythematous or nonpigment plaque with eczema-like appearance.
- 40% associated with GI, GU malignancy.
- Surgical resection with microscopic −ve margin.

Hernias

Inguinal Hernia
- 75% of abdominal wall hernias are in the groin.
- 90% of the patients are male, and 10% are female.
- Peak incidence in the fist year and after 40 years old.
- Femoral hernia is 30% in male and 70% in female.
- In female, inguinal: femoral hernias is 5:1.

Anatomy of Inguinal anal
- 4–6 cm in length.
- Spermatic cord passes through internal ring (deep), through transversalis fascia to external ring (superficial).
- Boundaries:

Anterior	External oblique aponeurosis
Posterior	Transversalis fascia, transversus abdominis, conjoint tendon
Superior	Internal oblique muscle
Inferior	Inguinal ligament

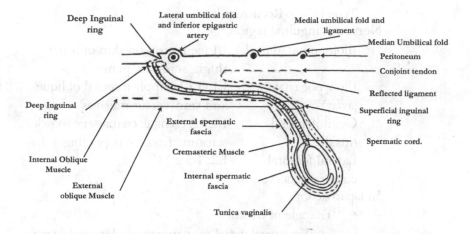

- Spermatic cord traverses the inguinal canal; it contains three arteries (testicular, cremasteric, deferential), three veins (pampiniform plexus), three nerves (ilioinguinal nerve, genital branch of genitofemoral nerve, and sympathetic nerves) and vas.

- Iliopubic tract: aponeurotic band from ASIS to Cooper's ligament.

  Lacunar ligament = Gimbernat's ligament.

- Cooper's ligament = pectineal ligament—lateral portion of lacunar ligaments.

- Conjoint tendon is the inferior fusion of internal oblique muscle and transversus abdominis.

- Indirect hernia (oblique) protrude lateral to the inferior epigastric vessel while direct hernia is medial to it, within Hesselbach's Δ.

- Hesselbach's Δ border:

Inferior	Inguinal ligament
Medial	Rectus sheath
Superior lateral	Inferior epigastric vessels

- Nyhus classification system:

Type I	Normal internal ring (indirect)
Type II	Enlarged internal ring (indirect), not reaching scrotum
Type IIIa	Direct hernia
Type IIIb	Indirect hernia, reaching scrotum, sliding
Type IIIc	Femoral hernia
Type IV	Recurrent hernia

- Nerves of inguinal region.

Ilioinguinal (outside)	L1 (sensation on skin of inner thigh, scrotum, penis)
Iliohypogastric (away)	L1, T12 (supply internal oblique and transversus muscles)
Genitofemoral (inside)	L1, L2 (genital: cremasteric muscle, scrotum; femoral: upper thigh)
Lateral femoral cutaneous nerve	L2, L3

- In laparoscopy:
  - Triangle of doom:

	Vas, lateral vessel of spermatic cord (gonadal vein)
Contents of space:	External iliac vessels, deep circumflex iliac vein, femoral nerve, genital branch of genitofemoral nerve

- Triangle of pain:
  - Iliopubic tract, gonadal vessels
  - Contents of space: LFCN, femoral nerve, femoral branch of GFN
- Circle of death:
  - Common iliac, internal iliac, obturator, inferior epigastric vessels

Pathophysiology

- The hernia either congenital or acquired.
- Congenital: impendence of normal development → failure of peritoneum to close → patent processus vaginalis (PPV)
- Increase incidence of indirect hernia in premature baby.
- Patent procesus vaginalis predisposes the hernia.
- Acquired: weak musculature wall (mesenchyme).
- Causes of groin hernia:
  - Family history, ↑ the risk eightfold
  - Cough, COPD
  - Constipation, obesity
  - Birth weight < 1,500 g
  - Valsalva maneuver, ascites
  - Collagen and connective tissue disease
  - Smoking and heavy lifting

Diagnosis

- Asymptomatic or groin pain, swelling, change in bowel habit, urinary symptom.
- Nerve compression → pressure, localized sharp pain, and referred pain.
- Hernia increases with time.
- Change in bowel habit, either sliding or obstructed.
- Patient often can reduce it by himself.

Physical Examination

- Full exposure.
- Standing position to increase IAP.
- Inspection and palpation → advancing index finger through scrotum toward external ring and ask the patient to performe Valsalva maneuver.

- Transmission cough impulse to the tip of finger → indirect, while impulse on the dorsum of finger → direct.
- Femoral hernia below inguinal ligament, lateral to pubic tubercle.
- Mid-point of inguinal ligament: ASIS to pubic tubercle.
- Mid-inguinal point: ASIS to symphysis pubis.

Image
- US, CT, MRI.
- US sensitivity and specificity, 86%, 77%.
- CT sensitivity and specificity, 80%, 65%.
- MRI sensitivity and specificity, 95%, 96%.

Treatment
- Surgical repair.
- When unfit patient, surgery deferred and surgical reserve for emergency.
- 72% of asymptomatic develops pain within 7.5 years.
- Truss relief pain up to 65% of patient.
- Femoral hernia has increased risk of complication.
- Strangulation, 3 months to 2 years; inguinal hernia, 2.5%–4.5%; femoral, 22%–45%.
- Recommendation: femoral hernia and symptomatic inguinal hernia should be repaired electively when possible.
- Preoperative IV antibiotic is controversial, but date trends routine preoperative IV antibiotic.
- Taxis should be attempted for incarcerated hernia, not strangulated → analgesia, light sedation, Trendelenburg position → content is milking with compression.
- Strangulation: surgical emergency—fever, high WBCs, hemodynamic instability, bulge is warm, tender, discoloration of overlying skin.
- No taxis in strangulation → NPO, IVF, IV antibiotic, NGT then OR.

Inguinal Hernia Repair
  - **Classic Bassini repair**
    - Incise the skin approximately 2–3 cm above and parallel to the inguinal ligament

- Subcutaneous dissection (camper's and scarpa's fascia)
- Open the aponeurosis of the external oblique muscle in the direction of its fibers.
- Protect the ilioinguinal nerve, and proceed with the scissors
- open the aponeurosis till the external inguinal ring, exposing and opening the inguinal canal and spermatic cord.
- Elevate the spermatic cord carefully and retract it.
- Identify the sac, located anteromedial to the spermatic cord.
- Dissect it at the internal ring and lateral to the inferior epigastric vessels
- Ligate and resect the sac.
- Open the transversalis fascia.
- Continues Suture of superior 3 layers (upper flap of Transversalis fascia + "Conjoint tendon" = Internal Oblique + Transversus Abdominus) to the inferior 2 layers (lower flap of Transversalis fascia and inguinal ligament)

- **Modified Bassini: Conjoint Tendon Repair**
- Transversalis fascia is not opened.
- Two superior layers (conjoint tendon = internal oblique + transversus abdominus) sutured to inferior one layer, which is the inguinal ligament.

- **Shouldice Repair: Four-Layer Repair**
- Open the transversalis fascia.
- First layer: lower flap free edge of transversalis fascia to the posterior aspect of the upper flap of transversalis fascia.
- Second layer: upper flap of transversalis fascia free edge to base of lower flap and inguinal ligament.
- Third layer: conjoint tendon to inguinal ligament.
- Fourth layer: conjoint tendon to posterior aspect of the external oblique aponeurosis.
- Close the external oblique aponeurosis over the cord.

- **McVay Repair**
  - Open transversalis fascia.
  - Expose and identify Cooper's ligament (iliopectineal ligament).
  - Interrupted sutures between the conjoint tendon to Cooper's ligament starting from the pubic tubercle until you reach the femoral vein, then perform the *transition stitch*, which is conjoint to Cooper's to inguinal ligament stitch.
  - Continue the rest of the sutures between conjoint and inguinal until the internal ring.
  - Make a relaxing incision in the anterior rectus sheath (2–3 cm) above the tubercle, extending for about 10 cm superiorly.

- **Lichtenstein Repair: (Mesh Repair) Tension-Free Repair**
  - A mesh prosthesis is positioned over the inguinal floor.
  - The mesh should be at least 15 cm × 8 cm.
  - The medial end is rounded to correspond to the patient's particular anatomy and secured to the anterior rectus sheath at least 2 cm medial to the pubic tubercle, then fix it with a superficial stitch to the tubercle.
  - A continuous suture through the lower end of the mesh to the shelving edge of the inguinal ligament. The suture is tied at the internal ring.
  - An incision is made at the lateral end of the mesh to create two tails, two-thirds above and one-third below.
  - The tails are positioned around the cord structures, and the upper tail is placed on top of the lower and sutured together to create a new internal ring.
  - Then fix the mesh to the conjoint tendon, rectus sheath.

- **Laparoscopic Inguinal Hernia Repair**
  - Transabdominal preperitoneal procedure (TAPP)
  - Total extraperitoneal approach (TEP).

Femoral Hernia
- Femoral ring:

Anterior	Inguinal ligament, IPT
Posterior	Cooper's ligament post
Medial	Lacunar ligament

- Femoral Δ:

Superior	Inguinal hernia
Medial	Adductor longus
Lateral	Sartorius muscle

There are three standard common approaches:

1. **High Approach (McEvedy) (Extraperitoneal)**
   - Vertical incision over the femoral canal, extending superiorly to the lateral pararectus plane and inferiorly below the inguinal ligament.
   - The anterior rectus sheath is incised, and the rectus muscle is retracted medially, exposing the fascia transversalis.
   - Locate the neck of the sac entering the femoral ring.
   - Once the sac is identified, it should be pulled back from the femoral canal, excised, and ligated.
   - Then the repair will be either by suturing the inguinal ligament to the Cooper's ligament or through suturing the conjoint tendon to the Cooper's ligament (McVay repair).

2. **Inguinal/Transinguinal Approach or (Lotheissen Approach)**
   - The external oblique is opened, the inguinal canal is explored, and the cord is retracted.
   - The transversalis fascia is divided, taking care not to injure the inferior epigastric vessels.
   - The preperitoneal fat is bluntly dissected to expose the hernia sac entering the femoral ring, and same as the high approach, the peritoneum is not opened.
   - The sac is pulled back, excised, and ligated, and the defect is repaired just like high approach.

3. **Infrainguinal Approach (Lockwood Approach)**
   - Skin incision of 1–2 cm below the inguinal skin crease.
   - All layers should be dissected until reaching the sac, which is freed from surrounding structures, opened at the funds to explore content, and pushed back to abdomen if viable.
   - The sac is ligated and resected, and the defect is closed with three sutures between the inguinal ligament and the Cooper's ligament or using a small mesh plug.

Ventral Hernia

Epigastric Hernia
   - Midline, between xiphoid process and umbilicus.
   - Small, may multiply.
   - Contains usually omentum and part of falciform ligament.
   - Could be congenital due to defective midline fusion.

Umbilical Hernia
   - Occurs in umbilical ring, can be present at birth or develop later (rare).
   - Present in 10% of all newborn and more common in premature infants.
   - Closed spontaneously at the age of 5.
        → If not → elective repair.
   - Adult with small symptom → follow up.
        → Surgery if enlarged, symptomatic, or incarcerated.
   - Treatment can be primary closure or with prosthesis if > 2 cm open or laparoscopy.
   - Patient with CLD or ascites requires special consideration.
        First, manage ascites with paracentesis and medical treatment.
        Complication after paracentesis: bowel and omentum enter the defect, leaking ascites → bacterial peritonitis.
        Patients with refractory ascites → TIPS or LTPx then hernial repair.

Paraumbilical Hernia
   - Differs from umbilical hernia that appears around the umbilicus; the bulge will give the umbilicus a crescent shape, while in umbilical hernia, the bulge is through umbilicus and is round.

Spigelian Hernia
- Occurs at lateral border of rectus abdominis, adjacent or through the linea semilunaris.
- Most common location is just above the arcuate line.
- To confirm diagnosis → US or CT.
- Risk of incarceration is 17%.
- Repair if diagnosed, using open or laparoscopic repair.

Incisional Hernia
- 10%–20% eventually develop hernia at incision site.
- Risk factor: obesity, wound healing defect, prior procedure, prior incisional hernia, tech error.
- Treatment: primary vs. mesh, open vs. laparoscopy.
- Primary repair = simple closure and component separation.
    → Primary repair by simple suture > 3 cm → recurrent.
- Component separation:
    → Large subcutaneous flap.
    → Bilateral incision of external oblique aponeurosis.
    → Incision of rectus sheath muscle.
    → Wound infection, 20%; recurrent, 18.2%.
- Mesh repair is standard.
    → Underlay (sublay): deep to fascia (preperitoneal).
    → Interlay (inlay): within the musculoaponeurotic layer.
    → Onlay: above the fascia.
- Laparoscopic repair is underlay.
- Biological mesh: porcine, bovine, or human collagen.
    → Overtime replaced by host tissue.
    → Usually used in infected field.
    → High recurrence.
- Laparoscopy recurrence is 3.4% within 2 years.
- Low risk of in infection than open but high cost, early return to work.

Obturator Hernia
- Hernia through the obturator canal.
- Symptom: tender medial thigh mass, can be present with intestinal obstruction if incarcerated.
- Howship-Romberg sign—inner thigh pain with internal rotation.

- Exacerbated by adduction and internal rotation of the thigh and relieved by leg flexion.
- Diagnosis by CT: bowel gas below superior pubic ramus.
- Tx by operative repair, may need mesh.

Other Types of Hernias
- Littre's hernia, Richter hernia Sciatic hernia, lumbar hernia,.

Complication
- Bleeding, seroma, wound infection, urine retention.
- Hernia recurrence
    - Seroma, cord lipoma, recurrence.
    - Common medial illness associated with malnutrition, low immunity, DM, steroid, smoking.
    - Technical issue: mesh size, ischemia, infection.
    - Extensive dissection → cord injury.
    - Better approach after recurrence is laparoscopic approach.

- Pain
    - Acute or chronic.
    - Three mechanisms: nociceptive (somatic), neuropathic, visceral.
    - Nociceptive is most common → ligament, muscular trauma → NSAIDs.
    - Neuropathic: direct damage of the nerve or entrapment → localized burning, tearing sensation → steroid or local anesthesia injection.
    - Visceral pain: autonomic, can be during ejaculation → sympathetic injury.
    - Identification of nerve is 70%–90%.
    - Pain can be treated with reoperation, pain catheter.
    - Selective ilioinguinal, iliohypogatric and GFN neurolysis or neurectomy, removal of mesh, and revision of repair.
    - When inguinodynia is refractory → triple neurectomy with removal of meshoma.

- Refractory inguinodynia and orchialgia → resection of para-vasal nerve.
- Other chronic pain: local entrapment of nerve, osteitis pubis → greater risk of entrapment in open II and IH and in laparotomy, GFN, and LCFN → NSAIDs, steroid, anesthesia.
- Avoid pubic periosteum to stitch or tack.

- Nerve injury: in open approach ilioinguinal most susciptible for injury whereas in laparoscopy → GFN.
- Cord and testis injury
  - Ischemic orchitis caused by pampiniform plexus, not testicular artery.
    - → Pain within 1 week, enlarged testis, indurated, painful → 1%.
  - US → blood flow.
  - Emergent orchiectomy if necrosis.
  - Injury to testicular artery → atrophy.
  - Treatment reassurance, NSAIDs → intraoperative proximal ligation of large sac.
  - Injury to vas → infertility.
    Early → urology consultation for primary anastomosis.
  - Chronic scarring → vas obstruction.
  - Pain during ejaculation → self-limiting.
  - Round ligament in female → maintain uterine anteversion → injury to artery or ligament → nothing.

- Laparoscopic complication
  - Urine retention caused by general anesthesia.
  - Ileus and bowel obstruction.
    - → TAPP → bowel obstruction through hernia.
  - Visceral injury
    Small bowel, colon, bladder → less common → cystotomy → repair in several layers with 1–2 weeks Foley's catheter for decompression → confirmatory cystogram.

- Vascular injury

    Iliac or femoral vessels → most severe.

    → Most common: inferior epigastric (often delayed → rectus sheath hematoma).

- Hematoma and seroma
    - Hematoma: any layer.
    - Seroma: warm compression to accelerate resolution, to avoid infection → no aspiration.

The Appendix

Embryology
-   In six weeks, it starts to develop as outpouching; in 5 months, it starts to elongate to form vermiform appendix.
-   Unequal growth → lateral wall grow more → posteromedial location below ileocecal valve.
-   Midgut malrotation and situs inversus, incomplete or failure to rotate around axis of SMA → appendix in LUQ.
    -   → In LLQ in situ inversus (abdomen and/or thoracic) transposition.

Anatomy
-   6–9 cm in length.
-   Diameter, 3–8 mm, and intraluminal, 1–3 mm.
-   Artery → appendicular artery → ileocolic artery → SMA (posterior to terminal ileum).
-   LN along ileocolic artery.
-   Innervation: superior mesenteric plexus (T10–L1).
-   Parasympathetic → vagus nerve.
-   Mucosa, submucosa, musculosa (not well), serosa (partial cover).
-   Position: retroceal, 64%; subcecal, 32%; pelvic, 2%.
-   Lymphoid aggregates in submucosa.
-   Neuroendocrine complex: ganglion cells, Schwann cell, renal fiber, and neurosecretory cells.

Physiology
-   Immunological organ, IgA.
-   If appendectomy is done before age of 20, protect against UC (reported)
-   Appendectomy increases risk of CD (meta-analysis).
-   Colonizes healthy bacteria.

Acute appendicitis
Epidemiology
-   Lifetime risk is 8.6% on male and 6.7% on female.
-   Higher in ages 20s–30s.

Etiology and Pathogenesis
- Obstruction of lumen by fecalith or hypertrophy of lymphoid tissue.
- Fecalith is 40% in simple acute appendicitis, 65% in gangrenous without rupture, and 90% in gangrenous with rupture.
- Proximal obstruction → closed loop obstruction → secretion of appendix mucus → distension → stimulate nerve ending of visceral fiber (visceral pain) → vague, dull, diffuse pain in mid abdomen or epigastrium.
- The inflammation reaches the parietal layer of peritoneum (somatic pain), i.e., localized in RLQ.
    - → Distension is higher → higher multiplication of bacteria.
    - → Nausea, vomiting.
    - → Pressure is higher → venous obstruction → congestion → infarction → perforation.

    NB: some episode will resolve spontaneously.

Microbiology
- Tissue culture reveals → E. coli, bacteroides.
- If gangrenous or perforated appendix → aggressive bacteria.

Clinical Picture
If GI symptom developed before pain → mostly gastroenteritis.
- Symptoms
    - Starts in the periumbilical then localized RLQ, sensitivity, 81%; specificity, 51%.

        Nausea   sensitivity, 58%   specificity, 36%
        Vomiting   sensitivity, 51%   specificity, 45%
        Anorexia   sensitivity, 68%   specificity, 36%
        Obstipation, diarrhea if perforated
        NB: most sensitive symptom is anorexia, and most sensitive sign is RIF tenderness.
- Signs
    - Early: minimal alter of V/S.
    - Pulse and temperature are slightly high.
    - Prefer to lie supine, to decrease irritation, move slowly.
    - On palpation: maximal tenderness at McBurney point.

- on deep palpation → guarding.
- When removed hand quickly → sudden pain (rebound tenderness) Blumberg's sign.
- Rovsing sign (palpation of LIF will induce pain in RIF) → strong indication of peritoneal irritation (indirect rebound tenderness).
- Anatomical variation, retrocecal → right flank pain when in pelvis → missing.
- Psoas sign: irritation when right leg is extended.
- Obturator sign: internal rotation of flexed thigh.
- Dunphy's sign: ↑ abdominal pain with coughing.

Laboratory

- WBCs > 11,000 (look for neutrophil shift, lymphopenia).
- Unusual if WBCs is 18,000, if higher → perforated appendicitis with or without abscess.
- ↑ CRP (strong indicator).
- Appendicitis is unlikely if WBCs, CRP, and proportion of neutrophil are all normal.
- Urine analysis—to rule out UTI.

Clinical Scoring System

- Alvarado score
- Appendicitis inflammatory response score

Imaging Study

- CXR—to rule out lower-right lobe pneumonia.
- AXR—appendicolith (7%–15%); displacement of cecum, evident of mural thickness, loss of psoas shadow, pattern of small bowel obstruction (functional) usually at RIF; scoliosis to the left side.
- Barium enema—if lumen is filled → no appendicitis.
- T^{99}-labeled leukocyte scan.
- CT more sensitive than US.

  - US
    - Blind ending, non-compressible structure.
    - Non-peristaltic bowel originates from cecum.
    - Thickening of appendix wall.

- Periappendicular free fluid.
- If diameter < 5 mm, appendicitis is unlikely.
  - Sensitivity 55%–96%
  - Specificity 85%–98% (operator dependent)

- CT
  - Dilated lumen > 5 mm, and wall is thickened. Periappendicular fat stranding, thickened mesoappendix or phlegmon, free fluid, fecalith can be visualized.
  - Sensitivity, 92%–97%; specificity, 85%–94%.
  - CT ↓ −ve appendectomy (appendectomy for normal appendix), 12%–19%.
  - But has S/E radiation, allergy, expensive,
    - oral contrast → nausea and vomiting
    - IV contrast → renal impairment, anaphylaxis.
  - Despite US and CT, misdiagnosis is 5%–15%.
  - Misdiagnosis is high in female in reproductive age.

Differential Diagnosis
- Other disease of acute abdomen
- Acute mesenteric adenitis
- PID, twisted ovary
- Rupture griffin follicle
- Acute gastroenteritis

- **Pediatric Population**
  - Acute mesenteric adenitis is frequent.
    - → URTI recently subsided.
  - Pain is diffused.
  - Guarding is usual, but rigidity is rare.
  - Generalized lymphadenopathy may be present.
  - WBCs are normal or high.
  - Observe for several hours; it's self-limiting.

- **Elderly Patient**
  - Diverticulitis—sigmoid overlies to RLQ.
  - Perforating CA.
  - CT is diagnostic.

- **Female Patient**
  - PID, twisted ovary, ruptured GF, endometriosis, ectopic pregnancy.
  - PID infection bilaterally 50%, nausea and vomiting → tender usually on lower and painful with movement of cervix.
    - → Purulent vaginal discharge.
      - → ↓ in early phase of menses and ↑ in luteal phase.
      - → Tenderness is diffused in ruptured graafian follicle
      - → US and CT.
  - Torsion requires emergent surgery → if left → thrombosis gangrene → resection.
  - Ectopic pregnancy: abdominal pain, high WBCs, low Hct, intra-abdominal hemorrhage, high beta HCG → surgery.

- **Immunosuppressed Patient**
  - HIV, 0.5%; it's higher than normal population, 0.1%–0.2%.
  - Symptom same as with normal population.
  - No ↑ WBCs.
  - ↑ rupture of appendix, 43%.
    - → Delayed presentation.
  - Typhlitis (neutropenic enterocolitis)—DDx.

Initial Management

- Operative vs. non-operative in uncomplicated appendicitis
  - Appendectomy is standard of care.
  - surgical intervention is warrented if the patient is going to area with no surgical facility (submarine).
  - Failure rate is 50%.
  - Recurrent appendicitis, 7%–14%.
  - ↑ hospital stay, ↑ morbidity, ↑ failure rate, ↑ antibiotics resistance.

- Urgent vs. emergent operation in uncomplicated appendicitis
  - No difference in wound infection, intra-abdominal abscess, or operative time.
  - But ↑ hospital stay in urgent intervention compare to emergent intervention.
  - Should consider available room and staff.

Complicated Appendicitis

- I.e., perforated → abscess or phlegm.
- 25%.
- Incidence of perforation is ↑ in less than 5 years and more than 65 years.
- Most perforations occur early before patient arrived in the hospital.
- Some studies showed increase risk with time, and some disagreed.
- ↑ risk of infertility → adhesion of tube, should be suspected in peritonitis and SIRS.
- 2%–6% form a mass (phlegm) in 5–7 days.
- Treatment: sign of sepsis and peritonitis → midline incision (lower).
- If mass phlegmon: operative vs. conservative → meta-analysis: non-operative (conservative) is superior to operative intervention.
- Morbidity with operative is 37% and non-operative, 11%.
- Failure of conservative management, 7.6%.
- Recurrent rate is 7.4%, does not mandate interval appendectomy.
- In pediatrics, early intervention is superior than conservative.
- Failure of conservative is 20%.

- **Interval Appendectomy**
  - No clear role, recurrence is 7.4%, almost the same with normal population.

Operative Intervention for Appendicitis

Laparoscopic vs. open appendectomy:

Laparoscopic → ↓ SSI, ↓ hospital stay, but ↑ intra-abdominal abscess (collection), ↓ pain, quick return to normal life, the cost is equal, benefit of diagnostic tool.

- Single-incision laparoscopic appendectomy
- Natural Orifice Transluminal Endoscopic Surgery (NOTES)

Open Appendectomy

- After induction of anesthesia, do time-out to make sure of the patient's name, procedure, and staff names, then position the patient.
- Gridiron or Lanz incision at McBurney's point.
- SC tissue (Camper's and Scarpa's fascia) is divided.
- The external oblique fascia is divided.
- The three muscle layers of the abdominal wall are split in the direction of their fibers and retracted.
- The peritoneum is opened transversely.
- Any fluid should be noted, aspirated, and if purulent, sent for C/S.
- Any remaining fluid is then suctioned from the field.
- The cecum is identified, grasped, and exteriorized through the wound using a gauze sponge or blunt bowel graspers.
- The base of the appendix is identified at the confluence of the taenia coli.
- If the appendix is retrocecal, the cecum should be mobilized medially by incising the lateral peritoneal attachments of the cecum.
- The mesenteric window is created in an avascular area of the mesoappendix.
- The mesentery of the appendix is divided. It is important to correctly identify the appendicular artery and assure that it is properly ligated.
- The appendix is divided approximately 5 mm from the cecal wall using a suture ligature.
- Using a sharp scalpel, the appendix is transected between the suture ligature.
- The mucosa of the appendiceal stump is lightly touched with electrocautery.

- The lower abdominal cavity is irrigated thoroughly with normal saline.
- Closure of the fascial layers of the wound is carried out using running or interrupted absorbable suture.
- SC tissue and skin are closed.

Laparoscopic Appendectomy

- The peritoneal cavity is accessed at the umbilicus (using either a Veress needle or a Hasson technique), and a 5 mm or 10 mm trocar and laparoscope are placed.
- Another 5 mm trocar is placed in the midline above the symphysis pubis.
- Third 5 mm trocar is placed in LLQ or RUQ.
- An additional trocar can be placed as needed to improve exposure.
- The patient is then placed in Trendelenburg position and rotated to the left to help expose the cecum.
- Instruments are placed and the appendix inspected.
- If the appendix is normal, a search for other sources.
- Appendix is elevated with an instrument and dissected free of any adhesions.
- The appendix is elevated with a grasper.
- The mesoappendix is isolated with a dissector by making a window between it and the appendix.
- The mesoappendix is divided with clips, harmonic shears, or a laparoscopic stapling device.
- The appendix is divided at its base with endo-loop, linear stapling device or ligatures.
- The appendix is placed in a specimen bag and removed through the largest port site.
- Irrigation and suction
- Removal of the trocars, deflate the air and closure.

Special Circumstances
Acute Appendicitis in Young

- To establish diagnosis is more difficult in children as history can't be taken properly.
- Inability to walk, describe the pain or percussion, cough.

- High incidence of perforation, omentum is small → minimally contained.
- < 5 years, the −ve appendectomy is 25% and perforation, 45%.
- In 12 years, the −ve appendectomy is 10% and perforation, 20%.
- Wound infection with perforation is 11% and with no perforation, 2.8%.
- Abscess collection with perforation is 6% and with no perforation, 3%.
- Treatment: appendectomy.
- IV antibiotics: 24–48 hrs in nonperforated and completed in perforated till WBC normalizes or 24 hrs off fever.

Acute Appendicitis in Elderly

- Atypical presentation.
- Many DDx.
- Increased incidence of perforation.
- Perforation in adult is 20%–30%, while in elderly, 50%–70%, and higher above 80s.
- Present in abdominal pain but no clinical sign.
- High index of suspicion if high temperature of 38°C, high WBCs, and anorexia.
- ↑ postoperative mortality and morbidity.
- Laparoscopy is preferred.

Acute Appendicitis in Pregnancy

- Most common surgical emergency in pregnancy.
- 1:766.
- Anytime but rare in third trimester.
- −ve appendectomy is 25%, i.e., higher than non-pregnant, usually in second trimester.
- Anatomic changes, pain in upper-right abdomen, 74%.
- Laboratory is not helpful, as WBC is usually 16,000.
- US or MRI.
- Laparoscopy in equivocal case but higher complication, 2.3 times of fetal loss.
- Overall, fetal loss, 4%; early delivery, 7%.
- Pregnant with ruptured appendicitis is 20%–25%.
- Needs careful history, physical examination, and diagnostic tool accuracy.

NB
- Valentino's syndrome: was first described when Rudolph Valentino, a famous American actor, presented with the signs and symptoms of acute appendicitis in New York City. He had an appendectomy but later went on to develop overt peritonitis and multiple organ failures and later he died.
- Autopsy went on to reveal he had been suffering from a perforated gastric ulcer.
- Contaminants from the perforated peptic ulcer had trickled down the right paracolic gutter to the right iliac fossa, causing the localized peritonism in the right iliac fossa, the presence of suppurative fluid, and a mildly inflamed appendix (chemical periappendicitis).
- Only two such cases of Valentino's syndrome have been reported in recent times where one of the patients was treated conservatively with antibiotics and the other one with laparoscopy.

Postoperative Care and Complication
- Uncomplicated, ↓ complication.
- Start diet at the same day of discharge or following day.
- IV antibiotics for 24 hrs if uncomplicated and for 4–7 days if complicated.
- Postoperative ileus may occur, and diet started is based on clinical evaluation.

Surgical Site Infection (SSI)
- Superficial or deep.
- Treatment: opening the incision and wound swab for C/S.
- In laparoscopy → port site is the more common site of infection.
- If patient with cellulitis → antibiotics.
- If postoperative collection with fever, high WBC, abdominal pain ileus, bowel obstruction, diarrhea:
    If small → IV antibiotics.
    If large → drainage by CT-guided or US + antibiotics.
    If interventional radiology not available → laparoscopy.

Stump Appendicitis
- Incomplete appendectomy.
- Usually 9 years after operation.
- No difference if done by laparoscopy or open.
- Usually complicated and requires colectomy.
- Use appendiceal critical view to avoid complication:
  - Appendix at ten o'clock.
  - Taenia coli at three o'clock.
  - Terminal ileum at six o'clock.

  When taenia coli disappears → ligation, remaining stump no larger than 0.5 cm.

Incidental Appendectomy
- Appendectomy performed to prevent appendicitis.
- Routinely in Ladd's procedure in malrotation.
- Nowadays, not warranted because of morbidity of the procedure.

Neoplasm of Appendix
- Less than 1%.
- Most common: appendiceal carcinoid, appendiceal adenoma.
- Mean age is 69.

Carcinoid
- Firm yellow bulbar mass.
- Most common site of gastrointestinal tract is appendix.
- Carcinoid syndrome is rare, but if widespread is present, 2.9%.
- Occasionally obstructing the lumen → acute appendicitis.
- If < 1 cm, rarely extension outside.
- Usually presented with localized disease, 64%.
- Treatment: if < 1 cm → appendectomy.
- If 1–2 cm at the base involving mesentery or LNs → right hemicolectomy.

Adenocarcinoma
- Rare.
- Three types:
  - a. Mucinous adenocarcinoma

     b.   Colonic adenocarcinoma

     c.   Adenocarcinoid

- Most common presentation is acute appendicitis.
- Can also be present with ascites, early perforation.
- Treatment: right hemicolectomy.
- Overall SR is 55%, 5 years.
- Increase incidence of synchronous and metachronous disease.

NB

Synchronous: two or more primarily coexist at the time of diagnosis.

Metachromous: developed consequently, sometimes after years of resection.

Mucocele
- Obstruction, dilation, intraluminal accumulation of mucoid material.
- Maybe caused by the following:
    a.   Retention cyst
    b.   Mucosal hyperplasia
    c.   Cystadenoma
    d.   Cystadenocarcinoma
- Symptom is nonspecific, usually intestinal obstruction.
- If intact mucocele → no future risk.

  If ruptured → escape to peritoneal cavity.

  If laparoscopy → open laparotomy is recommended.
- Presence of mucocele doesn't mandate right hemicolectomy but resection of appendix + wide mesoappendix resection + LNs and fluid cytology of internal peritoneal fluid.
- Right hemicolectomy or ileocectomy (preferable) is reserved for +ve margin at the base or +ve LNs.
- If ruptured neoplasm with gross spillage → refer to higher center for reexploration + HIPEC.

Pseudomyxoma Peritonei
- Diffuse collection of gelatinous fluid associated with mucinous implant on peritoneal and omentum.
- 3:1 = female:male.

- Caused by neoplastic mucus-secreting cells within the peritoneum.
- Difficult to classify as malignant because it may be a spare, widespread, low-grade cytology.
- Symptom: abdominal pain, distension or mass, ureteric obstruction, and venous obstruction can be seen.
- Progresses slowly and recurrence is 76%.
- LNS and metastasis are uncommon.
- Diagnosis:
    - CT—mucinous ascites deposit in diaphragm.
    - Right retrohepatic, left paracolic gutter, ligament of treitz, and ovary.
- Treatment:
    - → Surgical debulking (cytoreductive surgery), remove all gross disease of omentum, liver, stomach + appendectomy are routinely.
    - → TAH + BSO in female.
- SR high in R0 or R1 while worst in R2 (remaining disease).
- 5 years, SR is 30%.
- HIPEC + cytoreductive surgery.
- It takes 300–1,020 min.
- Mortality, 6%, and morbidity, 38%.
- CRS + HIPEC increase SR to 53%–78% at initial performance.
- Recurrent → surgery.
- Recurrent procedure → enterotomies, leak, fistula.

Lymphoma

- Uncommon, most frequently NHL, appendix lymphoma.
- Primary lymphoma from appendix, 1%–3%.
- Usually presented with intestinal obstruction.
- Finding on CT → appendix diameter is 2.5 cm and surrounding soft tissue thickening.
- Treatment: appendectomy.
    - → Right hemicolectomy if mesentery or cecum is involved.
- Staging postoperative if → limited to appendix → no additional adjuvant therapy.
- If beyond appendix → consider adjuvant therapy.

Soft Tissue Sarcoma

Introduction
- Arises from the mesoderm.
- Majority is soft tissue sarcoma.
- Other types of sarcoma include osteosarcoma, chondrosarcoma, angiosarcoma, leiomyosarcoma.
- Ewing sarcoma and primitive NET occur either on the bone or soft tissue.
- Most of the primary soft tissue sarcomas are in the extremities, 50%–60%; trunk, 19%; retroperitoneum, 15%; and head and neck, 9%.
- Soft tissue sarcoma includes fifty subtypes.
- The most common subtypes (historically), excluding Kaposi's sarcoma → fibrous histiocytoma, 28%; liposarcoma, 15%; leiomyosarcoma, 12%; synovial, 10%; peripheral nerve sheath, 6%.
- Today, malignant fibrous histiocytoma is classified as liposarcoma, leiomyosarcoma, undifferentiated pleomorphic sarcoma, or myxofibrosarcoma.
- Rhabdomyosarcoma is the most common sarcoma in pediatrics, whereas pleomorphic rhabdomyosarcoma occurs in adult.
  - → It differs in biology and treatment.
- 5 years, SR is 50%–60%.
- Patient who dies from sarcoma mostly succumb to lung metastasis → occurs 2–3 years after initial diagnosis.

Frequency of Histological Subtype of Soft Tissue Sarcoma
- Liposarcoma, 15%; leiomyosarcoma, 12%; unclassified, 11%; synovial, 10%; malignant peripheral nerve sheath, 6%; rhabdomyosarcoma, 5%; fibrosarcoma, 3%; Ewing sarcoma, 2%; angiosarcoma, 2%; osteosarcoma, 1%; chondrosarcoma, 1%.

Incidence
- 5–6 individuals per 100,000/year.
- Less than 1% of all malignancy in adult and 15% in children.

Epidemiology

- Sarcoma not resulting from progression or dedifferentiated liposarcoma of benign soft tissue tumor, except peripheral nerve sheath tumor in patient with neurofibromatosis.

Radiation Exposure

- External radiotherapy is rare but still associated with mutation among patients treated with radiation of breast CA, cervix, testis, lymph, lymphoma and has eight- to fiftyfold risk.
- most common histological type → osteogenic sarcoma, malignant fibrous histiocytoma, angiosarcoma, lymphangiosarcoma.
- The risk is increasing with the dose.
- Median time to develop 10 years postexposure.

Occupational Chemical Exposure

- Herbicide such as phenylacetic acid, wood preservative containing chlorophenols.

Chronic Lymphedema

- 0.07% underwent ALND.
- Lymphangiosarcoma is aggressive tumor, SR is 19 months.

Molecular Pathogenesis

- Classified into three groups:
    1. Specific translocation
    2. Gene amplification
    3. Complex genomic rearrangement
- Translocation causing over expression of autocrine growth factor.
- Oncogenic mutation → GIST classic example of sarcoma, mutation KIT receptor, or PDGFR-α → majority has mutation in exon II of KIT and responds dramatically to tyrosine kinase inhibitor (imatinib).

Initial Assessment

-   Clinical behavior determined by anatomic location (depth in relation to investing fascia), histological subtype, grade of aggressiveness, size.
-   Pattern of metastasis: hematogenous, primary to lung.
-   LNs is rare, < 5%.

Clinical Presentation

-   Asymptomatic mass.
-   Extremity sarcoma → DVT.
-   Tumor in distal extremity is small, but in proximal or retroperitoneal, it is large.
-   Can compress adjacent organ.
-   Infrequently, tumor impingement on bone or neurovascular bundle.
-   Less frequently, compress GI and produce symptom or compress lumbar or pelvic nerves.
-   DDx includes lipoma as it's a hundred times more than sarcoma.

Diagnostic Imaging

-   Should be performed before any invasive procedure.
-   MRI for extremities.
-   CT for retroperitoneum, intra-abdominal.
-   CT chest for lung metastasis with high-grade tumor > 5 cm.
-   MRI brain with alveolar soft part sarcoma and angiosarcoma.
-   US instead of MRI if not available.
-   MRI T1—equal or slightly high to adjacent skeletal muscle.
       T2—higher intensity than skeletal.
       T1—intratumoral necrosis.
-   MRI postresection Q3–4M for first 2 years, then Q6M for 3–5 years, then annually.
-   FDG-PET used to assess response to chemotherapy.

Biopsy Technique

-   FNA: at center, low diagnostic accuracy of 60%–90% than core biopsy and to establish histological type and grade.
    -   o FNA procedure of choice for metastasis focus or recurrence.

- Core needle biopsy:
  o Accuracy is 93%.
  o US, CT-guided prevent sampling from non-diagnostic necrotic or cystic area.
  o Complication is less than 1%.
- Incisional biopsy
  o Historically, it was the gold standard.
  o CNBx cannot produce adequate tissue for diagnostic or non-diagnostic.
  o Disadvantage: schedule, needs GA, high cost.
  o Complication: hematoma, infected dehiscence, tumor fungating.
  o Biopsy should be oriented longitudinally along extremities to allow subsequent WLE.
  o Adequate hemostasis to prevent dissemination of tumor cell.
- Excisional biopsy
  o For superficial extremity or truncal lesion < 3 cm.
  o Rarely performed.
  o No excisional biopsy in lesion in hands and feet.

Pathologic Assessment and Classification
  - Disagreement by pathologists (conflict), 25%–40%.
  - Pathologiests classified soft tissue sarcoma as follows:
    1. Tumor with limited metastasis potential: desmoid, well-differentiated liposarcoma, dermatofibrosarcoma protuberans.
    2. Tumor with intermediate risk of metastasis spread: usually has large myxoid component → myxoid liposarcoma, myxofibrosarcoma.
    3. Highly aggressive with metastasis: angiosarcoma, clear cell carcinoma, dedifferentiated liposarcoma, leiomyosarcoma, rhabdomyosarcoma.

  NB: Recently, it has been noted that fibrous histiocytoma is not a separate tumor entity → sarcoma subtype.
      → Most of retroperitoneal fibrous histiocytoma → reclassified as dedifferentiated liposarcoma.

Staging and Prognostic Factor
- AJCC staging system is based on the histological grade of aggressiveness, tumor size, depth, LNs, or distant metastasis.
    - → This system does not apply on GIST, fibromatosis (desmoid), Kaposi's sarcoma, infantile fibrosarcoma.

- Histologic grade of aggressiveness
  - Important for grade.
  - Tissue (adequate).
  - Differentiation (good, moderate, poor/anaplastic), cellularity, pleomorphism, necrosis (absent < 50%, > 50%), number of mitosis (< 10, 10–19, > 20) per HPF.
  - Tumor grade to predict metastasis:

Low	5%–10%
Intermediate	20%–30%
High grade	50%–60%

  - 5 years, SR is 90%, 70%, 40%, respectively.

- Tumor size and location
  - Classified to two groups   T1 < 5 cm

        T2 > 5 cm
  - Some author suggests   T3 > 15 cm

- Nodal metastasis
  - Rare, but in epithelioid sarcoma, pediatric rhabdomyosarcoma, angiosarcoma, clear cell sarcoma, synovial sarcoma can occur.
  - Sarcoma with LNs → stage III.
  - If suspicious LNs → FNA.

- Distant metastasis
  - Most often to lung, other liver, bone, visceral.

- Prognostic factor
  - Size, grade, depth, LNs, distant metastasis.
  - Old age and gender-associated recurrence and mortality.
  - +ve microscopic margin and early recurrence → low SR.
  - Ki-67, proliferative marker, correlated with poor clinical outcome.
  - ↑ CD100, E-cadherin, catenin → poor outcome.

- Prognostic nomogram
  - Accurate in predicting SR.

Treatment of Extremity and Trunk Wall Sarcoma
- Goal is to maximize recurrence-free.
- Overall, SR in all stage of sarcoma is 50%–60%, 5 years.
- For patient with extremities sarcoma, SR is 70%, 5 years.
- Most patients die from metastatic disease within 2–3 years, 80%.

- **Recommendation for Management of Soft Tissues Masses**
  1. If the mass > 3 cm → US, CT, and core needle biopsy.
  2. Once diagnosed as sarcoma → MRI for extremities, CT for other sites, and evaluate metastatic disease with CT chest in grade 2, 3, or large tumor T2.
  3. WLE with 1–2 cm −ve margin for T1.
  4. Radiation therapy for T2, intermediate, or high grade.
  5. Patient with locally advanced, high-grade or distant metastasis → chemotherapy.
  6. Aggressive surgery if isolated local recurrence or resectable metastatic disease.

  Surgery
  - Primary tumor with no distant metastasis → surgery alone.
  - when wide surgery margin not (cannot be) achieved → surgery + radiation.
  - When primary or recurrent tumor cannot be grossly resected → limb sparing < 5% → amputation is a treatment of choice.
  - If +ve margin → re-excision.
  - In microscopic residual disease → local control is unlikely even with postoperative radiation.

  - Wide Local Excision (WLE)
    - WLE with excision of biopsy site.
    - Successful by 1–2 cm −ve margin.
    - If major neurovascular → do not resect but remove adventitia or perineurium.

- Surgical clips in tumor bed for postoperative radiation.
- If bone involved → resection of bone.
- Hand and feet → limited preserving surgery + adjuvant radiotherapy, but amputation is the optimal choice.

• Locoregional Lymphadenopathy
- Improves SR in lymphadenopathy underwent lymphadenectomy.
- If clinically or radiologically +ve → FNA.
- SLNBx is controversial.

• Amputation
- Treatment of choice (5%) with primary or recurrence, which cannot grossly resected with limb sparing.
- Historically, local excision with large and aggressive tumor has 50%–70% recurrence.
- Today, additional radiation made limb salvage possible.
- Comparison of amputation vs. limb salvage with adjuvant radiation = no difference.

• Isolated Regional Perfusion
- Is a limb-saving technique in which soft tissue sarcoma perfuse with high dose of TNF-α and melphalan under hyperthermic condition.

NB

In HIPEC: cisplatin, mitomycin are used.
- Isolate main arteries and veins.
- Apply tourniquet or band to achieve complete vascular isolation.
- Perfusion for 90 min.
- 40°C.
- Response rate is 18%–80%.
- SR is 50%–70%, 5 years.

Radiation Therapy

- Standard therapy of high-grade extremities or trunk wall either neo or adjuvant therapy.
- Mode of therapy (EBR, brachytherapy, IMRT).
- Optimal radiation margin is 5–7 cm, some center > 15 cm.
- Preoperative radiation → wait 4–8 weeks then surgery.
- Brachytherapy → placement of multiple radioactive seeds through catheter, in bed for 4–6 days, better than radiation, 4–8 weeks → costs less than EBR → used for recurrent disease that was previously treated with EBR.
- IMRT → more specific to deliver radiation than EBR, low surrounding tissue exposure.
- Preoperative radiation → wound dehiscence, wound necrosis, infection, seroma, ulceration cellulitis.
- Preoperative radiation infection (13%–37%) vs. postoperative radiation infection (5%–20%).

Standard Chemotherapy

- Most patients poorly respond to chemotherapy.
- Chemosensitive sarcoma: synovial, myxoid / round cell liposarcoma, uterine leiomyosarcoma.
- Chemotherapy intermediate sensitive sarcoma: pleomorphic liposarcoma, myxofibrosarcoma, epithelioid sarcoma, leiomyosarcoma, MPNST, angiosarcoma, desmoplastic round cell.
- Chemotherapy-resistant: clear cell sarcoma, endometrial stromal sarcoma, alveolar soft part sarcoma, extraskeletal myxoid chondrosarcoma.
- Doxorubicin and ifosfamide for soft tissue sarcoma.
- Doxorubicin Q3W, 6 doses maximum → cardiotoxic.

- Novel Chemotherapy
  - Alkaloid bind to DNA affecting transcription.
  - For leiomyosarcoma, myxoid liposarcoma.

- Targeted Therapy
  - Thyroxine kinase inhibitor (imatinib) → for GIST.
  - Anti-VEGF antibody for MET, unresectable angiosarcoma.
  - PDGFR and c-KIT to inhibit angiogenesis.

- Benefits of Systemic Therapy
  - Pre- and postchemotherapy are controversial.
  - Failure to demonstrate improvement because of the following:
    1. Regimen was suboptical (only one agent).
    2. Small group of patient, no difference in SR.
    3. Most studies include patients with low risk of metastasis, low grade since size < 5 cm.
  - Meta-analysis: improves overall SR by 4%.

- Neoadjuvant Chemotherapy
  - Based on adjuvant chemotherapy, 30%–50% response rate.
  - Rationale: enable to differentiate what is chemotherapy sensitivity and restriction.
  - Advantage: tumor shrinkage.
  - Study: three-cycle neoadjuvant vs. three-cycle neo and two-cycle adjuvant = same.

- Concurrent Chemotherapy Radiation
  - Systemic chemotherapy + EBR → ↑ free survival.

Post treatment Surveillance
  - NCCN recommended:
    o History and physical examination + CXR or CT chest Q3–6M for 2–3 years.
    o MRI for extremity, CT intra-abdomen Q6M.
    o Recurrence is common after surgery for abdominal sarcoma → CT Q6M during first 2 years and CT Q6M for 3 years.
    o 18% recurrence after 18 months of completed treatment in extremity sarcoma.

Management of Recurrence
- Up to 20% of extremity sarcoma develops recurrence and is often accompanied by distant metastasis; all patients with recurrence should undergo full staging assessment.
- For patient with extremity sarcoma, achieving −ve margin on resection of recurrent disease requires amputation.
  → Alternative treatment: function preserving resection + radiation with or without chemotherapy = accepted control.
- Extremity sarcoma → metastasis to lung.
- Myxoid liposarcoma of extremity → metastasized to abdomen and pelvis.

Management of recurrent and Distant Metastatic Sarcoma
- Patient with metastasis → surgical resection of primary soft tissue sarcoma may be appropriate as palliative procedure, e.g., pain.
- Most common site is the lung.
  If < 4 metastasis (nodule) → can be resected surgically, ↑SR.
- 5 years, SR after metastesectomy (lung) is 38%.

- Chemotherapy for Distant Metastatic Sarcoma
  - Doxorubicin alone or combined.
  - Mostly not curable.
  - Some patients with limited disease → surgery + chemoradiation.
  - Prediction of outcome: good performance status, previous response to chemotherapy, young age, absence of liver metastasis → resection, RFA, chemoembolization.

- Palliative and Radiation
  - When patient is not fit for surgery.
  - To prolong survival.

Special Clinical Situation
Myxoid Liposarcoma
- Soft tissue sarcoma with lipomatous differentiation.
- Differs from other liposarcoma subtypes but respects morphology and clinical behavior.
- Deep tumor in Lower limb.
- Metastasis to other locations of soft tissue, e.g., retroperitoneum and extremities.
  - For this reason → CT CAP for staging.

Retroperitoneum Sarcoma
- Most are malignant, and ⅓ is sarcoma.
- DDx primary germ cell tumor, lymphoma, metastasis of testicular tumor.
- ⅔ is high grade (grade 2–3).
- Present with large mass, 70% is > 10 cm.
- Produces obstructive symptom.
- Excludes lymphoma (fever, night sweat).
- Examine all nodal basins and testicular examination.
- Laboratory is helpful.
- ↑ LDH → lymphoma.
- ↑ βHCG, αFP → germ cell tumor.
- Diagnosis and staging → CT abdomen and pelvis. To see location, size, liver metastasis.
- Arteriography, venography to delineate vascular anatomy.
- CT chest for lung metastasis (11%).
- CT-guided core needs biopsy to diagnose → −ve biopsy should not delay management.
- Complete surgical resection with en bloc resection and sacrifice structure, kidney, colon, spleen, pancreas, small bowel, IVC, aorta.
- Surgery is considered marginal even if complete macroscopic resection.
- Complete resection median (SR 108 months) vs. incomplete (SR 18 months).
- Generally, surgery is not offered unless radiological studies showed resectability.
  - → But can be palliative for obstruction symptom (debulking).

- Adjuvant Therapy
  - Chemotherapy → failed to increase SR and decrease local recurrence.
  - Radiation to treat microresidual following surgery.
  - Radiation is complex and difficult because large field is close to radiosensitive organs (bowel).
  - Preoperative and post-EBR, intraoperative radiation, brachytherapy are helpful.
  - Preoperative radiation → well tolerated and less toxic.
  - Large, high-grade retrosarcoma → preoperative radiation then complete resection → postoperative radiation is discouraged unless bed is away from vital structure.

- Treatment of Recurrence
  - Retroperitoneal sarcoma recurs more than extremity.
  - Retroperitoneal liposarcoma recurs in tumor bed and metastasized to lung and liver.
  - Spread in peritoneal cavity (sarcomatosis).
  - Resection of recurrent retroperitoneal sarcoma = recurrent in extremity.
    - First recurrent resection (ability) 57%
    - Second recurrent resection 20%
    - Third recurrent resection 10%.
  - 25% of well-differentiated liposarcoma recur as poorly differentiated with area of dedifferentiated which is more aggressive and more propensity for metastasis.

Gastrointestinal Sarcoma

- Obstructive symptom: early satiety, dyspepsia, tenesmus, and change in bowel habits.
- Presentation: bleeding, 44%; mass, 38%; pain, 21%.
- CT: size, location, dissemination.
- Scope: upper and lower, mainstay.
- US + EGD (EUS) + biopsy to distinguish adenocarcinoma from sarcoma.

- In GI sarcoma, LNs are rare so lymphadenectomy is not routinely performed.
- Recommendation based on resection with 2–4 cm margin.
- If invasion to adjacent organ → en bloc resection.
- For sarcoma in small bowel or colon → segmental resection.

Breast Sarcoma
- Rare, 1% of breast CA and less than 5% of all soft tissue sarcoma.
- It can be angiosarcoma, stromal sarcoma, fibrosarcoma, and malignant fibrous histiocytoma.
- Angiosarcoma is 50% and associated with radiation treatment range from 3–20 years.
        → Incidence of 0.3% at 10 years, 0.5% at 15 years.
- Cystosarcoma phyllode: not sarcoma because it originates from hormonally responsive stromal cells.
- As with any sarcoma, prognostic factors: site, size, history type.
- Tumor smaller than 5 cm = better OC.
- Complete excision with −ve margin is the primary therapy.
        → No LNs dissection routinely.
        → Neoadjuvant chemotherapy or radiation can be considered for large, high-risk tumor.

Uterine Sarcoma
- Less than 5% of uterine malignancy.
- Histological subtypes: uterine leiomyosarcoma, endometrial stromal sarcoma, carcinosarcoma, undifferentiated endometrial sarcoma.
- 5 years, SR 30%–50%.
- TAH is recommended for localized disease.
- BSO is mandatory in endometrial sarcoma.
- Adjuvant radiotherapy: no benefit of survival.

    • Leiomyosarcoma
        - 35%–40% of uterine sarcoma.
        - Can affect 20s age-group but more in 50s–60s.
        - TAH +/− BSO depends on patient's wish and menses.

- LNS metastasis < 5%.
  → Adjuvant radiotherapy in high risk.
  → Adjuvant chemotherapy is controversial.

- Endometrial Stromal Sarcoma
  - 7%–10% of uterine sarcoma.
  - Mitotic count used to classify it.
  - Express progesterone receptor → respond to hormonal.
  - Treatment: total abdominal hysterectomy with bilateral salpingo- oophorectomy (TAH-BSO).
  - Postoperative hormonal replacement is contraindicated.

- Malignant Mixed Müllerian Tumor
  - 50% of uterine sarcoma.
  - In postmenopause.
  - TAH +/− BSO.
  - Adjuvant radiotherapy.

Gastrointestinal stromal disease (GIST)
- Account majority of GI sarcoma.
- Arises from intestinal pacemaker ICC.
- Express CD34, GFR c-KIT.
- Incidence: 6–15:1,000,000.
- Resistant to chemotherapy.
- 80% of GIST has mutation in the gene-encoding KIT receptor tyrosine kinase.
- Most common location for GIST is the stomach, 60%; then small bowel, 30%.
- Gastric GIST has favorable prognosis than other site.
- Diagnosis by EGD and/or CT abdomen.
- Metastasis is frequently in liver and/or abdomen cavity.

- **Radiological Assessment**
  - FDG-PET preoperative is useful and detects metabolic activity and early metastasis → detects early response to imatinib.

- PET is not widely available, and lesion with poor glucose uptake cannot be detected by PET → CT.

- **Management of Localized Disease**
  - Complete resection with −ve margin.
  - No lymphadenectomy.
  - 5 years, SR to all GIST is 20%–44%.
  - 5 years, SR with complete resection in early stage is 75%.
  - As for sarcoma, tumor size is an important prognostic factor + mitotic activity 5, 5–10, > 10.

- **Management of Locally Advanced or Metastatic Disease**
  - Multidisciplinary Approach.
  - Treatment with imatinib (Gleevec), a selective inhibitor of c-KIT protein tyrosine kinase → impressive response in large percentage of patients with unresectable or metastatic GIST.
  - 400–600 mg daily for 2 years.
    - → 54% partial response.
    - → 40% disease progression.
    - → S/E nausea, diarrhea, muscle cramps, periorbital edema.
    - → 21% experience serious complications, e.g., bleeding.
  - Many patients develop resistance.
  - Imatinib improves SR in advanced GIST, but most patients are not cured.
  - Some patients develop resistance.
  - Surgical resection of residual metastasis + imatinib → ↑ SR of 70%–96%.

- **Post-operative Imatinib**
  - Promising for metastatic and locally advanced GIST.
  - Study: treatment with imatinib for 12 months showed high recurrence-free survival.
  - NCCN: imatinib for patient with intermediate or high risk of recurrence at least 36 months as adjuvant therapy.

- **Pre-operative Imatinib**
  - Patient with marginally resectable GIST or with high risk of operative morbidity.
  - To downstage and allow less aggressive intervention.

Desmoid Tumor
- Low-grade sarcoma, can be locally aggressive, but no metastasis.
- ½ arise from extremity, with the remaining located in trunk or retroperitoneal.
- Abdominal wall desmoid tumor associated with pregnancy (hormonal).
- Usually sporadic but many associated with familial disease such as FAP (Gardner syndrome) APC gene, germline mutation.
- Sporadic linked to mutation in CTNNB for β-catenin.
- Therapy: WLE with −ve margin.
- Local recurrence in ⅓.
- ⅔ with +ve margin, no recurrence, 50% can skip surgical intervention.
- Radiation for unresectable tumor or adjuvant therapy following surgery for recurrent disease.
- Hormonal therapy like tamoxifen, and steroid are effective.

Pediatric Sarcomas
Rhabdomyosarcoma
- 7%–8% of all pediatric CA.
- Pediatric sarcoma: rhabdomyosarcoma and non-rhabdomyosarcoma associated with skeletal muscle.
- Most common soft tissue tumor in pediatric patients younger than 15 years.
- 24% in genitourinary, 20% in extremity, 20% in head and neck, 14% in parameningeal region.
- Small round cell tumor.
- Embryonal, 70%; alveolar, 20%.
- Complete surgical resection is the treatment of choice.
- SR is 90%.
- Unlike soft tissue sarcoma → high LNs metastasis, 20%–30%.

- 15%–20% with distant metastasis, 40%–50% to lung, then bone marrow and bone.
    - → Chemotherapy is recommended to all patients.
    - → Radiation for patient with microscopic residual after resection.
- 5 years, SR is 65%.

Nonrhabdomyosarcoma

- 60% of soft tissue sarcoma is nonrhabdomyosarcoma.
- Four groups of histological subtypes:
    a. Fibrosarcoma
    b. Kaposi's sarcoma
    c. Others: synovial, angiosarcoma, extraosseous Ewing sarcoma.
    d. Unspecified
- Most common type is synovial then MPNST and fibrosarcoma.
- CT, MRI.
- CNBx for establishing diagnosis.
- Surgery is the main treatment.
    - → If high-grade → radiation.
    - → Chemotherapy → no clear result.

Upper GI Tract

Esophagus

Anatomy
- It starts at the sixth cervical spine = cricoid cartilage.
- Located in the midline, except in lower neck and upper chest, there is a left deviation then return to middle in cranial then return to left in lower chest and anterior to aorta.
- Three narrowing:
  - Upper cricopharyngeal muscle
  - Middle left bronchus and aortic arch
  - Lower hiatus of diaphragm
- Lumen diameter is 1.6–1.9 cm.
- Pharynx formed by superior, middle, and inferior pharyngeal constrictor muscles.
- Esophagus has cervical; thoracic, abdominal portion.
  - Cervical esophagus (5 cm in length) (C6, T1–2) posteriorly, suprasternal notch anteriorly, carotid sheath, thyroid laterally.
  - Thoracic esophagus (20 cm)— it is in intimate relationship with the posterior wall of trachea and prevertebral fascia. Just above the tracheal bifurcation, the esophagus passes to the right of the aorta

    RLNs passes at the lateral wall (left is closer).
    - Thoracic duct passes through hiatus (T12) between aorta and azygos.
    - From bifurcation of trachea to downward, vagus nerve and esophageal nerve plexus lie on muscular wall of esophagus.
  - Abdominal portion: 2 cm including LES, surrounded by phrenoesophageal ligament as continuation of transversalis fascia of the abdomen blind to esophageal adventitia.
- Musculature: the outer muscular layer is longitudinal and the inner is circular muscular layer.
- Esophageal motility disorder involves mostly the distal esophagus.

Blood Supply

A: Cervical   Inferior thyroid artery

Thoracic   Bronchial artery + two branches from aorta

Abdominal   Ascending left gastric + inferior phrenic artery

V: Cervical   Inferior thyroid vein (ITV)

Thoracic   Bronchial, azygos, hemiazygos veins

Abdomen   Coronary vein (left gastric vein)

- If portal vein is obstructed → collateral to superior vena cava (SVC) via azygos.
- Parasympathetic: vagus nerve.
- RLN injury results in vocal cord paralysis, loss of cricopharyngeal sphincter, and motility of cervical esophagus leads to aspiration.
- Lymphtics in submucosal layer.
- Lymph spreads upward and downward more than horizontal, as well as tumor spreads superior and inferior.
- The tumor can spread via lymph before local invasion of musculosa.
- Cervical LNs → drain from parahiatal to paratracheal to deep cervical LNs.
- Thoracic → subcranial LNs.
- Abdomen → superior gastric LNs.

Physiology

Swallowing Mechanism

- $\frac{1}{3}$ by mouth and hypopharynx, $\frac{2}{3}$ by esophagus.
- Three valves are in pharynx—soft palate, epiglottis and cricopharyngeus muscle.
- One valve in esophagus (LES).
- When soft palate is paralyzed (e.g., CVA), it results to food regurgitation in nasopharynx.
- During swallowing, it results to the hyoid bone moving up and down:

1. Elevation of tongue
2. Posterior movement of the tongue
3. Elevation of soft palate

4. Elevation of thyroid
5. Elevation of larynx
6. Tilting of epiglottis

- Anti-reflux mechanism:

  1. Effective LES
  2. Esophageal clearance
  3. Functioning gastric reservoir

Physiological Reflux
1. Relaxation of LES.
2. In erect position, the pressure of LES = 12 mmHg.
3. In supine position, pressure of LES is more than in erect position.

Assessment of Esophageal Function

A. **To Detect Structural Abnormality**
- **EGD: First Diagnostic Test**
  - Allow assessment and biopsy; length of esophagitis is recorded.
    Grade I   Small circular erosion
    Grade II   Linear erosion + granulation and easy bleeding
    Grade III Erosion with circumferential epithelial loss + mucosa (cobblestone)
    Grade IV   Stricture

  - Rule out pseudoachalasia, hiatal hernia, Barrett's esophagus and malignancy.
  - Evaluation of vocal cord.
  - At the level of aortic arch, straightened muscle, transition to smooth muscle.
  - Biopsy for eosinophilic esophagitis → looks corrugated (feline), trachealization of esophagus.
  - GERD → Barrett's esophagus (salmon-colored appearance).
  - Provide biopsy, should take four biopsies in every 2 cm.
  - Barrett's esophagus is transformation of squamous epithelium to columnar (intestinal metaplasia).

- Earliest sign: high-grade dysplasia or intramucosal adenocarcinoma.
- Abnormal gastroesophageal flap by retroflexion, Hill classified it to four grades.
- Hiatal hernia → gastric Rugal folds, 2 cm above the margin of diaphragm.

- **Radiological Evaluation**
    - Barium swallow—in case of hiatal hernia, it's better than EGD.
    - Displacement of EG junction.
    - Detect stricture, mass, hernia.
    - Barium alone can miss the lesion.
    - Video esophagram:
        o Sensitivity to detect achalasia, 94%; scleroderma, 100%.
        o Initial test for cricopharyngeal bar, esophageal web and diverticula.
    - CT for extraluminal staging if CA.
    - Videogram is the gold standard for esophageal leak.

B. **To Detect Functional Abnormality**
- **Manometry (Stationary, and HR)**
    - Gold standard for motility disorder.
    - Determine motor function, dysphagia, non-CVS chest pain (achalasia, DES, nutcracker, HTN LES).
    - Essential preoperatively of anti-reflux operation.
    - Eight sensors—four in esophagus and four in GEJ.
    - HRM is superior.

- **Esophageal Impedance**
    - To assess function conductivity in hollow organ.
    - Air has very low electrical conductivity, resulting to very low voltage.
    - Saliva and food ↑ conductivity.
    - Reflux: low pH to less than 4.
    - This technology is used in patients with symptoms despite of PPI.

- **Esophageal Transit Scintigraphy**
  - ^{99m}Tc + gamma camera.

- **Video and Cineradiography**
  - Good for diverticulum.

C. **To Detect High Exposure of Esophagus to Gastric Juice**
- **24-Hour Ambulatory pH Monitoring**
  - 96% sensitivity and specificity.

D. **To Test Gastric-Duodenal Function and Relation to Esophagus**
  - Gastric-emptying study such as gastric-emptying scintigraphy (milk scan).

Pathology
Gastroesophageal Reflux Disease (GERD)
  - Incidence 20% of general population.
  - Heartburn, acid regurgitation.
  - The pain can be caused by other disease—myocardial infarction (MI), gastritis, gallstones.
  - ↑ by spicy food, caffeine, fatty food.

- **Clinical Picture**
  - Risk factor: obesity, hiatal hernia, pregnancy, connective tissue disorder, delayed gastric emptying, scleroderma, and pulmonary interstitial lung disease.
  - The reflux usually nocturnal and in supine position.
  - Symptoms: typical (esophagus), atypical (extra-esophagus), and complication (alarm).
  - Typical: burning chest pain, regurgitation, sour taste (water brash), tightness on odynophagia.
  - Atypical: cough, wheezing, hoarseness, postnasal drip, dental erosion, ear pain.
  - Alarm symptoms: dysphagia, early satiety, hemostasis, melena, vomiting and weight loss → Barrett's, CA.
  - Workup → +ve pH study and manometry.
  - Mechanical defective LES diagnosed when one of three component:
    - pressures < 6 mmHg

- total length < 2 cm
- abdominal length < 1 cm
- GERD increases swallowing as neutralization by saliva, resulting to more distension and decrease gastric emptying.

- **Etiology of Reflux-Induced Respiratory Symptom**
  - Vagal-mediated bronchoconstriction during episode of reflux.
  - Studies support correlation between idiopathic pulmonary fibrosis and hiatal hernia.
  - Embryologic origin of trachea, esophagus, and vagus nerve.
  - Relation between hiatal hernia and GERD.
    - Collar sling attenuated → GEJ funnel → stretch the phrenoesophageal ligament → enlargement of hiatal hernia.

- **Diagnosis**
  - Symptoms: sensitivity and specificity, 60%.
  - PPI improves the symptoms.
  - Should rule out motility disorder.

- **Studies to Confirm Diagnosis**
  - **Upper GI Endoscopy**
    - Identify hiatal hernia, short esophagus.
    - Diagnose GERD, stricture, Barrett's, CA.
    - Los Angeles classification of esophagitis:

      Grade
      A One or more mucosal break < 5 mm
      B One or more mucosal break > 5 mm
      C One or more mucosal break that is involved twofold and < 75% circumference
      D One or more mucosal break that is involved > 75% circumference

  - **Ambulatory pH Study**
    - Gold standard.

- **Esophageal Manometry**
  - Important to decide type of fundoplication, complete vs. partial, esophageal dysmotility increases after complete wrap.

- **HR manometry**

- **Gastric Scintigraphy**
  - To rule out gastroparesis and to add procedure such as pyloromyotomy.

- **Complication**
  - Esophagitis (stricture), Barrett's esophagus (BE), repetitive aspiration resulting in pulmonary fibrosis.
  - Maximal injury when acid + pepsin + bile salt.
  - Study on animal showed bile reflux leads to ↑ risk of BE (severe damage).
  - Bile and gastric acid do more damage than acid alone.
  - Bile reflux develops recurrent and progressive mucosal damage despite meditation.
  - BE transforms to CA by 0.2%–0.5% per year.
  - Respiratory complication: laryngopharyngeal reflux, asthma, pulmonary fibrosis, 50% with asthma has esophagitis, i.e., GERD.

- **Treatment**
  - High dose of PPI or anti-reflux surgery (ARS).
  - Anti-reflux surgery success rate is 90% in pediatrics and 70% in adult.
  - Surgery improves respiratory symptom by 30%.
    Surgery vs. PPI → surgery is superior.
  - In motility disorder, surgery will not improve symptoms.

- **Medical Treatment**
  - Mild—take antacid (12 weeks), elevate head on bed, avoid tight clothes, eat small frequent meals, avoid coffee, alcohol, chocolate, and (peppermints → ↓ LES tone).

- If symptom persists, PPI 40 mg/day, resulting to lower acidity (80%–90%); response is 100% in mild esophagitis but only 50% healing in severe esophagitis.
- If mixed gastric and duodenal juice, stopping the medication will result to recurrence by 80%.
- Most of GERD ® PPI is lifelong.
- 25% postfundoplication will have persistent symptom.
- Laparoscopic surgery controls symptom by 80%–90%.

- **Surgical Therapy for GERD**
  - 35%–50% has persistent or progressive GERD.
  - Multidisciplinary approach to decide for antireflux surgery (ARS).
  - if symptoms of GERD persists despite of medication, i.e., failed medical treatment.
  - Young patients are unwilling to take medication lifelong.
  - Defective LES and loss of esophageal contraction.
  - Large hiatal hernia.
  - Silent GERD, i.e., atypical symptom with documented reflux by pH study.
  - Lung transplant.
  - Stricture (should be dilated first)—if dysphagia disappears and there's adequate contraction → surgery.
  - BE (but if high grade or carcinoma) → endoscopic ablation, resection, esophagectomy.

  - **Contraindication**
    - Unfit patient.
    - Previous major surgery.
    - Lack of inexpertise.
    - Morbid obesity.
    - Patient with morbid obesity will get benefit from Roux-en-Y bypass rather than sleeve.

- **Preoperative Evaluatiuon**
    - Manometry pre- and post-operative.
    - Patient with normal peristaltic contraction → complete (360-degree) Nissen fundoplication or partial if absent peristalsis (should rule out achalasia).
    - Shortening of esophagus → barium swallow to identify sliding hernia → gastroplasty + anti-reflux.

- **Surgical Technique**
    1. Reduction of any hiatal hernia.
    2. Tension-free restoration of intra-abdominal esophagus.
    3. Approximation of diaphragmatic hiatal crura.
    4. Fundoplication.
    5. The aim is to create anti-reflux valve and allow swallowing and relive gaseous distension.
    - Will increase resting pressure with 12 mmHg.

    Principles of the procedure:
    1. The wrap at least 3 cm in length.
    2. Create loose wrap.
    3. Measure adequate length of LES.
    4. Allow relaxation during deglutition with the following:
        - Only fundus of stomach is used.
        - Gastric wrap around sphincter as stomach does not relax during swallowing.
        - Don't damage vagus nerve → failure of sphincter to relax.

    5. 360 wrap should not be longer than 2 cm constructed over bougie, 50–60 F.
    6. Ensure that fundus in abdomen is without tension.
        - If in thorax → that will convert sliding to para-esophageal hernia.
        - If under tension → increase recurrence.

195

o **Deciding Type of Fundoplication**
  - Partial vs. complete = same but dysphagia and gas bloating are less common with partial fundoplication.

o **Deciding Approach**
  - The advantage of abdominal approach is to inspect other cause of abdominal pain + add procedure, e.g., vagotomy or Collis gastroplasty.
  - The advantage of thoracic approach is that it's good in obese patients; also, if patient has hostile abdomen → left thoracotomy.
  - Laparoscopy is used routinely, i.e., procedure of choice and is better than laparotomy.

o **Deciding to Use Mesh**
  - In diaphragm, biological mesh is the best, but John Hopkins Hospital prefer PTFE.

o **Addressing Surgical Technology**
  - Originally, in Nissen fundoplication, the short gastric artery is left intact then modified to be divided to allow mobilization → prevent dysphagia post-operative.
    → No difference, either division is done or not, but three trials → if ligation done → ↑ bloating, ↓bleach.
  - Complete vs. partial = same outcome, 90%.
    ▪ Nissen fundoplication, 360 degrees
    ▪ Posterior partial fundoplication (Toupet)
    ▪ Anterior partial fundoplication (Dor)—easier
    ▪ +/− Collis gastroplasty
  - Complete Nissen fundoplication vs. posterior or anterior partial wrap → less dysphagia, less flatus, otherwise equal.
  - Anterior vs. posterior—posterior has more side effects.

- Medical vs. Nissen fundoplication:
  - Esophagitis, stricture is 20% with medial treatment while it is 3%–7% with surgery.
  - With medical treatment 25% has persistent acid reflux, 75% caused by bilious reflux.

- o **New Approach to GERD**
  - LINX anti-reflux
  - Endoscopic Approach (Stretta procedure)

- o **Cause of Failure of Surgery**
  - Recurrent GERD.
  - Esophageal dysmotility.
  - Gastroparesis: vagal nerve injury
  - Anatomic failures:
    1. Herniated wrap (commonest)
    2. Slipped wrap
    3. Disrupted wrap
    4. Paraesophageal hernia

- **Reoperative of Failed Anti-Reflux**
  - Unable to swallow, abdominal distension, or persistent GERD.
  - Most common cause of failure → placement of the wrap in stomach → herniation of repair into chest wall.
  - When dysphagia + poor esophageal motility + multiple surgeries and fit patient ® esophagectomy.
  - Each reoperative results in damage, resulting in lower rate of success.

- **Postoperative Care**
  - NPO, analgesia, antiemetic, e.g., ondansetron.
  - NGT is not used routinely unless with symptoms like nausea and vomiting.
  - Esophagogastrogram the next morning.
  - Patient must stay on soft diet for 6 weeks.
  - Stop PPI.
  - Avoid straining.

- **Outcomes and Complications**
  - Success rate after laparoscopic fundoplication is 90%.
  - Relief symptoms → 80%–90% heartburn, dysphagia, ⅔ of respiratory symptoms.
  - Dysphagia: < 6 weeks and may persist by 3% → endoscopic dilation.
  - Gas bloating syndrome.
  - Temporary dysphagia resolves in 3 months to 1 year.
  - Inability to bleach or vomit, increases flatus.

Barrett's Esophagus (BE)

- Barrett's esophagus: presence of endoscopic visible segment of columnar-lined epithelium and goblet cells by histopathology replaced the squamous epithelium.
- Occurs in 10%–15% of patients with GERD.
- Should be distinguished from island of gastric fundus in upper half of esophagus (inlet patch), which is a long congenital segment of columnar mucosa without intestinal metaplasia.
- The hallmark of intestinal metaplasia are presence goblet cells.
- Anti-reflux surgery is curative and preventive.
- Gastric hypersecretion, 44%.
- PPI to relief symptoms.
- Complication: ulceration, 0.2%–0.5% per year develops esophageal CA, which is forty times than general population i.e. Precursor of esophagus adenocarcinoma.
- 1/3 of BE present with malignancy.
- Need PPI and ARS to prevent progression

- **Evaluation**
  - Prague classification.
  - Any lesion of columnar tissue, biopsy in four quadrants every 1–2 cm.
  - The pH study confirms reflux.
  - Before ARS → need to rule out esophageal motility disorder.

- **Barrett's Esophagus without Dysplasia**
  - Managed as GERD.
  - The goal is to improve symptom, to prevent progression to cancer.

- Should have EGD surveillance.
- Patient with dysmotility → partial fundoplication.
- Keep patient on PPI.

- **Barrett's Esophagus with LGD**
  - If EGD didn't include four-quadrant biopsy → repeat it.
  - Patient should be kept on PPI.
  - Rpeat endoscope + biopsy after 6 months.
  - Patient can be offered ARS → regress to non-dysplastic Barrett's esophagus.
  - If LGD persists after ARS → mucosal ablation.

- **Barrett's Esophagus with HGD**
  - First step to repeat EGD to see if associated nodule.
  - Small lesion → endoscopic mucosal resection (EMR)), leaving muscularis propria intact.
  - If the lesion is 1–2 cm → EUS for lesion depth, and LNs invasion.
  - Need to confirm whether it's a mucosa T1a or a submucosal T1b invasion.
  - LNs metastasis is 2% in T1a and 25% in T1b.
  - Poor differentiation → higher LNS metastasis.
  - If patient is classified as T1a → endoscopic resection, ablation of any columnar epithelium → then EGD surveillance or esophagostomy.
  - Advantage of esophagectomy → eradication of CA, no recurrence, no EGD surveillance, but higher mortality and morbidity.
  - Esophagectomy is considered if long segment of columnar epithelium with multifocal adenocarcinoma.

- **Outcomes of ARS in Barrett's Esophagus**
  - Failure of fundoplication in 3–5 years, 15%–20% compared to patients with no Barrett's esophagus, 5%–10%.
  - The aim is to regress LGD and to prevent CA.
  - If patient has large hiatal hernia, poor esophageal body function, previous failed ARS, complication and poor outcome → esophagectomy may be the best option.

- **Surveillance Endoscopy for Barrett's Esophagus**
  - To detect prognosis of Barrett's esophagus and to detect invasive disease.
  - Barrett's esophagus with no dysplasia, EGD Q3–5Y.
  - LGD → shorter interval, initial Q6M, then increase interval accordingly.
  - If HGD → EGD every 3 months.

Diaphragmatic (Hiatal) Hernia

Type I	Sliding LES into chest
Type II	Rolling = PEH (fundus in chest but normal LES)
Type III	Sling rolling (mixed) together
Type IV	Additional organ (colon)
Type I, II	May end by whole stomach in chest

Type II, III, IV are also referred as PEH

- **Incidence and Etiology**
  - Sliding hernia is seven times more than PEH
  - Thinning of phrenoesophageal membrane

- **Symptoms**
  - Hiatal hernia → heartburn.
  - PEH → dysphagia.
  - If hiatal accompanied with PEH → no heartburn.
  - Regurgitation, postprandial epigastric fullness or pain, vomiting, weight loss, dyspnea.
  - Respiratory complication → pneumonia.
  - PEH compresses left atrium → pulmonary edema.
  - Dangerous bleeding, volvulus or obstruction ischemia leads to perforation → sepsis.
  - Strangulation, 5%.
  - In sliding heartburn, GERD → surgery will improve symptom by 91%.

- **Diagnosis**
  - Chest x-ray.
  - Barium is mostly used for PEH than sliding.
  - Fiber optic, i.e., EGD → retroflexion.

- 24 hrs pH study → ↑ acid exposure to esophagus; 60% with PEH and 71% in sliding depending on LES pressure and length.

- **Surgical Indication**
  - Any symptoms: heartburn, regurgitation, postprandial epigastric fullness or pain, vomiting, weight loss, dyspnea.
  - Asymptomatic in elderly → conservative.
  - Asymptomatic in young age → repair to avoid complications.

- **Preoperative Evaluation**
  - Upper GI contrast study + CT scan + esophageal motility study.
  - No need for pH study as all patients will require Nissen fundoplication (360-degree wrap) with repair of hernia.
  - Perioperative cardiopulmonary assessment is done because usually the patient is old.
  - EGD to evaluate distal esophagus and stomach.

Surgical Technique
1. Reduction of herniated abdominal content into abdomen.
2. Excision of the sac.
3. Mobilization of intrathoracic esophagus.
4. Return of GEJ to the abdomen.
5. Repair of diaphragmatic defect.

Approach
- o Laparoscopic or Laparotomy repair
- o Left thoracotomy approach

- **Treatment**
  - Controversial aspects include the following:
    A. Indication for repair
      - Presence of PEH → surgery:
        1. As incidence of catastrophic complication.
        2. Emergency repair ↑ mortality.
           → Emergency repair ↑ hospital stay 48 days ↑ mortality whereas elective repair stay is 9 day and mortality is 1%.

201

- Transabdominal surgical approach → laparoscopy or open or transthoracic = same outcome.
- Transthoracic facilitates complete esophageal mobilization but increases pain post-operative.
  → use in case of volvulus.
- Laparoscopic repair is standard procedure.

B. Repair of diaphragm
- PEH has high recurrence of 10%–40% when crura are closed primarily by permanent suture.
- Most surgeons believe use of synthetic or biological mesh.
- Non-absorbable synthetic mesh.

C. Role of fundoplication
- Controversial.
- Fundoplication, ↑ operative time, ↑cost.
- but some authors are routinely use fundoplication, as the acid exposure is 60% in PEH and 71% in sliding hernias.

D. Treatment of short esophagus
- Giant PEH associated with short esophagus.
- Barium and EGD showed short esophagus.
- Definition: failure to achieve 2.5 cm of esophagus intra-abdominal → Collis gastroplasty, by creation of neo-esophagus using gastric cardia.

E. Laparoscopy should be considered as standard of care.

F. PTFE prosthesis has the lowest recurrence.

- **Result**
  - Outcome: relief is 90%.
  - Radiological recurrence is 25%–40%.
  - Diaphragm must be repaired +fundoplication, gastroplasty.
  - Asymptomatic recurrent PEH ® minimal complication.

- **Postoperative Consideration and Outcome**
  - Adequate pain control.
  - Next morning, contrast upper GI study to ensure adequate gastric emptying.
  - Discharge home D1 with clear liquid diet for 72 hrs, then soft diet for 1 week.

- OPD follow-up after 3 weeks, 6 months.
- Outcomes:
  o 90% durability.
  o 40% will have radiological recurrence.

Schatzki's Ring

- Thin submucosal circumferential ring in the squamocolumnar junction, often associated with hiatal hernia.
- Incidence, 0.2%–14%.
- The cause could be congenital mucosal fold or chronic reflux.
- Differs from hiatal hernia in symptom and investigation.
- Symptom: dysphagia of solid food.
- Treatment: varies—dilation alone and/or anti-reflux surgery alone, incision and excision.
- Progressive in 59% and ⁻ in 29%.
- Some respond to one-session dilation, while most require multiple sessions.
- Bonavina is a drug-induced injury (esophageal stricture), without history of reflux.
- Treatment without reflux → dilation.
- Treatment with reflux → dilatation + anti-reflux surgery.

Scleroderma (Distal Esophageal Squamocolumnar Junction)

- Systemic disease (autoimmune) accompanied by skin abnormality; blood vessels, heart, and esophageal abnormality (80%); and renal impairment.
- Age: third–fourth decade.
- Inflammation of small vessels → perivascular deposition of collagen that may compromise in gastrointestinal tract → atrophy.
- Primary neurogenic disorder.
- Methacholine → acts on smooth muscle receptor directly → LES.
- Edrophonium (cholinesterase inhibitors) → ↑ acetylcholine → given to the patient with scleroderma → ↑ LES pressure, suggest, it's neurogenic rather than myogenic.
- In early stage, reverse by reserpine.
- In advanced disease manifested by smooth muscle atrophy and collagen deposition, reserpine no longer produces this reversal.

- normal peristalsis in the proximal striated esophagus, with absent peristalsis in the distal smooth muscle portion.
- Diagnosis by manometry.
- GERD commonly occurs.
- Barium (distal stricture from esophagus) and proximal dilation.
- First treatment is antacid, then PPI + dilation, but the esophagitis and stricture is severe and shortened the esophagus.
- Surgery is controversial, but laparoscopic partial fundoplication is the procedure of choice.
- If esophagus is shortened → Collis gastroplasty.
- 50% will have a good outcome.
- If severe esophagitis + previous failed anti-reflux surgery + delayed gastric emptying → gastric resection with Roux-en-Y. (gastrojejunostomy).

Eosinophilic Esophagitis (EE)
- IgE is elevated, like asthma.
- Endoscopy + radiology → diagnosis.

- **Symptoms**
  - Chest pain (postprandial), dysphagia.
  - Confused with GERD.
  - Does not respond to PPI.
  - Barium (ringed esophagus) (feline esophagus) strips on house cat (trachealization).

- **Pathology**
  - Biopsy → must see minimum of 15 eosinophil HPF.

- **Treatment**
  - Test food allergy.
  - Inhalation or ingestion of corticosteroids.
  - if failed → dilation (rigid), Maloney or Savary, but easily injured as it's fragile (tear).

Motility Disorder of Pharynx and Upper Esophagus
It can be categorized into one or a combination of the following abnormalities:

  a. Inadequate oropharyngeal bolus transport

b. Inability to pressurize the pharynx
c. Inability to elevate the larynx
d. Discoordination of pharyngeal contraction and cricopharyngeal relaxation
e. Decreased compliance of the pharyngoesophageal segment

causes

- CNS (peripheral and central), CVA, brain stem tumor, multiple sclerosis, Parkinson's, pseudobulbar palsy, pure myopathy, e.g., myasthenia gravis or dystrophy or external compression of esophagus, LNs, thyromegaly, Zenker's diverticulum.

Zenker's Diverticulum

- Incidence 1:1,000.
- Affects white male.
- Due to compliance of skeletal muscle and swallowing incoordination.
- Herniation of mucosa through Killian triangle above cricopharyngeus muscle and below the inferior constrictor pharyngeal muscle.
- Usually because of impaired relaxation of UES.
- **Symptoms**: dysphagia with regurgitation of undigested food, choking, chronic cough, hoarseness, weight loss, aspiration, and Boyce's sign.
- **Diagnosis**: barium swallow, no endoscopy → dangerous.
- **Treatment**: cricopharyngeal myotomy → up to 64% success rate → myotomy ± diverticulectomy ± diverticulopexy.
- Incision under local anesthesia or general anesthesia in anterior border of left sternocleidomastoid, retract the SCM muscle and carotid sheath laterally and thyroid, trachea, and larynx medially; it's easy to localize the diverticulum just below inferior pharyngeal constrictor and above cricopharyngeal muscle.
  Under local anesthesia → swallowing benefit.
  Under general anesthesia → myotomy increases 2 cm of inferior constrictor muscle, decreases 4–5 cm in cricopharyngeal muscle.
- Be careful of hematoma (hemostasis).

- If large diverticulum → suture to prevertebral fascia (inverted), i.e., diverticulopexy.
- If excessively large → diverticulectomy.
- Complications: salivary fistula (common with surgical intervention), hematoma, abscess, RLN injury, Horner syndrome.
- Conclusion: open is better than endoscopic intervention.
- Recurrence is 5% with surgery vs. 21% with endoscopic intervention.
- Another approach: endoscopic stapling diverticulectomy, effective in large diverticulum > 2 cm.
- To decrease rate of fistula and abscess → diverticulopexy.

Motility Disease of Esophageal Body and Lower Esophagus

- Primary:
  - Achalasia, diffuse and segmental esophageal spasm, nutcracker esophagus, esophageal hypertension, LES, NEMD.

- Secondary:
  - Collagen and vascular disease, systemic sclerosis, polymyositis, neuromuscular, systemic lupus erythematosus, pseudo-obstruction.
  - Diagnosis by manometry.

Achalasia

- Incomplete relaxation of LES < 75%.
- Aperistalsis in the esophageal body.
- Elevated LES pressure ≤ 26 mmHg.
- 1:100,000.
- Studies showed no relaxation rather than increase pressure → ↑ frequency of wave and decrease contraction.
- There is pseudo-achalasia resulting from infiltrating tumor or stricture in distal esophagus or post-anti-reflux procedure (too tight).
- After myotomy → relieve symptom → it is primary disease of LES.

- **Pathogenesis**
  - neurogenic degeneration seen in vagus nerve and myenteric plexus → hypertension in LES, failure to relax → high esophageal pressure resulting to dilation and loss of peristalsis.
  - Dilation is caused by (1) retention of food (2) ↑ intraluminal pressure.

- **Diagnosis**
  - Barium swallow (bird beak).
  - EGD: dilated tortuous esophagus, retained food esophagitis resistance in LES to pass the scope.
  - Manometry is the gold standard.
  - There is a subgroup with high contraction (vigorous achalasia) now replaced by Chicago type III (distinguish by HR manometry).
  - Distinguishing it from DES is difficult as both has corkscrew.
  - DDx: esophageal ring or web, scleroderma, eosinophils esophagus, GERD, previous ARS or bariatric, malignancy, and amyloidosis.
  - Chicago classification:

    Type I   25%–40% low pressure contraction with minimal esophageal function, dilation of esophagus on esophagram

    Type II   Commonest, 65% (bird beak)

    Type III   10% uncoordinated activity in distal $\frac{2}{3}$ of esophagus → corkscrew on esophagram

- **Treatment**
  - No cure, the aim is to decrease pressure in LES.

  Medical
  - Nitrate, Ca^{++} channel blockers, and phosphodiesterase −5.
  - Sildenafil block effect of phosphodiesterase −5 → improved muscle contraction.

Endoscopic Therapy
o Botulinum toxin—blocks release of acetylcholine →
   paralysis.
   - Temporary, 3–4 months.

o Pneumatic dilation—if perforation ® CT scan.
   ⅓ recurrence in 5 years + GERD, 30%.

o Per-oral endoscopic myotomy (POEM)
   - Success rate is 90%.
   - Start nystatin for 5 days before intervention → to
     eradicate food candida.
   - Before procedure, antibiotic first, cephalic +
     fluconazole.

Surgery
o Laparoscopic Heller myotomy (LHM) + partial
   fundoplication is the gold standard.
   - Need rapid sequence intubation as risk of aspiration
     with achalasia.
   - The myotomy is 5 cm above GEJ and 2–5 cm
     into gastric cardia till large veins of transverse
     submucosal venous plexus are identified, 90%
     improvement.

o Transthoracic myotomy
   → Seventh intercostal space (left).

o Esophagectomy
   - If > 6 cm diameter.

• **Outcome Assessment of Therapy of Achalasia**
   - Difficult to judge as patients modify their diet.
   - Objective assessment such as LES pressure, esophageal
     pressure, scintigraphy, esophagus-emptying time.
   - Studies on outcomes:
       - Eckart: pneumatic dilation with achalasia →
         post dilation → remission by 70% within 2
         years.

- Bonavina: excellent result with transabdominal myotomy.
        - Malthaner and Pearson: achalasia underwent esophageal myotomy and Belsey hemi-fundoplication resulting to 2 recurrence, 2 GERD.
        - Ellis: transthoracic short esophageal myotomy with no anti-reflux resulting to 89% improvement within 9 years.
    - Laparoscopic myotomy + partial fundoplication—resulting to relief of dysphagia by 93%.
    - RCT → laparoscopic Heller myotomy vs. pneumatic dilation vs. botulinum toxin, surgery is superior.
    - Best treatment for achalasia: laparoscopic Heller myotomy + partial fundoplication.

Diffuse and Segmental Esophageal Spasm (SES)
    - Substernal chest pain and/or dysphagia.
    - Differs from achalasia as it is primarily a disease of the body of esophagus with decreased dysphagia and ↑ chest pain.
    - Esophagram + manometry can distinguish it from achalasia.
    - Rapid wave.
    - Hypertrophy of muscular layer + degeneration of nasopharyngeal branch of vagus nerve.
    - Usually confines to distal $\frac{2}{3}$ of the esophagus.
    - Manometry: high waves, multiple peeled contractions.
    - LES has normal resting pressure.
    - Can develop epiphrenic or mid-esophageal diverticulum between two area of high pressure.
    - Treatment: nitrate, sildenafil, valium, antidepressant, PPI. Myotomy, if medical treatment fails.

Nutcracker Esophagus
    - Super squeezer esophagus, hypertensive peristalsis.
    - High contraction, high pressure > 180 mmHg.
    - Long duration of shallow > 7 seconds.
    - LES relaxes normally.
    - Treatment aimed at treatment of GERD.

Hypertensive Lower Esophageal Sphincter (LES)
-   Chest pain, dysphagia.
-   Myotomy is indicated when not responding to medical treatment and dilation.
    → If in doubt → botulinum toxin.
    → → If responding → myotomy.

Ineffective Esophageal Motility
-   Low distal esophageal peristalsis or absence of esophageal contraction in 30% of wet swallowing.
-   Distinguished from achalasia by low LES pressure.
-   Associated with scleroderma.
-   No standard treatment.
        PPI, life style modification.

Non-specific Esophageal Motility
-   No name and feature of esophageal motility.
-   No dysphagia.
-   Retrograde contraction.
-   Associated with DM, hypothyroid eosinophilic esophagitis, and amyloidosis.
-   Also associated with shortness of esophagus (paraesophageal hernia).

Secondary Esophageal Motility
-   Connective tissue disorder, scleroderma.
-   In patient treated with esophageal atresia.
-   Heartburn, dysphagia.
-   Increases motility + decreases LES or absent.
-   Treatment is controversial → anti-reflux surgery (partial), as complete results to severe dysphagia.

Diverticula of Esophageal Body
-   Epiphrenic diverticula arises from terminal $\frac{1}{3}$ of thoracic esophagus associated with distal muscular hypertrophy.
-   Surgery depends on proximity to vertebra, either resection or suspension.

- If resection done → muscle closes over the resection + myotomy on the opposite wall from above diverticula LES, but increases risk of GERD.
- If hiatal hernia → repair.
- Mid-esophageal or traction diverticula → from mediastinal LNs inflammation, i.e., traction, such fungal infection of lung (aspergillosis), lymphoma sarcoidosis.
- Symptoms: asymptomatic but dysphagia, regurgitation or sometimes from tracheoesophageal fistula ® chronic cough with swallowing.
- Suspension → proximity to spine, but before, do manometry to exclude motor dysfunction.

Benign Tumor and Cyst
- Leiomyoma
    - 50% of benign lesion.
    - Male: female = 2:1, usually in the lower ⅓.
    - Great in size, oval in shape.
    - Protrudes to outer wall of esophagus.
    - Symptoms: dysphagia and pain.
    - Bleeding is rare, healthy mucosa.
    - Barium swallow → filling defect.
    - Endoscopy → no biopsy → will perforate.
    - EUS.
    - Growth is slow, and it has limited potential for malignancy.
    - Should be removed (enucleation).
    - Proximal and middle = through right thoracotomy.
    - Distal = left thoracotomy.
    - Success rate is 100%.
    - Large lesion in GEJ → esophageal resection.

- Cyst
    - Congenital: columnar ciliated (respiratory)
    - Acquired: glandular epithelium (stomach)
    - Enteric and bronchogenic are the most common.
    - Intramurally: middle or lower ⅓.
    - Surgical resection by enucleation.
    - During removal → fistula should be removed.

Esophageal Perforation

- Life-threatening.
- Mortality rate is 10%–40%, depending on patient condition, comorbid disease.
- Recent literatures focuses on non-operative management.
- Causes: iatrogenic (EGD), transesophageal Echo (60%), spontaneous (Boerhaave syndrome, 15%), foreign body (14%), trauma (10%), causative injury.

- **Diagnosis**
  - History: instrumentation (e.g., EGD), the pain is retrosternal (chest, epigastric, or vague pain).
  - Physical examination: may be stable or in sepsis, mediastinitis.
  - Spontaneous rupture → ↑ mortality → delay in recognition and treatment.
  - Mediastinal emphysema, 1 hr to be demonstrated and widening of mediastinum after 6 hrs.
  - CXR → air or effusion in pleural space is misdiagnosed with pneumothorax or pancreatitis, and high pleural amylase by saliva goes with pancreatitis.
  - If CXR is normal → misdiagnose with MI.
  - Spontaneous rupture in left pleura represent ⅔, usually above GEJ.
  - When esophageal pressure is 150–200 mmHg, rupture occurs.
  - When hiatal hernia and LES is exposed to IAP → Mallory-Weiss mucosal tear and bleeding rather than perforation.
  - Mediastinal widening (edema) after several hours.
  - In cervical perforation → cervical emphysema.
  - Air will be visible in erector spinae muscle.
  - ⅔ left side, ⅕ in right side, ¹/₁₀ bilaterally.

- **Investigation**
  - Laboratory: high WBCs.
  - X-ray: first sign is air in deep muscle of neck.
    - → Pneumomediastinum, pleural effusion, pneumothorax, SC emphysema.

o Esophagography
  - Contrast esophagram → extravasation (90%), use water-soluble contrast such as gastrografin or omnipaque, then barium for better resolution.
    - If in the pleura or abdomen → terminate the procedure.
    - If in mediastinum → give barium.
  - Barium in pleura or peritoneum → soiling and difficult to remove
  - 10% false −ve because erect (upright), so it should be in right lateral decubitus position.

o CT
  - To detect pneumoperitoneium, pneumothorax and free fluid.

o EGD
  - Diagnostic and therapeutic.
  - If image is non-diagnostic
  - rule out malignancy with biopsy.

• **Initial Management**
  - Physiological stability to determine if patient is a candidate for non-operative management or not.
  - If contained leak:
    - HR < 100.
    - WBC—12,000–14,000.
    - No evidence of ongoing sepsis → non-operative management should be in ICU for 2–3 days.
    - NPO, elevate head, broad-spectrum antibiotic, PPI, TPN.
    - If distal perforation → antifungal.
  - Repeat image in 72–96 hrs; if nothing, proceed to liquid diet.
  - Early diagnosis, the most favorable outcome.
  - Treatment: primary closure within 24 hrs, 80%–90% SR.
  - Commonest location of injury is left lateral wall.
  - The injury edges are trimmed and closed primarily.
  - Closure is reinforced with use of pleural patch or construction with Nissen fundoplication.
  - SR decreases to 50% After 24 hrs → need to resect of diseased part.

- Contamination of mediastinum is drained.
- feeding jejunostomy.
- Recovery from sepsis is dramatic.
- If the patient is stabilized, discharge and return for reconstruction with substernal colon interposition.
- Non-operative management usually follows dilation of stricture or pneumatic dilation of achalasia.
- Cameron criteria for non-operative management:
  1. Contain perforation within mediastinum and drain back to esophagus.
  2. Symptom is mild.
  3. Minimal clinical sepsis.
- Oral intake within 7–14 days, depending on radiographic exam.

- **Operative Management**
  o Cervical esophagus Perforation
    - Left-sided neck approach, drain all fluid.
    - Primary repair.
    - If delayed, single-layer repair.
    - May use strap muscle for interposition flap.
    - Gastrografin esophagram postoperative D5.

  o Thoracic esophagus Perforation
    Upper ⅔ right-side thoracotomy via fifth intercostal space:
      - Debridement.
      - If fresh perforation, single running absorbable suture, then irrigation + buttress intercostal flap + chest tube.
    Lower ⅓ left-sided:
      - Esophagectomy and gastrostomy are not recommended unless ongoing sepsis, malignancy perforation.

  o Abdominal esophagus Perforation
    - Upper midline incision.
    - May require left thoracotomy.
    - May require diaphragm rotational flap.

NB:

> If there's leak in esophagogastrostomy anastomosis site after esophagectomy or if gastric conduit is necrotic → right thoracotomy to reduce gastric remnant, cervical esophagostomy + gastrostomy, then delay reconstruction.

Caustic Injury

- Mainly in children, adults, or teenagers who attempted suicide.
- Alkaline is more frequent as acid ingestion is painful.

- **Pathology**

Acute	Potential for perforation
Chronic	Stricture
Alkalis	Dissolve tissue → deeper
Acid	Coagulative necrosis

  - Upper esophagus is more affected than lower.
  - Three phases:
    1. Acute phase in 1–4 days.
    2. Ulceration and granulation in 10–12 days → necrotic slough esophagus.
    3. Cicatrization and scarring during third week. Connective tissue begins to contract → pocket and bands.

- **Clinical manifestations**
  - Pain in the mouth, substernal, hypersalivation, dysphagia, fever resulting from esophageal injury.
  - Bleeding then disappears at second phase.
  - In third phase → dysphagia because of scarring, 60% in 1 month, 80% in 2 months.
  - Hypovolemia, acidosis resulting to renal damage.
  - Laryngeal spasm and edema, pulmonary edema (acidic) can be without oral cavity affection.
  - Early endoscopy, but don't introduce beyond the pathology.
    - Degree grading of corrosive esophagitis:
      - 1st Mucosal hyperemia and edema

2nd Limited hemorrhage, ulceration, pseudomembrane formation

3rd Sloughing of mucosa, deep ulcer, massive bleeding, obstruction resulting from edema, perforation

- If EGD is normal → stricture later.
- Radiography is not reliable but needed later on for follow up → stricture.
- Most common location of injury:
  o Pharynx 10%
  o Esophagus 70% (middle, 55%; upper, 13%; lower, 2%)
  o Stomach 20% (antrum, 91%)
  o Stomach and Esophagus 14%

• **Treatment**
- Immediate and late.
- Immediately administer neutralizing agent in first hr
  If alkaline → ½ strength, lemon, orange.
  If acidic → milk, egg white, or antacid.
- Don't give sodium bicarbonate → CO_2 → distention → perforation.
- Emesis resulting to reexposure of material and perforation.
- Consider feeding jejunostomy.
- IVF, antibiotic.
- In the past → wait till stricture.
- Now → dilation, complication includes perforation, which mandate ih resection.
- When extensive gastric involvement → partial or total gastrectomy.
- When air is within esophageal wall (necrosis) → esophagectomy.
- Esophagoscopy → first degree → observe for 1–2 days.
- Second, third degree → questionable → second look after 36 hrs.
- Second, third degree → extensive necrosis → options: stent, posterior gastric biopsy, esophagogastric resection, cervical esophagostomy, resection of affected organ, or jejunostomy.

- Stent is removed after 21 days and after barium → esophagoscopy → stricture → dilation (bougie).
- Dilation within acute phase success rate is 78% (excellent) whereas chronic is 21%.
- If dilation failed even with small size, surgery is considered.
- Indications:
  a. Complete stenosis, failure to establish lumen
  b. Irregularity or pocket in barium
  c. Periesophagitis, mediastinitis
  d. Fistula
  e. Failure to attempt lumen above 40 Francis bougie
  f. Patient unwilling to repeated dilation
- Stomach, colon, jejunum replace the esophagus via retrosternal or postmediastinum.
- → Retrosternal is chosen if fibrosis and previous esophagectomy.
- Don't perform sleeve resection.
- If esophagus left in place → blind sac → abscess.

Acquired Fistula
- Common in tracheobronchial tree.
- Mostly associated with esophagus or bronchial malignancy.
- Others: diverticulitis, trauma.
- Symptoms: Coughing with ingestion fluid.
- Recurrent pulmonary infection.
- Spontaneous closure is rare.
- Treatment of excision of fistula and underlying cause and closure of esophagus defect + pleural flap.
- Malignancy fistula → palliative → esophageal endoprosthesis or another option → salivary tube (spit fistula).

Carcinoma of the Esophagus
- Incidence is 20 per 100,000 in USA, UK and 160 per 100,000 in China.
- SCC is the commonest, then adenocarcinoma; adenocarcinoma now increases to 50% → because of ↑ BE and GERD.
- Transformation of Barrett's esophagus to CA → 10%–15%, i.e., forty to sixty times more than general population.

- Risk factors:
    - SCC:
      Tobacco (all types), alcohol, pickles, diet rich in nitrate, deficiency of zinc, hot liquid > 70°C, achalasia, chewing betel nut, HPV
    - Adenocarcinoma:
      GERD, BE, obesity, smoking, Caucasian, red meat, high iron intake

- **Clinical Picture**
  1. Dysphagia not developed till obstruct ⅔ of circumference.
     - Reflux history.
     - Hoarseness: LNs compress RLN.
     - Hiccup: phrenic nerve is involved.
     - If tumor is in cardia → anorexia, weight loss before dysphagia.
     - Systemic metastasis, jaundice, bone pain.
  2. By surveillance (biopsy) if history of reflux or Barrett's.

TNM classification

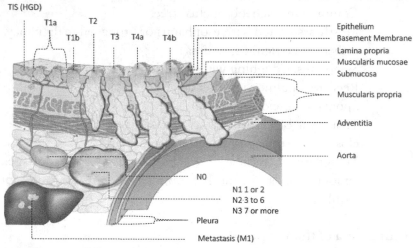

SR, 5 years	Tis	90%
	T1	75%
	T2	45%
	T3	30%
	T4	15%

SR with no LNs metastasis is 30%–60%

While SR with LNs metastasis is 15%–25%

- **Diagnosis**
  - EGD (gold standard), biopsy in 4 quadrants every 1-2 cm.
  - CT CAP for staging, LNs and distant metastasis.
  - can differentiate LNs involvement, whether it's malignant or inflammatory, by FDG-PET.
  - EUS is higher in sensitivity for staging (depth).
  - EMR if the tumor < 2 cm.
  - Bronchoscopy with FNA.
  - Prognosis does not depend on tumor size or invasion or LNs or metastasis → but cell type, degrees of differentiation, location of tumor are important in patient with advanced disease.
  - ≤ 5 LNs—better prognosis.
  - Histologic grade:
    - G1   Well differentiated
    - G2   Moderate differentiation
    - G3   Poor differentiation
    - G4   Undifferentiated
  - Tumor location:
    - Cervical   8%
    - Upper thoracic   3%
    - Middle thoracic   32%
    - Lower thoracic   25%
    - Cardia   32%

- **Pre operative consideration**
  - Age
    - Above 80 rarely indicates esophagectomy, but high performance with good cardiopulmonary reserve may consider esophagectomy through MIS or open.

  - Cardiopulmonary Reserve
    - FEV in 1 second should be > 2 L;
      If < 1.25 L → poor candidiate for thoracotomy.

- If poor cardiopulmonary reserve → transhiatal esophagectomy.
- ECG is not enough → echo to determine EF.
- Thallium image may require coronary angiography.
- Most semifit, who can climb three flights of stairs, can perform surgery.

o Nutritional State
  - Weight loss > 20 lbs, hypoalbuminemia < 3.5 g, should place feeding tube preoperative through jejunostomy, rich fish oil.

o Clinical Staging
  - Advanced disease → RLN paralysis, Horner, spinal pain, paralysis of diaphragm, fistula, pleural effusion, tumor > 8 cm, > 4 LNs, weight loss > 20%, loss of appetite.

- **Treatment**
  Tis T1a, Low-Risk T1b
  - Tis → no basement membrane invasion.
  - Option: intensive surveillance, EMR, esophagectomy.
  - HGD synchronous invasive CA (40%–60%) → so esophagectomy is standard of care.
      T1a   LNs +ve 2%, accepted esophageal sparing local therapy
      T1b   ↑ LNs invasion submucosal layer → esophagectomy + regional LNs resection
  - Esophageal sparing local therapy.
  - RFA, photodynamic therapy (PDT), cryotherapy, EMR, then PPI high dose + surveillance Q3M for 1 year with 4Q biopsy; if no risk, ↑ interval.

  T2–T4, Any N, M0
  - Neoadjuvant chemoradiotherapy + esophagectomy

Curative vs. Palliative Based on Location, Age, Health, Extent of the Disease

a. Cervical esophageal CA is always SCC with rare adenocarcinoma arising from congenital inlet patch. Usually unresectable → early invasion of larynx, great vessels, trachea

→ esophageal laryngectomy, but for most patients → stereotactic radiotherapy and chemotherapy.

b. Middle ⅓ → most common and LNs metastasis is common usually in thoracic LNs.

- Ti–T2 with no LNs → resection only.
- If LNs or T3 → neoadjuvant chemotherapy + radiation then surgery.
- Resection of tumor of midthoracic → direct vision, thoracoscopy (VAST) or thoracotomy.

c. Lower esophagus usually adenocarcinoma, curative resection requires a cervical division of the esophagus and > 50% proximal gastrectomy in most patients with carcinoma of the distal esophagus or cardia.

- Resection + LNs, because GI tumor spreads longitudinally in submucosal layer → grossly normal gastrointestinal with longitudinal LNs can result in skip area, so wide local excision, > 8 cm.
- Wong study → 10 cm margin at least, no barrier between esophagus and stomach.
- submucosal LNs invasion → 50% recurrence

Palliation of Esophageal CA

- Metastatic CA or T4b.
- Dysphagia from esophageal CA:
  Grade
  I   Eating normally
  II   Required liquid with meal
  III   Semisolid but no solid
  IV   Liquid only
  V   No liquid but able to swallow saliva
  VI   Unable to swallow saliva.

- Grade I–III—chemoradiation for 8 weeks; some are totally cured, but many recurrences in 1–5 years, and some are candidates for salvage esophagectomy.
- Grade IV—indwelling esophageal stent.
  If advanced (hopeless) → metal permanent stent.

Technique

- Ivor Lewis: laparotomy + right thoracotomy
- McKeown esophagectomy (three holes + esophagectomy)
- Transhiatal esophagectomy
- Left thoracoabdomenal esophagectomy

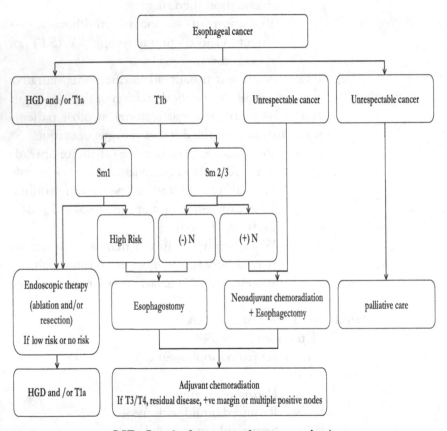

NB: Sm (submucosal penetration).
N (Lymph Node Metastasis).

Complication of Esophagectomy
- Respiratory complication → epidural catheter can help.
- Chyle leak.
- Leak from esophagus → esophagram with water-soluble contrast or CT or EGD (safe).

Comparative Studies of Esophagectomy Technique
- Transthoracic vs. transhiatal
    - Extensive dissection for LNs does not appear to add benefit.
    - Transhiatal → long-term survival and less mortality and morbidity.
    - MIS has less pulmonary complication than open but no difference related to mortality.

Alternative Therapies
- Radiotherapy
    - Primary treatment with radiotherapy does not produce result.
    - Radiotherapy is for patient who is not a candidate for surgery.
    - Radiotherapy alone for palliation of dysphagia, SR for 3 months.
    - Radiotherapy for hemorrhage from tumor.

- Adjuvant chemotherapy
    - Effective to treat micrometastasis.
    - To prevent hematogenous dissemination.
    - Disadvantages: immunosuppressant, blood flow decreasing.
    - Neoadjuvant is more effective—blood flow is good, decreases tumor size, less likely to develop resistance after surgery.
    - Not beneficial in SCC above the carina.

- Neoadjuvant chemotherapy
    - Adenocarcinoma → (5/FU) cisplatin as neoadjuvant is more effective than surgery alone.

- Postoperative complication: sepsis and respiratory complication.

- Preoperative chemotherapy radiation
    - Beneficial in adenocarcinoma and SCC.
    - Improves local response.
    - Time of surgery is 6–8 weeks after.
    - After 8 weeks, adenocarcinoma starts to form scar.
    - After chemoradiation → 17%–24% has no tumor when resected surgically.

Sarcoma of Esophagus
- Sarcoma and carcinosarcoma is rare, 0.1%–1.5%.
- Dysphagia and symptom according to location.
- Barium: large polypoid intraluminal esophageal mass.
- Esophagoscopy: intraluminal necrotic mass.
- Biopsy → not from necrosis, taken until bleeding.
- Superficial to muscularis propria.
- Unlikely to have LNs metastasis.
- Two lesions in sarcomatous lesion:
    1. Epidermoid carcinoma with spindle cell → carcinoma sarcoma
    2. True sarcoma, leiomyosarcoma, fibrosarcoma, rhabdomyosarcoma (two latest are rare)
- Surgical resection of polypoid sarcoma is the treatment of choice, as radiotherapy has little success and the tumor is deep.
- 5 years, SR is 50%.

Technique of Esophageal Reconstruction
- Gastric advancement
- Colonic interposition
- Jejunal free or advancement into chest

- Partial esophageal resection
    - Distal lesion with preserved proximal esophagus is the best treatment with jejunal interposition up to inferior border of pulmonary hilum; needs thoracotomy.

- Jejunum is dynamitic graft, while stomach and colon is conduit.
- Stomach is a poor choice → reflux.
- Colon is hypomotile → esophagitis.
- Replacement of cervical portion while preserved distal portion → free transfer of the jejunum → successful in majority by revisualization by use of internal mammary artery or vein or brachiocephalic vein.
- Removal of sternoclavicular joint in performing distal esophageal anastomosis.

- Reconstruction after esophagectomy
  - If stomach is contracted, reduced or had a previous surgery.
    → stomach is prohibited.
  - Presence of diverticula disease, CA, or colitis → colon is prohibited.
  - Colon is more affected by arterial disease than stomach.
  - Stomach provides only 1 anastomosis.
    → disadvantage: aspiration, reflux and postprandial pressure sensation.
  - 40%–50% dysphagia with stomach, but less in colon.
  - Colon with dysphagia 24% after 1 year.
  - Stomach in chest resulting to duodenogastric reflux but the reflux is less with colon.

- Vagal sparing esophagectomy with colon interposition
  - Traditionally esophageal surgery → bilaterally vagotomy → dumping, diarrhea, weight loss by 15%–20%.
  - Sparing → upper midline abdominal incision → vagus nerve bilaterally identified and circled with a tape.
  - Limited highly selected vagotomy.
  - Endoscopy GIA below GEJ.
  - Prepare colon.

- Neck incision on anterior border of left sternocleidomastoid and strap muscle is exposed, omohyoid divided.
- Retract carotid sheath (left) laterally and trachea medially. Left inferior thyroid A. is ligated.
- RLN preserved, esophagus dissected circumferentially to inferior direction.
- Esophagus is divided at thoracic inlet, leaving 3–4 cm cervical esophagus.
- Proximal esophagus retracted to prevent saliva contamination.
- Return to abdomen.
- Flush esophagus with povidone solution.
- Vein stripper passed up till neck.
- Seared distal end up in the neck with stripper.
- Stripper pulled back to abdomen → preserve esophageal plexus and vagus nerve.
- In case of achalasia, only mucosa is secured and stripped, leaving enriched blood supply → mediastinal tunnel.
- Prepared colon → passed behind stomach.
- End-to-end anastomosis with cervical esophagus using single-layer technology.
- Then anastomose of colon to stomach.
- Colon → end-to-end anastomosis.

Stomach

Anatomy
Blood Supply
- Arterial: via celiac axis.
    - Left gastric artery arises from the celiac axis.
    - Right gastric artery arises from the proper hepatic artery.
    - Right gastroepiploic artery from gastroduodenal artery which arise from common hepatic artery.
    - Left gastroepiploic artery is the largest branch of splenic artery.
    - Short gastric artery arises from splenic artery.
    - 20% of left gastric artery supplies an aberrant vessel that travels in lesser omentum to left liver; if injured, it can produce ischemia to the liver.

- Venous: parallel.
    - Left gastric vein or coronary vein drains to the portal vein (PV), sometimes to splenic vein.
    - Right gastric vein drains blood to the portal vein (PV).
    - Right gastroepiploic vein drains blood to the superior mesenteric vein (SMV).
    - Left gastroepiploic vein ends in the splenic vein.
    - Short gastric vein ends in the splenic vein.

Special consideration:
1. Can ligate two named vessels, right gastric and right epiploic arteries in esophageal replacement and two epiploic arteries in sleeve gastrectomy without any compromise.
2. In subtotal gastrectomy, ligation of four vessels except short gastric.
3. Angiography can control gastric ulcer bleeding.
4. Splenorenal shunt is used in portal hypertension.

- **Lymphatics**

  Generally parallel to blood vessels.
  - Cardia and medical ½ body → LNs in left gastric and celiac.
  - Lesser curvature of antrum → LNs in right gastric and pyloric.
  - Greater curvature ½ distally → LNs in right gastroepiploic.
  - Greater curvature ½ proximally → LNs in left gastroepiploic or splenic.
  - Node in lesser and greater curvature → celiac.
  - Because of unpredictability and rich LNs and venous network → wide resection margin needed → sometimes away LNs is +ve while beside tumor is −ve.
  - According to JRSGC, lymph nodes organized in D1 and D2.
    → D1 = LNs 3, 4a, 4b, 5, 6.
    D2 = LNs 1, 2, 7, 8, 9, 10, 11, 12.

- **Innervation**
  - Vagus = extrinsic parasympathetic to stomach, acetylcholine is the most important transmitter.
  - Vagus arise from floor of fourth cerebral ventricle → neck → carotid sheath → mediastinum → RLN → esophagus → left anterior + right posterior (LARP) → near GEJ, branch to liver in gastrohepatic ligament → continue in lesser curvature → anterior nerve of latarjet → similarly posterior latarjet → body → angularis incisura (crow's feet).
  - 50% of population have more than one nerve in the hiatus (criminal nerve of Grassi), this branch typically arises above the esophageal hiatus and is easily missed during truncal or highly selective vagotomy (HSV).
  - Vagal fibers originate in the brain synapse with neurons in Auerbach's or myenteric plexus and Meissner's submucosal plexus.
  - Vagus (cholinergic) → acid secretion, ↑mucosal blood flow, cytoprotective.
  - Sympathetic nerve is (adrenergic) T5–T10.

Histology
- Partial cell contains mitochondria.
- Parietal cell secretes HCI, intrinsic factor, enterochromaffin-like (ECL), bicarbonate.
  - ECL a type of neuroendocrine cell, secretes histamine.
  - Bicarbonate secreted through D cells.
- Chief cell → pepsinogen, activated at pH 2.5.
- G cell → gastrin (antrum).
- D cell → somatostatin.
- mucus-secreting surface epithelial cells (SECs)
- 13% parietal, 44% chief, 40% mucous, 3% endocrine.
- Musculosa consists of an incomplete inner oblique layer, a complete middle circular layer, and a complete outer longitudinal layer.
- In musculosa → Auerbach's or myenteric plexus and interstitial cell of Cajal (ICC).
- Serosa prevents tumor to metastasized (not present in esophagus and lower rectum).

Physiology
- **Acid Secretion**
  - Long-term PPI → C. difficile.
  - Parietal cell: stimulated via one of three: acetylcholine (vagus), gastrin (G), and (histamine ECL cell).
  - The enzyme is H^+/K^+ ATPase proton pump.
  - K^+ exchange with H^+ and accompany with Cl^-.
  - Normal human stomach → one billion parietal cells.
  - PPI irreversibly interferes with function → before or during meal.
  - If stopped → the function gradually returns as new cells.
  - Gastrin, acetylcholine, and histamine stimulate the parietal cell to secrete hydrochloric acid; gastrin binds to type B cholecystokinin (CCK) receptors, and acetylcholine binds to M_3 muscarinic receptors. Both stimulate phospholipase C via a G protein.
  - Three phases of secretion: cephalic, stomach, bowel (60%, 30%, 10%, respectively).
  - Interprandial secretion of 2–5 mEq/hr.
  - Acid decreases to 70%–90% by vagotomy or H_2 blocker.

- Histamine mediates gastrin and acetylcholine.
- Somatostatin inhibits histamine and gastrin.
- Somatostatin is inhibited by H. pylori.

- **Gastric Mucosal Barrier**
  - Any slough $\rightarrow$ replaced by restitution.
  - Mucosal barrier: bicarbonate secretion, epithelial barrier.
  - Important mediators of these protective mechanisms include prostaglandins, nitric oxide, intrinsic nerves, and peptides.
  - Protective reflexes involve afferent sensory neurons.
  - Important protective factors is saliva, duodenal secretions, and pancreatic or biliary secretions.
  - Sucralfate acts locally to enhance mucosal defenses.

- **Gastrointestinal Hormone**
  - Gastrin: G cell in antrum
    - Most stimulus is peptide, amino acid and HCl⁻.
    - Inhibited by somatostatin (D cell) blocked by H_2 antagonist.
    - Chronic hypergastrinemia $\rightarrow$ hyperplasia, carcinoid, pernicious anemia, PPI, gastrinoma, retained antrum, vagatomy.

  - Somatostatin: D cell
    - The major stimulus for somatostatin release is antral acidification.
    - Acetylcholine via vagus nerve inhibits it.

  - Gastric-releasing peptide
    - Body and antrum.
    - Stimulates acid secretion.
    - Gastric protective mediator, $\uparrow$ mucosal blood flow.

  - Leptin
    - In adipose tissue (adipocyte), chest wall; produces satiety hormone.

- Ghrelin
  - Pituitary but primary is stomach.
  - Stimulates appetite (hunger).

- Pepsinogen
  - Most stimulus is the food.
  - Acetylcholine → mediator.
  - Pepsinogen I is secreted by chief cells.
  - Pepsinogen Õ is secreted by SEC and gastrin.
  - Active if pH is 2.5.

- Intrinsic factor
  - Bind vitamin B12 → absorbed in terminal ileum.
  - Vitamin B12 ↓ in gastrectomy → pernicious anemia.
  - Also decreased by gastric bypass.
  - PPI does not inhibit intrinsic factor.

- **Gastric Motility and Emptying**
  - Acetylcholine → increases neurotransmitters.
  - Nitric oxide (NO), VIP, and histamine decrease neurotransmitters.
  - Specialized cell interstitial cell of Cajal (ICC) in muscularis propria has pacemaker property in term of ↑ motility; it is the origin of GIST.

- **Segmental Gastric Motility**
  - Proximal: tonic contraction, 5 mintues.
  - Gastroparesis—peacemaker.
  - During fasting, MMC = 100 min, with 4 phases:
    Phase I   No contraction
    Phase II   No propulsive contraction
    Phase III   Propulsive contraction
    Phase IV   Emptying to duodenum and jejunum
  - Initiation of phase III of distal stomach by motilin (mucosa of duodenum).
  - Chewing gum → increases antral motor activity.
  - Nitric oxide → pyloric relaxation.
  - CCK inhibits gastric emptying.
  - Half of liquid emptying in 12 min.

231

- Half of solid emptying in 2 hrs.
- Diabetic patients suffer from delay emptying.

- **Diagnostic Test For Gastric Disease**
  - Esophagogastroduodenoscopy (EGD)
    - Used for Weight loss, vomiting (recurrent), dysphagia, bleeding, anemia.
    - Offer biopsy, brush cytology.
    - If gastritis → biopsy to rule out H. pylori, sjould be treated → if not treated well → MALT, gastric CA.

  - Radiology
    - X-ray: perforation or delayed gastric emptying → large air fluid level.
    - Double contrast GI series → better than EGD in diverticula, fistula, stricture, hiatal hernia.

  - CT, MRI
    - Virtual gastroscopy by CT, MRI.

  - Angiography
    - To detect occult bleeding.

  - Endoscopic ultrasound (EUS)
    - Gastric lesion, staging.
    - Assesses response to chemotherapy.

  - Gastric secretory analysis
    - To measure gastric output.
    - Hypergastrinemia, ZES, refractory ulcer, or GERD.
    - Normal basal acid output (BAO) = < 5 mEq/hr.
    - Gastrinoma = ↑ BAO > 30.
    - Postvagotomy or gastric resection > 15.
    - BAO to MAO (maximum acidic output)ratio = 0.6.
    - Stop PPI, H_2 when performing the study.

  - Scintigraphy
    - Gastric-emptying scintigraphy (milk scan).

- Duodenal reflux diagnosed by IV hepatobiliary iminodiacetic acid (HIDA) scan, concentrated in the liver then executed in duodenum.
  → Ejection fraction of gall bladder (dyskinesia).
- PET or CT/PET for CA.

- Test for H. pylori
  - Serology (serum) and fecal antigen → active H. pylori (low sensitivity).
  - Biopsy and Histology examination is gold standard.
  - Urease, urea breath test to confirm eradication.

- Antroduodenal motility and electrogastrogram (EGG)
  - Anomalous epigastric symptoms.
  - EGG → transcutaneous recording of EGG.
  - Antroduodenal motility test → transnasally or orally to distal duodenum.
  - Combination of two tests + scintigraphy for gastric motility.

Pathology
Peptic Ulcer Disease (PUD)
- Imbalance between mucosal defense and peptic injury.
- Mortality rate (MR): duodenal, 3.7%; gastric, 2.1%.

- **Pathophysiology and Etiology**
  - The most common cause is H. pylori & NSAIDs.
  - H. pylori → acid hypersecretion + ↓ mucosal defense.
  - Generally,
    Duodenal ulcer → hypersecretion.
    Gastric ulcer → weak mucosa.
  - Others: gastrinoma (ZES), G cell hyperplasia, smoking, trauma, burn, cocaine, stress, steroid, aging.

  - H. pylori
    - Flagella, 50% is infected worldwide.
    - Predispose metaplasia, dysplasia, stomach CA (gastric lymphoma), IBD, GERD.

- The organism processes urease → ammonia and bicarbonate → created environment buffers the acid secreted by stomach.
- Ammonia damage the mucosa.
- H. pylori → disturbs acid secretion by inhibit D cells (somatostatin) to secrete, i.e., ↓ somatostatin which decreases gastrin + ↓ bicarbonate + ↑ cytokines.
  → ↑ gastrin, ↑ HCL.
  → Duodenal metaplasia → colonize in duodenal mucosa ↑ risk of ulcer fiftyfold.
  → Mucosal injury → toxin vacA and cag, ↑ cytokines
  → (IL-8), ↑ apoptosis, and inflammation.
- Causes 90% of duodenal ulcer and 70% of gastric ulcer.

- Acid secretion and PUD
  - Duodenal ulcer has BAO + MAO.
  - Duodenal ulcer—excessive gastric secretion and serum gastrin.
  - Duodenal ulcer— gastric emptying.
  Modified Johnson classification of PUD:

Type I	Near angularis incisura
Type II	Gastric and duodenal (normal or high acid)
Type III	Prepyloric (normal or high acid)
Type IV	Near GEJ.
Type V	Drug-induced (NSAIDs) Can be anywhere

- Non-steroidal anti-inflammatory drugs (NSAIDs)
  - ↑ fivefold, and UGIB, fourfold.
  - More than ½ with hemorrhage or perforation has history of NSAIDs.
  - In elderly, ten times.
  - NSAIDs + steroid + anticoagulant + over 60s.
  - Ranitidine is less effective than PPI.

- Smoking and others
  - ↑ gastric secretion and duodenogastric reflux.
  - ↓ prostaglandin and bicarbonate.
  - Curling's ulcer in burn patients.
  - Coca-Cola, alcohol, ↑ PUD.

- **Clinical Manifestation**
  - Epigastric abdominal pain, burning,.
  - Gastric ulcer → the pain ↑ with eating,
  ↓ chance of awaking from sleep.
  - History of PUD or NSAIDs.
  - Nausea, bloating, weight loss, +ve occult blood in stool.

- **Diagnosis**
  - Should rule out pancreatitis, hepatitis.
  - Start with x-ray supine, double contrast GI
  x-ray, CT.
  - Serum gastrin to rule out gastrinoma.
  - Definitive diagnosis with EGD.

- **Complication**
  - Bleeding, perforation, obstruction, respectively.
  - Melena or hematemesis → to determine whether positive or negative UGIB, introduce NGT till bilious aspirate.
  - Shock, pain are uncommon.
    → Resuscitation + EGD, +/− hematemesis therapy.
  - ¾ of bleeding will stop with PPI.
  - ¼ will continue bleeding or rebleed.
  - Use risk stratification to predict rebleed and death → Blatchford and Rockall scores.
  - Gastric outlet obstruction (5%)
    - acute (edema) swelling, and peristalsis dysfunction or chronic (cicatrix) symptom → non-bilious vomiting + hyperchloremic metabolic alkalosis, pain, weight loss, succession splash in epigastrium.
    - Initial treatment: NGT, IVF and correct electrolytes, PPI.
    - Diagnosis by endoscopy.

- Treatment: either balloon dilation or surgical; CA should be ruled out.

- **Medical Treatment**
  - PPI or H$_2$ blocker and sucralfate.
  - With ulcer complication, should start an IV PPI infusion and consider lifelong PPI unless the cause is eliminated, i.e., stop alcohol, NSAIDs.
  - Stop PPI after 3 months if H. pylori is eradicated
    → to confirm eradication in 4–6 weeks with urea breath test.
  - Follow-up endoscopy in 8–12 weeks.
    → If healed ulceration, discharge on PPI;
    → if after 12 weeks with medical treatment and no improvement → surgical intervention is warrented.

- **Surgical Overview**
  - Indication → bleeding, perforation, obstructions, refractory disease.
  - Most surgeon → oversewing of the bleeding vessel or simple patch for perforation.
  - Vagotomy is uncommon because of unfamiliarity.
  - The operation depends on:
    - Type of ulcer.
    - Patient conditions.
    - Intra-abdominal factor (scar, adhesion).
    - Surgeon experience, personal preference.
  - Generally, a resection operation has higher mortality and lesser recurrence, and an unresection operation has lesser mortality and higher recurrence.
  - Truncal vagotomy + drainage, selective vagotomy, highly selective vagotomy (HSV).
  - In HSV for proximal ⅔ of stomach, preserved vagal innervation of pylorus + hepatobiliary → decrease acidity by 75%.
  - In vagotomy, leave 6–8 cm before GEJ and 7 cm before pylorus intact to preserve pyloric function as well as hepatobiliary function.
  - For non-compliance or intolerance to medical treatment can consider surgery.

- Taylor procedure → posterior vagotomy + anterior seromyotomy equal to HSV.
- Gastric ulcer → biopsy.
- Vagotomy → denervated pylorus → drainage (pyloroplasty).
- Techniques for pyloroplasty:
  - Heineke-Mikulicz
  - Finney
  - Jaboulay
- Distal gastrectomy without vagotomy → 50% includes ulcer type I.
- Antrectomy leaves 60%–70% stomach.
- Subtotal is rarely used.
- Pylorus-preserving gastrectomy (PPG) → dumping, lesser reflux (duodenal).
- Reconstruction by Billroth I and II and Roux-en-Y.
- Anterior gastrostomy → inspect and oversew.
- Total gastrostomy considered if life-threatening bleeding or diffused.
- In setting of perforation → wedge out + primary repair ± graham patch rather than gastric resection, but if patient is already on H. pylori + PPI → acid-reducing operation maybe a burden.
- Vagotomy reduces 50% of acid secretion whereas Vagotomy + antrectomy 85%.

Vagotomy and Drainage
- Vagotomy to eliminate parasympathetic innervation of any acid hypersecretion.
- Truncal vagotomy (TV): anterior and posterior at level of distal esophagus, 4 cm proximal to GEJ requires mobilization of esophagus by 5–6 cm.
- Selective vagotomy (SV) (anterior): right and left vagus nerve just below postceliac branch then innervate pancreatic small bowel and anterior branch that supply liver and gallbladder. Postoperative diarrhea and dumping are lower than TV.
- High selective vagotomy (HSV): preserves latarjet nerves, to preserve motor function to pylorus, Crow's feet are not divided.
- Both TV + SV requires pyloroplasty (Heineke-Mikulicz).

Resection of Ulcer

- If formal acid-reducing operation is not done:
    1. Clear the edge for primary repair after Bx.
    2. Wedge out stapler and send it to histopathology.
- If no malignancy and no previous antacid treatment → the area of resection can be closed or patched → then patient should be put on antacid and H. pylori treatment.
- If formal resection (e.g., antrectomy), the ulcer location dictates extension of dissection or can send the specimen to histopathology to G cells and extent of resection.
- If in lesser curvature → Pauchet procedure.

Reconstruction

- Billroth I, II, Roux-en-Y.
- Billroth II → bile reflux → Roux-en-Y prevents it.
- Roux-en-Y limb should be at least 40 cm to prevent bile reflux.
- Complication: Roux stasis syndrome—abdominal pain, bloating from gastric artery.
- In retrocolic or antecolic types, retro provides more length.
- Laparoscopy vs. open:
    1. Stability of patient
    2. Expert surgeon
    3. Faster recovery

Bleeding Gastric Ulcer

- Most common cause of ulcer-related death.
- Corner stone: endoscopy + PPI.
- Surgery: suture ligation + any (HSV or vagotomy + Drainage) or gastric resection + vagotomy.
- Management of bleeding ulcer → resuscitation + IV infusion PPI will stop the bleeding in 75% and 25% will not, need endoscopic hemostatic intervention.
- EGD hemostatic modifiers → injection with epinephrine and cauterized.
- Exposed vessels → clip if it persists → surgery.
- Indication for surgical intervention:
    - failure of endoscopy
    - transfusion of 4–6 units, i.e., massive hemorrhage
    - no endoscopist

- no blood available
- repeated hospitalization
- concurrent perforation or obstruction.
- Massive bleeding from posterior duodenal ulcer → mostly gastroduodenal artery or from lesser curvature left gastric artery.
- Early operation mostly because old age, shock, transfusion more than 4 units within 24 hrs or 8 units in 48 hrs, rebleeding.
- MR → 20%.
- If rebleeding → repeat EGD and consider angioembolism if persistent or recurrent in patient with instability or requiring transfusion > 6 units
- Rockall and Forrest scores help stratify rebleeding risk. Mortality can be 40%.

Forrest classification

Forrest score	Endoscopic appearance	Risk of rebleeding
Ia	Ulcer with active pulsating bleeding	55%
Ib	Ulcer with active non pulsating bleeding	50%
IIa	Ulcer with a visible non bleeding vessel	43%
IIb	Ulcer with an adherent clot	22%
IIc	Ulcer with hematin on ulcer base	10%
III	Ulcer with clean base	5%

Rockall Score

Points	0	1	2	3
Age	< 60	61–79	80	
Comorbid	-	-	CHD, COPD	CRF, LF, Metastatic disease
Diagnosis	Mallory-Weiss	All other	GI CA	
Bleeding stigmata	-	-	Visible vessel	
Shock	-	P > 100 SBP > 100	SBP < 100	

Operation for Bleeding Gastric Ulcer
-   Oversewing without vagotomy.
-   Vagotomy + Antrectomy.
-   Oversewing alone ↑ risk of rebleeding but less mortality.
-   In re-operation for rebleeding → Vagotomy + antrectomy.
-   Unstable patient → no resection → pyloromyotomy → figure of 8 or U shape stitch → pyloroplasty, if stable → vagotomy.
-   If stable patient → vagotomy + Antrectomy.
-   Planned surgery is better than emergent surgery.
-   Distal gastrectomy with ulcer is the best choice.
-   Vagotomy + Drainage procedure with oversewing and biopsy, then PPI is another option.
-   Unstable patient → oversewing + PPI.

Perforated Gastric Ulcer
-   NSAIDs mostly.
-   Non-operative → stable, no peritonitis with radiological contrast study to decimate sealed perforation.
-   In stable patient < 24 hrs → patch + HSV.
-   USA and Europe trend → simple patch +Bx + PPI.
-   For gastric ulcer → distal gastrectomy; vagotomy for type II, III.
-   In unstable patients → patch closure with biopsy or local excision and closure or biopsy and closure + TV + drainage.

Obstructive gastric ulcer
-   Because of edema and/or motor dysfunction.
-   May respond to PPI, octreotide, NGT.
-   Endoscopic balloon dilation often provides transient respond but if fail → surgical.
-   Standard is vagotomy + antrectomy
-   Alternative:
    → vagotomy + Gastrojejunostomy.
    → HSV + Gastrojejunostomy = vagotomy + antrectomy

Gastric Outlet Obstruction
- Non-bilious vomiting, weight loss.
- Gold standard is vagotomy + antrectomy.
- Alternative is vagotomy + gastrojejunostomy.

Intractable or Non-healing Ulcer
- Causes: missed CA, not taking PPI, still on NSAIDs, still smoking, H. pylori in spite of −ve tests.
- Multiple, recurrent, large ulcer (> 2 cm), complication or malignancy (suspicion) → gastric resection.

Management of Duodenal Ulcer
- Risk factor same as gastric ulcer, CD.
- Duodenal ulcer is twice common in male than female.
- Symptoms: abdominal pain, nausea and vomiting, anemia.
- Duodenal ulcer → pain, 2–3 hrs after meal.
- ⅔ of duodenal ulcer patients → awakes from sleep.
- Presentation: bleeding, perforation, obstruction, abdominal pain.
- Most common cause of UGIB → 90% non-operative.
- Treatment: treat H. pylori, PPI, stop NSAIDs.
- Gastric resection in duodenal ulcer is not justified.

Perforated duodenal ulcer
- Presentation: acute abdominal peritonitis
- Mortality rate is 25%.
- NPO, IVF resuscitation, IV antibiotic, PPI, anticoagulant.
- Non-operative management if stable patient with sealed perforation.
- Treatment of choice: laparotomy for closure of defect and omental patch after wash, 5–10 liters
- No need for biopsy but send fluid for C/S.
- Drain.

Closure of Perforation
- Graham patch.
- Tension-free, well-vascularized omentum.
- Two to three sutures.
- Additional suture may be used.
- NGT, test it by free air or fluid or methylene blue.

- Rare: large defect, 2–3 cm → duodenal opening to Roux limb, better than serosal patch or truncal vagotomy.
- Pyloric exclusion can be considerd here.

Bleeding Duodenal ulcer

- Most common reason of hospitalization of duodenal ulcer is bleeding.
- ¾ of patient will stop bleeding with IVF and PPI.
- 25% rebleed or continue bleeding.
- Hemostasis can be achieved by endoscopy + PPI infusion.
- EGD epinephrine injection, clips, cautery.

Operation for Bleeding Duodenal Ulcer.

- Oversewing alone.
- Oversewing + vagotomy + drainage.
- Vagotomy + antrectomy→ less bleeding.
- Oversewn by long duodenostomy or pyloro-duodenotomy.
- Close as long as pyloroplasty.
- If patient is stable, vagotomy ± pyloroplasty or gastrojejunostomy.

To Decrease Recurrence after Emergency Duodenal Ulcer Operation

- Rule out gastrinoma.
- Treatment H. pylori + PPI.
- No smoking, no NSAIDs.
- Definitive ulcer operation.

Post-Operative and Long-Term Care

- ICU.
- ± NGT.
- Postoperative contrast study.
- Antibiotic + antifungal for 3–5 days.
- Remove drain after break from NPO in 24 hrs.
- Reoperative if persistent leak from perforation site or abdominal wall dehiscence.
- Anti–H. pylori, PPI, stop NSAIDs, smoking.

Zollinger-Ellison Syndrome (ZES)(Gastrinoma)

- Uncontrolled secretion of gastrin by duodenal or pancreas → severe PUD + diarrhea.
- Second most common functional NET (gastrinoma).
- 80% sporadic, 20% inherited = MEN I (parathyroid, pituitary, pancreas, or duodenal gastrinoma).
- Gastrinoma with MEN I, usually multiple → surgical cure is uncommon.
- Sporadic → single lesion.
- Location includes duodenum, pancreas (Bizaro triangle).
- Ectopic location: stomach, ovary, lung, heart, LNs.
- 75%–95% in duodenum, not pancreas.
- The duodenal gastrinoma spreads more to LNs than pancreatic gastrinoma.
- Malignancy rate is 60%–90%, and most has +ve LNs; 50%–80% of the metastasis → liver.
- 90% of sporadic disease is cured after surgery.
- 5 years, SR is 40%.

- **Diagnosis**
    - Epigastric pain, GERD, diarrhea.
    - 90% has peptic ulcer located in the proximal duodenum but can be in the distal duodenum, jejunum.
    - Should be suspected if refractory PUD.
    - MEN I Gastrinoma is diagnosed at age 20–30, and sporadic at age 40–50.
    - Important DDx is hypergastrinemia with ↑ BAO.
    - BAO > 15 mEq/hr or > 5 mEq/hr with previous surgery.
    - Should hold PPI for several days before measuring gastrin level.
    - Diagnosis by secretin stimulation test → IV bolus of 2 u/kg → increase gastrin to 200 pg/mL → gastrinoma.
    - For patient with gastrinoma, measure Ca^{++} + PTH to rule out MENI association.
    - 80% found in gastrinoma triangle (Bizaro)
    - Ultrasound-specific but not sensitive.
    - CT and MRI detect lesion > 2 cm.
    - EUS is most sensitive but misses smaller lesion.

- Somatostatin receptor scintigraphy is the diagnostic tool of choice (octreotide scan) → 100% sensitivity.
- Gastrinoma cells contain type II somatostatin.
- Now, angiolocalization → transhepatic selective venous sampling with IV secretin.
- An arterial catheter is selectively placed in a named vessel supplying the pancreas (e.g., GDA or splenic), and a venous catheter is placed in a hepatic vein.
  - → Secretin is injected into the artery, and gastrin is sampled in the hepatic vein.
  - → → A significant elevation in hepatic venous gastrin indicates that the tumor is supplied by the injected artery.
- This test is performed if pancreaticoduodenectomy is contemplated.
- All patients with sporadic gastrinoma → surgery.
- 90% preoperative localization.

- **Treatment**
  - Oral omeprazole and IV pantoprazole to normalize BAO.
  - ZES-MEN I parathyroidectomy first, then remove 3 ½ glands.
  - If the tumor size > 2 cm → liver metastasis.
  - Pancreatic enucleation of mass.
  - If exploration is not successful to find the tumor → longitudinal duodenotomy → inspection and palpation for resection+ LNs of portal and peripancreatic region is sampled.
  - Ablation or resection of hepatic metastasis.
  - If untreatable MEN I gastrinoma → HSV.
  - No gastrectomy in ZES.

Gastritis and Stress Ulcer

- Mucosal inflammation.
- Most common cause is H.pylori; others are PUD, Crohn's disease, TB, bile reflux.
- Immune cell and cytokines infiltration.
- Any ICU patient → should be protected with PPI.
- Stress, ICU, burn → ↓ blood flow to the stomach.

- Hemorrhagic stress ulceration → vagotomy + drainage procedure with oversewing or near-total gastrostomy.
- Angiography and endoscopic hemostatic treatment should be considered.

Mallory-Weiss Syndrome (MWS)
- Mucosal tear at GEJ.
- Acute upper GI bleeding following vomiting.
- 15% of severe upper GI bleeding.
- Mechanism is similar to spontaneous esophageal perforation.
- Acute↑ in IAP against closed glottis in patient with hiatal hernia.
- Arterial bleeding → massive.
- Diagnosis requires high index of suspicion.
- UGI endoscopy (diagnostic and therapeutic) → longitudinal fissure in mucosa of herniated stomach.
- Will stop spontaneously by 95%.
- PRBCs, NGT, antiemetics.
- Sengstaken-Blakemore tube will not stop it → as it's arterial.
- Endoscopic injection of epinephrine, if it doesn't stop spontaneously.
- Sometimes surgery is needed → laparotomy + high gastrotomy, oversewing of linear tear.
- Mortality is uncommon, and recurrence is rare.

Benign Gastric Condition
Leiomyoma
- Submucosal lesion and firm.
- if ulcerated → bleeding, it has umbilicated appearance.
- Lesion < 2 cm, usually asymptomatic.
- Lesion > 2 cm, causes pain and obstruction.
- Lesion < 2 cm, observe, or enucleation if FNA → smooth muscle tumor
- Large tumor with symptom → wedge resection (laparoscopic).
- If patient prefers to observe, tell the patient of the possibility of malignancy (foci).

Lipoma
- Submucosal fatty tumor.
- Excision is unnecessary unless symptomatic.

Gastric Motility Disease
- Delayed gastric emptying (gastroparesis), rapid gastric emptying, motor and sensory abnormalities (e.g., functional dyspepsia).
- Surgically relevant secondary disorders of gastric motility (e.g., dumping, gastric stasis, and Roux syndrome).
- Gastroparesis is mostly 80% in female, postprandial vomiting, ↓ glucose, following insulin.
- Upper GI series to delineate anatomy.
- Diagnosis: gastric-emptying scintigraphy.
- Treatment: antiemetic, botulinum injection to pylorus.
- Diabetic patient + gastroparesis, not a candidate for pancreatic transplant.
- Gastrostomy (decompression) and jejunostomy feeding.
- Other Treatment: implantation of peacemaker or gastric resection.

Isolated Gastric Varices
- In the absence of esophageal varices.
- Type I fundic, type II distal (duodenum).
- Associated with splenic vein thrombosis.
- Patient with bleeding is considered high risk.
- Octreotide, vasopressin infusion decreases the bleeding.
- Balloon tamponade, Sengstaken-Blakemore → temporary control → ETT intubation.
- EGD sclerotherapy or varix ligation, but less successful than esophageal.
- Interventional radiology for TIPS if Portal HTN.
- Splenectomy is effective for isolated gastric varices.
- Operative mortality rate is 5%.
- Liver TPx in cirrhotic liver is the Tx of choice.

Hypertrophic Gastropathy (Menetrier Disease) (MD)
- Two diseases with hypertrophy: ZES and MD.
- MD-associated protein losing gastropathy + hypochlorhydria.

- Large rugal fold in proximal stomach (antral sparing).
- Biopsy → hyperplasia.
- Mucus-secreting cells.
- Overexpression EGF in mucosa → increase EGFR and receptor tyrosine kinese.
- Some suggest treatment with EGFR blocking is successful.
- Epigastric pain, weight loss, diarrhea, hypoproteinemia.
- Usually, regress spontaneous.
- Gastric resection → if persistent bleeding, to ↓ protein loosing and ↓ risk of gastric CA.

Watermelon Stomach (Gastric Antral Vascular Ectasia)

- Parallel red strip atop mucosal fold.
- Histopathology: gastric antral vascular ectasia (GAVE)
- Blood vessels contain thrombus in lamina propria.
- Mucosal fibromuscular hyperplasia.
- Distal stomach is affected.
- GAVE in older female with anemia, associated with connective tissue disease (autoimmune).
- 25% has liver disease.
- Treatment: estrogen, progesterone, EGD with ND (YAG laser or argon plasma).
- Antrectomy to control bleeding.
- Patient with portal HTN and GAVE → TIPS.

Dieulafoy Lesion

- Congenital AVM, large submucosal artery → eroded → pulsatile bleeding.
- Middle-aged men + CLD.
- EGD with hemostatic agent, angioembolization, or surgery → oversew or resection.

Bezoar

- Indigestible matter, trichobezoar (hair).
- Young female → obstructive.
- Diagnosis by upper GI series and confirmed by EGD.
- Treatment: papain, cellulose, acetylcysteine, Coca-Cola.
- If persistent → EGD removal or surgery.

Diverticula
- Solitary, congenital / acquired.
- Congenital → true, bulge of muscular layer.
- Acquired → no muscular layer → because of pulsion.
- Mostly in posterior cardia or fundus.
- Usually asymptomatic but can produce pain or bleeding.
- Laparoscopic removal if symptomatic.

Foreign Body (FB)
- EGD and removal for body packer, battery, corrosive object.
- If not a harmful object (e.g., coin) and passed the pylorus → it will pass spontaneously.

Volvulus
- Associated with large hiatal hernia but can be without it.
- Types
    o Mesenteroaxial: bisects the lesser and greater curvature i.e. the antrum rotates anteriorly and superiorly (flip up)
    o Organoaxial: the stomach rotates around an axis that connects the GEJ and the pylorus.
- Often chronic and asymptomatic.
- Complications: strangulation and infarction (common with organoaxial.
- If symptomatic → NGT → emergent surgery.
- Resection or not, gastropexy or not, depending on the situation.
- For elective reduction of stomach, repair of hiatal hernia, gastropexy through laparoscopy is the procedure of choice.

Gastrostomy
- Drainage or decompression or feeding.
- Technique: PEG, laparoscopic-assisted, open (Stamm, Witzel, Janeway).
- Janeway is created as a permanent stoma.
- Most commonly used is Stamm (open or laparoscopy).
- Complications: infectious, dislodgement, leak.

Upper Gastrointestinal Bleeding (UGIB)
- More common than LGIB.
- 90% identified by EGD.
- Common causes: PUD, neoplasm, CD, NSAID-induced erosion, esophageal varices (CLD), vasculitis, intussusception, gastritis, MWS, esophageal varices.
- Less common: benign, malignant neoplasm, angiodysplasia, dieulafoy lesion, menetrier disease, and watermelon stomach.
- Obscure bleeding → 10% (angiodysplasia, 75%; neoplasm, 10%).
- Meckel's diverticulum is the most common of obscure GI bleeding in pediatrics.
- Presentation: hematemesis, anemia, occult blood in stool or melena, hematochezia.
- Diagnosis: NGT, EGD, enteroscopy, intra-operative push enteroscopy, capsule and Sonde enteroscopy.
  - Push: allow visualization of 60 cm of jejunum, diagnostic (3%–65%).
  - Sonde: thin fiber-optic (50%–70%) visualization of small bowel, no therapeutic advantage or biopsy.
- Capsule identifies 90% of the bleeding.
      If all above not identified the bleeding → enteroclysis.
      If still not identified → angiography.
      ^{99m}Tc RBC scanning if +ve angiography.

- Management:
  - ABC.
  - History and physical examination.
- Need to ask the following:
  a. What is the magnitude and acuity of bleeding—high BP, low BP, low Hb—mental status, hematemesis?
  b. Any chronic illness?
  c. Is patient on anticoagulant or immunosuppression?
  d. EGD, varices, active bleeding, visible vessels, deep ulcer.
- NGT to determine the cause of bleeding, i.e., upper or lower.
- PPI, octreotide, antibiotic (↓ risk of bleeding and rebleeding).
- Crossmatching, ICU, surgeon, gastroentrology consultation → EGD within 12 hrs after resuscitation and correction of coagulopathy.

- EGD (diagnostic and therapeutic) → offer injection of epinephrine, hemoclips, cauterization, banding.
- If the source is esophageal or gastric, varices can temporarily introduce Sengstaken-Blakemore tube (consider TIPS) and definitive treatment by liver TPx.
- If still no source identified → tagged RBC scan.
- Angiography is diagnostic and therapeutic by embolization.
- If still bleeding or concomitant perforation or obstruction → operative intervention, intra-opetaive enteroscopy + multiple bowel clamping + bowel transillumination, then resection and anastomosis.

Premalignant Condition
- Atrophic gastritis, 90%; adenoma, 2.5%; verrucous gastritis, 1.5%; hyperplastic polyps, 0.53%; chronic ulcer, 0.68%.

- Polyps
    1. Neoplastic
        - Adenoma has 10%–20% risk of malignancy (villous > tubular).
        - Fundic gland polyp.

    2. Non-neoplastic
        - Hyperplastic
        - Hamartomatous
        - Inflammatory
    - In general, non-neoplastic has no risk.
    - Fundic gland polyp → long PPI use → not premalignant unless associated with FAP.
    - Large hyperplastic > 2 cm → dysplasia or CIS.
    - Adenomas are premalignant like colon.
    - FAP → ↑ risk tenfolds to develop CA.
    - Patient with HNCRC → stomach CA.
    - Polyps > 1 cm → excision or biopsy.

- Atrophic gastritis
    - Caused by H. pylori, PPI medication.

- Intestinal metaplasia
  - Precursor lesion, goblet cells, if treating H. pylori → ↓ metaplasia.

- Benign gastric ulcer
  - The ulcer is malignant until proven otherwise.

- Gastric CA remnant
  - Develops 10 years after resection.
  - High with simple-loop gastrojejunostomy ↓in Roux-en-Y

- Other premalignant state
  - Mutated E-cadherin has ↑ risk of malignancy → prophylactic gastrectomy.
  - 10% is familial stomach CA.
  - 10% is HNPCC stomach CA.
  - 10% mucosal hyperplasia of Menetrier disease, needs periodic EGD.
  - Glandular hyperplasia associated with gastrinoma, not premalignant but ↑ ECL + carcinoid.

Malignant Neoplasm of Stomach
- Adenocarcinoma, 95%; lymphoma, 4%; GIST, 1% (rare); angiosarcoma; carcinosarcoma.
- From another hematogenous metastasis (melanoma, breast).
- Invasion by adjacent organ (colon, pancreas).
- Peritoneal seeding.

Adenocarcinoma
- Fifth most commom GIT CA.
- Third leading to death.
- 5 years, SR is 26%.
- Black: white = 2:1.
- In young age, aggressive, poorly differentiated, and may infiltrate all layers (linitis plastic).
- Affects low socioeconomic.
- Common in China, Japan, and Korea.

Etiology
-   Pernicious anemia, blood group A^+, family history (50%).
-   When patients migrate from a high-incidence region to a low-incidence region, the risk of gastric cancer decreases in the subsequent generations born in the new region.
-   Diet: pickled, salted, smoked, nitrate food.
-   Smoking, atrophic gastritis, HNCRC (Lynch syndrome), CDH mutation, FAP, Menetrier disease ↑ risk of stomach CA.
-   With H. pylori, the risk is threefold.
-   EBV predispose 10% of stomach CA
-   Aspirin, fresh fruit, vitamin C and E, ↓ stomach CA.
-   Bone marrow–derived stem cells play a role in pathogenesis and lower risk of esophageal CA (distal) and proximal stomach CA.
-   Genetic aneuploidy:
    -   Most common genetic abnormality with stomach CA → P53, COX-2 genetic (⅔).
    -   Overexpression COX-2 → more aggressive.
    -   Germline CDH1 gene-encoding E-cadherin → prophylactic gastrectomy should be considered

Pathology
-   Dysplasia
    -   Precurser for gastric adenocarcinoma.
    -   Gastric resection for severe dysplasia and multifocal.
    -   EMR if localized.
    -   If mild → follow-up EGD surveillance + biopsy + H. pylori treatment.

-   Early gastric CA
    -   Limited to mucosa and submucosa regardless of LNs.
    -   10% will have +ve LNs.
    -   70% well differentiated, 30% poorly differentiated.
    -   Cure rate with gastric resection and lymphadenectomy → 95%.

- Japan picks up 50% of cases in early stage, while in USA, 20%.
- Small intramucosal → EMR.

Types:

Type 0-I	Protruded, polypid
Type 0-IIa	Elevated
Type 0-IIb	Flat
Type 0-IIc	Depressed
Type 0-III	Excavated

- **Gross and microscopic:**
  - Four gross forms polypoid, fungating, ulcerative, scirrhous.
  - Scirrhous → infiltrates all layers (linitis plastica) → poor prognosis, is technically resectable but microscopic infiltration to esophagus and duodenal → recurrence within 6 months, but chemotherapy increases survival.
  - 40% distal, 30% middle, 30% proximal.

- **Pathology (histology)**
  - Prognosis factors: LNs, depth, tumor grade (degree of differentiation).
  - Lauren classification: intestinal, 55%; diffuse, 33%; unclassified, 14%.
  - Intestinal: less aggressive.
  - Ming classification: expanding, 67%; infiltrative, 33%.
  - Diffused: poorly differentiated with young patient.
  - HER2 overexpression → 15%–25% unfavorabl prognosis → trastuzumab → improves SR.
  - IHC stain for HER2 is mandatory.

- **Pathological staging**
  - TNM
    - Tis Mucosa, no invasion to lamina propria, dysplasia
    - T1   Invades lamina propria, muscularis mucosa

T1b	Invades submucosa
T2	Invades musculosa
T3	Invade serosa
T4a	Perforated serosa
T4b	Invades adjacent structure
N1	1–2 LNs
N2	3–6 LNs
N3	N3a, 7–15 LNs; N3b > 16 LNs
M0	No metastasis
M1	Metastatic disease

Symptoms

- Mostly advanced stage III, IV when diagnosed.
- Pain, ↓ appetite, weight loss, anorexia, nausea and vomiting.
- GI bleeding (5%) (acute) but chronic → anemia.
- Physical examination is unremarkable but can have epigastric fullness or Sister Mary Joseph's nodule, Virchow's LNs (left supraclavicular), or Blumer's shelf (prerectal metastasis) deposition of tumor is rectovaginal pouch.
- Trousseau (thrombophlebitis), acanthosis nigricans → pigmentation of axilla and groin.
- Metastasis to lung → pleural effusion. •
- T4 large. tumor, i.e. ↑ chance of liver metastasis, carcinomatosis → to ovary (Krukenberg tumor)
- Malignant ascites.

Diagnosis and Staging

- Screening not recommended in Europe.
- EGD is the diagnostic tool of choice.
- EGD + biopsy if −ve with high suspicion clinically or endoscopic → re-EGD with aggressive biopsy.
- LNs +ve in 60%–75%.
- CT for metastasis.
- +ve peritoneal cytology = stage IV.
- Double contrast barium → 75% sensitive.
- Magnifying endoscopy → NBI (microvisualization) for mucosa.

- Preoperative staging with CT chest, abdomen, and pelvis or MRI.
- Best to stage locally EUS, shows also LN > 5 mm.
- Some center: T3 or +ve LNs → neoadjuvant chemotherapy.
- PET whole body → distant metastasis and local regional, but PET-CT is best.
- Laparoscopic staging and peritoneal cytology → cytology +ve (micro carcinomatosis).
- Poor prognosis can be improved by aggressive adjuvant therapy → systemic chemotherapy or HIPEC → but currently no change in management, and you should have −ve margin.
- If laparoscopic exploration is performed and you find impressive carcinomatosis → change operative plan and avoid futile procedure.

Treatment

- **Endoscopic Mucosal Resection (EMR)**
  - Early stage, no LNs.
  - According to Japan gastric cancer association, for differentiated mucosal CA < 2 cm, no ulceration, no LNs metastasis → endoscopic resection.
- **Endoscopic submucosal dissection (ESD)**
  - Tumor smaller than 3 cm confined to mucosal, ↓ LNs (3%), no ulcer, no pigmentation.
  - Additional laparoscopic LNs sampling in selected patient.

  NB
  R0 −ve margin
  R1 microscopic +ve margin on tumor (ink)
  R2 +ve margin

- **Surgical Excision: Main Concern**
  - Surgical resection is only curative in gastric CA.
  - The goal is (R0) resection, to all margins.
  - Subtotal or total gastrectomy= no difference.
  - Grossly −ve 5 cm, if diffused > 5 cm.

- Frozen section to confirm −ve is important.
- Fifteen LNs are adequate for staging.
- En bloc resection with adjacent structure (colon, spleen, pancreas) if involved.
- If R1 → poor prognosis.
- NCCN does not recommend re-operation after R1.
- Extent for gastrectomy:
  - → Subtotal radical gastrectomy unless R0 cant be achieved → total gastrectomy.
- Ligate left and right gastric and gastroepiploic + en bloc removal of distal (75%) + pylorus + 2 cm of duodenum + greater and lesser omentum + all associated LNs → > 15 LNs.
- Reconstruction by Billroth II, but if gastric remnant is too small → Roux-en-Y.
- In Japan, they perform Billroth 1, i.e., one anastomosis.
- Operative mortality is 2%–5%.
- Proximal tumor → total gastrectomy + esophagogastrostomy + vagotomy + pyloroplasty → if the pylorus is left intact → bile reflux esophagitis, decrease gastric emptying.

- **Lymphadenectomy**
  - Still controversial.
    - D0 Not effort to remove LNs
    - D1 Excision of perigastric nodes
    - D2 D1+ LNs located along main trunk of celiac axis
  - D1 = 1, 2, 3, 4a–b, 5, 6, 7.
  - D2 = D1+ 8a, 9, 10, 11, and 12a.
  - Dutch and British showed no difference in D1 vs. D2 lymphadenectomy, but D2 has increased postoperative morbidity. In this trial, distal pancreatectomy + splenectomy included with D2.
  - In the USA and many Western countries, remove only D1.
  - In Japan (SRGC) and Asia, the standard is D2 = remove peritoneal layer over anterior mesocolon

+ node along hepatic and splenic artery + crural LNs.

- Splenectomy + distal pancreatectomy is not routinely performed.
- D2 LNs resection has ↑ mortality and morbidity.
- But if D2 is performed → perisplenic LNs resection + splenectomy (to fulfill criteria of D2).

- **Chemoradiation for CA**
  - 5 years SR of resected adenocarcinoma for stages I, II, III, 75%, 50%, 25%, respectively.
  - Chemotherapy (5-FU and leucovorin), radiotherapy (4,500 cGY) → SR.
  - To benefit from adjuvant therapy→ should have adequate operation, i.e., R0.
  - Japan: stage T2b, T3, T4 → surgery alone + D2 → 5 years, SR is 69%.

  - **Neoadjuvant**
    - Neoadjuvant chemotherapy, survival.
    - Neoadjuvant for T3 or N1.
    - USA and Europe, R0 with neoadjuvant chemo- radiation.
    - It is recommended with locoregional advanced disease.

  - **Adjuvant**
    - Unfortunately, even with R0, it has high recurrence in 2 years.
    - Adjuvant chemotherapy and radiation, survival.
    - Adjuvant therapy is standard of care in USA.

Palliation
- Palliative with advanced disease is 50%.
- Palliative chemotherapy.
- Palliative procedure = stent, jejunostomy feeding.

Prognosis
- 5 years, SR is increased from .15% to 22% in USA depending on TNM.

Screening surveillance
- Periodic EGD + biopsy.
- Patient with FAP, HNPCC, Menetrier disease needs to shorten the interval.

Gastric Lymphoma
- 4%–50% is NHL.
- Most common site of primary lymphoma.
- Most common type is B cell, a type of mucosa-associated lymphoid tissue (MALT).
- ½ is low grade.
- Risk factors: Chronic gastritis, H.pylori.
- If H.pylori eradicated and lymphoma persists → stage I.
- Chemotherapy without radiotherapy for advanced disease III, IV.
- Lymphadenopathy and organomegaly suggest the diagnosis.
- EUS, CT, bone marrow biopsy.
- Most high-grade treatment → chemotherapy + radiation.
- Radical gastrectomy + D2 lymphadencetomy if bulky, perforation, or bleeding.

Gastrointestinal Stromal Tumor (GIST)
- GIST is the most common sarcoma of GIT, 1% of GIT neoplasm.
- Mutation of proto-oncogenes c-KIT.
- Arises from interstitial cell of Cajal (ICC).
- Differ from leiomyoma and sarcoma as they are not arise from smooth muscle.
- 75% mutation in c-KIT, 10% with mutation PDGRF-α, other BRAF.
- Prognosis depends on size, mitosis, metastasis.
- Metastasis by hematogenous.
- Any lesions > 1 cm behave as malignant.
- All GIST should be resected with −ve margin.
- Express c-KIT (CD117).

- Smooth muscle tumor expresses actin and desmin.
- ⅔ GIST in the gastric body.
- Submucosal tumor slowly growing.
- Metastasized to liver, lung, and sometimes LNs.
- Diagnosis by endoscopy and biopsy.
- Metastatic workup by CT CAP.
- Wedge resection is suffiecient unless it is large or invading → en bloc resection.
- 5 years, SR is 50%, high grade, 30%.

- **Clinical Picture**
  - Disease of old people, 60s.
  - Stomach, 40%–60%; small bowel, 25%–35%; majority in jejunum and ileum.
  - Median size is 5–7 cm.
  - Bleeding ¼ of patient from mucosal erosion or if intraperitoneal rupture.
  - LNs involvement is rare, 5%.
  - In pediatric population: male, multifocal, frequent LNs, and imatinib resistance.

- **Workup**
  - CT is test of choice.
  - For periampullary and rectum → MRI.
  - FDG-PET for metastasis.
  - Can be diagnosed incidentally during EGD, FNA sensitivity is 70%–80%.
    → Spindle cells c-KIT positive by IHC.
    → Core biopsy is required as FNA is inconclusive.
  - If radiologically appears GIST, biopsy is not required.

- **Risk Stratification**
  1. Tumor size
  2. Mitotic rate
  3. Location
  4. Classification

Very low	< 2 cm	< 5/50 HPF
Low	2–5 cm	< 5/50 HPF
Intermediate	< 5 cm	6–10/50 HPF

High   5-10 cm> 5-10/50 HPF

- Size > 5 cm, mitosis > 5/50, non-gastric → poor outcome.

- **Surgery for Primary Disease**
  - NCCN recommends that if tumor > 2 cm → resection.
  - Reasonable to resect < 2 cm lesion by EGD.
  - At the time of surgery, inspect peritoneum, liver surface.
  - Avoid spillage.
  - R0 is the goal, no wide margin, no LNs.
  - No difference between -ve margin 1 cm vs. 5 cm.
  - Open surgery is preferred.
  - If large and huge, it may require extensive resection such as gastrectomy; splenectomy requires en bloc resection → if recognized preoperative → neoadjuvant imatinib.
  - If the tumor in the small bowel → resection and anastomosis.
  - If the tumor near ampulla → pancreaticoduodenectomy.
  - Neoadjuvant considered in duodenum and rectum.

- **Neoadjuvant Imatinib**
  - Imatinib (Gleevec) tyrosine kinase inhibitor (TKI) and PDGFR-α
  - Neoadjuvant, ↑ resectability.
  - Used in locally advanced large tumor, difficult location.
  - CT followup after initial treatment by 4 weeks.

- **Adjuvant Imatinib**
  - In metastatic disease or unresectable tumor → result is dramatic.
  - ↑ survival, SR 5 years.
  - If ≥ 5 mitosis 150 HPF or any non-gastric > 5 cm.
  - Should prolong the course to decrease recurrence.
  - Imatinib prolongs survival in metastatic disease, > 5 years.

-   Surgery R0 + imatinib ↑ recurrence-free survival (RFS).

Gastric Carcinoid Tumor

-   Rare (1%), arises from gastric enterochromaffin–like (ECL) cells, potentially malignant.
-   Increase incidence → ↑ use of EGD, ↑ PPI.
-   ↑ PPI, ↑ gastrin → ↑ ECL.
-   It's a subtype of neuroendocrine tumor (NET).
-   Three types:
    -   Type I—75% with chronic high gastrin secondary to pernicious anemia or atrophic gastritis < 5% metastasis.
    -   Type II—with MEN I and ZES, 10% metastasis.
    -   Type III—sporadic, Solitary > 2 cm, no increase in gastrin, most have nodal or distant metastasis.
-   Diagnosis by EGD and biopsy; EUS is helpful for submucosal lesion.
-   CT and octreotide scan are useful for staging.
-   Treatment: resection.

    Type I, II—EMR.

    Large → gastrectomy + D1 or D2.

-   SR with −ve LNs is 95% and with +ve LNs, 50%.
-   Somatostatin analogue (Octreotide) useful to control symptom, but doesn't increase SR.

Subtotal Gastrectomy

-   After induction of anesthesia, do time-out to make sure of the patient's name, procedure, staff names, then position the patient.
-   A midline incision is made from the xiphoid to below the umbilicus.
-   A bilateral subcostal incision may also be used if the patient has a shallow costal angle.
-   If operating for cancer, the entire omentum is mobilized superiorly en bloc with the stomach.
-   Kocher maneuver is performed to mobilize the duodenum.
-   The right gastroepiploic vessels are divided beyond the pylorus.

- The right gastric vessels should be divided at the left edge of the porta hepatis.
- The duodenum is circumferentially dissected about 2 cm distal to the pylorus and divided with a linear stapler.
- The lesser omentum is divided close to the liver.
- The left gastric artery is divided and ligated.
- Any remaining short gastric vessels on the greater curvature of the stomach are ligated and divided up to the level of the gastroesophageal junction.
- The stomach is divided using two linear staplers.
- The first stapler is applied at approximate right angles to the greater curvature.
- The second firing of the stapler should be angled up to the top of the lesser curvature of the stomach, within 1–2 cm of the esophagus.
- The proximal jejunum is brought up to the stomach in either an antecolic or retrocolic position for reconstruction (Billroth II).

Postgastrectomy Problem
Dumping

- Destruction or bypass of the pylorus.
- 5%–10% after pyloplasty, pyloromyotomy, distal gastrectomy.
- Abrupt delivering of hyperosmolar load into small bowel after 15–30 min.
- Tachycardia, diaphoresis, weakness.
- It can be produced by NS infusion.
- Crampy abdominal pain and diarrhea.
- Late dumping, 2–3 hrs postprandial → relieved by administering sugar.
- Early dumping due to increase in VIP, CCK, neurotensin, renin-angiotensin-aldosterone, low ANP, and peripheral hormone peptide YY.
- Late dumping due to ↓ glucose, ↑ insulin.
- Treatment: medical, dietary, and octreotide; avoid fluid with meal, milkshakes (hyperosmolar).
- Octreotide 100 ug SC BID up to 500 daily → and restoration of fast MMC.
- Alpha-glucosidase decreases symptom.

- Few require surgery.
- Treatment: reverse segment (10 cm) interposition between stomach and small bowel (Henley loop)
- In refractory cases → Roux-en-Y + vagotomy + hemigastrectomy is considered.

Diarrhea
- Post-truncal vagotomy, dumping, malabsorption, blind loop.
- Tx: cholestyramine, codeine, loperamide, octreotide.
- Fat malabsorption, ↑ stomach motility, bacterial overgrowth.
- 10 cm reverse jejunal interposition.
- Both procedures → obstructive and bacterial overgrowth.

Gastric Stasis
- Vagotomy or resection of main peacemaker.
- Stricture, efferent limb kink, retrograde peristalsis.
- EGD, GI series, gastric-emptying scan.
- EGG, manometry.
- Treatment: diet, promotility, antibiotic for bacterial overgrowth.
- If following vagotomy + drainage → subtotal gastrectomy and simple-loop gastrojejunostomy.
- Billroth II is preferable than Roux-en-Y.
- If following distal gastrectomy → near-total 95% or total with Roux-en-Y.
- Gastric pacing is promising.

Bile Reflux Esophagitis
- Resection of pylorus → bile to esophagus.
- DDx: afferent or efferent loop obstruction, dysfunction of cardia.
- Diagnosis: x-ray, GI series, CT scan.
- Esophagus impedance, scintigraphy (bile reflux scan).
- After distal gastrecotmy:
  1. Roux-en-Y gastrojejunostomy.
  2. Interposition of 40 cm iso-peristaltic jejunal loop between remnant stomach and duodenal (Henley loop).
  3. Billroth II.

- Roux limb should be > 45 cm, preferably 60 cm, if too long, obstruction and malabsorption.
- Marginal ulcer → generous distal gastrectomy.
- If gastrojejunostomy with reflux (bile) → take down the anastomosis → Roux en Y.

Roux Syndrome
- Pain, vomiting, weight loss.
- GI series → delayed gastric emptying.
- Treatment: promotility.
    - Surgical resection of the remnant stomach, if severe, total gastrectomy.
    - Roux limb should be resected if dilated and flaccid → short bowel syndrome.

Gallstone
- Secondary to vagal denervation.
- If gallbladder stone → incidental cholecystectomy.

Weight Loss
- Vagotomy and gastric resection.
- Alter dietary intake and malabsorption.
- Anorexia due to loss of ghrelin.

Anemia
- Intrinsic factor impaired after gastrectomy which is important to vit B12 absorption.
- Also gastrectomy impair the iron metabolism → Fe^{+++} + HCL + vitamin C → Fe^{++} to be absorbed.
- Treatment: vitamin B12, folate, iron.

Bone Disease
- Gastric surgery → disturb Ca^{++} + vitamin D.
- Ca^{++} absorption in duodenum, which is bypassed by GJ.
- Fat malabsorption → blind loop → bacteria ↓ vitamin D, fat-soluble vitamin
- Treatment: Ca^{++} + vitamin D.

Small Bowel

Anatomy

- 4–6 meters in length.
- Duodenum, jejunum, and ileum.
- Jejunum, 40%; ileum, 60%.
- Internal mucosal fold plicae circularis or valvulae conniventes (concertina) more in proximal bowel (jejunum).
- Jejunum is wider, thicker, has less fat, long vasa recta, and prominent plicae cirulares, but ileum has more prominent lymphoid follicles.
- Blood supply:
     Proximal duodenum → celiac and SMA.
     Jejunum and ileum → SMA.
- Venus → SMV.
- LNs → cisterna chyli → thoracic duct → left subclavian vein.
- Nerve supply: parasympathetic, vagus; sympathetic, splanchnic nerve.

Histology

- Mucosa: (epithelium, lamina propria, muscularis mucosa)
    - Villi and crypt
    - Enterocyte, goblet, enteroendocrine, Paneth cell
    - Villus and crypt life span is 2–5 days then apoptosis/ exofoliation
    - Enterocyte: absorption, microvilli, surface area 40 times
    - Goblet: mucin (defense)
    - Enteroendocrine: secretory granules
    - Paneth cells → secretory, digestion, antimicrobial
- Submucosa: strongest layer, contains blood vessels, LNs (Meissner plexus).
- Musculosa: outer → longitudal, inner → circular (Auerbach's or myenteric plexus)
- Serosa

Development
- Endoderm in the fourth week.
- On the sixth week, vitelline duct → obliterate at the end → if incomplete → Meckel's diverticulum.
- Mesoderm split → adhere to endoderm → visceral peritoneum.
- Mesoderm split → adhere to ectoderm → parietal peritoneum.
- Fifth weeks GA → herniate outside the abdominal cavity → at tenth week, retracted back.
- Organogenesis completed in 12 weeks.

Physiology
- Digestion and absorption
  - Active and passive transport, transcellular, paracellular.
  - Passive: diffusion active by energy through cell.
- Water and electrolyte absorption + secretion
  - Daily, 8–9 L enter small bowel, 80% get absorbed and leave 1.5 L to the colon.
- Carbohydrate
  - 45% amylase (salivary and pancreas).
- Protein
  - 10%–15% endogenous, pepsin at stomach.
  - Trypsinogen → trypsin.
  - Glutamine: major source of energy of enterocyte.
- Fat
  - 40% start in proximal jejunum.
  - Long-chain triglyceride. (Reminder: phospholipid, lecithin, fatty acid, cholesterol, fat-soluble vitamin.)
  - Fat starts to absorb in proximal jejunum.
  - Lipolysis → fatty acid and monoglyceride start in lipase of stomach then pancreas catalyzed.
  - Bile acid → lipolysis.
  - Bile salt → absorption at terminal ileum.
- Vitamins
  - Vitamin B12 + intrinsic factor absorption at terminal ileum.
  - Water-soluble vitamins: vitamin C, folate, vitamin B complex.
  - Fat-soluble vitamins: KEDA.

- Ca^{++} absorption occurs in duodenum, better formula is calcium citrate.
- Mg^{+++}, Cu^{++}, and iron absorbed in duodenum + proximal jejunum.

- Barrier and immune function
  - IgA, GALT (gut-associated lymphoid tissue) like Peyer's patch, mesenteric LNs, lymphoid follicle.
  - Communication of microbiota + host defense and prevention of inflammatory response → such as Crohn's.
- Motility
  - Two pattern of motion:
    - Following the meal: segmentation contraction and peristalsis
    - The interdigestive period: also known as the migrating motor complex (MMC)
  - Excitatory transmitter: acetylcholine, substance P.
  - Inhibitory transmitter: NO, VIP, ATP.
- Endocrine
  - Secretin family: glucagon, GIP, VIP.
  - Somatostatin.
- Adaptation
  - Villi lengthening, ↑ absorption area.
  - Takes 1–2 years.
  - Stimulates intergrowth: peptide, pancreatic secretion, fiber, fatty acid, glutamine.
  - Jejunal resection → tolerate; ileal, compensate.

Pathology
Small Bowel Obstruction
Epidemiology
  - Intrinsic:
    - Intraluminal: foreign body, gallstone, meconium.
    - Intramural: tumor, Crohn's disease.
  - Extrinsic: adhesion, hernia, carcinomatosis.
  - Intra-abdominal adhesion related to prior surgery account, 75% of small bowel obstruction.
  - Intestinal malrotation and midgut volvulus are important DDx in pediatrics.

- Rare cause: SMA syndrome.

Pathophysiology
- Gas + fluid accumulates proximal to the obstruction.
- Swallowed air represents 70% and gas fermentation, 30%.
- Fluid from swallowed saliva + intestinal juice.
- ↑ distension, ↓ motility.
- Translocation of bacteria.
- ↑ pressure → ischemia (strangulation).
- Partial obstruction → portion of lumen occluded → allowing gas and fluid to pass.
- Closed loop obstruction (volvulus), exaggerated symptom.

Clinical Presentation
- Cardinal symptoms: pain, distension, vomiting, and obstipation.
- If proximal obstruction → vomiting.
- If distal obstruction → distension.
- Hyperactive motility initially, then ↓.
- Laboratory → ↓ volume, ↑ WBCs.
- Feature of ischemia: tachycardia, abdominal tenderness (localized), fever, ↑↑ WBCs, acidosis.

Diagnosis
- Distinguish mechanical obstruction from ileus.
- Partial or complete obstruction.
- Simple or strangulation.
- Prior abdominal surgery.
- Examination: → rule out hernia.
- Radiological: AXR supine and erect, CXR erect.
- Findings: dilated small bowel > 3 cm; air fluid level: little air in the colon (70%–80%), but specificity is low because of ileus + colon obstruction.
- CT: sensitivity and specificity, 80%–90%.
- Transition zone, dilated proximally and collapsed distally; contrast not passing the transition zone.
- Can detect closed loop or strangulation U- or C-shaped dilated bowel.

- Strangulation: thickening of bowel wall, pneumatosis intestinalis, portal vein gas, mesenteric haziness, ↓ enhancement of the wall.
- CT with oral water soluble or dilated barium water soluble → diagnostic and therapeutic as laxative effect, within 24 hrs, but doesn't ↓ surgical intervention.
- Low sensitivity (50%) in partial bowel obstruction.
- Fecalization of small bowel → chronic obstruction.
- Gastrografin in case of perforation.
- Enteroclysis: 200 mL of barium followed by 1–2 L of methylcellulose in water to distal jejunum by long NGT (double contrast), better assessment of mucosal surface (small lesion) (parietal obstruction), superior to AXR and CT with contrast.

Treatment
- Fluid resuscitation → Foley for UOP.
- CVP or PAC monitoring.
- Broad-spectrum antibiotics.
- NGT.
- Standard for complete obstruction → surgery.
- Non-operative management (some advocators).
- Early intervention to minimize complication.
- Conservative treatment in the form of NGT, IVF for the following:
    - Partial obstruction
    - Post-operative ileus
    - Crohn's disease
    - Carcinomatosis
- 61%–81% success rate in patient with partial obstruction.
- If patient doesn't improve within 24 hrs → surgery.
- Ileus—0.7% after laparotomy.
    - Function returns in 3–5 days.
    - AXR: air fluid level → 30% will not have.
    - Non-operative treatment → 2–3 weeks; NPO, IVF, TPN, but if peritonitis → exploration.
- In patient with Crohn's disease → bypass.
- Treat accordingly as follows:
    - Adhesions are lysed.

- Tumor is resected.
- Hernia is reduced and repaired.
- Viability criteria:
  - Normal colon and peristalsis, mesenteric artery pulsation, can use Doppler for perfusion → IV fluorescein, UV illumination.
- If not viable → resection and anastomosis.
- Uncertain viability → second look in 24–48 hrs.
- Role of laparoscopy (adhesive band) → conversion to open, 17%–33%.

Outcome

- For a patient with adhesive intestinal obstruction, the treatment is conservative; 20% of them will have readmissions over subsequent 5 years.
- Mortality rate (MR) for non-strangulated surgery is 5% and with strangulated, 8%–25%, and after colorectal surgery, 30%, within 10 years.

Prevention

- Good surgical technique, careful handling of tissue, minimal use and exposure of peritoneum.
- Use of laparoscopy when possible as open has four- to fivefold higher risk.
- Use of hyaluronan-based agent (Seprafilm).
- Do not wrap anastomosis with any material e.g. Surgicel.

Paralytic Ileus

- Ileus + pseudo-obstruction.
- Most cause of morbidity and delayed discharge.

Pathophysiology

- Causes: abdominal surgery, infection, inflammation, electrolyte, drugs.
- Abdominal surgery → stress-induced sympathetic reflexes → ↑ inflammatory mediator release anesthetic/analgesic will decrease motility.
- Small bowel return to normal within 24 hrs; colon, 48 hrs to 3–5 days.

- Listening is not reliable → passing flatus is more reliable.
- Chronic pseudo-obstruction → smooth muscle and myentric plexus → degeneration and fibrosis of muscular propria has the following causes:
  - Primary cause
    - Familial visceral myopathy
  - Secondary cause
    - Smooth muscle disorder: collagen disease (scleroderma), amyloidosis
    - Neuro disorder: Parkinson's disease, spinal cord injury
    - Endocrine: hypothyroidism, DM
    - Radiation enteritis
    - Drugs: phenobarbital, antidepressant

Clinical Presentation
- ↓ appetite, nausea and vomiting, ↓ flatus, distension.
- Bowel sound: low or absent.

Diagnosis
- If it persists for 3–5 days or occurs in absence of abdominal surgery → further evaluation to r/o mechanical obstruction.
- Review drugs.
- Electrolyte abnormalities.
- Radiography; in post-operative patients, it's better to be evaluated with CT scan.
- Chronic pseudo-obstruction needs radiological study and manometry.
- Diagnostic laparoscopy or open for full-thickness biopsy.

Therapy
- NPO, IVF, electrolyte.
- Correct underlying cause.
- NGT.
- May need TPN if prolonged.
- Early ambulation, decrease ileus but new evidence showed feeding protocol → ↑ motility.
- Use NSAIDs instead of opioid; use epidural (thoracic).

- Studies showed limiting the intra- and postoperative IVF → decreases ileus.
- The most useful method is chewing gum to enhance GI motility.
- Alvimopan, an oral opioid antagonist.
- Lipid-rich nutrition → CCK → vagovagal reflex.
- Prokinetic has poor efficiency.
- Cisapride → cardiac toxicity.
- May require decompressive gastrostomy or small bowel resection (rare).

Crohn's Disease (CD)

- Chronic idiopathic transmural chronic inflammation mostly affects distal ileum, but any part can be affected in gastrointestinal tract (from mouth to rectum).
- Incidence 3.3–8 per 100,000 and increasing dramatically.
- High in Eastern Europeans and Ashkenazi Jews by two- to fourfold.
- In China, 1.38 per 100,000.
- Female > male.
- The 30s age-group is the highest peak, and 60s is another peak, but it can affect any age-group.
- Genetic and environmental factors play an important role.
- First degree relative with CD ↑ the risk by fourteen- to fifteenfold.
- In monozygote twins, 67%.
- Simple Mendelian inheritance pattern.
- ↑ in high socioeconomic class.
- Breastfeeding is protective.
- Smoking has ↑↑ need of surgery and chance of relapse.

Pathophysiology

- Stimulus is unknown.
- Hypothesis: environmental and genetic factors.
- Infection: listeria, pseudomonas, mycobacteria, paratuberculosis.
- Abnormal epithelial barrier or immune dysregulation.

- Poor epithelial barrier → exposure of lamina propria lymphocyte to antigenic stimuli derived from the intestinal lumen.
- Chromosome 16 (IBD 1 locus) = NOD2 gene → fortyfold high.
- Earliest lesion → aphthous ulcer—3 mm ulcer halo of erythema.
- Granuloma is 70% of specimen → non-caseating in active disease and normal tissue (bowel layer and LNs).
- Linear ulcer → multiple ulcers fuse parallel to longitudinal axis (cobblestone appearance).
- Advanced disease → transmural → fibrosis stricture, intra-abdominal abscess, fistula, perforation (rare).
- Characterized by Skip lesion.
- Fat wrapping (mesenteric fat to serosa).
- In ulcerative colitis (UC) → mucosa and submucosa are involved and continuous and affect rectum, but usually, the rectum is spared in CD.
- UC → can affect ileum as backwash ileitis.

Clinical Presentation
- Abdominal pain, diarrhea, weight loss.
- Can be any of the following:
  a) Fibrostenotic disease
  b) Fistulizing disease
  c) Aggressive inflammatory disease
- Constitutional symptoms.
- Affects small bowel by 80%; colon alone, 20%.
- Mostly in the ileocecal valve area.
- Isolated perineal disease and anorectal account, 5%–10%.
- Uncommon location: stomach, duodenum.
- ¼ has extraintestinal manifestation:
  • Dermatologic
    o Erythema nodosum, pyoderma gangrenosum
  • Rheumatologic
    o Peripheral arthritis, ankylosing spondylitis, sacroiliitis
  • Ocular
    o Conjunctivitis, uveitis/iritis episcleritis

273

- Hepatobiliary
  - Hepatic steatosis, cholelithiasis
  - Primary sclerosing cholangitis, pericholangitis
- Urologic
  - Nephrolithiasis, ureteral obstruction
- Miscellaneous
  - Thromboembolic disease
  - Vasculitis
  - Osteoporosis
  - Endocarditis, myocarditis, pleuropericarditis, interstitial lung disease
  - Amyloidosis
  - Pancreatitis
- Erythema nodosum, peripheral arthritis → severe disease.

Diagnosis

- endoscopy and Histopathology is the mainstay.
- DDx: IBS, mesenteric ischemia, UC, SLE, lymphoma, typhoid enteritis (salmonella), typhi infection, mycobacterium tuberculosis, diverticular disease, campylobacter, yersinia, CMV.
- Diagnosis → colonoscopy with intubation of terminal ileum is the main diagnostic tool and can reveal focal ulcerations adjacent to areas of normal-appearing mucosa, along with polypoid mucosal changes that give a "cobblestone appearance."
- Skip areas of involvement are typical finding, with segments of normal-appearing bowel interrupted by large areas of obvious disease; this pattern is different from the continuous involvement in UC.
- CT → for intra-abdominal collection, abscess.
- EGD for proximal disease, can use capsule.
- Histopathology: crypt abscess, destroyed mucosa, transmural inflammation deep to serosa.
- Antibody: perinuclear antineutrophil cytoplasmic antibody (P-ANCA) and anti–saccharomyces cerevisiae antibody (ASCA).
- P-ANCA −ve and ASCA +ve in CD.
- P-ANCA +ve and ASCA −ve in UC.

Therapy
- No curative therapy.
- Medical treatment for induced remission.
- Surgery for specific consideration.

- **Medical Therapy**
  - Antibiotic, aminosalicylate (5-ASA), mesalamine (Pentasa), corticosteroids, and immunosuppressants.
  - Antibiotic for infection and complication → perianal disease, enterocutaneous fistula, active colonic disease.
  - Oral glucocorticoid, IV used in severe active disease → but ineffective to prevent relapse → taper when remission, some are steroid dependent (i.e., recurrent when tapered) and some are not respondent (steroid resistant).
  - Thiopurine (6 mercaptopurine) to maintain remission for 3–6 months, S/E: bone marrow suppression.
  - Some studies → ↓ relapse when resection of the involved intestine.
  - If the patient is not responding → methotrexate IM.
  - Cyclosporine (little role).
  - Infliximab and anti-TNF-a → ↑ closure of enterocutaneous fistula → can be used in sepsis.
  - Biologic therapy like infliximab (Remicade); the newer agent is adalimumab (Humera).
  - Perianal disease = antibiotics such as flagyl or ciprofloxacin for 2–4 weeks.
  - In case of relapse = azathioprine.

- **Surgical Therapy**
  - General principle of operation in CD:
    o Midline incision → avoid stoma as possible.
    o Can be by laparoscopy.
    o Length of bowel removed → minimized.
    o Resection till grossly normal bowel.
    o Creation of stoma in ill patient, otherwise, if stable → primary anastomosis.
  - 50%–70% require at least one surgery.
  - In acute severe disease, Crohn's colitis, toxic megacolon.

- Failure of medical treatment.
- Complications: obstruction, perforation, hemorrhage, fistula.
- Complications of medication: cushinoid, growth retardation by 30% in children.
- Most common indication is obstruction.
- Abscess → interventional radiology.
- Less common: hemorrhage, perforation.
  - Segmental intestinal resection with primary anastomosis.
    - Grossly free margin, 2 cm = 12 cm.
    - No difference between stapler and handsewn.
  - Strictureplasty
    - Bowel is opened longitudinally and closed transversely.
    - Any ulcer → biopsy.
    - Heineke-Mikulicz pyroplasty if the segment < 12 cm.
    - Finney if < 25 cm.
    - For longer segment > 50 cm → side-to-side enteroenterostomy.
    - Strictureplasty marked with clip → radiological identification.
    - If stricture occurs after strictureplasty, i.e., recurrence → resection.
    - Contraindication of strictureplasty → intra-abdominal abscess or fistula.
    - Gastrojejunostomy bypass → if duodenum is involved.
    - Laparoscopy is good option, ↓ stay, ↓ pain, ↓ ileus, but recurrence = open.

Outcome

- Complication (15%–30%): wound infection, leak, intra-abdominal abscess.
- Recurrence is 70% within 1 year, 90% within 3 years.
- Reoperation in 7–10 years.
- Clinical recurrence is 60% within 5 years, 95% within 15 years.

Intestinal Fistula

- Fistula—abnormal communication between two epithelialized surfaces.
- Internal or external fistulas.
- Enterocutaneous   < 200 cc/day → low output fistula.
                     > 500 cc/day → high output fistula.
- 80% of enterocutaneous fistula is iatrogenic, enterotomies anastomosis, and wound dehiscence.
- If spontaneous → CD, cancer.

Pathophysiology

- Enteroenteric fistula → malabsorption.
- Enterovesical → UTI.
- Enterocutaneous fistula → irritation → excoriation.
- High otput fistula → dehydration, electrolyte disturbance.
- Fistula potentially closes spontaneously unless FRIENDS: foreign body, radiation, inflammation, epithelialization, malnutrition, distal obstruction, neoplasm, drugs (steroid).

Clinical Picture

- History iatrogenic insult, 5–10 days → fever, leukocytosis ileus, tenderness, wound infection.

Diagnosis

- CT with oral contrast.
- Abscess → percutaneous drainage.
- If fistula is not clear → small bowel series, enteroclysis to rule out distal obstructions.
- Fistulogram.

Therapy

- Stabilization: IVF, TPN, control of sepsis, antibiotics, drainage, skin protection by stoma bag.
- Definitive treatment.
- Rehabilitation.
- Oral feed can be attempted to distal fistula and low output.
- Somatostatin (octreotide) can be helpful in high-output fistula.

Timing of Surgical Intervention
- 2–3 months of conservative treatment.
- 90% will close at fifth week.
- Fistula tract with segmental resection.
- Simple closure → high recurrence.
- Studies on biological sealant reported.

Outcome
- Over 50% spontaneous closure, inhibit (FRIENDS) to accelerate healing.
- 30% recurrence if no resection.

Radiation Enteritis
- Radiation-induced injury.
- Transient condition (acute), 75%.
- Chronic, 5%–15%.

Pathology
- If received radiation > 4,500 cGy.
- Generation of free radicals.
- Induce cell death → free radicals → break double standard DNA.
- Mucosal sloughing, ulcer, hemorrhage.
- Associated complication: HTN, DM, CHD.
- ↑ incidence if concomitant chemotherapy doxorubicin, 5FU.
- In acute, resolve after cessation of radiotherapy, but in chronic → progressive occlusive vasculitis → ischemia, fibrosis → stricture, abscess, fistula.

Clinical Presentation
- Nausea and vomiting, diarrhea, crampy abdominal pain; these subside after finish the radiotherapy.
- Chronic → after 2 years of radiotherapy → partial obstruction, nausea and vomiting, distension, crampy, weight loss → terminal ileum mostly affected.

Diagnosis
- History.
- Enteroclysis, 90% specific.

- CT → no specificity or sensitivity.

Therapy
- Acute: self-limiting.
- Diarrhea → admission → IVF.
- No role for surgery unless with complication.
- Role of surgery: resection of diseased segment and anastomosis of healthy segment. Difficult to distinguish between healthy and diseased segment.
- Leak, 50%.
- If limited resection is not achievable → bypass.
- If aggressive resection → short bowel syndrome (SBS).

Outcome
- Mortality and morbidity → 10%.

Prevention
- Keep radiotherapy below 5,000 cGY.
- Multibeam radiation technique in ↓ area of maximal radiotherapy exposure.
- Oral sulfasalazine can decrease the insult.
- In patient known to receive radiotherapy post-operative, keep bowel out of pelvis → absorbable mesh to separate pelvis.

Meckel's Diverticulum
- Rule of 2: 2% of population, 2:1 male, 2 feet proximal to ileocecal valve (ICV), ½ of symptomatic patients is under age of 2 years.
- True diverticulum.
- Found within 100 cm from ICV.
- Contains heterotopic mucosa, 60% contain gastric mucosa, pancreatic mucosa is the next common (Brunner gland), pancreatic island, colonic mucosa, endometrium, hepatobiliary.

Pathophysiology
- At 8 weeks gestational age, failure of obliteration of omphalomesenteric (vitelline) duct or incomplete.

- Other abnormality → omphalomesenteric fistula enterocyte, fibrous band connecting to umbilicus.
- Bleeding from ulceration of gastric tissue.
- Intestinal obstruction: volvulus around fibrous band attacking diverticulum to umbilicus.
- Entrapment, intussusception, stricture.
- Can be found in hernia, inguinal and femoral (Littre's hernia).
- Asymptomatic unless with complication.
- Complication, 4%–6%.
- Most common presentation: bleeding, obstruction diverticulitis.
- Bleeding is the most common presentation in ages below 18 (50%), while obstruction is the most common in adults.
- Diverticulitis, 20%.
- Mimic to acute appendicitis.
- Neoplasm (carcinoid), 0.5%–3.2%.

Diagnosis
- Incidentally.
- CT is not accurate.
- Enteroclysis, 75%.
- Radionuclide ^{99m}Tc (Meckel scan), 90% sensitive in pediatrics, 50% in adult.
- Angiography to locate the bleeding.

Therapy
- Diverticulectomy with band.
- If bleeding → resect the segment.
- Incidentally: resection is controversial but most surgeons recommended not to interfere.

Acquired Diverticulum
- False diverticulum.
- Most common in duodenum near ampulla.
- 75% arise from medial wall of duodenum.
- The other is jejunoileal diverticula, most of it in jejunum, 15%, and ileum, 5%.
- Incidentally during ERCP, 5%–27%.

Pathophysiology
- Weak muscularis layer, bacterial overgrowth, low vitamin B12, megaloblastic anemia, malabsorption.
- Can compress biliary system → obstructive jaundice.

Clinical Picture
- Asymptomatic
- Complication: 6%–10% obstruction, bleeding, perforation, malabsorption.
- Periampullary: cholangitis, pancreatitis, sphincter of Oddi dysfunction.
- Some pain, diarrhea, bloating.

Diagnosis
- Incidentally.
- US and CT → mistaken as pancreatic pseudocyst.
- Enteroclysis: identify the diverticulum.

Therapy
- Asymptomatic → leave alone.
- Bacterial overgrowth → antibiotics.
- Other complications → resection (segment).
- If located in lateral duodenal → diverticulectomy.
- But if medial is too difficult → so non-operative management.
  - If bleeding is related to medial → lateral duodenotomy and oversew the blood vessel.
  - If perforation → drainage.
  - Diverticulectomy by hepatobiliary surgeon.

Mesenteric Artery Disease
- Vascular occlusive disease of the mesenteric vessels is relatively uncommon.
- Potentially affects over 60 years of age and is three times more frequent in women.
- The incidence of such a disease is low and represents 2% of the revascularization operations for atheromatous lesions.
- The most common cause of mesenteric ischemia is atherosclerotic vascular disease.

- Autopsy studies have demonstrated splanchnic atherosclerosis in 35% to 70% of cases.
- Other etiologies exist and include FMD, panarteritis nodosa, arteritis, and celiac artery compression from a median arcuate ligament.
- Chronic mesenteric ischemia is related to a lack of blood supply in the splanchnic region and is caused by disease in one or more visceral arteries: the celiac trunk, SMA, IMA.
- Mesenteric ischemia is thought to occur when two of the three visceral vessels are affected with severe stenosis or occlusion.
- This disease process may evolve in a chronic fashion, as in the case of progressive luminal obliteration due to atherosclerosis. On the other hand, mesenteric ischemia can occur suddenly, as in the case of thromboembolism.
- Most catastrophic vascular disorders have mortality rates ranging from 50% to 75%.
- Delays in diagnosis and treatment are the main contributing factors in its high mortality.
- It is estimated that mesenteric ischemia accounts for 1 in every 1,000 hospital admissions.
- Causes of mesenteric ischemia:
  1. Acute ischemia (thrombosis, embolus)
  2. Chronic ischemia
  3. Non-occlusive mesenteric ischemia (NOMI) (vasospasm)
  4. Venous thrombosis

Types of Mesenteric Artery Occlusive Disease
- Acute thrombosis occurs in patients with underlying mesenteric atherosclerosis.
- In acute embolic mesenteric ischemia, the emboli typically originates from a cardiac source and frequently occurs in patients with atrial fibrillation or following myocardial infarction.
- Non-occlusive mesenteric ischemia (NOMI) is characterized by a low flow state in otherwise normal mesenteric arteries and most frequently occurs in critically ill patients on vasopressors.

- Chronic mesenteric ischemia is a functional consequence of a long-standing atherosclerotic process that typically involves at least two of three main mesenteric vessels.
  - The gradual development of the occlusive process allows the development of collateral vessels that prevent the manifestations of acute ischemia.
  - Chronic mesenteric ischemic symptoms can occur due to extrinsic compression of the celiac artery by the diaphragm, which is termed median arcuate ligament syndrome.

Clinical Manifestations

- Acute: severe abdominal pain out of proportion, colicky, mid-abdominal pain, nausea, vomiting, diarrhea, distension, pass bloody stool.
- Chronic: abdominal pain, postprandial (food fear), weight loss.

Diagnostic Evaluation

- Laboratory: leukocytosis, metabolic acidosis develops as a result of anaerobic metabolism. ↑ amylase may indicate a diagnosis of pancreatitis but is also common in the setting of intestinal infarction.
- Increased lactate levels, hyperkalemia, and azotemia.
- Plain abdominal radiographs may provide helpful information to exclude other causes of abdominal pain, such as intestinal obstruction, perforation, or volvulus, which may exhibit symptoms mimicking intestinal ischemia.
- Pneumatosis intestinalis and gas in the portal vein may indicate infarcted bowel.
- Upper endoscopy, colonoscopy, or barium radiography does not provide any useful information when evaluating acute mesenteric ischemia.
- Barium enema is contraindicated if the diagnosis of mesenteric ischemia is being considered. It also can obscure accurate visualization of mesenteric circulation during angiography.
- CT scan of the abdomen should be performed.
- Duplex ultrasonography is a valuable non-invasive means of assessing the patency of the mesenteric vessels.

- Duplex has been successfully used for follow-up after open surgical reconstruction or endovascular treatment of the mesenteric vessels to assess recurrence of the disease.
- The definitive diagnosis of mesenteric vascular disease is made by biplanar mesenteric arteriography (gold standard)

Differential diagnosis
- Mesenteric emboli typically lodges at the orifice of the middle colic artery, which creates a "meniscus sign" with an abrupt cutoff of a normal proximal SMA several centimeters from its origin on the aorta.
- Mesenteric thrombosis, in contrast, occurs at the most proximal SMA, which tapers off at 1–2 cm from its origin.
- In chronic mesenteric occlusion, the appearance of collateral circulation is typically present.
- Non-occlusive mesenteric ischemia (NOMI) produces an arteriographic image of segmental mesenteric vasospasm with a relatively normal-appearing main SMA trunk.

Endovascular Treatment
Chronic Mesenteric Ischemia
- Endovascular treatment of mesenteric artery stenosis or short segment occlusion by balloon dilatation or stent placement represents a less invasive therapeutic alternative to open surgical intervention, particularly in patients whose medical comorbidities place them at a high operative risk category.
- Also used in case of restenosis post–open surgical repair.

Acute Mesenteric Ischemia
- Catheter-directed thrombolytic therapy is a potentially useful treatment modality for acute mesenteric ischemia, which can be initiated with intra-arterial delivery of thrombolytic agent into the mesenteric thrombus at the time of diagnostic angiography.
- Various thrombolytic medications includes urokinase, Abbokinase, Activase.
- Electively to correct the mesenteric stenosis.

Non-occlusive Mesenteric Ischemia

- The treatment of non-occlusive mesenteric ischemia is primarily pharmacologic with selective mesenteric arterial catheterization followed by infusion of vasodilatory agents, such as tolazoline or papaverine.
- Once the diagnosis is made on the mesenteric arteriography → intra-arterial papaverine is given at a dose of 30–60 mg/hr.
- This must be coupled with the cessation of other vasoconstricting agents.
- Concomitant intravenous heparin should be administered to prevent thrombosis in the cannulated vessels.

Surgical Treatment
Acute Embolic Mesenteric Ischemia

- Initial management is fluid resuscitation and systemic anticoagulation with heparin to prevent further thrombus propagation.
- Significant metabolic acidosis should be corrected with sodium bicarbonate.
- A central venous catheter, peripheral arterial catheter, and Foley catheter should be placed.
- Appropriate antibiotics are given prior to surgical exploration.
- It is helpful to obtain a preoperative mesenteric arteriogram to confirm the diagnosis and to plan appropriate treatment options.
- The primary goal is to restore arterial perfusion with removal of the embolus from the vessel.
- The abdomen is explored through a midline incision.
- The transverse colon is lifted superiorly, and the small intestine is reflected toward the upper-right quadrant.
- The SMA is approached at the root of the small bowel mesentery, usually as it emerges from beneath the pancreas to cross over the junction of the third and fourth portions of the duodenum.
- Once the proximal SMA is identified and controlled with vascular clamps, a transverse arteriotomy is made to extract the embolus, using standard balloon embolectomy catheters.

- In the event the embolus has lodged more distally, exposure of the distal SMA may be obtained in the root of the small bowel mesentery.
- Following the restoration of SMA flow, an assessment of intestinal viability must be made and non-viable bowel must be resected.
- A second-look procedure should be considered if questionable segment and performed 24–48 hrs following embolectomy.

Acute Thrombotic Mesenteric Ischemia

- Thrombotic mesenteric ischemia usually involves a severely atherosclerotic vessel, typically the proximal celiac artery and SMA.
- Therefore, these patients require a reconstructive procedure to the SMA to bypass the proximal occlusive lesion and restore adequate mesenteric flow.
- The saphenous vein is the graft material of choice.
- Prosthetic materials should be avoided in patients with non-viable bowel, due to the risk of bacterial contamination if resection of necrotic intestine is performed.
- The bypass graft may originate from either the aorta or iliac artery.

Chronic Mesenteric Ischemia

- The therapeutic goal in patients with chronic mesenteric ischemia is to revascularize mesenteric circulation and prevent the development of bowel infarction.
- Mesenteric occlusive disease can be treated by either transaortic endarterectomy or mesenteric artery bypass.

Miscellaneous Condition
Small Bowel Perforation

- GI endoscopy is the most common cause, then infections such as tuberculosis, typhoid, CMV, CD, ischemia, radiological reduction for Meckel's, neoplasm, foreign body.
- Among iatrogenic injuries → duodenal perforation during ERCP, 0.3%–2.1%.

- Diagnosis: CT—pneumoperitoneum, free perforation, free retroperitoneal air, contrast extravasation, paraduodenal collection.
- Retroperitoneal air is 30%, but majority is asymptomatic.
- Treatment: non-operative, in the absence of sepsis.
- Intraperitoneal duodenal perforation → surgical repair + pyloric exclusion and gastrojejunostomy or tube duodenostomy.
- Small bowel perforation (iatrogenic) → endoscopic repair (clips); if failed → surgical repair.

Chylous Ascites

- Accumulation of triglycerides-rich peritoneal fluid with milky, creamy apperance caused by intestinal lymph.
- Causes:
  - Malignancy (abdominal).
  - Abdomen or thoracic operation or trauma
  - Operation such as AAA repair, retroperitoneal LN dissection
  - IVC resection, liver transplant
  - Congenital lymphedema abnormality, radiation, pancreatitis, right-sided HF

- Diagnosis:
  - by paracentesis, fluid glyceride, 110 mg/dL.
  - CT scan to look for LNs or masses.
  - Lymphangiography or lymphoscintigraphy → to localize.

- Treatment
  - Treat underlying cause.
  - Administration of high-protein, low-fat diet → if not responding → TPN.
  - Octreotide, ↓ flow of LN.
  - Therapeutic paracentesis → for dyspnea, distension.
  - Surgical repair after localization.
  - Poor surgery candidate → peritoneovenous shunt, S/E → occlusion.

Intussusception

- Usually in pediatrics → start with radiologic reduction, if failed → surgical reduction.
- In adult →½ of the pathology is malignancy.
- Diagnosis by US, barium enema, or CT scan.
- Treatment: resection and pathological evaluation.
- Patient with Roux-en-Y → increase incidence.

Pneumatosis Intestinalis

- Gas within the bowel wall.
- Can be idiopathic or intestinal or non-intestinal, such as pulmonary disease and asthma.
- Most secondary to identifiable cause, 15% idiopathic.
- Surgical cause, ischemia, infarction.

Short Bowel Syndrome (SBS)

- Defined as less than 100 cm of residual small bowel length in absence of ileocecal valve or less than 80 in presence of ileocecal valve.
- Cause: Mesentric ischemia, malignant, CD, chronic TPN.

Pathophysiology

- 50% resection is tolerable.
- 50%–80% → malabsorption.
- TPN dependent, will persist if < 100 cm.
- In infant, can wean from TPN even if 10 cm only.
- The prediction depends on colon, competent ileocecal valve; healthy remnant bowel resection of jejunum is tolerable than ileum (B12, bile salt).
- Adaptation within 1–2 years.
- Exacerbation ↑ by gastrin → ↑ HCL as absorption better in alkaline media.

Therapy
Non-transplant Therapy
Therapeutic Goal

- Maintain fluid and electrolyte, nutritional supplement.
- Maximize and improve function of intestinal.
- 180 cm, no TPN needed.

- If 90 cm with colon, usually needs TPN < 1 year.
- 60 cm require permanent TPN.
- S/E of TPN → sepsis, venous thrombosis, liver cirrhosis and failure, renal failure.
- Initial diet, high carbs, high protein, medium-chain fatty acid.
- Slow gut motility such as the following:
  o Slow transit
    Loperamide, narcotic
  o Reduce GI Secretions
    H_2 blocker
    PPI
    Octreotide
  o Treatment of bacterial overgrowth
    Antibiotic, probiotics, prokinetic

Surgical Strategies
- Preservation of intestinal remnant.
- Surgical therapies for SBS:
  1. Strictureplasty
  2. Tapering enteroplasty
  3. Reversed segment
  4. Segmental reversal of SB
  5. Interposition of colon between small bowel
  6. LILT procedure
  7. STEP procedure

Intestinal Transplant
- 80% survives.

Alternative Therapy
- Biological therapy → expand mucosa.
- GLP-2 + glutamine + GH, high-carb diet.

Outcome
- 50%–70% with SBS → TPN.
- Prognosis is better in pediatrics.
- 2–5 years, SR is 86%–45%, respectively.

Small Bowel Neoplasm
- Adenoma is the most common benign neoplasm; others are fibroma, lipoma, hemangioma, lymphangioma, neurofibroma.
- Autopsy: incidence, 0.2%–0.3%.
- Usually asymptomatic.
- Incidentiallly during EGD, 0.3%–4.6%.
- Benign, 30%–50%.
- Primary CA is rare adenocarcinoma (35%-50%), carcinoid (20%–40%), lymphoma (10%–15%).
- GIST is the most common mesenchymal tumor, then leiomyoma, leiomyosarcoma.
- Small bowels frequently affected by metastasis (melanoma).
- Age-group: 50–60.
- Risk factors: red meat, smoked food, CD, HNPCC, FAP, Peutz-Jeghers syndrome.

Pathophysiology
- Small bowel contains 90% of mucosal surface of GI but only 1.1%–2.4% of GI malignancy because of the following:
    a) Diluted carcinogens in liquid chyme
    b) Rapid transit of chyme (limit the contrast)
    c) ↓ bacteria
    d) Mucosal protection by IgA
    e) Efficient epithelial apoptosis
- Adenocarcinoma arises from preexisting adenoma:
    - Tubular least for malignancy
    - Villous most for malignancy
    - Tubulovillous
- Malignant degeneration has been reported to be present in up to 45% of villous adenomas by the time of diagnosis.
- FAP → 100% to develop to duodenal adenoma → malignant transformation → duodenal cancer by a hundredfold, leading cause of death in patient with FAP who underwent colectomy.
- Peutz-Jeghers syndrome, hamartomatous polyp → malignant transformation.
- GIST: mutation of proto-oncogenes KIT (kinase I tyrosine) → activating mutation in c-KIT; KIT expression is assessed mutation by staining the tissue for CD117 Ag.

Clinical Picture
- Mostly asymptomatic.
- Pain, distension, nausea and vomiting.
- Obstruction by narrowing of lumen or intussusception.
- Hemorrhage, is the second presentation.
- 25% palpable abdominal mass.
- Fecal occult for blood may be +ve.
- Jaundice, cachexia, hepatomegaly.

- **Adenocarcinoma**
  - mostly in duodenum, except for CD → ileum
  - If the lesion is periampullary → obstructive jaundice or pancreatitis.

- **Carcinoid**
  - Usually diagnosed after metastasis, more aggressive than most common carcinoid tumor (appendiceal carcinoid)
  - 25%–50% of liver metastasis will develop carcinoid syndrome manifestation, such as diarrhea, flushing, low BP, tachycardia, fibrosis of endocardium and valves.
  - Mediator: serotonin, bradykinin, substance P.
  - Symptoms of carcinoid is rare in the absence of liver metastasis.

- **Lymphoma**
  - Primarily located in ileum.
  - 10% will present with perforation.

- **GIST**
  - 60%–70% in stomach.
  - Small bowel is the second most common, 25%–35%.
  - Hemorrhage comes with GIST more than any other small bowel malignancy.

Diagnosis
- ↑ serum 5 hydroxyindoleacetic acid (5-HIAA), chromogranin A in carcinoid tumors.
- ↑ CEA in adenocarcinoma.
- Enteroclysis → sensitive, 90%.

- UGI follow-through, 30%–44%.
- CT scan.
- Hemorrhage → angiography or radioisotopes tagged RBC scan.
- EGD → duodenal lesion.
- Colonoscopy → distal ileum.
- Intra-operative enteroscopy.

Therapy
- **Benign neoplasm with Symptoms**
    - Resection, surgically or endoscopically.
    - Adenoma → biopsy and removal because of malignancy potential.
    - Tumor < 1 cm → endoscopically.
            > 2 cm → surgically.
    - Transduodenal polypectomy or segmental resection.
    - If tumor is in second part of duodenum (D2)→ Whipple procedure.
    - Endoscopic polypectomy = surgical and less mortality and morbidity of benign periampullary duodenal + surveillance endoscopy.
    - Duodenal adenoma in FAP → need aggressive treatment → endoscopic removal, then surveillance for 6 months then annually if surgery is required → Whipple procedure.

- **Adenocarcinoma of Duodenum**
    - D1–D2 → Whipple.
    - D3–D4 → local resection.
    - For metastatic disease → bypass.
    - Chemotherapy is not proven in adenocarcinoma.

- **Carcinoid**
    - Resection + lymphadenectomy.
    - LNs < 1 cm, rarely to be involved but usually 75%–90% > 3 cm.
    - 30%–50% respond rate to chemotherapy.
    - Octreotide for carcinoid syndrome to decrease symptom.

- **Localized Lymphoma**
  - Resection.
  - If diffused → chemotherapy.
  - Adjuvant chemotherapy after resection is controversial.

- **GIST**
  - Segmental resection. Avoid lymphadenectomy as it's rarely involved.
  - Resistant to chemotherapy.
  - Imatinib (Gleevec) is a tyrosine kinase inhibitor and has potent activity against KIT.
  - 80% of irresectable GIST → imatinib → 50%–60% reduction in tumor.

Outcome

- Resection of adenocarcinoma in duodenum → 5 years SR is 50%–60%.
- SR in ileum or jejunum is 20%–30%.
- Carcinoid 5 years SR is 75%–95% if (localized), but with liver metastasis is 19%–54%.
- Lymphoma 5 years SR is 20%–40%, if localized → 60%.
- GIST recurrence is 35% in 5 years, SR is 35% 60%, correlated with size and mitotic index.

Colorectal

Colon

Embryology
- In fourth week, GIT starts to develop.
- at Sixth week the midgut herniation outside the abdomen and rotate anticlockwise (90 degrees) around SMA then return back to complete rotation 180 degrees, total of 270 degrees.

Anatomy and histology
- Five layers: mucosa, submucosa, two layers musculosa (inner circular, outer longitudinal), serosa.
- Outer longitudinal = taenia coli.
- Inner circular = complete to distal rectum to form internal anal sphincter.
- Colon and proximal ⅓ of the rectum covered by serosa.
- Colon is 3–5 ft.
- Rocoto-sigmoid level of sacral promontory.
- Cecum is widest (7.5 cm, 8.5 cm), thinner muscular layer → not obstructed but can be perforated.
- Ascending and descending colon is is fixed to retroperitoneum.
- Sigmoid is narrowest part, redundant → can reach RLQ → volvulus.

- **Blood Supply of Colon**
    - All small bowel + ascending and proximal transverse colon is supplied by SMA.
    - The distal of transverse colon, descending, sigmoid colon and upper rectum supplied by IMA.
    - SMA → ileocolic (absent in 20%) right, middle colic.
    - IMA → Left colic, sigmoidal arteries then continue to form superior rectal A
    - Marginal artery of Drummond (complete in 20%) communicates with SMA and IMA.
    - Vein is parallel but IMV → ascends in retroperitoneum over psoas muscle → posterior pancreas to join splenic

vein → during colectomy ligation of this vein at inferior edge of the pancreas.

- Watershed areas, i.e., dual blood supply from separated arterial supply, are as follows:
    - Griffiths' point (splenic flexure), arc of Riolan, and marginal artery of Drummond.
    - Sudeck's point (rectosigmoid junction), superior and inferior rectal artery.

NB: these two areas are more liable to ischemia because they are supplied by the most distal branch of the artery, it is the least area receive sufficient blood during systemic hypoperfusion.

- **Lymph Nodes**
    - Originates from muscalaris mucosa.
    - Bowel wall (epicolic), adjacent to artery arcade (paracolic), around named vessels (intermedia) at the origin of Superior and inferior mesenteric arteries.
    - SLND → in colon is controversial.

- **Nerves**
    - Sympathetic (inhibitory) and parasympathetic (stimulatory).
        Sympathetic: T6–12 and L1–3.
        Parasympathetic: right vagus, left S2–4.

Congenital Anomaly
- Failure of midgut to rotate at 10 weeks → intestinal malrotation and colonic non-fixation.
- Failure of canalization → colonic duplication.
- Incomplete descent of urogenital septum → imperforate anus.
- Many of hindgut anomaly → genitourinary anomaly.

Physiology
Fluid and Electrolyte
- The colon is the major site for water absorption.
- 90% 1–2 L/day, but can be up to 5 L.
- Na^+ absorption via Na^+/K^+ ATPase → water → passive.
- K^+ actively secreted and passively absorbed by diffusion.

- Bacterial degradation of protein and urea → ammonia → liver.
- ↓ bacteria by antibiotics or ↓ intraluminal pH (lactulose) → ↓ ammonia.

Short-Chain Fatty Acids
- SCFA (acetate, butyrate) produced by bacterial fermentation of carbohydrates.
- It is an important source of energy to colonic mucosa (active transport Na^+).
- Diversion → mucosal atrophy → diversion colitis.

Colonic Microflora and Intestinal Gas
- 30% dry weight of feces is bacteria 10^{12}.
- Aerobic(E. coli 10^9), anaerobic and bacteroid.
- Microflora for breakdown of carbohydrate, protein, bilirubin, bile acid, estrogen, cholesterol, and vitamin K and suppress of C. difficile.
- GI contains 100–200 cc of gas.
- Flatus, 400–1,200 cc/day.

Motility
- No MMC.
- Intermediate contraction, low or high amplitude.
- Branch of pudendal nerve → internal and external sphincter.

Clinical Evaluation
- History and physical examination →general and abdominal examination + digital rectal examination.

  - **Pain (abdomen)**
    - Result from obstruction, inflammation, neoplasm, perforation, or ischemia.
    - Sigmoidoscopy or colonoscopy → diagnose ischemic colitis, IBD, colonic mass, but if perforation or obstruction is contraindicated.

- **Pelvic pain**
  - Pain from distal colon and rectum or from urological problems.
  - Tenesmus: proctitis or rectal mass.
  - Cyclic pain → endometriosis.
  - PID.
  - Pelvic abscess from diverticulitis.

- **Anorectal pain**
  - Mostly fissure, perianal abscess, thrombosed piles → need physical examination.
  - Proctalgia fugax → levator ani spasm.

- **Constipation**
  - Colonoscopy, barium enema, virtual colonoscopy.
  - Either slow transit constipation or outlet obstruction.
  - Manometry, EMG → non-relax puborectalis (outlet obstruction).
  - Absence of anorectal inhibitory reflex.
  - rectal biopsy → Hirschsprung's disease.
  - Defecography → rectal prolapse, intussusception.
  - Treatment: fiber, high fluid, and laxative; surgery for rectocele or prolapse.
  - Slow transit constipation (colonic inertia) → subtotal colectomy.

- **Diarrhea and Irritable Bowel Syndrome (IBS)**
  - Bloody → colitis (ischemic or infectious).
  - Infectious → culture.
  - Sigmoidoscopy or colonoscopy → IBD or ischemia; if tenderness (i.e., peritonitis), colonoscopy is contraindicated.
  - Chronic diarrhea, UC, CD, short gut syndrome, rarely carcinoid, VIPoma, large villous lesion.
  - IBS: crampy abdominal pain, bloating, constipation, and urgent diarrhea → bulking agent, stop coffee, smoking, antispasmodic.

- **Incontinence (leaking gas or stool)**
  - Neurogenic or anatomic such as rectal prolapse.
  - Most traumatic cause → during delivery.
  - Pudendal nerve terminal motor latency → neuropathy.
  - Defecography is useful.
  - Anal manometry → resting and squeeze pressure.
  - Treatment: antidiarrhea.
  - Some patients may respond to biofeedback.
  - Surgery → sphincteroplasty.
  - Innovative technologies such as sacral nerve stimulation and the artificial bowel sphincter are proving useful in patients who fail other interventions.
  - Radiofrequency energy to anal canal (Secca procedure).
  - Injection of bulking agent.
  - Stoma for persisting and severe incontinence.

Laboratory
- **Fecal occult blood test (FOBT)**
  - Non-specific: ↑ with red meat and vitamin C intake.

- **Stool study**
  - Helpful in the evaluation of diarrhea.
  - Stool culture.
  - C. difficile → toxin in stool.

- **Serum**
  - CBC, chemistry, INR, LFT.

- **Tumor marker**
  - CEA 60%–90% elevation in colon CA → effective in follow-up after surgery.
  - Urokinase.

- **Genetic testing**
  - FAP, HNPCC → APC gene.

Imaging

- **Plain x-ray erect and supine**

- **Contrast study**
  - Gastrografin is not like barium that provides more mucosal detail but is used in case of suspected perforation or leak.

- **CT**
  - Insensitive of intraluminal lesion.
  - Ticking of bowel wall and fat stranding inflammation.

- **Virtual colonoscopy**
  - Intraluminal lesion.
  - Needs bowel preparation with oral and rectal contrast → increase sensitivity.
  - Can detect lesion (polyp) of 1 cm or larger.

- **MRI**
  - Pelvic lesion.
  - Rectal CA and mesorectum.
  - Detects fistulous tract.

- **PET**
  - Anaerobic glycolysis.
  - Detects metastasis and staging.
  - Provides PET-CT.

- **Angiography**
  - Bleeding, 0.5–1 mL/min.
  - Therapeutic infusion of vasopressor or embolization.

- **Endorectal/endoanal ultrasound**
  - Depth of invasion of lesion in rectum.
  - Normal rectal wall is five layers.
  - LNs enlargement.

- **Pelvic floor manometry**
  - Resting pressure reflects internal sphincter by 40%–80%.
  - Squeezing pressure reflects external sphincter by 40%–80%.

- **Neurophysiology**
  - Function of pudendal nerve, puborectalis.
  - EMG.

- **Rectal evacuation study**
  - Balloon expulsion test.
  - Defecography differentiates non-relaxing puborectalis from obstruction.

Endoscopy

- **Anoscopy**
  - Length: 8 cm, anal canal.
  - Therapeutic rubber band ligation of piles.
  - Rotates 90 degrees and inspects four quadrants.

- **Proctoscopy**
  - 25 cm, 15–19 mm diameter.
  - Can perform polypectomy as can reach the distal sigmoid.

- **Flexible sigmoidoscopy and colonoscopy**
  - Sigmoidoscopy, 60 cm (need fleet enema).
  - Colonoscopy, 100–160 cm (need bowel preparation).
  - Both diagnostic and therapeutic.

- **Capsule endoscopy.**

General Surgical Consideration

Resection
- Curative resection → proximal ligation of vessels.
- Benign, no wide mesenteric clearance needed.

Emergency Resection

- Obstruction, perforation, hemorrhage, mostly, patient is unstable.
- Bowels are always not well prepared.
- If the right colon or proximal transverse colon → right or extended right hemicolectomy with primary ileocolic anastomosis if healthy bowel and stable patient.
- For left colon: resection of involved bowel and end colostomy without mucus fistula.
    - → Some studies showed primary anastomosis without bowel preparation or with on-table lavage with or without diverting ileostomy is safe.
- If subtotal colectomy → small bowel to rectosigmoid anastomosis.

Minimally Invasive Technology of Resection

- Laparoscopy or hand-assisted or robotic.
- Improves cosmesis.
- ↓ post-operative pain.
- Earlier return of bowel function.
- Less immunosuppressive → ↑ outcome.
- ↓ hospital study.
- ↓ complication.
- Robotic has short learning curve.

Colectomies

Ileocolic Resection

- Limited resection of terminal ileum, cecum, appendix, right colectomy.
- Ileocolic artery + right colic, right branch of middle colic artery.
- 10 cm of ileum.
- Primary anastomosis is generally possible.

Extended Right Colectomy

- As above + ligation of middle colic at the base.
- Plus primary anastomosis.
- Can be extended if not healthy.

Transverse Colectomy
- Ligation of middle colic vessels, i.e., resection of transverse colon + colocolonic anastomosis can be performed or instead extended right hemicolectomy.

Left Colectomy
- Left branch of middle colic + left colic + first branch of sigmoid vessels, colo-colonic anastomosis.

Extended Left Colectomy
- Lesion in distal transverse colon.
- Right branch of middle colic is involved.
- Sigmoid colectomy—ligation of sigmoid branch of IMA, anastomosis of descending and rectum.
- Full mobilization of splenic flexure is required to create tension-free anastomosis.

Total and Subtotal Colectomy
- Fulminant colitis, attenuated FAP, or synchronous colon carcinoma.
- Ligation of iliocolic, right colic, middle colic and left colic arteries
- Preserved superior rectal artery.
- If preserved sigmoid → subtotal colectomy with ileosigmoid anastomosis.
- If sigmoid is involved → (total colectomy) with ileorectal anastomosis.
- If anastomosis is contraindicated → ileostomy is created and the remaining of sigmoid/rectum is managed as mucus fistula or Hartmann's pouch.

Proctocolectomy
- Colon, rectum, and anus canal + brook ileostomy.

Restorative Proctocolectomy
- Resection of the colon + rectum, but anal sphincter muscle and distal anal canal are preserved.

- Bowel continuity is restored by anastomosis of ileal reservoir to anal canal i.e. ileal pouch anal anastomosis (IPAA)
- Original technique → transanal mucosectomy and handsewn ileoanal anastomosis.
- Risk of incontinence ↑ after mucosectomy.
- Double staple has better function outcome.
- Neorectum aligned as J-S-W shape.
- J pouch is simplest of all = equal outcome.
- Most surgeons perform proximal ileostomy, then closed 6–12 weeks after confirming integrity of pouch.
- There is a report without diverting ileostomy (primary anastomosis)

Anterior Resection
- Historically, posterior resection → now obsolete.
- Anterior resection of rectum from the abdomen.
- Three types:
  1. High anterior resection
     - Distal sigmoid and upper rectum.
     - For benign lesion.
     - Pelvic peritoneum not divided.
     - IMA and vein are ligated at the base.

  2. Low anterior resection
     - Lesion in upper or mid rectum.
     - Rectosigmoid mobilized, pelvic peritoneum opened.
     - IMA ligated.
     - Rectum mobilized from sacrum by sharp dissection within endopelvic fascial plane.
       • Distal to anorectal ring.
       • Posteriorly through rectosacral fascia to coccyx.
       • Anterior through Denonvilliers' fascia.
     - Rectum and its mesorectum.
     - Require mobilization of splenic flexure and ligation and division of IMA and vein just inferior to pancreas.

- Circular stapler → anastomosis extraperitoneal.

3. Extended (ultra) low anterior resection
   - Lesion in distal rectum above sphincter, 1–2 cm.
   - Dissection till rectovaginal septum in women and distal to the seminal vesicles and prostate in men.
   - With creation of J colon or T coloplasty.
   - Temporary ileostomy is preferable.
   - Pelvic radiation preoperative → sphincter damage.
   - If with sphincter damage or history of incontinence → end colostomy.

Abdominoperineal resection (APR)

- Removal of rectum, anal canal, and anus + permanent colostomy.
- Perineal dissection in lithotomy or in prone position after closure of abdomen and creation of stoma.
- For benign → proctocolectomy → inter-sphincteric dissection between internal and external sphincter.

Hartmann's Procedure and Mucus Fistula

- Colonic or rectal resection without anastomosis with colostomy or ileostomy and blind pouch (rectum). If distal end of the colon is long → mucus fistula.

Anastomosis

- End → end, end → side, side → end, side → side.
- Handsewn or stapler.
- Submucosal layer (strongest) should be incorporated.
- Well-vascularized, tension-free, well-nourished.
- Highest risk of leak → distal rectum or anal canal prior radiation, peritoneal spillage, malnourished.

Anastomosis Configurations

E → E: in small bowel, colon and rectal anastomosis.

E → S: when one limb is larger than the other

S → E: when proximal is smaller (ileorectal)

S → S: ileocolic anastomosis

Anastomosis Techniques

- Handsewn: single or double layers, continuous or interrupted, permanent or absorbable sutures.
- Stapler:
    - Linear S → S
    - Circular E → E, E → S, S → E

Stomas

- Temporal or permanent.
- End or loop.
- Consultation with enterostomal therapist (ET) for education.
- Should be placed within rectus abdominis below belt line.
- Skin, SC → rectus sheath cruciate incision, can introduce two fingers for small bowel stoma and three fingers in colostomies.
- Taken care of inferior epigastric vessels.
- As small as possible.
- Everting the bowel.
- 3–4 absorbable through edge of the bowel then serosa, 2 cm from edge, then skin.
- Mucocutaneous junction is sutured circumferentially with interrupted absorbable suture.

Ileostomy

- **Temporary**
    - To protect anastomosis (lower rectum), during emergency, malnourished patient.
    - Segment of distal ileum is brought as loop.
    - Loop ileostomy secured with or without rod.
    - Incomplete diversion.
    - Advantage closure without laparotomy.
    - Gastrografin before closure (recommended).
    - Closure is delayed till chemotherapy is completed.

- **Permanent**
    - With proctocolectomy or patient with obstruction.
    - Easier than temporary.

Complications of Ileostomy
1. Necrosis (limited) → nothing → if extended below fascia → revision.
2. Retraction (obesity) → revision.
3. Dehydration, electro-abnormalities → output > 1,500 → loperamide or opioid, octreotide.
4. Skin irritation, excoriation.
5. Obstruction.
6. Parastomal hernia, if symptomatic → repair.
7. Prolapse → rare.

Colostomy
- Colostomy prolapse is more than with ileostomy.
- Most in the left side.
- Should be done in Brooke fashion.
- Distal → mucus fistula or Hartmann's pouch.
- Tacking distal end of colon to abdominal wall.
- Usually, closure requires laparotomy.

Complications of Colostomy
1. If necrosis → ileostomy.
2. Retraction occur but less than ileostomy.
3. Less irritant.
4. Obstruction.
5. Parastomal hernia (common than ileostomy).
6. Dehydration is rare.

Functional Result
- Usually, colonic segmental resection with primary anastomosis is excellent.
- Some of ileosigmoid or ileorectal → diarrhea, if longer length of small bowel resection or if proctitis.

- Some patients after right colectomy →
  diarrhea, because of bile acid malabsorption
  (cholestyramine).
- Physical and psychological problem.
- Pouch failure, 5%–10%.
- Patient with CD pouch failure is 50%; colitis,
  15%–20%.
- Pouchitis (50%), diarrhea, hematochezia, abdominal
  pain, fever, malaise, because of fecal stasis.
  o Diagnosis → biopsy.
  o Treatment: antibiotics such as metronidazole
    +/− ciprofloxacin + oral, prep or enema,
    aspirin.
  o Steroid is good option and probiotics is
    somewhat good.

Ureteric Stent
- To identify ureter intraoperative.
- Should multidisciplinary team approach.

Anesthesia Consideration
- **Local**
  - Many anorectal diseases can be done under local
    anesthesia → IV sedation + lidocaine + bupivacaine
    to perianal skin and sphincter around pudendal
    nerve, add epinephrine to ‾ bleeding and prolong
    time.

- **Regional Anesthesia**
  - Epidural, spinal, caudal anesthesia in severe comorbid.
  - Post-operative epidural increases pulmonary function.

- **General Anesthesia**
  - Pre-operative CVS evaluation.
  - Positioning.
  - Most colectomy → supine.
  - APR → lithotomy + pad under sacrum, taking care
    of peroneal nerve.
  - Anorectal → lithotomy or jackknife prone.

Pre-operative Bowel Preparation—Is It Warrented?
- Bowel contains 100 trillion microbes.
- Before routine antibiotic prophylaxis, infection rate was 40% and decreased to 25%.
- SSI is a hospital-acquired infection.
- Several large observational databases suggest true benefit from mechanical preparationand oral antibiotic in combination.

Rationale for Preparation
- The goal is to decrease bacterial and fecal load to ¯ the infection.

Mechanical Bowel Preparation (MBP)
Types:
1. **Irritant and Stimulant**
   - Senna tab
   - Dulcolax
   - Castor oil

2. **Bulk Laxative**
   - Methyl cellulose

3. **Osmotic Laxative**
   - Magnesium citrate saline
   - Lactulose
   - polyethylene glycol (PEG)(Movicol)

4. **Stool Softener**
   - Dulcolax
   - Correctol
   - Fleet enema

5. **Lubricant**
   - Glycerin suppository

6. **Chloride Channel Activator**
   - Lubiprostone

Data for Mechanical Preparation
- No difference between bowel preparation or no preparation.
- Another reviews meta-analysis: no difference but ↑ complications such as discomfort, electrolyte imbalance, dehydration, mucosal injury → ↑ contamination at surgery (liquid stool).
- Conclusion: MBP alone is not recommended for routine colorectal surgery.

Data on Oral Antibiotic
- Cochrane review: oral + IV Antibiotic lower SSI by 40% when compared IV antibiotic alone.
- Also, oral + MBP decrease anastomotic leak, lower SSI, ileus by 45%–77%.

Conclusion
- Recommendation is MBP + oral antibiotic + IV antibiotic.
- No MBP alone.
- No data for oral antibiotic alone.

Management of LGIB
1. Resuscitation (ABCD)
   - History and physical examination.
   - correct Coagulopathy.

2. Identify the source
   - Identify local cause by examination and anoscopy → piles, fissure.
   - Most common cause of LGIB is UGIB → NGT → till bilious stain.
   - If bloody stain → EGD.
   - The common causes of LGIB are diverticulosis, angiodysplasia, UC, and colon CA.
   - If patient is stable, colonoscopy → preparation 4–6 hrs.
   - Angiography, detect bleeding rate 0.5mL/hr
   - Tagged RBCs 0.1 mL/hr, if +ve → angioembolization.
   - Segmental colectomy if the source is identified.
   - If bleeding persists → blind subtotal colectomy → rare (unstable, the source is not identified).

Pathology

Inflammatory Bowel Disease (IBD)
General consideration
- UC, DC, indeteminenet colitis.
- UC is 8–15 per 100,000, low in Asia, Africa, non-white whereas CD is lower in africa, 1–5 per 100,000, high in Northern Europe and white.
- increase in ages 30 and 70.
- Two peaks: 15–30, 55–60.

Etiology
- Diet, infection, alcohol, and OCP.
- Smoking exacerbates CD but is protective against UC.
- Family history → 15%–30%.
- Autoimmune (immune and mucosal barrier).
- Bacteria → mycobacterium, paratuberculosis, listeria, measles.
- Defect in mucosal barrier → bacteria + toxin, pro-inflammatory.

Pathogenesis and DDx
- Ulcerative colitis (UC):
  - mucosa and submucosa involvement
  - colonoscopy: mucosa is friable, atrophic, and crypt abscess (UC more than CD) + pseudopolyps.
  - In long-standing → scar.
  - Can affect rectum (proctitis), rectum and sigmoid, left colon or pancolitis.
  - Can inflame distal ileum (backwash ileitis).
  - Symptoms: bloody diarrhea, crampy abdominal pain, proctitis → tenesmus.
  - If severe abdominal pain + fever → FC or TM distension with minimal to frank tenderness.
  - Diagnosis → colonoscopy and biopsy.
  - ASCA −ve, P-ANCA +ve.

- Crhons disease (CD)
  - affects any gastrointestinal from mouth to anus.

- Transmural inflammatory process, mucosal ulceration, non-caseating granuloma → chronic → fibrosis and stricture, fistula
- Rectal sparing or skip lesion.
- Deep serpiginous (cobblestone appearance).
- Symptom depends on severity of inflammation/ fibrosis and affected area.
  Diarrhea, crampy abdominal pain, stricture → obstruction, weight loss.
- Perianal disease: pain, abscess.
- ↑ CRP, ESR, albumin, anemia.
- ASCA +ve, P-ANCA −ve.

- indeteminenet colitis:
  - 15% cannot differentiate UC from CD
  - Same picture grossly and microscopically, so serology P-ANCA and ASCA are useful.
  - DDx: infection, E. histolytica, C. difficile, salmonella, shigella, N. gonorrhoeae.

Extraintestinal Manifestations

- Liver is the most common site, fatty infiltration, 40%–50%; cirrhosis, 2%–5%.
- Primary sclerosing cholangitis (PSC) is progressive, intrahepatic and extrahepatic bile duct fibrosis and stricture.
- 40%–60% of patient → with UC → no improvement after colectomy → liver TPx is the ideal.
- Bile duct cancer associated with IBD (long-standing), 20 years younger in usual age of cholangiocarcinoma.
- Arthritis is twenty times greater and usually improves with colectomy, but sacroiliitis and ankylosing spondylitis are not.
- Erythema nodosum, 5%–15%. Three to four times more in female than male (lower leg) mostly.
- Pyoderma gangrenosum: pretibial region or near stoma → ulceration → painful.
- Ocular lesion (10%), uveitis, iritis, conjunctivitis.

Non-operative Management

- Focus on ↓ inflammation and alleviating symptom.

- Mild to moderate flare → OPD.
- Severe symptoms → hospitalization.
- Limited distal large bowel (proctitis) with or without sigmoid involvement → topical therapy with ASA (salicylate) or corticosteroid suppository; systemic treatment is rarely used.

- **Salicylate**
  - Sulfasalazine, 5-acetylsalicylic acid, 5-ASA.
  - First line, mild to moderate disease.
  - ↓ inflammation by inhibit cyclooxygenase and 5-lipoxygenase.
  - Requires direct contact.
  - Pentasa, Asacol, Rowasa.

- **Antibiotics**
  - ↓ intraluminal bacterial load.
  - Metronidazole → ↓ Crohn's colitis and perianal disease.
  - Fluoroquinolones can be used instead.
  - If no toxic megacolon (TM) or fulminant colitis (FC) in IBD, antibiotics are not used.

- **Steroids**
  - Oral or IV.
  - Treatment of acute exacerbation in UC or CD.
  - 70%–90% improved.
  - Be cautious in children.
  - Failure to wean → relative indication for surgery.
  - Enema for local → proctitis.

- **Immunomodulating Agent**
  - Azathioprine, 6-mercaptopurine (6-MP) → antimetabolite → ↓ proliferation of inflammatory cells.
  - If failed 5-ASA and the patient is dependent or refractory to steroid.
  - Action in 6–12 weeks + concomitant use of steroid is required.
  - Cyclosporine → anti–T lymphocyte 80% with flare UC used → used to treat CD exacerbation.

- ⅔ of CD responds within 2 weeks → S/E → nephrotoxic, hirsutism.
- Methotrexate → 50% will improve.

- **Biologic Agent**
  - Inhibit TNF-a, IV, if failed steroid.
  - Infliximab, 50% of moderate to severe disease will improve.
  - Useful in perianal disease.
  - New agent: certolizumab.
  - Adalimumab in case of refractory steroid on UC.

- **Nutrition**
  - TPN in malnourished.
  - Measure albumin, prealbumin, transferrin.

Ulcerative Colitis (UC)
- Characterized by remission and exacerbation.
- Low grade can progress to fulminant disease.
- Bloody stool, severe diarrhea, and bleeding.
- The disease starts in the rectum then extends to sigmoid colon or whole colon.
- Inflammation of cecum → inflammation of ileum → backwash ileitis.
- Family history is the most prominent factor.
- 75% has +ve P-ANCA.
- Risk factors: high sugar consumption, low fiber diet, no breastfeeding.
- Smoking is protective for UC but is a risk factor of CD.
- Symptom depends on degree of involvement.
- Anemia.
- Diagnosis → endoscopically + biopsy; usually, proctoscopy establishes the disease as it starts in rectum, but complete colonoscopy should be performed to rule out CD and malignancy.
- Early → mucosal edema; late → friable ulcerated mucosa, pus and mucus.
- Colonoscopy and barium are not used in an acute setting because risk of perforation.

313

- Long-standing → shortened colon and loss of haustral marking (lead pipe) appearance in barium.
- Because it's a disease of mucosa → stricture is rare, any stricture → highly suspicious of malignancy.
- Surveillance colonoscopy at 1, 2, 8 years → four-quadrant biopsy at 10 cm interval ≈ 32 biopsies.
- Colonoscopy at acute phase is contraindicated and can proceed with limited colonoscopy rectum + sigmoid.
- DDx of other cause of bloody diarrhea: C. difficile, salmonella, E. coli.
  → Rule out by stool C/S.

- **Indication for Surgery**
  - Emergency or elective.
  - Indication of emergency surgery:
    - Hemorrhage, toxic megacolon (TM), fulminant colitis (FC), failure to respond to medical treatment.
  - Indication of elective surgery:
    o Intractability to medical therapy.
    o High risk to develop complication, e.g., aseptic necrosis of joint.
    o Poorly controlled symptom, poor quality of life, growth failure, or long-term therapy (steroid).
    o ↑ risk for CA.

- **Fulminant Colitis and Toxic Megacolon**
  - Severe colitis, 10%–15%.
  - Symptoms: bloody diarrhea, weight loss, volume depletion, fever, severe anemia.
  - Fulminant colitis: severe colitis + symptom of toxicity.
        → Bowel rest, TPN, IV steroid, broad-spectrum antibiotic.
        → If the disease has progressed to fever, leukocytosis, distension despite medical treatment → toxic colitis.
  - Failure to improve within 24–48 hrs → surgery.
  - Toxic colitis triad of fever, tachycardia, leukocytosis in patient with UC.

    $\rightarrow$ When distension of transverse colon
    $\rightarrow$ > 8 cm in x-ray $\rightarrow$ toxic megacolon $\rightarrow$
      impending colonic perforation $\rightarrow$ urgent
      resection is required.

- If patient with FC does not improve within 48–96 hrs $\rightarrow$ second-line therapy or surgery.
- 90% of patient with toxic megacolon refractory to steroid will respond to biologics (infliximab).
- 20%–30% of patients with fulminant colitis require surgery.
- If perforation is ensured $\rightarrow$ mortality rate after surgery is 57%.

- **Bleeding**
  - Massive bleeding with UC, 4%–5%.
  - 10% of colectomies (urgent).

- **CA**
  - o Risk of CA increases with time: 2% after 10 years, 8% after 20 years, then add 1% for each year, i.e., 18% after 30 years.
    Another meta-analysis:

Cumulative	Risk
10 years	2%
20 years	10%
30 years	50%
40 years	75%

  - Usually developed from flat dysplasia, so colonoscopy surveillance with 40–50 biopsies.
  - Use chemoendoscopy dye to mucosa at time of endoscopy $\rightarrow$ Lugol's solution, methylene blue $\rightarrow$ highlight between normal and dysplastic epithelium.
  - 20% with low-grade dysplasia has CA, so any patient with dysplasia $\rightarrow$ colectomy.
  - Controversy on prophylactic proctocolectomy in young age with no dysplasia.
    - $\rightarrow$ the recommendations is surveillance colonoscopy + biopsy.

- Endoscopic surveillance should begin after 8 years of the diagnosis and/or sooner depending of the age of patient.
- If patient has PSC and family history of CRC → surveillance interval should be shortened to annually.
  → Colonoscopy performed after remission to ↓ confusion in recognizing CA.
- If biopsy → HGD → elective prophylactic proctocolectomy → unrecognized synchronous CRC, in 20% of patients.
- For LGD → perform colectomy → if patient declines surgery → surveillance Q3–6M.
- Stricture, 5%–12%, and 25% being malignant.
  → Usually located at splenic flexure (86%).
  → Malignancy obstruction, 100%; benign, 14%.
  → Oncologic resection for colon and rectum is recommended for patient present with stricture.

- **Extracolonic Manifestation**
  - Hepatobiliary disease is most likely to inflow surgical management of colon and rectum.
  - Patient may require Liver TPx in primary sclerosing cholangitis (PSC).
    → If colectomy is required → stroma is contraindicated as ileostomy varices from Portal HTN.
  - Proctocolectomy is beneficial for erythema nodosum (most response), arthritis, and for eye disease but does not affect the outcome of PSC, ankylosing spondylolysis, sacroiliitis.

- **Growth Failure in Children**
  - Surgery is required.

Operative Management

Surgical Options

- Consider comorbidity, functional and continence status, and urgency of operation.
- Patient should have counseling for possible stoma.
- May require staged procedure.
- Today, MIS, ↓ use of stroma, cosmesis, fast recovery, ↓ incisional hernia, ↓ adhesion.
- Proctocolectomy + end ileostomy (gold standard).

- **Subtotal Colectomy + End Ileostomy (Hartmann's Procedure)**
  - Least morbid operation.
  - Operation of choice in emergency situation such as FC, TM, perforation,
  - first-stage process in patient desiring fertility.
  - Need surveillance proctoscopy for remnant rectum.

- **Total Proctocolectomy and End Ileostomy**
  - Low morbidity rate.
  - Comorbid patient.
  - Option in patient with high risk of pouch failure (impaired anal sphincter, previous anoperineal disease).

- **Total Proctocolectomy and Ileal Pouch-Anal Anastomosis (TPC-IPAA)**
  - Procedure of choice for many patients with UC in elective manner.
  - Morbidity, 19%–27%; mortality, 0.2%–0.4%.
  - 8–12 motions/day at the beginning then decrease.
  - Contraindicated in metastatic disease → adjuvant radiation therapy before pouch creation → because of postoperative pouchitis (radiation enteritis) and failure.
  - Can be done as two or three stages.
    - Two Stages
      1. TPC + IPAA and diverting loop ileostomy
      2. Reversal of ileostomy

    - Three Stages
      1. Subtotal colostomy + end ileostomy

2. Proctectomy + IPAA and diverting loop ileostomy
3. Reversal of ileostomy.

- Laparoscopic approach with one stage showed similar mortality and morbidity and stay.
- Double stapler pouch is preferred in J pouch anastomosis unless CA → mucosectomy + handsewn.
- Mobilization of SMA from retroperitoneal to ensure and achieve good length of ileum.
  → Ileocolic can be divided to increase length.
  → Wait 15 min to see vascularity of the pouch.

- **Colectomy with Ileorectal Anastomosis (IRA)**
  - Rarely used.
  - For IC, young, good rectal compliance for those who want to preserve fertility and avoid stoma, minimal rectal inflammation.
  - Risk of malignancy.
  - Disadvantage: can leave cancer behind.
  - Its contraindications if severe inflammation in rectum, perianal disease, known case of anal incontinence.
  - Need proctoscopic surveillance with biopsy.

- **TPC + Ileostomy (Kock Pouch)**
  - The procedure is abandoned when IPAA has good outcome.
  - Dysfunction, obstruction, slippage (50%).
  - Pouchitis, 25% → end ileostomy.

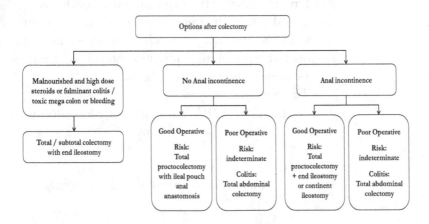

Crohn's Disease (CD)

- Characterized by remission and exacerbation.
- Diagnosis by colonoscopy or EGD, barium.
- Skip lesion is different from UC.
- Rectal sparing, 40%.
- Most common site is terminal ileum and cecum.
- Isolated perianal disease → complex fistula and/or abscess with skin tag, 5%.

Indication of Surgery

- As affecting any part, not like UC which can cured after resection of colon and rectum; CD is not.
- Surgery is for complication.
- CD → acute inflammation or chronic fibrotic disease.
- Acute intestinal inflammation.
- Complication: with fistula or intra-abdominal abscess.
- Treatment: anti-inflammatory, antibiotics, and NPO, TPN if malnourished.
- Most intra-abdominal abscess → CT-guided drainage.
- Once stabilized → resection of fistula with diseased part.
- Secondary fistula → no resection → simple closure.
- Stricture and fibrosis, resection, or strictureplasty.

Ileocolic and Small Bowel CD

- Ileum and cecum, 40%.
- Small bowel, 38%.
- Most common indication of surgery → fistula; abscess, 38%; obstruction, 35%–37%.
- Psoas abscess → from ileocolic disease.
- Short segment of small bowel is removed with right colon.
- Isolated chronic stricture → remove.
- If multiple fibrotic strictures, remove → strictureplasty.
  Short → transverse strictureplasty.
  Long → side-to-side bowel anastomosis.
- Risk of recurrence after resection of ileocolic or small bowel is high, 50% within 10 years.

Crohn's Colitis

- May present with TM or FC.
- Treatment is same as TM, FC in UC.
- Resuscitation, IVF antibiotics, IV steroid, if fail → total colectomy + end ileostomy + elective proctectomy required if CD involved rectum.
- Other indication → intractability, complication of medical treatment, risk of malignancy.
- Segmental colectomy is appreciated if the remaining part is normal.
- Isolated stricture → segmental colectomy.
- Now recognized that CD, especially with pancolitis → ↑ risk of cancer.
- Annul surveillance of colonoscopy and biopsy after 7 years.
- If dysplasia → proctocolectomy.
- Ileal pouch-anal anastomosis (IPAA) is not recommended because of complication.

Anal and Perianal CD

- Common, 35%.
- Isolated, 3%–5%.
- Most common lesion: skin tag + fissure.
  Fissure is deep and broad, multiple, located in lateral rather than anterior or posterior.
- Fistula is complex with multiple tracts.
- Treatment: alleviation of symptom.
- Skin tag and hemorrhoid should not be excised unless symptomatic → chronic non-healed wound.
- Fissure → responds to medical treatment usually lateral sphincterotomy, relatively contraindicated as non-healing + ↑ incontinence.
- Anal ulcer → EUA → to exclude deep abscess or fistula.
- If fissure without CD proctitis → partial lateral internal sphincterotomy.
- Seton to control fistula and avoid division of sphincter.

- Endoanal advancement flap may be considered if rectal mucosa is not involved.
- Intractable perianal sepsis → proctectomy.
- Rectovaginal fistula → rectal or vaginal mucosal advancement flap if healthy rectum, otherwise → proctectomy is the best option.
- Metronidazole is considered if active inflammation.
- Anti-TNF-a is effective in chronic fistula, secondary to CD.
- Pro-inflammatory IL-12 and interferon-d are used to inhibit immune cell migration.

Indeterminate Colitis (IC)

- 15% of IBD.
- Indication of surgery as UC.
- If diagnosis suggests UC → IPAA.
- If CD or indeterminant → completion proctectomy + end ileostomy.
- IPAA can be considered but failure rate is 15%–20%.

Diverticular Disease

- Diverticulosis refers to the presence of diverticula without inflammation.
- Diverticulitis refers to inflammation and infection associated with diverticula.
- Diverticular bleeding can be massive but usually is self-limited.
- It is pseudodiverticulum in which mucosa and muscularis mucosa herniate through colonic wall, at the point of penetration of nutrient artery (vasa recta), between the teniae coli, because of high pressure.
- True diverticula, which comprise all layers of the bowel wall, are rare and are usually congenital in origin.
- New suggestion of diverticulitis miminc IBD histopathology → most cells in mucosa → release of pro-inflammatory cytokines.
- Bleeding can be massive but self-limiting.
- Affects mostly the older people > 50.
- Sigmoid colon is the most commonly affected site, but in Asia, ascending colon, is commonest site 70%.
- Acquired cause → lack of dietary fiber increases radial pressure.

Evaluation

- Initial: laboratory, urine analysis, usually high WBC.
- Historically: barium with double contrast (air insufflation).
- CT: thin cut with oral and IV contrast; sensitivity and specificity, 98%–99%.
- Colonoscopy.
- CT colonography is not for acute phase, reserved for long-standing recurrent disease.
- US HR, 97%.
- MRI, 92%–94%.

Management

- Depends on presentation, stage, and complications.
- Asymptomatic diverticulosis is discovered at the time of colonoscopy or abdominal image managed by diet modification.
- 4% will develop diverticulitis; affects young and old populations.

- **Symptomatic Uncomplicated Diverticular Disease (SUDD)**
  - Lower-left quadrant (LLQ): pain and tenderness, fever.
  - Physical examination: tachycardia, tender LIF, ↑ WBCs.
  - CT: pericolic soft tissue stranding, colonic wall ticking, and/or phlegmon.
  - Can be managed as OPD with oral broad spectrum antibiotic for 7–10 days.
  - 10%–20% of patient with severe pain, fever, high WBCs are treated with bowel rest and IV antibiotics.
  - First dose of IV antibiotic, then oral antibiotic vs. hospitalization with IV antibiotic = same.
    - → Comorbid patient usually needs hospitalization.
    - → Otherwise, oral (aerobic + anaerobic) antibiotic such as ciprofloxacin or metronidazole for 7–10 days and bowel rest.
  - Some studies suggest diverticulitis is an inflammatory process rather than infection.
    - → Antibiotic or not = no difference, but ASCRS recommended antibiotic.
  - Deterioration and development of peritonitis → OR.
  - NSAIDs, 5-ASA, probiotics, rifaximin can be used and alleviate the disease.

- Medical therapy's success rate is 75%–91% as outpatient.
- Risk of complication is higher with recurrent disease.
- Immunosuppressed patient → colectomy after first episode.
- Colonoscopy after 4–6 weeks.
- Sigmoid colectomy + primary anastomosis is procedure of choice.
- Resection extended till rectum distally because risk of recurrence is higher for remnant sigmoid.
- Use of laparoscopy is encouraged.

- **Complicated Diverticulitis**
  - Abscess, obstruction, peritonitis (free perforation).
  - Fistula: colovesical, colovaginal, coloenteric.

Hinchey Classification
Stage I   Colonic inflammatory + pericolic abscess
Stage II   Intra-abdominal or retroperitoneal or pelvic abscess
Stage III   Generalized purulent peritonitis
Stage IV   Generalized fecal peritonitis

Modified Hinchey Classification
Stage 0   Mild clinical diverticulitis phlegmon
Stage Ia   Pericolic inflammation
Stage Ib   Pericolic abscess
Stage II   Intra-abdominal or pelvic retroperitoneal abscess
Stage III   General purulent peritonitis
Stage IV   General feculent peritonitis

Treatment of Complicated Diverticulitis
According to Hinchey classification:
- **Hinchey I, II**
  - Small abscess (3–4) cm will resolve spontaneously.
  - Large abscess or no clinical improvement → percutaneous drainage under CT or US guidance + IV antibiotic, bowel rest.
    - → 57.74% will avoid urgent operation.

> $\rightarrow$ Drain left in place till clinical improvement and output is minimal, < 30 mL/day.
> $\rightarrow$ Can be assessed by CT before removal of the drain.
> $\rightarrow$ Surgery considered if no improvement or inaccessible collection for drainage.

- Some suggest diverticulectomy (not supported).
- Immunosuppressant patient at risk if surgery was delayed, so threshold for surgery should be low.

- **Management of Free Perforation (Hinchey III, IV)**
  - Typically has sepsis.
  - Purulent vs. feculent, mortality rate is 6% vs. 35%.
  - Aggressive resuscitation.
  - Broad-spectrum antibiotic (IV).
  - Emergency surgery options:
    1. Historically, Hartmann's procedure
       Colostomy is taken down after 3–6 months
       $\rightarrow$ mortality, 10%–18%; morbidity, 43%; and stoma complication, 10%.
         - $\rightarrow$ It requires second operation for closure of colostomy.
         - $\rightarrow$ Nearly 35% will end with permanent colostomy.
    2. Laparoscopic peritoneal lavage (LPL) to control sepsis then elective definitive surgery.
       Hartmann's procedure vs. LPL = no difference, but reoperattion, 5.7% vs. 20%.
       Guidelines do not supports this.
    3. Resection with primary anastomosis + on-table lavage ± diversion (ileostomy).
         - $\rightarrow$ No need for second laparotomy, avoid stroma complication.
         - $\rightarrow$ Morbidity—31%, 23%, 49%.
         - $\rightarrow$ Mortality—3.8%, 7.2%, 17.4%.
           Still controversial in three studies.
  - Placing ureteric stent preoperatively is helpful.
  - Suspicion of malignancy $\rightarrow$ en bloc wide excision.

Evaluation after Recovery from Acute Diverticulitis
- After successful non-operative treatment →
  recommendation → colonoscopy after 6–8 weeks to
  confirm diverticular disease and to exclude IBD and CA.
  - → 3%–5% who has diverticulitis has CA in
    colonoscopy.
  - → Can use CT colonography.
- Fistula is a late complication, 12%, commonest
  colovesical fistula.
  - → Diagnosis by CT, cystogram or cystoscope.
  - → Can be by CT and rectal contrast.
- Fibrosis → stricture → biopsy to exclude CA.

Role of Surgery after Recovery from Acute Diverticulitis
- Traditional teaching → elective sigmoid colectomy after
  two episodes of uncomplicated diverticulitis or one
  episode of complicated diverticulitis, the mortality rate
  at first episode is 4.7% and 7.8% on second episode.
- Rate of recurrence after uncomplicated treated
  diverticulitis is 13%–23%, and only 6% with
  complicated diverticulitis.
- ASCRS do not consider the number of episodes in
  indication for colectomy, as chance of perforation at first
  episode is 25%; second, 12.7%; and third, 5.9%.
- Patient with comorbid disease, immunosuppression, has
  risk of perforation.
  - → Needs definitive intervention at first hospitalization.
- In complicated diverticulitis, elective sigmoid colectomy
  should be done after recovery.
- If patient with late complication, such as fistula, stricture
  → elective surgery is indicated.

Surgical Consideration
- Entire sigmoid is resected along with proximal rectum.
  - → More extension with low rectal anastomosis may
    be required if disease is extensive.
  - → Proximal extension till healthy descending colon.
  - → Mobilized splenic flexus mandate divides IMA
    and vein.

- No routine ureteric stent.
- MIS: conversion rate is 19%, ↓ stay, ↓ blood loss, ↓use of analgesia, decrease 30% of ileus, less anastomotic leak.
- Mortality after elective surgery of diverticulitis is 1%–2%. Morbidity, 25%–55%.
  Recurrence, 2.6%–12% → incomplete resection.

Diverticular Bleeding
- Most common causes of severe PR bleeding are bleeding diverticulosis, UC, angiodysplasia.
- Risk factors: HTN, atherosclerosis, smoking, alcohol, aspirin, Plavix, NSAIDs.
- Abrupt passage of red blood.
  → Melena can happen with slowly oozing from right colon diverticulum.
- Will stop spontaneously at 70%–80%.
- 3%–5% severe bleeding.
- Treatment: fluid and blood transfusion.
- 10%–15% have UGIB cause → should be ruled out.
- Several diagnostic procedures: colonoscopy, radionuclide, mesenteric angiography, CT angiography.
- For mild tomoderate → colonoscopy is diagnostic and therapeutic hemostasis by epinephrine injection or bipolar cautery or endoscopic band ligation. Disadvantage: bowel is not prepared.
- Radionuclide scan: non-invasive, detects bleeding, rate of 0.1 mL/min. Disadvantage: only for localization, not therapeutic.
- Mesenteric angiography, 0.5 mL/min → selective infusion of vasopressin, control is 90%, but recurrent bleeding in 50%.
- Can use coil embolization, 25% rebleed, 10% ischemia.
- CT angiography detects bleeding rate of 0.3—0.5 mL/min.
- After non-operative management → recurrence, 25% (lifetime).
  → Elective surgery is not warranted.

- Indication of surgery:
  → Failure of endoscopic or radiological intervention.

→ Requires blood transfusion of 4–6 units within 24 hrs.

→ Continuous bleeding after 72 hrs.

→ Rebleed after 1 week.

- If the source has been identified → segmental resection → rebleeding, 6%.

→ If bleeding site could not be identified → subtotal colectomy.

→ In the absence of comorbidity → primary anastomosis is safe.

→ Patients who receive massive transfusion do not have high risk of anastomosis leak.

Megacolon

- Chronic, dilated, elongated, hypertrophied colon.
- Congenital or acquired.
- Degree reflated to duration of obstruction.
- Evaluation by scope or radiation to exclude mechanical.

• Congenital Megacolon

- Caused by Hirschsprung's disease → failure of migration of neural crest cells to distal colon → absence of ganglionic cells in distal colon → failure of relaxation → dilation.
- Surgical resection of ganglionic segment is curative.
- Usually with infant and children → in adulthood also → if extremely short segment.

• Acquired Megacolon

- Infectious or chronic constipation.
- Infection by Trypanosoma cruzi (changes diagnosis) → destroys ganglion cells and produces megacolon and megaesophagus.
- Chronic constipation from medication (anticholinergic) or neurological disease (paraplegia, poliomyelitis, amyotrophic, lateral sclerosis, MS).
- Treatment: diverting ileostomy or subtotal colectomy with ileorectal anastomosis.

Toxic Megacolon (TM)

Sequale of colitis:
- Moderate colitis
    - Pulse > 90, SBP > 100, temp is 100°F–101.5°F, WBC is 12,000–15,000.
    - Pseudomembranous on colonoscopy, ↑colonic thickening on CT.
    - Colon diameter > 6 cm, Oliguria responsive to volume replacement, normal lactate.
    - Mild abdominal tenderness, mild tachypnea.
- Severe colitis
    - Moderate colitis + any of the following:
    - Pulse > 120, SBP < 100, WBC > 15,000
    - Renal failure, respiratory distress or intubation, albumin < 2.0.
    - Lactate > 2.0, mental status changes, moderate abdominal tenderness.
- Fulminant colitis (FC)
    - severe colitis with toxicity with or without colonic dilatation + of the following:
    - no improvement after 12–24 hrs of treatment, need vasopressors.
    - Ventilator dependence, abrupt rise in WBC
- Toxic megacolon (TM)
    - segmental or total colonic distension in presence of acute colitis and systemic toxicity or progression from fulminant colitis.
        → Cecal diameter > 12 cm or entire colon > 6 cm
    - Distinguished from pseudo-obstruction and Hirschsprung's disease by systemic toxicity.
    - Life-threatening, result of UC, CD, C. difficile infection.
    - Transverse colon is the area of concern in TM.
        → > 10 times bloody diarrhea
          HR > 90, T > 37.5
        → Requirement of blood transfusion
          ESR > 30
        → Abdominal distension and tenderness and dilated colon in x-ray.

Causes, Incidence, Pathogenesis

- Most common causes: UC, C. diff, associated colitis.
- Less common causes: CD, salmonella, shigella, CMV, ischemic colitis, chemotherapy, colonoscopy, barium enema, drug, low mortality, narcotic, antidiarrhea.
- TM with UC = 5%.
- C. diff historically 3%, now ↑ to 23%.
- Severe inflammation of colon → release of inflammatory mediator → smooth muscle relaxation.
- Acute severe mucosal inflammation → transmural.
  - → Inflamed smooth muscle produces nitric oxide (NO) → loss of motor tone and paralysis → toxicity from bacteria translocation.
  - → Also low K^+, low Mg^{++}, opiate, antidepressant.

Diagnosis

- History, physical examination, radiological.
- High index of suspicion with diarrhea, distension, and toxicity.
- Presence of peritonitis → ? perforation.
- Steroid masks the abdominal signs.
- Criteria:
Fever	> 38.5
HR	> 120
WBCs	> 10.5 (or anemia)
- Dehydration, mental changes, electrolyte disturbance, hypotension.
- X-ray typically shows air fluid level, thickening of colonic wall, and ascending colon; transverse colon vary ≈ 6–15 cm.
- If more than 8 cm, that means impending perforation.
- CT is useful to examine other cause of obstruction.
- Laboratory: ↑WBCs, anemia, ↑ ESR, ↑ CRP, ↓ K^+, Mg^+, and albumin.
- Stool C/S.

- Blood C/S as 25% of TM has bacteremia → cell cytotoxicity assay (best) and cell culture neutralizing therapy.
- Limited colonoscopy if patient is not a known case of UC and IBD, also to r/o pseudomembranous colitis.

Therapy

- Aggressive medical therapy, if failed → surgery.

Medical Therapy

- No evidence to use NGT → does not decompress colon.
- Rectal tube rarely helpful.
- Frequent repositioning > prone, let gas go to descending and rectum (no evidence).
- Bowel rest, NPO, IVF.
- Correct electrolytes (K$^+$, Mg^{+++}).
- Correct anemia.
- Stop antimotility drug (narcotic).
- Anti-DVT, antigastric ulcer.
- Broad-spectrum antibiotic.

- Treatment of TM and UC
  - Steroid IV hydrocortisone 100 mg IV Q6H.
  - 5-ASA, TNF-α.

- Treatment of TM and C. difficile.
  - If confirmed:
    - Oral vancomycin, 125–500 mg PO Q6H.
    - Or metronidazole, 500 mg PO Q8H or (IV).
      → Vancomycin, PR or NGT, if patient does not tolerate orally.

Surgical Therapy

- Timing of surgery, decreases mortality and morbidity.
- Medical treatment is effective in 50%–70%.
- If perforation or abdominal compartment syndrome (ACS) → mortality rate is 9%–40%.
- Discuss with patient and family for possible stroma.

- Absolute indication from surgery.
    - → Progressive colonic distension, uncontrolled hemorrhage, perforation, clinical deterioration, i.e., progressive sepsis (tachycardia, hypotension, needs pressor).
- Lack of improvement within 48 hrs is a relative indication for surgery.
- Mechanical bowel preparation is contraindicated.
- MIS is unsuitable because of fragile tissue, distended bowels.
- Standard: total colectomy + end ileostomy.
    - → No rectal resection even if inflamed.
    - → Divide mesentery close to bowel.
    - → If the rectum is severely inflamed → bring remnant of sigmoid colon as mucus fistula.
    - → If rectal stump left intra-peritoneum → rectal tube decompression to decompress and frequent vancomycin enema.
- Drain left at top of rectal stump → leak 5–7 days post-operative → emergent washing.
- Postoperative: ICU, continuous monitoring, IV antibiotic, taper steroids.
- There is another less invasive approach → loop ileostomy → colonic lavage and rectal tube.
    - → Lavage with 8 L warm NS and PEG with post-op vancomycin enema → colon is preserved 93%; colectomy, 7%.
    - → Not considered in patient with sepsis and pressor.

Outcomes
- Overall mortality rate is 19%.
- Mortality: medical vs. surgical = 27% vs. 19.5%.
- Progression to perforation, ↑ mortality, 40%; without perforation, 8.8%.
- Mortality after colostomy, 2%–5%.
- Complications: stricture, 15%; chronic segmental ischemia, 20%.
- Colonoscopy after recovery to rule out IBD, malignancy.

- Failure to improve within 2–3 days → surgery → necrotic bowel should be resected → sometimes second look may be necessary.

Ischemic Colitis

- Result from low flow and/or small vessel occlusion, i.e., when blood supply to colon does not meet cellular metabolic demand or result of occlusion of small blood vessels of the colon.
- Ranging from self-limiting form up to severe transmural colitis and gangrene.
- 1:1,000 of hospital admissions.
- Distinguish ischemic colitis from acute mesenteric ischemia by sudden severe pain.
- 20% of ischemic colitis require surgery.
- Commonly in old age with comorbidities.
- Predisposition: patient underwent abdominal surgery with ligation of IMA, septic shock, or heart failure.
- Other causes:
  - CVS/chest — Atherosclerosis, AF, COPD, HTN
  - GI — Constipation, diarrhea, IBS
  - Low flow state — Septic shock, CHF, H. shock, low BP
  - Surgery — Abdominal surgery, aortic (AAA) surgery, Cardiovascular surgery
  - Invasive procedure — Post-vascular stent (abdomen), postcolonoscopy
  - Metabolic — DM, RA, SLE, dyslipidemia
  - Miscellaneous — Hypercoagulability, SCD
  - Drugs — Constipating drug (opioid) antidiarrhea, immunomodulators, OCP, antibiotic, pseudoephedrine, diuretics, chemotherapy
- Anatomic consideration:
  - o Watershed: splenic flexure, rectosigmoid junction.
  - o Ileocolic is susceptible to embolic occlusion based on straight takeoff from SMA.

Clinical Presentation
- Crampy abdominal pain, bloody diarrhea, hematochezia, tenesmus (50%).
- Abdominal tenderness over affected area.
- Nausea and vomiting, low-grade fever.
- History focusing over risk factor.
- Left colon (splenic flexure) is more common followed by sigmoid colon.
- 25% isolated right side (AF, CHD, CRF).
- Most episodes are self-limiting.
- Recurrence is 10%.
- Chronic ischemic colitis up to 3 months.
- Colonoscopy → biopsy.

Diagnosis
- X-ray: rounded densities with gas-filled colon (thumb printing), mural thickening (mucosal edema and submucosal hemorrhage).
- CT: most common initial diagnostic tool, IV and oral contrast → pericolic fat stranding, ascites, pneumatosis, PV gas ± megacolon.
- CT angiography to r/o mesenteric ischemia.
- If ischemic colitis is diagnosed, no need for further vascular imaging.
- US can be used with Doppler flow.
- MRI does not provide additional information.
- Flexible colonoscopy is the gold standard in ischemic colitis, i.e., colonoscopy or sigmoidoscopy.
    - → Within 48 hrs.
- Single longitudinal ulcer (single strip) specific to ischemic colitis.
    - → If more severe ischemia → dusky submucosal hemorrhage and ulceration.
    - → Biopsy → mucosal infarction and ghost cells.
- Laboratory: ↑ WBCs, ↑ urea, ↑ lactate, ↑ LDH, ↓ Hb, ↓ albumin.
- DDx: mesenteric ischemia, IBD, diverticulitis, colon CA.
    - → Mesenteric ischemia most commonly affects small bowel.

Treatment
- Determine severity of ischemic colitis.
- If suspected acute mesenteric ischemia → CT angiography.
- If peritonitis or perforation → surgery (laparotomy).

- **Non-surgical Management**
  - 80% of ischemic colitis will respond to medical treatment → resolution of symptom over a few days.
  - NPO, IVF, and broad-spectrum IV antibiotic empirically at least for 1 week.
  - If nausea and vomiting → NGT.
  - Steroid is not recommended, unless used as therapeutic for SLE, RA, IBD.
  - In critically ill patient, limit the pressor.
  - Optimize COP.
  - Patient with Hx of AAA surgery or stent is at risk of IMA occlusion, fever, high WBCs, bloody diarrhea, abdominal pain, and distension after AAA repair + acidosis → urgent flexible endoscopy to evacuate colonic ischemia.

- **Surgical Management**
  - Mortality rate is 50%.
  - Indication for acute surgery:
    - Peritonitis, pneumoperitoneum, massive hemorrhage, sigmoid of transmural necrosis or pneumatosis intestinalis or portal vein gas.
    - If patient has worsened abdominal pain, high WBC, ↑ acidosis → exploration.
  - Right side appears to be more severe with increased need for surgery and high mortality compared to left, as well as pancolitis.
  - Intraoperative → IV fluorescein followed by illumination with UV light (Wood's lamp), helpful to assess bowel viability.
    - → Also, infra-red (light) angiography is a new method → ICG (IV).
  - Most cases require urgent exploration → resection.
  - Usually, stoma as primary repair is not advisable.

- If extension or patchy involvement → second look after 24 hrs.
- If entire colon is involved or massive bleeding → subtotal colectomy and end ileostomy.
- If patient underwent non-operative management and continues to have symptom > 2 weeks → reevaluation for colonic resection.
- Stricture is a consequence of ischemic colitis.
- If symptom continues → repeat colonoscopy + biopsy.

Infectious Colitis

- **Pseudomembranous Colitis (C. Difficile infection)(CDI)**
    - Gram +ve anaerobic bacillus.
    - Nosocomial infection.
    - Range from watery diarrhea to fulminant colitis (life-threatening).
    - Bacterial overgrowth because of prolong use of antibiotics, mostly clindamycin, risk of three- to fourfold.
    - Even single-dose antibiotics can produce the disease.
    - Prolonged hospitalization, low immunity.
    - Colonization of 20%–50% after hospitalization and can survive weeks to years.
    - The most frequently identified hypervirulent strain is known as NAP1/B1/O27, which is associated with mortality and resistance to antibiotic.
    - Bowel preparation and chemotherapy can alter colonic microflora.
    - Toxin alters enterocyte and disrupts tight junction.
    - Risk factors:
        - Primary risk factors: age > 65 years, antibiotic use within the previous 3 months, and hospitalization.
        - Secondary risk factors: female gender, double-occupancy rooms, ICU admission, post-pyloric tube feedings, chemotherapy, PPI or H2 blockers, gastrointestinal procedures, organ transplantation, HIV, autoimmune disease, IBD.

Clinical Picture
- Ranging from diarrhea to fulminant colitis (antibiotic-associated diarrhea).
- Worsening symptom → surgical intervention.
- SIRS, mortality, 30%–90%.
- Varies from moderated to FC.

Diagnosis
- C. difficile produces two toxins: toxin A (enterotoxin), toxin B (cytotoxic).
- Most useful tests are stool C/S, image, colonoscopy.
- Enzyme immunoassay for toxin A, B establishes definitive diagnosis.
- Laboratory: ↑ WBC, ↓ albumin, ↑ lactate.
- Plain x-ray: may reveal megacolon.
- CT sensitive with FCDI.
- Endoscopy → pseudomembranous, ulcer, plaque. Can be used as decompression, placement of tube, or irrigation with vancomycin.

Test	Sensitivity	Specificity
Cell cytotoxicity assays	60% - 100%	96% - 99%
Cell culture neutralization assays	67% - 86%	97% - 100%
Enzymatic detection of glutamate dehydrogenase	71% - 91%	76% - 98%
Enzyme immunoassay tests for toxins and B	39% - 76%	84% - 100%
Nucleic acid amplification test for toxins A and B	84% - 100%	94% - 100%

Medical Treatment
- Stop antibiotic, antidiarrhea, and narcotics.
- First line of treatment is oral vancomycin or IV or oral metronidazole.
- Progressive or recurrent infection → fecal microbiota transplantation (MTPx) → 90% effective.

Surgery
- 20% of critically ill with CDI will need surgery.
- Classic indication:
    → TM, FC, perforation, failure of medical treatment within 48–72 hrs, with sign of toxicity.
- TM with cecal diameter > 12 cm or entire colon > 6 cm.
- Total colectomy + end ileostomy.
    → No segmental resection.
    → Anastomosis is not recommended.
    → No laparoscopy.
    → CVP, arterial line, fluid resuscitation.
    → Stoma reversal after full recovery, 20%–55% with median interval closure in 234 days.
- Mortality after colectomy is 34%–57%.
- Alternative procedures → stoma from ileostomy, irrigation with PEG and NS and catheter, ± vancomycin enema.
    → lower mortality, ↑ stoma closure.

Recurrence
- 6%–47% within first week.
- First recurrence → oral vancomycin ± IV flagyl or oral, vancomycin enema.
- If subsequent recurrence → antibiotic, fecal TPx.

- **Other Infectious Colitides**
    - Bacteria, fungi, parasite, virus.
    - Bacteria: E. coli, yersinia, salmonella, shigella, MTB.
    - Parasite: amoeba.
    - Viral: mostly HIV, herpes simplex, CMV.
    - Symptoms: diarrhea with or without blood, crampy abdominal pain.

Management of Large Bowel Obstruction
1. Mechanical
    - Large bowel often due to neoplasm

- Colorectal cancer (CRC) is 50% of large bowel obstruction, ⅓ of CRC is near or total obstruction.
- Volvulus is the second most common cause.
- Diverticular disease is the third most common cause (stricture), 10%.
- Other: IBD, intussusception.

2. Functional or Adynamic
   - Colonic pseudo-obstruction (inertia), post-operative ileus, narcotic.

General Approach
- Abdominal pain, distension, obstipation, vomiting is late presentation.
- Hypovolemia, electrolyte imbalance.
- Clinical sign suggests perforation, strangulation, or ischemia with fever, tachycardia, peritonitis, pain out of proportion, shock.

Diagnosis
- History / physical examination
  - If disease is chronic and progressive, period of bloating, constipation, or acute such as volvulus.
  - Change in bowel habit, weight loss.

- Laboratory
  - CBC, anemia, leukocytosis.
  - Electrolyte imbalance.

- Image
  - X-ray: air fluid level; sensitivity, 84%; specificity, 72%.
  - Can distinguish cecum from sigmoid obstruction.
  - Distended bowel.

- CT (gold standard)
  - Sensitivity, 98%; specificity, 96%.
  - Cause, site, diameter of bowel.
  - Such cecum $\geq$ 12 cm $\rightarrow$ impending perforation.

- Endoscopy
    - Flexible sigmoidoscopy or colonoscopy.
    - Allow biopsy, can be therapeutic to reduce volvulus → risk of perforation is 1%.

Treatment

- Laparotomy if perforation, closed loop obstruction with ischemia.
- Because of IV volume depletion and fluid sequestration → aggressive fluid resuscitation + correction of electrolytes.
- UOP.
- NGT.
- Pre-operative IV antibiotic.
- Pre-operative stoma marking.

Surgical Technique

- Colostomy
    - Proximal to obstruction if patient is unstable, ill, septic, gross contaminated, malnourished.
        - → Loop colostomy is used because of distal blind loop.
    - ↑ morbidity: pararectal hernia, low quality of life. Re-operation.

- Segmental Colectomy
    - If right-side obstruction → right hemicolectomy + primary anastomosis.
        - → Can be by laparoscopy if stable and not overdilated.
        - → Decreases leak.
    - If left side → debate as there's 20% chance of leak.
    - If unstable left side → Hartmann's procedure, resection of distal obstruction + end colostomy.
        - → Morbidity is 35%.
        - → 45% of patients will remain with permanent colostomy.
    - If left side can perform resection with primary anastomosis as retrospective study showed right =

left resection + primary anastomosis is the same risk of leak.
- But if high-risk patient → protective loop ileostomy.
- Even if anastomotic leak or sepsis post-operative → percutaneous drainage.
- Loop ileostomy reversal is easier than colostomy.

- Subtotal Colectomy
    - With ileosigmoid or ileorectal anastomosis or end ileostomy and Hartmann's pouch.
    - This is an operation of choice for failed medical treatment with refractory functional large bowel obstruction.
    - Rarely used in mechanical bowel obstruction.

- Endoscopic Stent
    - Palliative with stent is used for patient who is not a candidate for surgery for advanced CA.
    - Or if benefitting from neo-chemotherapy and/or radiotherapy.
    - Success rate is 90%.
    - Bridge to surgery.
    - Allow decompression.
    - Surgery mortality is low, 5%–20% in elective surgery compared to emergency, ↑ primary anastomosis, ↓ stoma usage.

Volvulus
- Air-filled segment of colon twists about its mesentry.
- Sigmoid, 90%; cecum and colon, 10%.
- Chronic constipation, large redundant colon predisposed the volvulus especially if narrow mesentry.

- **Sigmoid Volvulus**
    - Distiguish from others by x-ray (bent inner tube or coffee bean) appearance.
    - Gastrografin → bird beak.
    - CT scan: swirl sign or whirlpool sign.

- Treatment: IVF (resuscitation) → then endoscopic deterioration by flexible sigmoidoscopy or colonoscopy → then rectal tube inserted to maintain decompression (majority cases), 85%–95%.
- If critical patient, clinical deterioration or signs of perforation or gangrene → OR.
- If scope → necrotic mucosa, ulceration, dark blood in endoscope → OR.
- If laparotomy → dead bowel → sigmoid colectomy with end colostomy (Hartmann's procedure).
- Recurrence is 40%–60%.
- Elective sigmoid colectomy should be performed.
- It is recommended to do sigmoid resection at same admission.

- **Cecal Volvulus (Bascule)**
  - Non-fixation of right colon.
  - Rotation around ileocolic vessel.
  - 10%–30% cecal fold around itself.
  - X-ray kidney shape with air-filled structure at upper-left quadrant (LUQ).
  - 20% gangrenous.
  - Cecal volvulus is never detorted; colonoscopy reduction success rate is 30%.
  - Gold standard is resection + primary anastomosis.
  - Right hemicolectomy + ileocolic anastomosis.

- **Transverse Colon volvulus**
  - Rare.
  - Gastrografin → proximal obstruction.
  - Endoscopic deterioration can occasionally be successful → most patients require OR (resection).

Pseudo-Obstruction (Ogilvie Syndrome)

- Functional disorder obstruction → massive dilated in absence of mechanical obstruction.
- Autonomic dysfunction and severe adynamic ileus.

- Associated with a number of conditions such as hospitalization, bed rest, post-operative, use of narcotic, comorbid disease like cardiopulmonary disease.
- Diagnosis by massive dilation of colon (right or transverse) in the absence of mechanical obstruction.
- CT: dilated colon without transitional zone.
- Initial treatment: conservative such as NPO, IVF, correct electrolytes, stop opioid and anticholinergic drugs.
- Rectal tube decompression is rarely effective, because of the distention in right and transverse colon.
- If failed → neostigmine (acetylcholinesterase inhibitors) after 24–48 hrs of conservative treatment, 2 mg IV STAT with cardiac monitor for bradycardia, may be inappropriate for cardiopulmonary diasease.
  → Next is colonic decompression (colonoscopy).
- Crucial to exclude mechanical obstruction by gastrografin enema prior to medical treatment and endoscopy.
- If failed to decompress → subtotal colectomy + end ileostomy after 6 days on conservative treatment.
- Can use percutaneous cecostomy before surgery.

Management of Radiotion Injury to Small and Large Bowel
- Common with cancer of abdomen, pelvis, retroperitoneum.
- Effect on bowel may be acute and self-limiting.
- Chronic manifests after months to year after therapy.

Therapeutic and Toxic Effect of Radiotherapy
- Direct cellular damage secondary to inflammatory and immunity response.
- Tissue with high cell turnover such as skin and bowel are sensitive to acute effect of radiation.
- In normal circumstances, reactive O_2 oxidation from cell antioxidant in radiotherapy overwhelms the process.
- Other tissues such as brain and lung have acute toxicity.
- DM, atherosclerosis, collagen disease → high susceptibility to chronic radiotherapy toxicity and also smoking and decrease weight.
- New modality such as SBRI, IMRI → high dose of radiotherapy to the tumor to decrease toxicity.

- Brachytherapy: placement of radioactive material around tumor to maximize the effect.

Radiation Injury to the Bowel

- Terminal ileum, cecum, rectum are most common sites of injury.
- Presence of adhesion from previous surgery is high risk.
- Acute phase by activated O_2 radicals → mucosal inflammation and stimulation of pro-inflammatory cytokines → infiltration of inflammatory cells to mucosa.
- Chronic: fibrosis → vasculitis → chronic ischemia → mucosal atrophy.
- Acute GI toxicity occurs mostly at week 5, resulting in diarrhea, cramping, minor bleeding.
- Treatment: supportive, antimotility, rehydration.
- Late: months to years → stricture, fistulation, telangiectasia.
- Symptom of acute bowel toxicity occurs in 60%–90% who underwent radiotherapy for abdomen.
- Prostate CA → EBR → 40%–60% rectal acute toxicity.
- Another late complication → bowel malignancy, 1.7 %.

Prevention

- Good position, prone, full UB, elevate hips, isolate the bowel.
- Modern delivery: SBRI, IMRI.
- Use of clips intraoperative or PET-CT to localize the tumor bed to minimize radiation.
- ACE inhibitor, statin, arginine, probiotics, ↓ severity of radiotherapy-induced bowel injury.
- One of the best ways is to use radiotherapy preoperatively rather than postoperatively, especially in retroperitoneal, pelvis (as bowel enters the field post-proctectomy).

- **Indication of Surgery**
  - If acute, no role.
  - Chronic obstruction, perforation, fistula, and bleeding → generally, resection and anastomosis are better than bypass, except if single-loop adherent in pelvic area.

- Proctitis (very common):
  - diarrhea, bleeding, mucus discharge.
    Acute: no role of surgery, self-limited.
    Chronic: bleeding, sucralfate enema, short-chain fatty acid.
    → Formalin solution.
    → Endoscopic option: cautery, laser.
  - In severe uncontrollable bleeding, APR or intersphincteric proctectomy.

- Fistula
  - Upper and mid rectum → resection anastomosis.
  - The interposition of a well-vascularized tongue of omentum or a pedicled rectus muscle between the anastomosis and the affected organ may be considered.
  - Temporary proximal diversion should be performed.
  - Lower rectum → fecal diversion and/or urinary before reconstruction, then reconstruction with flap.

Iatrogenic Injury of Colon
- **Intra-Operative**
  - During pelvic procedure.
  - Early recognition.
  - Majority of injuries are closed primarily.
  - If delayed recognition → peritonitis → fecal diversion is almost always required.

- **Barium Enema**
  - Rare, but ↑ mortality and morbidity if unrecognized early, especially if intraperitoneal → spillage of barium → peritonitis.
  - If early recognized → primary closure, abdominal irrigation.
  - If patient developed sepsis → fecal diversion.
  - Small extraperitoneal: rectum → bowel rest, IV antibiotics, and close observation.

- **Colonoscopic Perforation**
  - 1%, either by tip, shear force, barotrauma, biopsy, fulguration, polypectomy results in post-polypectomy syndrome → abdominal pain, fever, leukocytosis, peritonitis.
  - Treatment: depends on size and underlying diasease.
  - Large → surgical exploration, as bowel is prepared, usually little contamination → repair primarily.
  - If delayed, unstable, high contaminant → proximal diversion.
  - If underlying neoplasm → definitive resection.
  - Usually, patient has microperforation → NPO, IVF, IV antibiotic, close observation.

Surgical Management of Constipation
- Constipation, 28% of general population.
- Small percent is due to surgical issues.

Definition and Scoring
Rome III criteria:
- Requires two or more criteria at least 3 months.
  1. Straining at 25% of defecation.
  2. Lumpy or hard stool at least 25% of defecation.
  3. Sensation of incomplete for at least 25% of defecation.
  4. Sensation of anorectal blockage at least 15%.
  5. Manual maneuver to facilitate 25% of defecation.
  6. Less than 3 motion/week.
- To diagnose IBS, recurrent abdominal pain or discomfort for at least 3 months + three criteria:
  1. Pain discomfort released by defecation.
  2. Change in stool frequency.
  3. Change in stool appearance.
- Bristol stool scale.
- Wexner constipation score.

Classification and Surgery Selection
- Colonic or extracolonic, functional or non-functional, primary or secondary.

- Selection of patient for surgery:
    1. Slow transit constipation or colonic inertia.
    2. Pelvic floor dysfunction.
    3. Mixed
    4. Norma transit constipation
- Treatment of NTC IBS is non-surgical.

Steps for Treatment
1. Colonoscopy or contrast enema, flexible sigmoidoscopy, proctoscopy to rule out mechanical blockage.
2. If no anatomical cause → fybogel (fiber) BID.
3. If no improvement → PEG or lactulose.
4. If no improvement → 5-HT serotonin agonist.
      → If no improvement within 6 months → anal manometry and defecography.

- **Transit Studies**
    - Ingest 24 radiopaque markers in single capsule.
    - Normal transit time is 31 hrs in male and 39 hrs in female
      → x-ray obtained in day 3, 5.
    - Also, colonic transit can be assessed by nuclear scintigraphy.
    - Defecography: dynamic evaluation of pelvic floor during active defecation + fluoroscopy or MRI.
    - Manometry and HRAM are new techniques.

Surgical Option and Technique
- **Subtotal Colectomy**
- **Pelvic floor dysfunction (PFD)**
    - Includes obstructed defecation syndrome, and paradoxical puborectalis → diagnosed by defecography.
    - Rectocele, enterocele, sigmoidocele → STARR.

- **Mixed**
    - Total abdominal colectomy with biofeedback for PFD.
    - Adult Hirschsprung's disease
      → History of lifelong constipation, anal manometry, and full-thickness rectal biopsy.

Colon Cancer and Polyps

- Colorectal cancer (CRC)→ most common malignancy in gastrointestinal tract.
- 140,000 new cases annually; 50,000 dies annually.
- Male = female.

Etiology

- Age ↑ after 50s–90s → screening above 50.
- Sporadic, 80%; hereditary (family history), 20%.
- Environment and dietary
  - ↑ animal fat and red meat, ↓ fiber.
  - Fish oil, coconut, olive oil do not increase the risk.
  - Fat toxic to colonic mucosa.
  - Alcohol ↑ the incidence.
  - Obesity and sedentary life ↑ the risk.
  - Vitamins A, C, E ↓ incidence.
- IBD
- Others:
  - Smoking for 35 years.
  - Ureterosigmoidostomy.
  - Acromegaly.
  - Pelvic irradiation.

Pathogenesis

- **Genetic Defect**
  - CA developed from adenomatous polyps.
  - Defect in APC gene (tumor suppressor genes) → initiation of polyps → responsible also for FAP (APC → dominant).
  - One of mostly gene-involved K-RAS (EGER) proto-oncogen.
  - BRAF.
  - P53 → apoptosis irreversible genetic damage, 75% of CRC.
  - MYH mutations have been associated with an AFAP (recessive).
  - PTEN: hamartomas polyps, Cowden syndrome, juvenile polyps.

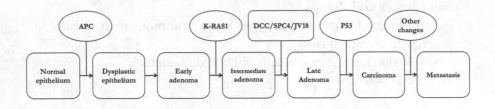

- **Genetic Pathway**
  LOH, MSI, CpG, CIMP

Polyps

- Overgrowth of epithelium lining mucosa.
- Carcinoid and lipoma are not polyps.
- Usually asymptomatic but can bleed, tenesmus if in the rectum.
- Majority of CRCs are arise from adenomatous polyps.

Types

- **Neoplastic**: adenoma (tubular, villous, tubulovillous), serrated (sessile serrated adenoma).
- **Non-neoplastic**: hyperplastic, inflammatory, hamartomatous.

- **Adenoma**
  - Adenomatous polyp—occurs in 25% of above 50s, 50% at age 70, but only 1%–4% at age 20.
    - Tubular adenoma, 5% risk of malignancy.
    - Tubulovillous adenoma, 22%.
    - Villous adenoma, 40%.
  - Invasive CA is rare in polyps < 1 cm.
  - Represent > 50% of all colonic polyps.
  - Risk increases with size.
  - 80% of CRC developed from adenoma.
  - Risk of CA if > 2 cm, 35%–50%.
  - Pedunculated or sessile.
  - Pedunculated → colonoscopic snare excision.
  - For rectal sessile → transanal excision (OR).
  - First mutation leading to sporadic adenoma polyps is APC.

$\rightarrow$ Followed by deleted in colorectal carcinoma (DCC) $\rightarrow$ advanced adenoma.

$\rightarrow$ Final step, P53.

- Average time for development of adenoma to CA is 7–10 years.
- Incidence of synchronous adenoma in colon CA is 30%.
- Risk of unresectable polyp to have CA is 4% at 5 years, 14% at 10 years.

  $\rightarrow$ If adenoma found in sigmoidoscopy should converted to colonoscopy for biopsy or polypectomy and subsequent surveillance.

- Risk of metachronous colon CA, $\uparrow$ numbers of advanced adenomas.
- Sessile $\rightarrow$ saline lift, piecemeal snare, EMR $\rightarrow$ Indian ink for follow-up colonoscopic biopsy.
- Colectomy for large, flat, or if invasive CA is confirmed.
- Complication of polypectomy $\rightarrow$ perforation and bleeding.
- Small perforation $\rightarrow$ NPO, IV antibiotics, close observation. If sepsis, peritonitis $\rightarrow$ laparotomy.
- Bleeding during intervention $\rightarrow$ resnare, cauterization if delayed angiography with infusion of vasopressin.

- **Serrated Polyp**
  - Uncommon, 0.5%–4%.
  - $\uparrow$ risk of malignancy.
  - Usually > 5 mm, affects right colon and male gender.
  - Separated pathway: B-RAF, CPG, MLH1.
  - Rapid progression than adenoma.

- **Hyperplastic Polyps**
  - Results from accumulating cells on mucosal surface.
  - Small < 5 mm, hyperplasia with no dysplasia.
  - Most common non-neoplastic type.
  - 50% of polyps are 1–5 mm; 28%, 6–9 mm, 14%, > 10 mm.

- Typically, sessile adenoma is found in sigmoid and rectum.
- Not premalignant but cannot be distinguished from adenomatous polyps endoscopically.
- Large hyperplastic > 2 cm → premalignant may have foci of dysplasia tissue.
- Should not shorten standard recommended screening interval of 10 years.

- **Hamartomatous Polyps**
  - Polyps of childhood but can occur at any age.
  - Bleeding is the most common presentation, then intussusception and/or obstruction.
  - Treatment → polypectomy.
  - Sporadic and non-sporadic.
  - Non-sporadic is found in three syndromes → familial juvenile polyposis, Peutz-Jeghers syndrome, Cowden syndrome.
  - Not premalignant.
  - in non-sporadic (syndromic) → can develop to CA.

- Juvenile Polyposis Coli
  - Autosomal dominant → 10–100 polyps in GIT (mostly colon and rectum).
  - 50% are associated with CRC.
  - If patient has family history → familial juvenile polyposis.
    - → Repeat colonoscopy Q3 Years if no polyps, annually if there are polyps.
  - Extraintestinal manifestations: lip and palate anomalies, polydactyly, intestinal malrotation, CHD, hydrocephalus, AVM in GI, lung, brain, GI bleeding.
  - CRC is higher than gastric, duodenal, and pancreatic CA.
  - Screening colonoscopy if symptomatic or at age of 10–15.
  - If no polyp is reported asurviellence 2–3 years.

- if polyp is reported → annually.
- EGD at age 25.
- Usual treatment if rectum is spared → colectomy (total), ileorectal anastomosis + close surveillance to rectum.
- If rectum is involved → proctocolectomy—IPAA.

- **Peutz-Jeghers Syndrome**
  - Mutation of LKB1 (STK11) tumor suppressor genes.
  - Polyposis of small bowel and less frequent in colon and rectum.
  - Melanin spot in buccal mucosa and lips and mucosal hyperpigmentation.
  - It's hamartomatous and has no malignancy risk.
  - can develope a carcinoma of gastrointestinal tract, 2%–13%.
  - Start colonoscopy if symptomatic or at 15–20 Q3Y, then annual flexible sigmoidoscopy.
  - Can lead to intussusception, bleeding, obstruction.

- **Cronkhite-Canada Syndrome**
  - Gastrointestinal polyposis + alopecia + cutaneous pigmentation, atrophy of finger and toenail.
  - Symptoms: diarrhea, vomiting, malabsorption, protein-losing enteropathy.
  - Many patients die from this disease.
  - Surgery for obstruction.

- **Cowden Syndrome**
  - Autosomal dominant: hamartoma of all three layers of embryo.
  - Facial trichilemmomas, breast CA, thyroid disease, GI polyps.

- Treatment is based on symptom, should be screened.
- 16% risk of CRC.
- Colonoscopy at age 45 then Q5Y.

- **Inflammatory Polyps (Pseudopolyps)**
  - Associated with IBD but can occur in amebic colitis, ischemic colitis, schistosomal colitis.
  - Not premalignant but cannot be distinguished from adenomatous polyps.
  - Microscopic → normal regenerated mucosa (polyps) surrounded by area of mucosal loss.
  - Can be extensive → mimic to FAP.

Guideline for Colonoscopy Screening and Surveillance

- General population at age 50 and 10 years interval.
- First-degree relative with CRC, start 10 years younger than youngest age at the time of diagnosis and 5 years interval.
- After 85, stop surveillance.
- Other modality: virtual colonoscopy, stool DNA testing.
- Patient with small hyperplastic polyp, 10 years interval.
- If 1–2 tubular adenoma < 10 mm or LGD → 5–10 years interval.
- High-risk adenoma:
  1. 3–10 adenomas.
  2. 1 tubular > 1 cm.
  3. villous or HGD.
     → Repeat after 3 years.
- If large sessile polyp is removed → repeat colonoscopy 3–6 months.
- If single Serrated sessile adenoma < 10 mm with no dysplasia → repeat 5 years.
- If multiple serrated sessile adenoma > 1 cm, with dysplasia → repeat after 3 years.

NB: for screening guidelines of any disease, please visit: www.uspreventiveservicestaskforce.org.

Management of Polyps
- Relative contraindications for polypectomy are coagulopathy, acute colitis, malignancy such as ulcerative hard-fixed lesion, necrosis, inability to raise the lesion.
- forceps polypectomy for smaller < 2–5 mm.
- Snare polypectomy:
    - For large polyp > 4 mm.
    - Short stalk.
    - Injection of normal saline with or without epinephrine in the submucosa if large sessile polyp.

- If large > 2 cm or giant > 3 cm:
    - Endoscopic Mucosal Resection (EMR)
        - By snare, injection of submucosal plane by saline
            → If incomplete excision → argon plasma coagulation.
        - Surveillance should be 3–6 months.
    - Endoscopic Submucosal Dissection (ESD)
        - Offer en bloc excision.
        - Injection of saline in submucosa at the edges.
            → Incise the edge, dissection, then remove en bloc.
        - Removal achievement is 85%, and −ve margin, 75%.

    NB: it's important to tattoo area of excision with Indian ink.

Complications
- Bleeding
    - 0.5%–2.25%.
    - Hemostatic clip or epinephrine injection.
- Perforation
    - 0.1%.
        → With EMR, 1%; ESD, 4%.
        → Conservative treatment.
        → If any sign of deterioration → laparoscopy or laparotomy.

- Postpolypectomy syndrome
  - 0.3% due to electrocautery.
  - Pain, fever, high WBCs.
  - CT: fat stranding but no pneumoperitoneum, only microperforation and bacteria translocation.
  - Treatment: NPO, IVF, IV antibiotic, observation.
- Large polyp in rectum
  - Combined endoscopic and laparoscopic surgery.

Approach to Malignant Polyps
- Up to 5% of polyp contain invasive component, the risk is ↑ with increasing polyp size.
- Depth of submucosal invasion predicts LNs metastasis.
- Risk of LNs +ve in polyps (malignancy) is 11%, and it's 20% if single feature and 36% if two features.

Haggitt level

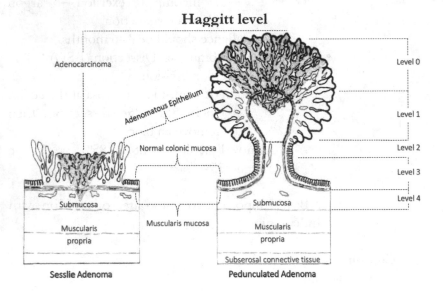

Pathologic Feature of Malignant Polyp

1. mucosal invasion	Head 1, neck 2, stalk 3, base or sessile 4
2. Submucosal invasion	Upper ⅓ SM1, middle SM2, 1 cm SM3
3. Tumor grade	Well, moderate, poor differentiation
4. Tumor budding	presence of clusters of malignant cells in the submucosa

Management

- The adequacy of endoscopic resection is dependent on the risk of nodal metastasis, as endoscopic resection does not remove or sample the LNs drainage basin.
- Many studies have shown that the incidence of nodal metastasis is < 1% for polyps completely removed endoscopically with a Haggitt level 1, 2, or 3 invasion.
- Cranley and colleagues suggest a 0.3% incidence of nodal involvement in pedunculated polyps with favorable criteria.
- For Haggitt level 4 lesions with favorable histology or sessile lesions with SM1 or SM2 depth without additional unfavorable histologic features, it is felt that these lesions are low risk and can be favorably managed with endoscopic polypectomy alone, provided margins are > 2 mm.
- Pedunculated polyps with Haggitt level 4 lesions exhibiting unfavorable histology, sessile lesions with SM1 or SM2 depth and poor histologic features, and sessile lesions with SM3 depth have a much higher incidence of lymph node metastasis and ranges from 12%–25%, indicating a formal oncologic resection.
- Unfavorable features that define poor histology include: lymphovascular invasion, poor differentiation, and negative resection margin < 2 mm.
- Close observation and surveillance after polypectomy.
- Apart from all the above, formal oncologic resection should be recommended in fit patient because of risk of LNs metastasis.

Inherited Colorectal Cancer
Familial Adenomatous Polyposis (FAP)

- Autosomal dominant, 1% of all CRC.
- Mutation in APC gene located in chromosome 5q21 (tumor suppressor gene).
- APC mutation +ve in 75%.
- Most have +ve family history; 25% do not.
- Defines as > 100 adenomas or < 100 with family history.
- 100 to 1,000 adenomatous polyps after puberty.

- 100% CA risk lifetime by age 40–50.
- Present by 15% at age 10 and 75% at age 20.
- APC gene testing for all family members.
- Flexible sigmoidoscopy for first-degree relative at age 10–15 annually until 24, then every 2 years until 34, then every 3 years until 44, and then every 3–5 years.
- At risk to develop adenocarcinoma at any part of GIT, especially in duodenum (periampullary).
  - Extraintestinal manifestation
    - 80%–90% gastric, fundic, hyperplastic polyps have less malignancy potential.
    - Gastric edema, 10%.
    - Duodenal adenoma around ampulla.
      - → CA in 5%–10%.
      - → EGD at age 20, then every 1–3 years.
      - → Spigelman classification:

Stage I	0%	no dysplasia→ biopsy and observation
Stage II	2.3%.	Mild dysplasia, tubular 1-4 mm → PPD or PD if CA
Stage III	2.4%	moderate dysplasia, tubulovillous 5-10 mm → PPD or PD if CA
Stage IV	36%	HGD, villous > 1 cm, PPD or PD if CA

      PPD: pancreas-preserving duodenectomy
      PD: pancreaticoduodenectomy
    - Chemoprevention: NSAIDs.
  - Another manifestation: osteoma, epidermoid cyst, congenital hypertrophy of rectal pigmentation, desmoid tumor (Gardner syndrome).
  - Mandibular osteoma, medulloblastoma, CA liver and biliary, thyroid nodule.
- Once diagnosed with FAP + polyps developed → surgery.

- Desmoid tumor:
  - 15%–30% myofibroblastic tumor.
  - ↑ in male.
  - Treatment: excision with −ve margin 1 cm, recurrence 20%–50%, bypass if for palliative.
  - Medical treatment: COX-2 NSAIDs, tamoxifen helps in regression.
- Four factors affecting the choice of operative intervention:
  1. Age of patient
  2. Presence of severe symptom
  3. Rectal polyposis
  4. Location or desmoid tumor
- There are three options of operation:
  1. Total proctocolectomy + end ileostomy (Brooke)
  2. Total abdominal colectomy + ileorectal anastomosis
  3. Restorative proctocolectomy + ileal pouch-anal anastomosis (IPAA) with or without temporary ileostomy
- Most elect to have IPAA in the absence of distal rectal CA or mesenteric desmoid tumor or poor sphincter.
- Mucosectomy in patient undergoing IPAA → to prevent neoplasia of transitional zone, 50% → incontinence.
- In case of colectomy and ileorectal anastomosis, need to do annual proctoscopy with frequent biopsy.
- COX-2 delays and decreases the development of polyps.

Attenuated FAP

- Late presentation at 30–40 of age, 10–100 polyps in the right colon.
- CRC → in 50% but occurs later in 55 years.
- At risk of duodenal polyps.
- APC mutation present in 30% autosomal dominant.
- Most are Autosomal recessive.

- Risk of malignancy is 100% at age 60.
- Family members are at risk as well.
- Colonoscopy at age 13–15, then every 4 years till age 28, then every 3 years.
- Prophylactic COX-2 is appreciated.
- Should rule out HNPCC.

Hereditary Non-Polyposis Colorectal Cancer (HNPCC) (Lynch Syndrome)

- More common than FAP, 1%–3% of all CRC.
- Mismatch repair MSI.
- Autosomal dominant.
- CRC at age of 40–45.
- 70% affected.
- Mostly affects proximal colon, better prognosis than sporadic.
- Synchronous or metachronous lesions, 40%.
- Extracolonic malignancy; endometrial, ovary, pancreas, stomach, small bowel, biliary, and urinary cancers.
- Diagnosis is based on family history.
- Amsterdam criteria to diagnose HNPCC:
    - Three affected relatives, one must be a first-degree relative in two successive generations + one diagnosed before 50.
- Tumor testing for mismatch repair gene IHC and/ or MSI.
- Screening colonoscopy annually begins at 20–25 or 10 years younger than youngest age at the time of diagnosis.
- Endometrial CA → transvaginal US or endometrial biopsy after age 25–35.
- Risk at 40 to develop another CA → total colectomy with ileorectal anastomosis once adenoma or CA. → Annual proctoscopy.
- TAH-BSO is recommended after childbearing age.

Mutation Y Homolog–Associated Polyposis

- MYH or MAP.
- Autosomal recessive.

- Polyps are variable but median ≈ 50 polyps.
- Left colon CA risk is 80% at age 40.
- Colonoscopy, EGD at age 25–30 years; if no polyps, repeat 3–5 years.

Familial Colorectal CA

- Non-syndromic familial CRC, 10%–15%.
- Average risk population is 6%.
- 12% if +ve 1, first-degree relative.
- 35% if +ve 2, first-degree relative.
- If CA incidence before 50 → increase risk of family member.
- Screening colonoscopy every 5 years beginning at 40 or 10 years earlier than diagnosis of the patient's relative.
- Defect in LOH or MSI may be present.

Prevention (Screening and Surveillance)

- **Fecal Occult Blood Test (FOBT)**
  - Reduce CRC mortality by 33% and metastasis by 50%.
  - Missing adenoma, 50%.
  - Specificity is low, i.e., 90% with false +ve test.
  - Increases with red meat, vitamin C intake.
  - Guideline → annually for symptomatic above 50.

- **Flexible Sigmoidoscopy**
  - Every 5 years → ↓ 60%–70% of CRC mortality.
  - Proximal colonic lesion → cannot be identified.
  - Usually paired with air contrast barium enema.
  - Any polyps → colonoscopy.
  - ACS recommendation→ annual FOBT + flexible sigmoidoscopy every 5 years; addition of ACBE improves sensitivity.

- **Colonoscopy**
  - Most accurate and most complete even for polyp < 1 cm.
  - Allow biopsy, polypectomy, control hemorrhage, dilatation.

- Require bowel preparation and sedation.
- Complication: perforation, 0.2%–0.3%.

- **Air Contrast Barium Enema (ACBE)**
  - Polyp > 1 cm (90% sensitive).
  - Compromised in sigmoid in presence of diverticulosis.

- **CT Colonography (Virtual Colonoscopy)**
  - Less invasive.
  - Accurate.
  - Helical CT technology 3D reconstruction.
  - Requires bowel preparation.
  - Colon insufflated with air.
  - Detects lesion > 1 cm, if +ve → colonoscopy.
  - False +ve from stool, haustral folds, flat lesion.

- **Guidelines of Screening (ACS)**
  - If no symptom or family history, no polyps beginning at age 50
  - Yearly FOBT, flexible sigmoidoscopy every 5 years or a combination of both.
  - ACBE every 5 years.
  - Colonoscopy every 10 years.

Routes of Spread and Natural History

- Affects 1 million worldwide; 50% will die from the disease.
- Second leading cause of death.
- Carcinoma arises from mucosa, then invades adjacent layer.
- Bulky and circumferential → obstruction
- nodal metastasis with increase in size of tumor and depth (most predictor).
- Tis, there is no invasion to basement membrane of the mucosa, i.e. high-grade dysplasia → no risk of LNs metastasis.
- T1, T2, 5%–20% +ve LNs metastasis.
- T3, T4, 50% +ve LNs metastasis.

- Number of LNs correlates with presence of distant disease.
- Four or more +ve LNs → poor prognosis.
- Nodal spreading along inferior rectal vessels to internal iliac node or groin is rare unless obstructive of proximal LNs by tumor or anal canal tumor.
- Most common metastasis (distant) is the liver via hematogenous spread via portal vein.
- Liver metastasis increases with tumor size.
- Carcinomatosis (diffused peritoneal metastasis) by peritoneal seeding → dismal prognosis.

Staging and Preoperative Evaluation
- **Clinical Picture**
  - Most common presentation in abdominal pain: bleeding per rectum, anemia, constipation, or diarrhea, i.e., change in bowel habit, weight loss, ¯ appetite.
  - Right-side CA: anemia could be obstructed at ileocecal valve.
  - Left-side CA: obstruction as small-caliber firm stool.
  - Rectal: bleeding, tenesmus, pain.

- **TNM Classification**
  Old Dukes or modified Astler-Coller has been replaced by TNM.

Tx	Cannot be assessed
T0	No evidence of CA
Tis	Carcinoma in situ (high-grade dysplasia)
T1	Tumor invades submucosa
T2	Tumor invades mucosa
T3	Tumor invades subserosa
T4	Tumor invades adjacent organ
Nx	Cannot be assessed
N0	No LNs
N1	Metastasis 1–3, pericolic or perirectal
N2	Metastasis +4, pericolic or perirectal
N3	Metastasis to any along named major vessels
M0	No metastasis
M1	Metastatic disease

- **Staging**

I	T1–T2	N0
II	T3–T4	N0
III	any T with	N1
IV	any T with	any N with M

  - In colon, staging depends on examination of specimen.
  - Minimum of twelve LNs to adequately assess nodal status and accurate staging.
  - In rectal CA → endorectal US or MRI may be used for prediction.
  - Survival rate per stage: I, 93%; II, 80%; III, 60%; IV, 16% or less.
  - Nodal involvement is the single predictor factor.
  - degree of differentiation and mucinous or signet ring is the most important predictors.

- **Pre-operative Evaluation**
  - Liver function test.
  - ↑ CEA in advanced disease but not prognostic factor → it is useful for follow-up after resection.
  - Colonoscopy, as 5% for colon CA has synchronous lesion.
  - CT chest, abdomen, pelvis (CAP).
  - For rectal: rigid sigmoidoscopy or proctoscopy + biopsy. EUS or MRI is helpful.
  - PET is not routinely recommended.

Therapy for Colonic CA

  - Remove primary with its lymphovascular supply, i.e., pericolic LNs removed with regional LNs located along the course of major vessel.
  - Synchronous: two or more primary CA can coexist at the time of diagnosis.
  - Metachronous: CA developed consequently, sometimes years after resection.
  - Twelve LNs needed minimum for assessment (staging).
  - Needs at least 5 cm free margin.

- If distant metastasis is low volume, may proceed with resection (metastasectomy).
  → If large volume → abort the procedure → for neoadjuvant therapy.
- Some centers use diagnostic laparoscopy.
- No evidence of the bowel preparation will improve outcomes, but bowel preparation + oral antibiotic and IV antibiotic preoperative before skin incision decrease SSI.
- The outcome depends on stage.
- Two categories: amenable to resection and palliative.
- If resectable, surgery then adjuvant chemotherapy.
- If advanced disease → Neoadjuvant chemotherapy; then re-assessment → resection or palliative.
- 80%–90% are candidates for colonic resection.
- Should assess the liver by intraoperative U/S.
- Do more extensive resection if LNs are involved, even if subtotal colectomy.
- Tumor in cecum or ascending → right hemicolectomy (can extened accordingly) + high ligation of ileocolic and right colic to provide adequate lymphadenectomy.
- Tumor in transverse colon → either right or left, colectomy depends on proximal or distal.
- Tumor in descending → left hemicolectomy and high ligation of left colic artery.
- Sigmoid colon → either left hemicolectomy or sigmoid resection.
- Open vs. laparotomy vs. robotic = same outcome.
  → → Robotic— ↑ time, ↑ cost, but same outcome with laparoscopy.
  → → Laparoscopy—↓ stay, ↑ outcome, ↑ early recovery, ↓ need for analgesia.
- Enhance recovery after surgery (ERAS): improves the outcome.

Stage 0: Tis, N0, M0
- Carcinoma in situ (no risk of LNs metastasis).
- Excision with free margin.

- Many by endoscopy (resection) and followed with frequent colonoscopy.
- If polyps can't be resected completely → segmental resection.

Stage I: Malignant Polyps (T1, N0, M0)

- Risk of LNs depends on the depth of the tumor.
- If invasive component at the head of pedunculated with no stalk involvement → risk of LNs metastasis is 1% → can be by endoscopy resection.
- If lymphovascular invasion, poorly different or tumor in 1 mm of margin → segmental colectomy.
- Sessile with extension to submucosa → segmental resection.

Stage I, II: Localized Colon CA (T1–3, N0, M0)

- Surgical resection.
- Few developed either local or distant recurrence.
- Adjuvant chemotherapy will not improve survival.
- 46% of patient with completely resected stage II will die.
- Adjuvant therapy for selected patient (young, high grade).

Stage III: T any, N1, M0

- Adjuvant chemotherapy is recommended routinely to decrease recurrence.
- 5 FU, FOLFOX.
- MSI predicts the good prognosis.

Stage IV: Distant Metastasis (T any, N any, M1)

- 15% with liver metastasis (isolated).
- All patients require adjuvant chemotherapy.
- With resection: 5 years Survival rate is 20%–40%, whereas SR is less with no resection.
- Hepatic resection of synchronous metastasis at the same time of OR or next.
- Second most common metastasis is lung, 20%, then ovary and retroperitoneum.

- Remind patient with stage IV cannot be cured with surgery → palliative treatment:
  - Colonic stent
  - Diverting stomach or bypass
  - Hemorrhage in unresectable tumor → angioembolization

Adjuvant Treatment

- Patient with node +ve, i.e., stage III → adjuvant chemotherapy FOLFOX for 6 months.
- Stage II is controversial but for high risk patient:
  - → Poorly differentiated, LNs and vascular invasion, bowel perforation, +ve margin.
- Colon is not like rectal CA → radiotherapy is rarely indicated.
- No neoadjuvant therapy except for respectable metastasis.

Management of Obstructive or Perforated Colon CA

- Proximal obstruction tumor → right hemi with primary anastomosis.
- Distal obstruction → proximal dilation → after resection table lavage.
- Perforation → fecal contamination → resection + proximal colostomy or ileostomy (Hartmann).

Surveillance and Follow-Up

- Aim:
  1. Identify recurrent disease.
  2. Identify metachronous polyps.
  3. Reassure patient.
- According to NCCN:
- T3 or T4: history, physical examination, CEA Q3M for 2 years, then Q6M for next 3 years.
- Colonoscopy, within 1 year postoperatively.
  - → If no polyp, repeat it Q3Y.
  - → If polyp → repeat it after 1 year
  - Annual CT CAP.
    - → If ↑ CEA → colonoscopy or image (CT)

Subtotal Colectomy

- After induction of anesthesia, do time-out to make sure of the patient's name, procedure, staff names, then position the patient supine or modified lithotomy.
- Lower midline incision.
- Assess the liver and peritoneum for any signs of metastasis.
- Bookwalter or Thompson retractor is very helpful to retract the bowel cephalic away.
- Mobilize the left colon starting at the level of sigmoid or rectosigmoid junction distally.
- Retract the colon medially; start mobilizing along the white line of Toldt.
- The ureter and the gonadal vessels should be identified.
- The left kidney and Gerota's fascia should be visible, then divide the colorenal attachment.
- Free the omentum from transverse colon.
- IMA is easily identified by palpation at its origin from the aorta.
- Divide the IMV.
- Divide either the left colic or the inferior mesenteric artery.
- Use suture ligation or LigaSure to mesocolon to divide all the way through transverse colon; ligate middle colic artery.
- Then start to mobilize the right colon.
- 10 cm of ileum will be resected due to common blood supply with cecum.
- Retract the colon medially; start mobilizing along the white line of Toldt.
- Identify the ureter (crossing the common iliac artery), duodenum, and the gonadal vessels.
- Continue with hepatic flexure mobilization, and avoid excessive traction on the duodenum.
- Once colon is fully mobilized, identify the lymphovascular pedicles by retracting the small bowel to the left side to expose the root of the mesentery.
- Identify the SMA.

- Incise the peritoneum over the vascular pedicle and ligate the vessels.
- Divide the ileal mesentery between artery hemostats applied serially, proximal and distal.
- Options for restoring bowel continuity include ileorectal anastomosis or ileostomy and closure of rectal stump in case of instability or peritonitis.
- Irrigated with sterile saline with/without drain.
- Hemostasis is confirmed, and omentum is positioned over the anastomosis, followed by closure.

Management of Peritoneal Surface Malignancy of Appendix or Colorectal Origin

- Encompasses with many gynecologic and GI malignancy (ovarian, stomach, appendiceal, CRC).
- Mucin-secreting tumor (by goblet cells); the worst is signet ring tumor.
- Needs cytoreductive surgery (CRS) remove all deposit + hyperthermic interperitoneal chemotherapy (HIPEC), then systemic chemotherapy.
- Classified Low grade, high grade.
- Low grade such as PMP → laparotomy: CRS + HIPEC.
- High grade → systemic chemotherapy then CRS + HIPEC.
- should evaluate and inspect diaphragm, lesser omentum, porta hepatis, proximal and distal small bowel, pelvic organ, and peritoneum.

Peritoneal Surface Severity Score (PSDSS)

- Primary tumor (G), peritoneal dissemination (P), extent of peritoneal dissemination (E)

- **Primary Neoplasm (G)**
  - Five groups:
    1. —non-rupture
    2. —rupture, low risk of recurrence
    3. —rupture, high risk of recurrence
    4. —low grade
    5. —high grade

- **Evaluation of Peritoneal Dissemination (P)**
  - P0 No Peritoneal dissemination identified
  - P1 Only extracellular mucin
  - P2 Extracellular + epithelial cells
  - P3 Tumor identified with well, moderate differentiation.
  - P4 Tumor identified with poor differentiation.
- **Extent of Peritoneal Dissemination (E)**
  - Associated with volume of tumor by peritoneal CA Index (PCI) at the time of surgery or by CT.
    - E0 No peritoneal dissemination
    - E1 Low volume, PCI ≤ 10
    - E2 Moderate volume, PCI < 20 but > 10
    - E3 High volume, PCI > 20

Survival of Patient with Mucinous Appendiceal Neoplasm
- With CRS + HIPEC 3 & 5 years, SR is 73% & 57%.
- SR with CRS only is 43%.

Peritoneal Metastasis at Time of Elective Surgery
- 8% of CRC will have peritoneal metastasis, usually detected by CT, MRI, PET, but few can present at theater.
- Proceed to colon resection only if perforation, obstruction, or bleeding; if not → Bx and close.

Outcomes
- 90% will be treated with palliative chemotherapy + biologics.
- Avoid surgery in patient with large tumor volume, poor differential, or signet ring.
- Some studies show CRS + systemic chemotherapy vs. CRS + HIPEC are the same.

Rectum

Rectal Landmarks
- Rectum is 12–15 cm in length, three submucosal folds (valves of Houston)
- Posteriorly: presacral fascia (between rectum and sacral plexus) S1-S3, at S4 (Waldeyer's fascia), posterior to anorectal junction.
- Anterior: Denonvilliers' fascia separates rectum from prostate and seminal vesicles in male and vagina in female.
- Lateral ligament supports lower rectum.

Blood Supply
A: Upper: Superior Rectal A. → continuation of IMA
Middle: Middle Rectal A. → internal iliac artery
Lower: Inferior Rectal A. → internal pudendal artery fom internal iliac artery.

V: Upper: Superior Rectal V. → IMV → portal vein
Middle: Middle Rectal V. → internal iliac vein
Lower: Inferior Rectal V. → internal pudendal → internal iliac vein

- Submucosal plexus deep to column of Morgagni form hemorrhoidal plexus drain → three veins.

Lymph
- Upper and middle → inferior mesenteric LNs.
- Lower → inferior mesenteric LNs + lateral aspect to internal iliac LNs.

Anorectal Nerve Supply
Sympathetic: L1–L3
Parasympathetic: S2–S4

- Internal anal sphincter supplied by sympathetic and parasympathetic.
- External anal sphincter and puborectalis muscle supplied by inferior rectal branch of internal pudendal nerve.

- Other levator ani muscle supplied by internal pudendal nerve and S3 to S5.
- Sensory of anal canal distal to dentate line → inferior rectal branch of pudendal nerve.
- Rectum and proximal anal canal relatively insensible.

Benign Rectal Condition
Rectal Prolapse
- Circumference full-thickness protrusion of rectum through anus.
- Types:
    - Partial: only mucosa (radial fold).
    - Complete: all layers (circular, mucosal fold).
- Internal rectal intussusception: rectum descends within itself but no protrusion outside the anus.
- Female: male = 6:1.
- Affects mostly above 70.

Risk Factor
1. Deep Douglas Pouch.
2. Laxity of pelvic floor and anal canal.
3. Weakness of internal and external anal sphincter.
4. Pudendal neuropathy.
5. Lack rectal fixation with redundant rectosigmoid junction.

Symptom
- Tenesmus, protrusion of tissue may or may not be reduced, mucus discharge, ulceration, fecal incontinence, constipation, tenesmus, urine incontinence.

Evaluation
- History, physical examination
- Examination: prone jackknife position, often reduced, resting tone.
- Colonoscopy to exclude colonic disease.
- Manometry to assess sphincter function and pudendal nerve for terminal motor latency, EMG.
- MRI defecography used for occult or intestinal intussusception.

Treatment
- Surgery is the only definitive treatment.
- There's more than a hundred procedures.
- If patient is not a candidate → stool softener.
- Surgery goal includes the following:
  1. Narrowing of anal orifice.
  2. Obliteration of Douglas pouch.
  3. Restoration of pelvic floor.
  4. Low rectosigmoid redundancy (bowel resection).
  5. Fixation of rectum to sacrum.
- Classified to abdominal or perineal approach.
- Perineal reserved for patient who is not a candidate for abdominal surgery:old age, or has comorbid disease.

- **Preoperative Management**
  - Bowel preparation, oral antibiotic.
  - Preoperative IV antibiotic, VTE prophylaxis.

- **Perineal Approach**
  o STARR procedure used for internal intussusception.
  o Mucosal sleeve resection: resection of mucosal (Delorme's procedure).
  → Complication: morbidity, 4%–33%; mortality, 0%–2.5%; leak; stricture; diarrhea; recurrence, 6%–26%.
  o Perineal rectosigmoidectomy with J pouch or Altemeier procedure.

- **Abdominal Procedure**
  - Fixation of rectum, it could be by prosthesis.
  - Resection of sigmoid colon and some cases combined with rectal fixation.

- **Ripstein Procedure**
  o Reduction of hernia (perianal) and closure of cul de sac (Moschcowitz repair).
  o Abdominal suture rectopexy and sigmoid resection.
  o Abdominal suture rectopexy.
  o Ventral rectopexy.

- Best and durable → abdominal rectopexy with or without sigmoidectomy, recurrence is low, 10%.
- Perineal rectosigmoidectomy in high-risk patient, higher recurrence.
- Anal encirclement is abandoned.

Recurrent Prolapse
- Most important part is remaining blood supply.
- If perineal rectosigmoidectomy is done, perineal resection can be repeated.
- If Delorme's procedure or abdominal rectopexy is done → additional sigmoid resection can harm rectum → redo rectopexy with or without resection or perineal rectosigmoidectomy.

Solitary Rectal Ulcer Syndrome (SRUS)
- Either ulcer or nodule.
- Pathology is still unknown but
  1. Puborectalis contraction
  2. Internal or external full-thickness rectal prolapse
     → Repetitive injury to rectum during defecation.
     → Nodular scarring and others such as ergotamine suppository (VC), radiotherapy, anal intercourse.

Presentation
- Excess rectal mucus, bleeding, anismus, tenesmus, difficult evacuation.
- Diagnosis by presence of the following:
  1. Staining and feeling of incomplete evacuation with passage of blood and mucus.
  2. Internal or external rectal prolapse.
  3. Solitary or multiple erythematous ulcerated lesions.
  4. Histological evidence of muscularis mucosa distortion.

Evaluation
- History (sexual behavior), physical evaluation.
- Endoscopy.

- Usually lacerated 5–12 cm from anal verge → Bx must be done.
- Radiography: defecating proctography.
- EMG activity.
- Endoanal US.

Treatment

- Behavior modification.
- Biofeedback (most important).
- High-fiber diet.
- Botulinum toxin, success rate is 50%.
- Surgery if failed medical Tx or associated with rectal prolapse → abdominal rectopexy with or without sigmoid resection.
- Proctectomy in difficult cases.

Therapy for Rectal CA

- Rectal CA is ⅓ of colorectal cancer (CRC).
- Rectum starts fusion of taenia coli into a single longitudinal smooth muscle (rectosigmoid) to anal canal.
- Length of the rectum is 12 cm.
- Three parts: upper, middle, lower.
- Same biology of colon CA.
- It is radiosensitive.

Preoperative Evaluation

- **History, Physical Examination, Laboratory Investigations**
  - History: bleeding PR, change in bowel habit (stool, flatus), tenesmus, incontinence, previous colonoscopy, family history.
  - Should be educated for stoma therapy.
  - Examination: abdomen, DRE, proctoscopy.
  - Full colonoscopy as 5% will have synchronous lesion.
  - If full colonoscopy is not possible → virtual colonoscopy, CT.
  - Complete laboratory, CBC, chemistry, CEA.

- **Preoperative Image Study**
  1. Delineate depth of tumor.
  2. Assess locoregional LN.

3. Distant metastasis.

- MRI to differentiate the stages, i.e., rectum from perirectal fat.
    - Best modality to differentiate T2 from T3.
    - Inner hyperintense: mucosa, submucosa
    - Middle hypointense: muscularis propria
    - Outer hyperintense: perirectal fat
    - MRI provides relation between tumor and mesorectal fascia to achieve −ve circumference resection margin (CRM).
    - Sensitivity, 77%; specificity, 94% to identify mesorectal fascia.
    - Sensitivity, 77%; specificity, 74% to identify LNS.
- ERUS: better than MRI in distinguishing T0, T1, and T2.
- CT for intra-abdominal metastasis.
- PET or PET-CT: helpful in suspicious lesion on CT in distant metastasis.
- Sensitivity, 94%; specificity, 99%.

TNM Classification
    Tx Cannot be assessed
    T0 No evidence of primary tumor
    Tis CIS—intraepithelial (mucosa) or invade lamina propria
    T1 Tumor invades submucosa
    T2 Tumor invades muscularis propria
    T3 Tumor invades through muscularis to perirectal fat
    T4 Tumor penetrates:
        (a) visceral peritoneal or (b) adjacent organ
    N1 1–3 regional LNs
    N2 4 LNs
    N3 4–6 LNs
    N4 > 7 LNs

- General principle in staging:
        T1–T2   = Stage I
        T3   = Stage II
        Any T with N1 = Stage III
        Any N with M   = Stage IV

- Minimum 12 LNs to adequately assess nodal status and accurate staging.

Management
- Multidisciplinary approach, i.e., tumor board.

Principle of Surgery
- **Local Therapy**
  - Transanal excision (TAE) of adenoma, transanal endoscopic microsurgery (TEM), and transanal minimally invasive surgery (TAMIS) are used for adenoma and benign lesions, also used for selected T1 and same T2 but does not allow pathological examination.
  - ↑ Local recurrence after local excision.
  - Ablation, electrocautery, endocavity radiation.
  - Fulguration for high-risk patient with limited life span.

- **Radical Resection**
  - Removal of involved segment of rectum + lymphovascular supply.
  - 2 cm −ve margin.
  - Total mesorectal excision during low and extended low anterior resection.
  - For upper rectum of rectosigmoid → partial mesorectal excision of at least 5 cm distal to tumor.
  - Total mesorectal excision (TME) → ↓ recurrence, ↑ SR, ↓ bleeding, ↓ injury to pelvic nerve and presacral plexus.
  - In recurrence (involve pelvic organ) → need pelvic exenteration = same APR but en bloc of ureters, bladder, prostate, uterus, vagina → permanent colostomy + ileal conduit + sacrectomy up to level S2–S3.
  - When radial margin is involved or threatened → neoadjuvant chemotherapy and radiation.
  - Endorectal US, MRI to assess the response, then surgery.

- **Stage-Specific Therapy**
  Stage 0: Tis, N0, M0; stage I: T1, N0
    - Local excision with −ve margin of 1 cm.
    - Can be managed by local excision.
    - The goal is to excise the tumor with −ve margin.
    - Advantage: low morbidity, preserves anorectal function, and avoids permanent colostomy.
    - Recurrence is 11%–29% with strict selection criteria:
        - Tumor Location
        - Within 15 cm from anal region. Tumor involves < ⅓ of circumference of rectum, mobile, not fixed, T1, N0 by MRI, ERUS.
        - Histopathology Feature
        - Well or moderately differentiated,
        - no lymphovascular invasion.
        - No mucinous or signet cell component, T1 on final histopathology.
        - Usually 30% will achieve R0.
    - In recurrence, 33% require multivisceral resection, 5% require pelvic exenteration.
    - Radical excision is strongly recommended.
    - If patient refuses radical surgery as permanent colostomy → local excision + neoadjuvant or adjuvant chemotherapy and radiation.

  Stage II: T2, N0
    - Invades muscularis propria but not perirectal tissue.
    - Standard treatment: total mesorectal excision (TME).
        → If +ve LNs → adjuvant chemotherapy + radiation.
    - Can be considered neoadjuvant chemotherapy + radiation if bulky tumor in upper part of anorectal sphincter to preserve sphincter.
        → Downstage of 64% to T1 or T0.
        → Can use local excision.
        → 44% is completely cured.

Stage IIIa: Locally Advanced CA:T3-T4/Nx

- Distal rectum → ↑ recurrence.
- Either neoadjuvant chemoradiation then surgery or surgery then adjuvant chemoradiation.
- Advantage of neoadjuvant therapy: downstage of tumor size.
- Disadvantages: overtreatment of early stage, slow wound healing, pelvic fibrosis.

Stage IIIb: LNs Metastasis (T any, NI, M0)

- Standard treatment: neoadjuvant chemotherapy + radiation then TME (LAR or APR) then adjuvant chemotherapy.
- Post-operative chemotherapy radiation doubles stricture formation but decreases recurrence by 6%–12%.

Stage IV: Distant Metastasis (T any, N any, M1)

- Up to 60% of CRC developed liver metastasis.
- Survival is limited.
- Local therapy can be adequate to control bleeding and obstruction → stent → diverting colostomy + mucous fistula.
- Systemic chemotherapy is initial modality then restaging
- Mostly palliative.
- Pelvic exenteration should be avoided.

Surgical Consideration
Transanal Excision

- Most accessible and located below peritoneal reflection ≈ 6–8 cm.
- Full-thickness excision with −ve margin, 1 cm margin till perirectal fat.
- TEM, TAMIS.
- Mid and upper rectal lesion.

Radical Resection

- Resection of tumor + rectum en bloc with its blood supply and LNs and surrounding mesorectum.
- LAR preserve the sphincters.
  - → Contraindicated to LAR is invasion of tumor to anal sphincter or levator ani muscle.
  - → Impaired anorectal function is a relative contraindication.
- Should consider the following:
  1. TME
  2. Autonomic nerve preservation
  3. −ve circumference and distal image
  4. Sphincter preservation

Total Mesorectal Excision (TME)

- Complete resection of rectum + mesorectum + lymphatic with preservation of pelvic nerve.
- Avascular plane (holy plane)
- Result en bloc (package) resection → −ve margin, low recurrence.
- Sharp dissection.
- Associated with increase −ve CRM.

- Autonomic Nerve Preservation
  - Sympathetic nerve of pelvis T12–L3, which forms superior hypogastric plexus → gives hypogastric nerves.
  - Parasympathetic nerve of pelvis S2–S4 (nervi erigentes) → joins sympathetic to form inferior hypogastric nerve.
  - If injury to autonomic → genitourinary dysfunction.
    - → Damage to sympathetic → i.e., hypogastric → ↑ UB tone, low capacity + retrograde ejaculation in male.
    - → Damage to parasympathetic → difficult voiding from neck of UB tone + ED in male and ↓ lubrication in female.

- Distal Resection Margin
  - 2–5 cm traditionally.

- At least 2 cm, and in final histopathology
- Some centeres accept $\geq$ 1 cm.

Low Anterior Resection (LAR)
Procedure:
- Modified lithotomy under GA.
- Lower midline incision.
- Bookwalter retractor for full exposure and to retract the small bowel cephalic.
- Assess the liver and peritoneum for any signs of metastasis.
- Mobilization of the left colon until the rectosigmoid junction.
- Identify the ureter and gonadal vessels.
- Start dissection proximally to expose the inferior mesentericartery and distally to the right side of the rectum.
- Ligate the inferior mesenteric artery distally to left colic artery.
- Transect the colon at the sigmoid colon by GIA 60 stapler.
- Use the transected sigmoid as guide by superior traction to guide your dissection toward the rectum and the presacral fascia.
- Incise the peritoneum surrounding the rectum from both sides until both incisions meet.
- The posterior dissection is started first by sharp dissection to include the mesorectum with the rectum, which is identified by the avascular loose areolar tissue (the holy plane).
- Watch the hypogastric nerve plexus at the sacral promontory.
- Retract the bladder anteriorly and start the lateral dissection, will encounter the lateral stalk containing the middle rectal vessels, then ligate and divide it.
- The anterior dissection is the most difficult due to lack of planes. Divide the Denonviller's fascia and avoid injuring the bladder, prostate in males, or vagina in females.
- Reassess the tumor and the distal margin.
- If there is negative margin achieved → transect and prepare for the anastomosis using circular stapler 28 or 30.
- Make sure there's no tension and there are good vascular healthy edges.

- Test the anastomosis by checking the doughnut, airtight, and by sigmoidoscopy to assess from inside.

Abdominoperineal Resection (APR)
- Combined abdominal and perineal approach to resection rectum, mesorectum, anus, surrounding perineal, soft tissue, and pelvic floor musculature en bloc.
- Permanent end colostomy.
- If direct invasion to sphincter muscle or if adequate margin could be obtained or if patient has already fecal incontinence.

Neo-adjuvant and Adjuvant Therapy
- In locally advanced tumor.
- Short-course radiotherapy 5 Gy × 5 days → surgery within 1 week.
- Long-course chemo-radiation over 5–6 weeks → surgery after 4–8 weeks.
- Guideline after resection: all patients with stage III and high-risk stage II → adjuvant therapy.

Follow-Up and Surveillance
- High recurrence once first pathology is developed, either locally or systematically or metachronous.
- Colonoscopy within 12 months after diagnosis of original CA.
- If normal → repeat it every 3 years to 5 years.
- Patient treated with local excision → frequent colonoscopy every 3–6 months for 3 years, then 6 months for 2 years.
- CEA every 3–6 months for 2 years.
- CT annually for 5 years.
- Intensive surveillance for HNPCC.

Treatment of Recurrent CRC
- 20%–40% of cured patient → recurrent within 2 years but pre-operative chemoradiation → delay recurrence.
- If patient does not receive chemotherapy radiation → neoadjuvant chemotherapy radiation prior to salvage surgery, i.e., metastasectomy of lower limb.

- CT CAP, PET.
- Radical surgery can prolong SR in some patients but may require pelvic exenteration +/− sacrectomy.

Other Neoplasm
Carcinoid
- 25% in rectum, mostly benign, and SR is 80%.
- Risk of malignancy increases with size.
- 60% greater than 2 cm → metastasis.
- Less likely to secrete vasoactive substance than carcinoid in other location, and carcinoid is uncommon in absence of liver metastasis.
- Small tumor can be resected transanally.
- Large tumor with muscularis invasion → radical excision.
- Carcinoid in proximal colon is less likely to be malignant and majority present with bulky lesion.
- ⅔ of liver metastasis → radical excision.
- Symptoms of carcinoid syndrome.
- Treatment: octreotide and/or interferon alpha.

NB Carcinoid tumor:
- Is a neuroendocrine tumor.
- Appendix, ileum are commonly affected, then cecum, lung, rectum, stomach.
- 10% secrete excessive 5-HT serotonin.
- Usually, symptoms start after liver metastasis, such as flushing, diarrhea, wheezing, abdominal cramp, pulmonary edema.
- ⅔ found in gastrointestinal tract and arise from ECL.
- 6% will have carcinoid syndrome.

Carcinoid Carcinoma
- Carcinoid + adenocarcinoma.
- Carcinoid carcinoma in colon and rectum → same adenocarcinoma.

Lymphoma
- Rare, 10% of gastrointestinal lymphoma.
- Cecum is the most common.

- Bowel resection is treatment of choice.
- Adjuvant therapy may be given based on stage of disease.

Leiomyoma and Leiomyosarcoma

- Leiomyoma is benign tumor originated from smooth muscle.
- Difficult to be distinguished from sarcoma → lesion should be resected.
- Small lesion by local resection, larger by radical resection.
- Sarcoma is rare in GI tumor rectum is commonly affected.
- Symptoms: bleeding, obstruction → radical resection.

GIST

- Rare, common in stomach and small bowel.
- Colon and rectum, 10%.
- 50% lesion should be resected.

Retrorectal/Presacral Tumor

- Lies between upper ⅔ of rectum and sacrum above retrosacral fascia, lateral: endosacral fascia → (lateral ligation).
- Retrosacral space contains embryonic remnant (neuroectoderm, notochord).
- Neurogenic, osseous, inflammatory.
- Common in pediatrics.
- Inflammatory (solid or cystic), usually abscess.
- Scimitar sign.
- Solid: teratoma, chordoma, neurogenic.
  - Teratoma, 30% malignant.
  - Chordoma is the most common tumor in this region → bony destructive lesion.
  - Neurogenic neurofibroma, sarcoma, ependymoma.
- X-ray, CT, MRI for diagnosis.
- Treatment: surgical excision.
- If high → abdominal approach, if low → transanally.
- SR is excellent after resection.
- Biopsy is controversial → historically not done → infection.
- if large sarcoma → neoadjuvant therapy.
- Recent study → needle tract seeding.

Anal Canal

- Anus begins when rectum passes puborectalis portion.
- Surgical anus, 2–4 cm.
- anorectal ring is 1–2 cm above the dentate line (DL).
- Dentate (pectineal) line is a transition between columnar rectal mucosa to squamous.
- → Divide into proximal to DL and distal to DL.
- Dentate line surrounded by longitudinal mucosal fold → columns of Morgagni (anal crypt).
- → This crypt is the source of cryptoglandular abscess.
- In the distal rectum, the inner smooth muscle thickened to forms internal anal sphincter surrounded by superficial and deep external sphincter.
- Deep external sphincter → extension of puborectalis muscle.
- Puborectalis, iliococcygeus, and pubococcygeus form the levator ani muscle (pelvic floor).
- Blood supply.

  Arterial: Above DL—Middle rectal artery
                Below DL—Inferior rectal artery

  Venous: Above DL—Internal hemorrhoidal plexus → PV
                Below DL—Extenal hemorrhoidal Plexus → systemic veins.

  Lymphatic: Above DL and mesorectal → internal iliac LNs
                Below DL → inguinal LNs

- Microscopically:
  Three zones of mucosa with different histological type.
    → Glandular, anal transitional zone (ATZ), non-keratinizing squamous.
- ATZ contains mucin, melanocyte.
- Aanal CA represent 1.5% of GI CA.
- CA developed according to arising epithelium such as squamous, adenocarcinoma, melanoma, NET, lymphoma.

Benign Anal Disease

- Workup for the patient with anal, perianal symptoms:
    → History and physical exam, DRE, defecography, manometry, CT, MRI, contrast enema, endoscopy, endoanal US, EUA.

Hemorrhoid

- Cushions of submucosal tissue containing venule, arteriole, smooth muscle fiber.
- Three locations: left lateral, right anterior, right posterior (3, 7, 11 o'clock).
- Straining, ↑ abdominal pressure, hard stool, ↑ venous engorgement of hemorrhoidal plexus → prolapse hemorrhoid.

- **External Hemorrhoid (peri-anal hematoma)**
  - Distal to dentate line and covered by anoderm, because anoderm is rich in Nerves → thrombosis → severe pain.
  - Skin tag—redundant fibrotic skin at anal verge (residual of thrombosed external piles).
  - May be itchy.
  - Acutely thrombosed (perianal hematoma) increases pain and palpable perianal mass, if early presentation:
    - → elliptical incision → (single is not effective → loculated) evacuation of clots.
    - → After 72 hrs, clots start to resorb → excision is unnecessary → sitz bath, analgesia, stool softner and lubricant.

- **Internal Hemorrhoid**
  - Proximal to dentate covered by anorectal mucosa.
  - May prolapse and bleed, but no pain unless thrombosis and necrotic.
  - Grades:
    - o First degree: bulges into anal canal and may prolapses below the dentate line.
    - o Second degree: prolapses through anus but reduces spontaneously.
    - o Third degree: prolapses through anus and requires manual reduction.
    - o Fourth degree: cannot be reduced → high strangulation.

- **Combined Internal and External—Straddle**
    - Hemorrhoidectomy for symptomatic, complicated, or combined.
    - Postpartum hemorrhoid because of straining.
    - Portal HTN → bleeding (portosystemic anastomosis), i.e., rectal varices (middle and upper hemorrhoidal plexus) → treatment of Portal HTN, suture ligation if massive bleeding → no surgery → severe hemorrhage.

Treatment
- **Medical**
    - First, second degree → usually responds to dietary fiber, stool softener, ↑ fluid intake, avoid strain, sitz bath
    - Daflon to support venous wall:
    - 6 tablets/day for 4 days then 4 tablets /day for 3 days.

- **Rubber Band Ligation**
    - Persistent bleeding on first, second degrees, selected patient with third degree.
    - Mucosa located 1–2 cm above dentate line → scarring.
    - Only 1–2 rubber ligations per visit.
    - If distal to DL → severe pain.
    - Complication: urinary retention, infection, bleeding.
    - Necrotizing infection → uncommon, pain, fever, infection → EUA → debridement, incision, and drainage → antibiotics for 7+ days.
    - Bleeding after slough mucosa → self-limiting.
    - If it persists → EUA and ligation.

- **Infrared Photocoagulation**
    - For first, second degree.
    - Coagulation, all three piles at the same time.
    - Large and prolapse are not effective.

- **Sclerotherapy**
  - For first, second degree.
  - sclerosing agent into submucosa.
  - Complication if infection: fibrosis.

- **Operative Hemorrhoidectomy**
  1. **Closed Submucosal Hemorrhoidectomy**
     - Parks or Ferguson → resection of hemorrhoidal tissue and closure of the wound with absorbent suture.
     - Prone or lithotomy.
     - Elliptical incision, distal to anal verge and extended to anorectal ring.
     - Identify internal sphincter fiber (dissection).
     - Excision of hemorrhoid and closure with absorbent suture in running.
     - Three piles can be removed by this technique.

  2. **Open Hemorrhoidectomy**
     - Milligan-Morgan hemorrhoidectomy.
     - Excision as above, wound healed by secondary intention.

  3. **Whitehead Hemorrhoidectomy**
     - Circumferential excision of hemorrhoidal cushion, just proximal to DL → advanced suture of mucosa to DL.
     - Abandoned → risk of ectropion (whitehead deformity).

  4. **Procedure for Prolapse and Hemorrhoid (Stapler Hemorrhoidectomy)**
     - PPH was replaced by the name stapler hemorrhoidectomy, after excision of hemorrhoid instead of pexes.
     - The redundant mucosa above DL → PPH removes short segment of rectal mucosa (circumference) using circular stapler.

- Safe, effective, less post-operative pain, low disability.
- No complication.

5. **Doppler-Guided Hemorrhoidal Artery Ligation**
   - Called transanal hemorrhoidal dearterialization.
   - By Doppler → ligation.
   - Promising procedure.

- **Complication of Hemorrhoidectomy**
  - Post-operative pain → oral narcotics, NSAIDs, muscle relaxant, sitz bath.
  - Urine retention is a common complication, 10%–50% → limited by intra-post-operative IVF, and analgesia.
  - Fecal impaction limited by bowel preparation and enema.
  - Bleeding → inadequate ligation of pedicle vessels, if after 7–10 days post-operative from necrotic mucosa.
  - Infection → necrotizing fasciitis.
  - Long-term incontinence, ectropion, stenosis, whitehead deformity, transient incontinence to flatus.

Anal Fissure
- Tear in the anoderm distal to DL.
- Trauma, hard stool, prolonged diarrhea.
- Tear → spasm of internal anal sphincter → pain and increased tearing, ↓ blood supply.
- Majority in posterir-midline, 15% anteriorly.
- If not located in midline → CD, TB, CA, HPV, HIV, syphilis, and leukemia.

Symptom
- Tearing pain with hematochezia (stool with blood streaks), pain lasts for hours, then bowel movement after.

- Gently separate buttocks → tender DRE.
- Acute fissure healed with medical treatment.
- Chronic → ulceration and heaped-up edges with white fiber, associated with skin tag.

Medical Therapy
- Break vicious cycle of pain, spasm, ischemia.
- Minimize trauma by bulk agent, stool softener, warm sitz bath, lidocaine gel.
- Nitroglycerin ointment → increases blood flow
  → or oral and topical Ca^{++} channel blockers (nifedipine). S/E: headache.
- Botulinum toxin: blocks acetylcholine release and causes temporary muscle paralysis.
- Anginine (nitric oxide) or muscarinic agonist → 50% healing.

Surgical Therapy
- If failed medical treatment which is gold standard.
- 90% success rate.
- Open or close technique.
- EUA and lateral internal sphincterotomy (LIS)→ ↓ spasm of internal sphincter by dividing a portion of the muscle (60-70%).
- Recurrence, 10%; incontinence, 5%–15%.
- Alternative: advanced flap, fissurectomy ± advancement flap.
- If failed → repeat LIS from other side, but ↑↑ fecal incontinence.

Anorectal Sepsis
Relevant Anatomy
- Majority result from infection of anal canal (cryptoglandular infection) found in intersphincteric plane.
- Their duct traverses and empties in anal crypt at level of dentate line.
- Infection of anal gland → abscess → enlarged and spread to several planes → perianal and perirectal.
  1. Perianal space—surrounds anus.

2. Intersphincteric space—separates internal sphincter and External sphincter, surrounded by perianal space and proximally by rectal wall.

3. Ischiorectal space (fossa): wedge shaped, fat filled space, situated on each side of anal canal below pelvic diaphragm.
   - Medially: external sphincteric muscle.
   - Laterally: obturator fascia, obturator internus muscle
   - Superiorly: levator ani muscle, inferior fascia of pelvic diaphragm
   - Inferiorely: perianal fascia.
   - Two spaces connected above anococcygeaus below levator ani muscle.

4. Supralevator abscess—above levator ani muscle.
   - Perianal abscess—spreads through ES below puborectalis → ischiorectal abscess → EUA.
   - Intersphincteric → EUA.
   - Pelvic and supralevator abscesses are rare.

Diagnosis
- Examination.
- Atypical presentation → CT, MRI.

Treatment
- Incision and drainage under anesthesia.
- If delayed → massive necrosis and septicemia.
- Antibiotics if scar cellulitis or low immunity, DM, valvular heart disease.

- **Perianal Abscess**
  - Can be under LA, incision and drainage, disk of skin excised to prevent closure, packing, then sitz bath the next day.

- **Ischiorectal Abscess**
  - if two sides connected → horseshoe.

- Incision and drainage if two sides drainage deep postanal space by incise anococcygeal ligament, and it may require two incisions.

- **Intersphincteric Abscess**
  - Pain is deep inside.
  - Can be felt in the anus if coughing.
  - EUA, drained by limited post-internal sphincterotomy.

- **Supralevator Abscess**
  - Uncommon.
  - DRE: indurated bulge above anorectal ring.
  - If extension of intersphincteric abscess → drainage through rectum.
    - → If draining it through ischiorectal fossa → suprasphincteric fistula.
  - If extension of ischiorectal abscess → incision and drainage through ischiorectal fossa.
    - → If draining it through rectum → extrasphincteric fistula.
  - If secondary to intra-abdominal disease → drainage from most direct route (transabdominal, rectum, ischiorectal fossa).

- **Perianal Sepsis (Immunocompromised)**
  - Because of leukopenia → several infections.
  - Antibiotics (broad spectrum).
  - Should not delay EUA because of neutropenia.
  - Incision and drainage and biopsy.

- **Fournier's gangrene**
  - Necrotizing fasciitis of perineum and external genitalia.
  - Polymicrobial and synergistic effects.
  - Causes: undrained or inadequate drain of abscess or UTI, diabetes mellitus, low immunity.
  - Physical examination: necrotic skin, bullae or crepitus involved the perineum and scrotum + systemic toxicity.

- Diagnosis: clinically or by x-ray, US, CT (gas below the skin).
- Treatment: extensive debridement (could be multiple), with assistance of urology team.
- IV antibiotics.
- Colostomy if extensive debridement and excision of sphincter.
- Mortality rate is 50%.

Fistula in Ano

- Originates from infected crypt (internal opening) and tracks to external opening, usually the site of drainage.
- Develops after 50% of anorectal abscess after incision and drainage.
- Majority are cryptoglandular in origin → trauma, CD, actinomycosis, tuberculosis can produce fistula → complex, non-healing, recurrent, high suspicion of these disease.

Diagnosis

- Drainage from internal opening to external opening
- Goodsall's rule:
  - Fistula with external opening in anterior—connect by short radial tract.
  - Fistula with external opening in posterior—track in curvilinear to posterior midline.
  - Exception if an anterior external opening is away for greater than 3 cm from anal margin → track to posterior midline.

Goodsall's rule

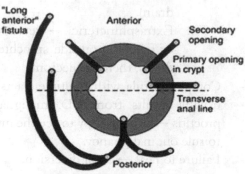

Fistula Classified in Relation to Anal Sphincter Complex

1. Intersphincteric tract: distal internal sphincter → intersphincteric space → to external sphincter near anal verge.
2. Transsphincteric: tract through internal and external sphincter to ischiorectal fossa.
3. Suprasphincteric: tract originally from internal sphincter plane and tract around external sphincter.
4. Extrasphincteric: originates from rectal wall and tract around both internal and external sphincter and exits laterally usually in ischiorectal fossa.

Treatment

- Aim: eradication of sepsis without sacrificing continence.
- Fistula tract that encircles sphincter complex of external sphincter is red in color, but internal sphincter is difficult to identify.
- Inject with H_2O_2 or methylene blue; don't create artificial tract.
  1. Intersphincteric → fistulotomy, curratage, and healing by secondary intention.
  2. Trans-sphincteric depending on location of sphincteric complex, if includes less than 30% of sphincteric muscle → sphincterotomy, but if high → initial seton (if the portion of fistula outside spinchter → open and drain).
  3. Suprasphincteric → seton (if the portion of fistula is outside spinchter → open and drain).
  4. Extrasphincteric → seton (if the portion of fistula is outside spinchter → open and drain), then fistulectomy.
- Complex fistula with multiple tracts is challenging, usually results from CD, malignancy, radiation, proctitis → proctoscopy to see the mucosa → biopsy to rule out malignancy.
- Failure to heal → fecal diversion.

- Seton aims to induce fibrosis by gradual cutting through the sphincters, usually by vessel loop (non-cutting).
- Higher fistula: endorectal advancement flap.
- New modality: fibrin glue (sealant) and collagen plug.
- Recent technique → ligation of intersphincteric fistula tract (LIFT) by placement of (lacrimal probe) to identify the plane → then divide and two ends are ligated.

Rectovaginal Fistula

- Low: proximal to DL and vaginal opening in fourchette, from obstetric trauma, foreign body (FB).
- Middle: vaginal opening between fourchette and cervix, severe obstetric trauma, surgical trauma (rectal neoplasm), radiation.
- High: vaginal opening near cervix, operative or radiation, diverticulitis, CD.

Diagnosis

- Flatus or stool from vagina.
- Complication: vaginitis.
- Diagnosis: barium enema, vaginogram, ERUS.

Treatment

- Size, location, etiology.
- As 50% result from obstetric injury will heal spontaneously, wait 3–6 months.
- If result from abscess → incision and drainage allow spontaneous closure.
- Low and middle: endorectal advancement flap, fecal diversion is rarely required.
- High: trans-abdominal approach → diseased tissue, small bowel, colon, rectum resected and hole in vagina closed → interposition of omentum or muscle between bowel anastomosis to decrease recurrence.
- If fistula is caused by CD, radiation, malignancy → heal spontaneously.
   → Treatment: drainage of sepsis, endorectal advancement flap.

- If previous: radiation damages the tissue → trans-abdominal approach with interposed healthy tissue.
- Malignancy → resection of neoplasm → any of the previous disease → biopsy.

Pilonidal Disease

- The word *pilonidal* is derived from the Latin words *pilus* (meaning "hair") and *nidus* (meaning "nest").
- Can affect umbilical axilla, finger web (barber).
- Once acute attack is resolved, recurrence is common.
- Acute abscess → incision and drainage in clinic or ER under local anesthesia; because healing is poor, some surgeons recommend incision lateral to intergluteal cleft (natal cleft)

Treatment

> Control sepsis and avoid definitive surgical treatment during acute state.

> Disease severity and operation approach should match.

> Avoid too much excision; if too deep → high recurrence and failure of treatment.

Non-operative

Hygiene and hair removal.

Operative Treatment

- Abscess is drained off midline under local anesthesia.
- Pit-picking and simple Bascom procedure: off midline.
- Excision with or without primary wound closure is the gold standard, to heal with secondary intervention.
- Unroof tract, curate the base and marsupialized wound, keep open in frequent visit.
- Small lateral incision and pit excision.
- Complex or recurrent → extensive resection and closure with Z-plasty, advancement flap, rotational flap, Karydakis flap, SC flap, cleft lift procedure, rhomboid flap.

Perianal Dermatitis

- **Pruritus ani**
    - Primary: idiopathic by exclusion, 20%–75%, fecal incontinence, poor hygiene or neurogenic or psychosis
    - Secondary: 15%
        - Infectious: bacterial (syphilis), fungal (candida), parasite (pinworms, scabies), viral (HPV).
        - Anorectal: piles, anorectal sepsis.
        - Malignancy: anal CA, Brown's, and Paget's disease.
        - Dermatologic: seborrhea, psoriasis, dermatitis.

Evaluation

- History, physical examination: detailed history, travel, food.
- DRE for any mass, FB, fistulas.
- Stage I, II, III (Washington criteria).

Treatment

o Good perianal hygiene, topical steroid.
o Removal of irritant, hygiene, no scratch → biopsy to rule out infection or malignancy.
o Hydrocortisone ointment to relief symptom, but not prolonged → dermal atrophy.
o Sitz bath, then keep dry and clean.
o Skin barrier, systemic antihistamine, SSRI, capsaicin.

- **Non-pruritic lesion**
    - Perianal skin conditions.
    - Leprosy, amebiasis, actinomycosis.
    - Neoplasm, Paget's disease, invasive CA.
    - Biopsy then proceed.

Sexually Transmitted Disease

- **Bacterial**
    - Proctitis is the most common symptom.
    - Neisseria gonorrhoeae: proctitis, bleeding, tenesmus.

- Chlamydia trachomatis.
- Treponema pallidum, syphilis: antibiotics or atypical fissure → inguinal LNs is a characteristic.
- Donovania granulomatis: shiny red mass in perineum.
- Diarrhea, illness: shigella can be be transmitted sexually. Treatment: antibiotics.

- **Parasitic**
  - Entamoeba histolytica: ulcer of gastrointestinal tract. Symptoms: diarrhea, abdominal pain.
  - Giardia lamblia.

- **Viral**
  - Herpes simplex: proctitis (type II).
  - Anal pain and tenesmus, vesicles → EUA → it could be abscess → diagnosis by biopsy or fluid from vesicles.
  - HPV: condyloma acuminata (anogenital warts) associated with IEL and SCC.
    → Thirty serotypes.
      Type 16 and 18 appear to predisposed malignancy.
      Type 6 and 11 cause warts.

  Treatment: Small: office treatment—bichloracetic acid, imiquimod.
  Large and numerous: excision with or without fulguration → biopsy to rule out malignancy.
  Vaccine presents anogenital condyloma.

Hidradenitis Suppurativa
- Infections of cutaneous apocrine sweat gland (axilla, buttocks).
- Infected gland rupture → tract.
- Treatment: incision and drainage of acute abscess and debridement for fistula and granulation.
- Radical excision and skin graft are not necessary.
- Now, promising treatment: TNF-a (Humira).

Anal Sphincter Injury and Incontinence
- Mostly during vaginal delivery.
- Risk of incontinence increases with sphincter injury by laceration that extends to rectum (fourth degree).
- Infection of episiotomy, laceration repair, prolonged labor, and use of midline episiotomy.
- Sphincter damage, post-hemorrhoidectomy, sphincterotomy, abscess incision and drainage, and fistulectomy.
- Diagnosis:
    - Anal manometry, EMG, pudendal nerve motor latency.
    - Endoanal ultrasound.
- Treatment:
    - Mild: dietary moderation observation.
    - Severe: surgical repair.
- Surgical repair:
    - → Wrap around sphincteroplasty (commonly used)—mobilized and divided muscle and reapproximation without tension.
      Internal and external sphincter overlapped together or separately.
    - → Postanal intersphincteric levatorplasty (less common)—use if rectal prolapse concomitantly.
      Levator ani is approximated to restore anorectal ring angle.
      Puborectalis and external sphincter are tightened.
      Colostomy is usually not required.
- If prior repair failed or complex injury → gracilias muscle transposition, remove it from insertion → tunnel it from perineum and wrap around anal canal.
- Artificial anal sphincter.
- Sacral nerve stimulation in case of neurogenic disease.

Foreign Body (FB)
- History and physical examination.
- Plain x-ray.
- If FB is low in rectum → removed under conscious sedation.
- If high → GA.
- Laparotomy is rarely required, after removal, proctoscopy or sigmoidoscopy.

- If hematoma → conservation; if perforation → laparotomy.

Immunosuppressed Patient
- **HIV**
    - Diarrhea by opportunistic pathogen.
    - Salmonella, shigella, chlamydia.
    - Fungi, protozoa: toxoplasmosis.
    - Virus CMV, HSV.
    - C. diffecile
    - Lymphoma (NHL).
    - Dysplasia is common (HSIL).
    - Abscess, fistula → EUA.

- **Immunosuppressant for TPx**
    - Common post-TPx.
    - Infection and medication → diarrhea.
    - CMV is the commonest.
    - C. diff is also the next common.
    - Kaposis is also common.
    - Post-TPx lymphoproliferative in GI tract.
    - TPx does not increase CRC compared to general population, but anal SCC has increase incidence post-TPx.

- **Neutropenic Patient**
    - Neutropenic enterocolitis (typhlitis)
        - Life-threatening, MR (50%), abdominal pain, distension, fever, bloody diarrhea, nausea and vomiting.
        - CT → dilated thickend cecum and pericolic stranding.
        - Treatment: some respond to NPO, IV antibiotics, TPN, granulocyte infusion, but if deterioration and peritonitis → OR.
    - Perianal pain → IV antibiotics → EUA (not delayed) if with pain and fever.
        - → Any indurated area, incision and drainage + biopsy (leukemia) + C/S.

Human Papilloma Virus (HPV)
- 15% of the population is a carrier of this virus.
- Has 100 types.
- Type 16, 18 associated with anal CA.
- 93% of anal SCC associated with HPV.
- Also predispose uterine (cervical) CA.

Anal Wart (Condyloma Acuminatum)
- HPV-infected people are 15–20 times at risk to develop anal CA than unaffected people.
- Treatment: antimitotic, local cytokines, antimetabolite (effective 40%–50%).
- Ablative, cryotherapy or surgical resection if medical treatment failed.

- **Squamous Intraepithelial Lesion**
  - Anal intraepithelial neoplasm (AIN).
  - Three grades:
    - I. Low grade dysplasia
    - II. Moderate dysplasia
    - III. High grade dysplasia
  - High grade intra-epithelial lesion (HSIL) precursor of invasive SCC (epidermoid CA) may appear as plaque lesion.
  - Perianal skin + anal canal.
    - → Anal canal alone is very unusual.
  - Associated with type HPV 6, 11, 16, 18.
  - Diagnosis: history of homosexual, anal mapping, Pap smear.
  - Prevention: vaccination against HPV → low incidence in the future.
  - Treatment:
    - Watchful waiting to surgery.
    - Ablation → 50% recurrence.
    - Topical immunomodulator (Aldara) → regression.
    - Topical 5FU.
  - Extensive disease → excision and flap closure.

- **Epidermoid Carcinoma (SCC)**
  - SCC, cloacogenic, transitional, basaloid.
  - Symptoms: pain, bleeding (mostly mass).
  - Slow-growing tumor.
  - Slow-growing inter- or perianal mass.
  - Bleeding, 45%; pain, 30%; asymptomatic, 20%.
  - Need to aske for sexual History.
  - Groin pain → LNs (inguinal).
  - If HIV, contraindication for chemotherapy, radiation, or radial surgery.

  o **Staging**

Tis	Brown disease, AIN IIK, III, high-grade dysplasia
T1	< 2 cm
T2	> 2 cm < 5 cm
T3	> 5 cm
T4	Invades adjacent organ
N1	Perianal LNs
N2	Internal iliac or inguinal LNs.

  - Historically:
    → Treatment: APR + inguinal LNs, dissection.

  o **Treatment: Nigro Protocol**
  - Continuous 5-FU infusion over 1–4 days + mytomycin in day 1 with full pelvis dose radiation (3,000) 15 × 200 over 3 weeks.
    → Complete response, i.e., medical treatment.
  - 5 years, SR is 92%.
    → If inguinal LNs +ve → 5 years, SR ↓ to 58%.
  - Some favor inguinal radiation.
  - Distant metastasis, 10%–15%.
    Liver, lung → chemotherapy.

  o **Role of Surgery**
  - Reserved for recurrent disease after chemoradiation.
    → APR is the only appropriate option.

o **Role of Inguinal LNs Dissection**
  - No prophylactic dissection.
  - For recurrent or persistent groin disease.
  - S-shaped skin incision.

o **Metastasis**
  - Combined chemotherapy 5-FU, cisplatin.

o **Perianal Skin CA (Mucocutaneous)**
  - Standard treatment: electron beam radiation.
  - If tumor extends to anal canal → chemotherapy radiation or APR.

- **Verrucous CA—Aggressive Form of Condyloma Acuminata**
  - Giant condyloma, verrucous carcinoma between normal condyloma and SCC.
  - Not a metastatic disease but locally extensive destruction
  - WLE with flap.
  - Role of chemoradiation is unclear.

- **Basal Cell Carcinoma**
  - Like skin (raised, pearly edges, central ulcer).
  - Slow-growing tumor, rare metastasis.
  - WLE, recurrence is 30%.
  - Radical resection and/or radiation may be required in large tumor.

- **Adenocarcinoma**
  - 10% of anal CA.
  - Arises from anal gland or from chronic anal fissure.
  - Stage I—surgery (APR).
  - Stage II, III—neoadjuvant chemotherapy → surgery (APR) → chemotherapy.
  - For T1 and favorable histological → local excision.

- **Melanoma**
  - Rare, 1% of CRC.
  - 4% of anal CA.
  - 1% of melanoma.

- Poor prognosis.
- 5 years, SR is low, 10%.
- APR or WLE + adjuvant chemotherapy, biological therapy, and radiation.
- Poor prognosis.

- **Paget's Disease**
    - Treatment: surgery.
    - Recurrence, 30%–70% after surgery.
    - Can use chemotherapy radiation or adjuvant as primary treatment.

- **NET**
    - WLE.
    - Neoadjuvant chemoradiation for high-grade NET.

- **Brown Disease**
    - It is carcinoma in situ → Biopsy in four quadrants then WLE.

- **Lymphoma**
    - Chemotherapy + radiation.

- **Mesenchymal Tumor (GIST)**
    - Neo-adjuvant chemotherapy or radiotherapy.
    - WLE to APR.
    - Adjuvant radiotherapy if +ve margin.

Hepatobiliary

Liver

Anatomy
- Largest organ in the body weighing 1,500 g.
- Surrounded by Glisson's capsule.
- The liver is held by several ligaments (7):
    1. Round ligament: obliterated umbilical vein → enters the left liver hilum at front edge of falciform.
    2. Falciform: separates left lateral and medial segments along umbilical fissure and anchors liver to anterior abdominal wall.
    3. Fibrous ligamentum venosum: between caudate and lateral segment.
    4. Right triangular ligament → attaches the liver to diaphragm, then extends anteriorly to become coronary ligament.
    5. Left triangular ligament.
    6. Hepatoduodenal ligament.
    7. Gastrohepatic ligament → just left of gallbladder fossa.

    NB: ligament numbers 1, 2, 4, 5 can be divided (bloodless) for mobilization.
- Hepatoduodenal ligament (porta hepatis) Content: bile duct, hepatic artery, portal vein, epiploic foramen (DAVE)
    - → foramen of Winslow (epiploic foramen) (omental foramen), this passage connects directly to the lesser sac, useful in Pringle maneuver.
        - o Boundaries of foramen of Winslow
            - Anterior: lesser omentum (hepatoduodenal ligament).
            - Posterior: peritoneum covering (IVC).
            - Superior: liver.
            - Inferior: duodenum.

Segmental Anatomy

- Grossly separated to right and left lobes by plane from IVC and gallbladder fossa (Cantlie line).
- Right lobe, 60%–70% of the liver, left lobe and caudate make the reminder.
- Caudate lobe located left and anterior to IVC and has three subsegments: Spiegel, paracaval portion, caudate process.
- Falciform separates left lobe to medial and lateral segments (sections).
- Eight segments of liver → clockwise:
  o Caudate lobe: I
  o Left lateral: II, III
  o Left medial (quadrate lobe):
    IV(A) cephalad just below diaphragm
    IV(B) gallbladder fossa.
  o Right lobe: V, VI, VII, VIII
- Hepatic vein divides the liver to four sectors.

Hepatic Artery

- 25% of blood supply and portal represents 75%.
- Celiac gives left gastric, splenic, common hepatic.
- Common hepatic gives GDA then becomes → proper hepatic artery proper.
- Proper hepatic gives right gastric, then divided to right and left (classic 76% of population), 24% variable.
- 10%–15% replaced or accessory right hepatic arises from SMA.
- 3%–10% replaced or accessory left hepatic arises from left gastric.
- 1%–2% complete replaced right and left hepatic artery come from SMA.
- Cystic artery comes from right hepatic.

Portal Vein

- Formed by SMV + splenic vein (IMV + splenic).
- Right and left branches, divided outside the liver parenchyma, the left branche with sharp bend and gives left lobe with caudate lobe whereas right PV divided higher in the hilum, may be inside the liver parenchyma.
- 25%–35% trifurcation or the left PV supplies right lobe.

- PV drains stomach, spleen, pancreas, small bowel, majority of colon.
- Pressure is 3–5 mmHg; in PHTN → 20–30 mmHg.
- Valveless.
- Portacaval anastomosis: coronary veins (left gastric) vein which produced esophagus and gastric varices.

Hepatic Vein and IVC
- Three Hepatic veinss: right middle, left → IVC.
    Right: drains V, VI, VII, VIII
    Middle: drains IV also V and VIII
    Left drains: II, III
    Caudate is unique and drains directly to IVC.
    Left and middle—common trunk before IVC, while right is separate.
- Large inferior accessory right HV → 15%–20%.

Bile and Hepatic Ducts
- Hepatic duct supplied by hepatic artery→ ligation of hepatic artery → ischemia to ducts.
- Right anterior branch enters liver above the hilum.
- Left duct is longer extrahepatic duct.
- Variation, 30%–40%.
- Gallbladder is adherent to segment IV-B (left lobe) and V (right lobe).

Neural Innervation and Lymphatic
- Parasympathetic: left vagus → anterior, right vagus → posterior.
- Sympathetic: greater thoracic splanchnic nerve and celiac ganglion.
- Denervation after liver TPx → same function.
- Pain in right shoulder, scapula, and back → right phrenic nerve.
- Lymphatic: perisinusoidal space of Disse → hilum.
    Cystic duct LNs (Calot's, Lund's node).

Physiology
- Largest gland in the body.
    • Storage: glycogen.
    • Metabolism: carbohydrates, fat, protein and detoxification, glycolysis, immunity in reticulo-endothelial system.

- Production: coagulation, glucose (energy), plasma protein (albumin), gluconeogenesis.
- Secretion: (digestion) bile, insulin-like GF.

Bilirubin Metabolism

- Hemoglobine is divided into Heme and Globin.
- The globin is further broken into amino acid.
- Heme is broken into iron + Biliverdin (Heme oxygenase).
- The iron gets recycled.
- Bilivirden is reduced to creat unconjugated bilirubin then bind to albumin to facilitate transpot to the liver.
- Once in liver, Glucoronic acid added to unconjugated bilirubin by (Glucuronyl transferase) to form conjugated bilirubin.
- The bilirubin secreted by the liver into duodenum, but it is impermeable to absorbed.
- Once in the colon, colonic bacteria deconjugate bilirubin and convert it into urobilinogen.
- 80% of urobilinogen is further oxidise by intestinal bacteria to form sterocobilin then excreted in feces.
- 20% of urobilingen is reabsorbed into blood stream as a part of enterohepatic circulation.

Formation of Bile

- Water (97%), electrolyte, bile salt, bile pigment, phospholipid (lecithin and cholesterol).
- Lipid-soluble vitamin (KEDA).
- Daily bile out put = 1 L.
- Bile salt + lecithin → absorption of fat.
- Bile salt is (Na^+ + K^+) salt of bile acid conjugated to amino acid.
- Bile salt absorption in small bowel: terminal ileum, 90%–95%.

Drug Metabolism

- Drug is lipophilic to facilitate absorption → in liver fat-soluble elimination → hydrophilic product.
- Acetaminophen is conjugated by liver to harmless glucuronide and sulfate (water soluble) to be excreted in urine.

- during overdose, the metabolic pathway overwhelmed →
  glutathione decreases → toxicity.
- Treatment: glutathione replenishing by sulfhydryl
  (N-acetylcysteine).

Liver Function Test

- AST, ALT, ALP, GGT, and bilirubin.
- These tests measure cell damage rather than function.
- Most accurate measurement for liver function is PT (INR)
  and albumin (long).

Radiological Evaluation of the Liver

US

- Using B mode.
- Useful in trauma → FAST.
- Doppler US can detect blood flow + direction and velocity.
- But limited at dome beneath the ribs, obese patient, bowel gas.
- Advent of contrast-enhanced US → injection of gas
  microbubble to increase sensitivity and space in liver lesion,
  taken by RES → accumulates in liver.
- Intraoperative US is the gold standard for detection of liver
  lesion → tumor staging, visualized intrahepatic vasculature
  + provides biopsy guidance.
- US elastography → degree of fibrosis and cirrhosis,
  sensitivity and specificity, 87% and 91%, unlike liver biopsy
  which is invasive.

CT scan

- Large series of x-ray.
- Spiral-improved capabilities compared to axial.
- HR submillimeter section thickness, ↑ radiation dose.
- In liver → contrast dual or triple.
- Majority of primary liver tumors → the feeding vessels is
  hepatic artery.
- Majority of liver metastasis is feeds by venous supply.
- Phases:
  - Arterial phase, 20–30 seconds after contrast delivery.
  - Venous or portal phase, 60–70 seconds.
  - Delayed phase after 3 minutes.

- Arterial phase → detects tumor (enhancement) (HCC).
- Venous phase → liver parenchyma as portal venous, 75%.
- CT cholangiography: contrast secreted by hepatocyte to bile. For hepatocyte, flow and biliary tree.

MRI

- Magnetic field, H^+ atoms.
- Different organs = different absorption.
- T1—how quickly tissue becomes magnetized.
- T2—how quickly it loses it.
- Good for soft tissue and excellent in fluid.
- MRI with contrast for liver lesion.
- MR elastography.
- MRCP used for pancreatic duct and biliary tree for biliary obstruction.

PET

- Image of metabolic activity, nuclear medicine test.
- Fluorodeoxyglucose (FDG).
- Offers functional imaging rather than anatomic.
- Better in sensitivity and specificity than CT in detection of metastasis.
- PET-CT is the best.
- More than 20% of CRC has liver metastasis.
- For tumor staging, follow-up, occult metastasis.
- In HCC degree of differentiation, correlate with FDG uptake, high-grade increase FDG, low-grade decrease FDG.

Pathology
Hepatocellular Injury

- AST (SGOT) found in liver, cardic and skeletal muscle, kidney, brain, pancreas i.e. not specific.
- ALT (SGPT) is mostly in liver (more specific).
- Common cause of ↑ LFT → viral hepatitis, alcohol abuse, medication, genetic (Wilson's disease) → Cu^{++} in brain, liver, hemochromatosis, autoimmune disease.
- Types:
    • Mild elevation (↑ LFT double or triple): alcohol, fatty liver, chronic viral hepatitis, drugs.

- Moderate elevation: acute hepatitis (viral).
- Severe elevation: ischemia, toxin (acetaminophen), fulminant hepatitis, ↑ LFT > 1,000

Abnormal Synthetic Function

- Albumin evaluate liver function (↓ if prolonged starvation) → the Liver produces 10 g/day and level depends on nutrition, kidney function, protein-losing enteropathy.
- Not a marker in acute hepatic dysfunction as half-life (HL) is 15–20 days.
- Most clotting factors are synthesized in liver, except VIII.
- PT (INR) is the best test for hepatic function.
- PT measures conversion of prothrombin to thrombin.
- Vitamin K is involved in factors: II, VII, IX, X
  → if decreased or using warfarin → ↑INR.

Cholestasis

- Bile from liver to duodenum, in some situation the pathway is impaired.
- Intra- or extrahepatic cause.
- Cholestasis → ↑ alkaline phosphatase (ALP), ↑ GGT.
- Total bilirubin is higher or normal in patient with liver disease.
- Normally, unconjugated bilirubin is 90%.
- In general, ↑ indirect bilirubin → intrahepatic cholestasis.
- ↑ direct bilirubin → extrahepatic cholestasis.
- Hemolysis → ↑ bilirubin (mainly indirect).
- ALP: in liver, bone and biliary ducts, HL is 7 days.
- GGT: found in hepatocyte and released from bile duct epithelium; also ↑ in alcoholism, pancreatic disease, MI, CRF, COPD, so not reliable, but if ↑ GGI + ↑ AP → mostly liver disease.

Jaundice

- Yellowish discoloration of sk, sclera and mucus membrane due to ↑ bilirubin.
- Detectable when bilirubin > 2.5–3 mg/dL.

Causes

- **Prehepatic**
  - Insufficient conjugation (excessive heme), i.e., hemolytic anemia.
  - Congenital spherocytosis, SCA, thalassemia, G6PD.
  - Acquired:
    1. Immune-mediated +ve Coombs test
    2. Non-immune −ve Coombs test (drug and toxin) → damage RBCs, e.g., trauma (heart valve), microangiopathy + infection.
  - Also, failure of transport of unconjugated bilirubin to liver by albumin (poor nutritional state).

- **Intrahepatic**
  - Ischemia, hypoxia.
  - Gilbert disease (hyperbilirubinemia): it is a genetic defect of glucuronyl transferase → ↓ conjugation of bilirubin to glucuronide, 4%, 7% → symptom starts with stress, fasting.
  - Crigler-Najjar syndrome.
  - Rotor and Dubin-Johnson syndromes → disrupt excretion of bile from hepatocyte to bile duct.
  - Inflammation, viral hepatitis.
  - Alcohol, sepsis, autoimmune.
  - Adol, OCP, anabolic steroid.

- **Posthepatic**
  - Intrinsic: CBD stone, GB stone (Mirizzi), biliary stricture, biliary atresia, cholangiocarcinoma, cholangitis, disorder of the ampulla of Vater.
  - Extrinsic: compression of biliary → pancreatic lesion.

NB: Nowadays → post ERCP, operative (clips), ischemia (interventional radiology).

Acute Liver Failure (ALF)
- Occurs when rate extent of hepatocyte death exceeds liver regeneration.
- Classifiedas follows:
  → Fulminant: development of encephalopathy within 8 weeks after development of symptoms without history of liver disease
  → → Subfulminant: development of encephalopathy within 26 weeks of patient having liver disease.
- Symptoms: cerebral edema, hemodynamic instability, bacterial or fungal infection, renal failure, coagulopathy, and metabolic disturbance.
- ALF → coma (hepatic) resulting to death.
- Most common cause of death is ICP due to edema; second most common are sepsis and MOF.
- Previously, SR is 20%, but now with liver TPx, 5 years, SR > 70%.

Etiology
- In the developing world or third world → viral hepatitis B, C, E.
- 65% in developed world is due to drug and toxin with acetaminophen.
- Others: autoimmune hepatitis, ischemic hepatitis cardiogenic shock, pregnancy related, Wilson's disease, Budd Chiari syndrome, 20% indeterminate.

Clinical Picture
- 73% female, median age of 38.
- Patient is ill before 6 days of encephalopathy and 2 days before onset of jaundice and development of encephalopathy.
- 40% has high creatinine, more than 2 mg/dL, pH < 7.3 14%.

Diagnosis and Clinical Management
- History of drug, viral, toxin, liver disease.
- Document patient's mental status.
- Identify any symptoms of CLD.

411

- Need Laboratory investigation.
- Liver biopsy to identify the cause, autoimmune, lymphoma, if coagulopathy → tissue biopsy via transjugular.
- Admit to hospital (ICU).
- Contact liver TPx center and transfer.
- If acetaminophen suspected → ↓ volume from GI tract → NGT or lavage, then administer N-acetylcysteine (NAC) antidote.
- Also can be administered to any suspected patient.
- NAC is administered either orally (140 mg/kg initial dose followed by 70 mg/kg Q4H × 17 doses) or IV (150 mg/kg loading dose followed by 50 mg/kg Q4H × 12 doses as maintenance).
- If suspected drug-induced → take all the patient's prescriptions.
- Majority of patients admitted to ICU → IVF, ulcer prophylaxis, monitoring, electrolyte, and treatment of the infection.
- Phosphate helps liver regeneration, thus hypophosphatemia is a sign of hepatic regeneration → IV phosphate.
- Avoid sedation.
- Elevate head by 30°.
- Frequent neurologic examination.
- ICP monitoring.
- CT head to rule out mass or hemorrhage.
- Administer blood product as ↓ platelet and prolonged PT.

NB: prostaglandin E, I, and phosphate enhance liver regeneration.

Prognosis
- Prognostic scoring system in King College Hospital.
- Other models such as Acute Physiological and Chronic Health Evaluation II (APACHE II).

Liver Transplant

- Liver TPx is the definitive therapy in patient who is unable to regenerate sufficient hepatocyte.
- SR is 20%–70%; in some center, 80%–90%.
- 10% die because there are no liver donors.
- Support device to minimize risk during waiting.

Liver Cirrhosis

- Definition: diffuse hepatic process, characterized by irreversible degeneration and fibrosis and scarring with loss of normal liver architecture into structurally abnormal nodules.
- 40% are asymptomatic.
- Cirrhosis → ESLD → needs TPx or death.
- Complications of ESLD: hyperbilirubinemia, malnutrition, coagulopathy, PHTN (ascites, varices), encephalopathy.
- ESLD → 5 years, mortality rate is 50%–70%.

Morphologic Classification of Cirrhosis

- Micronodular, macronodular and mixed.
- Morphologic pattern: right lobe atrophy, caudate, and left lateral hypertrophy, recanalization of umbilical vein, nodular surface, dilation of Portal V, gastroesophageal varices, splenomegaly.
- Microscopic: hepatitis, hepatocyte necrosis, Mallory body, neutrophil infiltration, perivenular inflammation.

Etiology

- Alcohol.
- Viral Hepatitis:
  - Hepatitis C is the most common cause of CLD, and most require TPx.
  → Identify by hepatitis C antibody as its RNA.
  - Hepatitis B diagnosis by HBsAg 4–6 months after initial infection as its DNA.
- Autoimmune:
  - primary biliary cirrhosis (PBC) → fatigue, pruritus, skin pigmentation (not jaundice),

antimitochondrial antibody → +ve, high cholesterol and late higher bilirubin.

- primary sclerosing cholangitis (PSC) → chronic cholestasis disease associated with UC and CD, pruritus, steatorrhea, decrease fat-soluble vitamin, metabolic bone disease diagnosed by imaging to biliary tree → diffuse multifocal stricture with focal dilation of bile duct → beaded appearance. Complication: biliary stricture cholangitis, cholelithiasis, and cholangiocarcinoma.

- Autoimmune hepatitis → high globulin, particularly gamma.

  Biopsy → mononuclear cell infiltrate with presence of plasma cells, treatment: prednisolone with or without azathioprine.

- Cholestasis.
- Drug induced.
- nonalcoholic steatohepatitis (NASH), usually history of DM, metabolic disease.
  - Diagnosis of NASH → Bx steatohepatitis.
  - In the past, ⅓ of liver cirrhosis without cause; now → NASH.
- Hereditary hemochromatosis
  - Most common metabolic disease causing cirrhosis.
  - Symptoms: skin pigmentation, DM, pseudogout, cardiomyopathy, family history, +ve for cirrhosis.
  - ↑ plasma ferritin, ↑ iron saturation (overload). Diagnosis: liver biopsy.
  - Uncommon metabolic disease: Wilson's, alpha-1 antitrypsin deficiency.

Clinical Manifestation

- Symptoms Fatigue, anorexia, weight loss, jaundice, abdominal pain, ascites, peripheral edema, GI bleeding, hepatic encephalopathy.
- Signs: spider angiomata, palmar erythema, alter in sex metabolism, finger clubbing → hypoalbuminemia, white nail bed, Dupuytren's contracture.

- Male → feminization, gynecomastia, loss of axillary hair, testicular atrophy.
- Splenomegaly, liver may increase or decrease or normal.
- Ascites and pleural effusion.
- PHTN with caput medusae with or without Cruveilhier-Baumgarten murmur, venous hum in epigastrium results from collateral between PV and remnant of umbilical vein.
- Jaundice if bilirubin is 2–3 mg/dL.
- Asterixis in patient with hepatitis, hepatic encephalopathy.
- Fetor hepaticus, malnutrition, decrease in weight, loss of temporal muscle.
- Muscle cramp, low muscle to fat ratio.
- Umbilical hernia and repair should be:
  → Elective with well-compensated cirrhosis or repair at the time of TPx or after TPx.
- HCC can occur with any cause of cirrhosis → so screening of HCC every 6 months via US and serum alpha-fetoprotein.
- Cardiac: ↑ COP, ↑ HR, ↓ SVR, ↓ BP.
- Easily infected because impaired phagocytic activity of reticuloendothelial system (RES) of the liver.
- Spnotaneous bacterial peritonitis occurs in patient with ascites.
- ↓ drug metabolism.

Laboratory Finding
- Depends on degree of compensation.
- Normocytic anemia.
- ↓ WBCs, ↓ platelet, bone marrow macroplastics.
- PT prolonged and not responding to vitamin K.
- ↓ albumin.
- Urobilinogen is present and ↓ excretion of Na^+ if ascites is present.
- LFT: AST, ALT, AP → increase.

Liver Biopsy
- To confirm cirrhosis → biopsy.
- Can be percutaneous, transjugular, or laparoscopy or CT, US-guided.

- Can use US elastography by inducing (elastic shear).

Hepatic Reserve Association of Surgical Risk
- Patient with liver disease is at risk of anesthesia and surgery.
- Emergency cardiac operation, abdominal, especially cholecystectomy, is at risk.
- Laboratory tests to assess hepatic reserve: indocyanine green, sorbitol, galactose elimination capacity, carbon 13 galactose breath test.
- MEGX: measure MEGX after lidocaine administration.
- Child A can undergo elective surgery, while child B can go with caution (better not). Child C, no elective surgery.

Child-Turcotte-Pugh (CTP) Score
- This score is developed to evaluate risk of portacaval shunt for PHTN.
- It shows to predict risk of intra-abdominal surgery.

Scoring	1 Pt.	2 Pts.	3 Pts.
Bilirubin	< 2	2–3	> 3
Albumin	> 3.5	2.8–3.5	< 2.8
INR	< 1.7	1.7–2.2	> 2.2
Encephalopathy	none.	Controlled	uncontrolled
Ascites	none.	controlled	uncontrolled

- Class A   5–6 pts. mortality, 10%
- Class B   7–9 pts. mortality, 30%
- Class C   10–15 pts. mortality, 75%–80%

Model for End-Stage Liver Disease (MELD) Score
- INR, bilirubin, creatinine.
- Developed for TIPS but can be used to determine performance before liver TPx.
- Predictor for 30-day mortality → now predicts perioperative mortality.
- Mortality rate is 1% for each point till 20; above 20, each point is 2%.

Essential Notes in General Surgery

- MELD below 10 can safely go to elective procedure, 10–15 undergo with caution, > 15 should not go for elective procedure.
- Calculation:

$$[0.957 \times Log_e (Cr) + 0.378 \times Log_e (bili)$$
$$+ 1.120 \times Log_e (INR) + 0.643] \times 10$$

MELD	Three-Month Mortality (%)
7	1
20	8
24	10
26	15
29	20
31	30
33	20
40	90

Portal Hypertension (PHTN)
- Defined as high Portal vein pressure more than 5–7 mmHg.
- Very limited shunt occurs normally.
- Portal vein supplies 75% of liver blood supply and 72% of O_2.
- 1,000–15,000 mL/min in adult.

Etiology
- Presinusoidal
  - Extrahepatic: splenic vein thrombosis, splenomegaly, splenic AVF.
  - Intrahepatic: schistosomiasis, sarcoid, coagulation, hepatic fibrosis.
- Sinusoidal
  - Cirrhosis, viral infection, alcohol, cirrhosis, PSC, autoimmune hepatitis.
- Postsinusoidal
  - Vascular occlusive disease, Budd-Chiari syndrome, CHF, pericarditis, IVC web.

417

Clinical presentation
- Development of collateral between portal and systemic venous system.
- Collaterals: GEJ → coronary vein
    Anal canal → superior hemorrhoidal vein
    Falciform ligament → paraumbilical veins (caput medusae)
    Splenic vein bed, left renal, and retroperitoneum + vein of Retzius and sappy.
- Most common site is coronary and short gastric to azygos vein → esophageal varices.
- Causes classified into prehepatic, intrahepatic, posthepatic.
- Most common causes are cirrhosis, hepatitis C.
- 50% in cirrhotic liver will develop esophageal varices and Most common causes are cirrhosis, hepatitis C. will bleed from it.
- Splenomegaly → associated with hypersplenism, causing pancytopenia.
- Ascites if ↑PHTN.
- Umbilical vein recanalization.
- Anorectal involvement is 45% of cirrhotic patient.
- Shunt (spontaneously) between PV and left renal vein or IVC.
- Can present with complication: esophageal varices bleeding.

Imaging for Portal Vein and Measurement of PV Pressure
- US: Doppler US → anatomy, if associated thrombosis, direction of flow and TIPS.
- CT, MRA.
- Angiography and portal venography.
- Most accurate method for PHTN is portal venography.
- Placing the catheter to Hepatic vein with deflated balloon to measure free hepatic venous pressure (FHVP).
- And with inflated ballone to occlude hepatic vein and measure WHVP.
- Hepatic venous pressure gradient:
  (HVPG) = WHVP − FHVP
    → which is difference between hepatic sinusoidal pressure and Portal pressure.
- If exceeding 10 mmHg → PHTN.

Management of gastroesophageal Varices

- Most common manifestation, common cause, and leading cause of death in PHTN is variceal bleeding.
- 30% of compensated and 60% of uncompensated liver failure will have esophageal varices.
- ⅓ of patients will experience variceal bleeding.
- Each episode, 20%–30% mortality → if untreated, 70%.
- Recurrent of variceal hemorrhage → within 2 years.

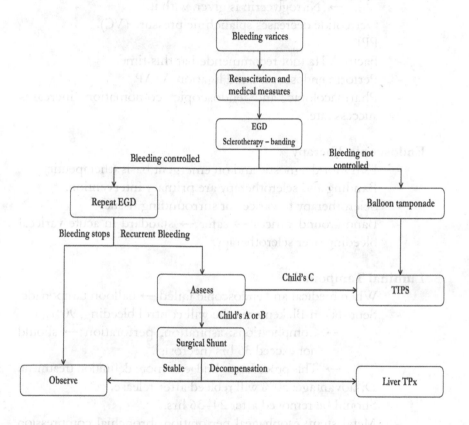

Management of Acute Variceal Hemorrhage

- ABC.
- Resuscitation, keep Hb ≈ 8 g/dL.
- Hb > 7–8 g/dL, over resuscitation and SBP > 100 mmHg worsen variceal bleeding.
- Over-resuscitation with blood and IVF increase mortality, morbidity, and rebleeding.
- ICU, resuscitation.

- High incidence to develop bacterial infection → ↑ mortlity and morbidity → 50% will develop spontaneous bacterial peritonitis (SBP) from bacterial infection, then UTI, pneumonia.
- Prophylactic IV antibiotics such as ceftriaxone or ciprofloxacin increase SR.
- FFP and platelet if coagulopathy.
- Vasoactive medication:
  - → Vasopressin → may increase HTN, MI, arrhythmia.
  - → Nitroglycerin is given with it.
- Octreotide decreases splanchnic pressure (VC).
- PPI.
- Factor VIIa (not recommended at this time).
- Perform endoscopic band ligation ASAP.
- Pharmacologic and endoscopic combination increases success rate.

Endoscopic Therapy
- EGD for diagnostic and on emergent basis (therapeutic).
- Banding and sclerotherapy are primary intervention.
- Sclerotherapy to varices or surrounding tissue.
- Band around varices → safer → standard in acute variceal bleeding over sclerotherapy.

Luminal Tamponade
- When medical and endoscopic failed → balloon tamponade.
- Sengstaken-Blakemore tube will control bleeding, 90%.
  - → Complications: aspiration, perforation → should not exceed 36 hrs (necrosis).
  - → This procedure is bridge to more definition treatment.
- Disadvantage: 50% will rebleed after release.
- Should be removed after 24–36 hrs.
- Metal stent: esophageal perforation, bronchial compression remains if place up to 2 weeks.

Transjugular Intrahepatic Portosystemic Shunt (TIPS)
- Metalic stent between intrahepatic branch of PV and hepatic vein.
- Percutaneous, usually right jugular → right hepatic vein, then hepatic parenchyma to PV (right PV) → parenchyma tract is balloon dilated, and after portography → stent.

- Needle track is dilated until pressure 12 is achieved.
- Success rate is 95%, stops 90% of refractory bleeding.
- Frequent follow-up for dilation and restenting.
- MR is 5%–40%.

- **Indication**
  - Variceal hemorrhage not responding to medical therapy or endoscopic therapy.
  - Ascites refractory to medical treatment
  - Budd-Chiari syndrome not responding to anticoagulant
  - Hepatic hydrothorax
  - child B, C
  - Hepatopulmonary syndrome
  - Hepatorenal syndrome

- **Contraindication**
  - Right side heart failure
  - Severe tricuspid regurgitation
  - Pulmonary HTN, CHF, encephalopathy
  - Active bacterial infection
  - Biliary obstruction
  - Relative: hepatic vein thrombosis, poor liver function

  NB: TIPS can be accepted as first-line treatment in advanced liver disease.

- **Complications of TIPS**
  - Dysfunctional occlusion or stenosis, 18%–78%; thrombosis, 10%–15%
  - Encephalopathy: compensated, 12%; uncompensated, 50%
  - Bleeding, 5% (haemobilia)
  - Sepsis, 2%–10%
  - Infarction, 2%–4%
  - Biliary infection, respiratory failure

Balloon-Occluded Retrograde Transvenous Obliteration (BRTO)
- Management of gastric variceal bleeding in patient with spontaneous gastrorenal or splenorenal shunts.
- Use transjugular or femoral vein to obliterate left renal vein with sclerosing agent.

- No encephalopathy.
- S/E: exacerbate PHTN, increase esophageal varices, ↑ ascites.

Surgical Shunts
- Reserved for chronic or recurrent hemorrhage.
- Decreased popularity after TIPS and liver TPx.
- Now shunt is considered for MELD < 15, for patient who is not a candidate for liver TPx or has limited access to TIPS.
- Aim is to decrease PV pressure and maintain hepatic blood flow and avoid encephalopathy.
- Failed TIPS.
- Types:

   o Nonselective: diverts all portal flow away from liver
      - Portacaval (distort anatomy): PV to IVC (end to side) or side to side to maintain blood flow to liver.
        Currently rarely performed as ↑ encephalopathy.
      - Mesocaval: SMV to IVC, easier and doesn't violate the anatomy for subsequent liver TPx, less encephalopathy but thrombosis and rebleeding.
        Usually uses 8–10 mm (PTFE) graft to connect between them.

   o Selective: decompresses porto-azygos system with preserve portal inflow
      - Distal splenorenal (Warren-Hassab shunt).
        Most currently used.
        Division of gastroesophageal collateral then splenic vein to left renal vein (end to side).
        Lower encephalopathy.
        Not used for intractable ascites.
        Does not interfere for further liver TPx.

Nonshunt Surgical Management for Refractory Variceal Bleeding
- If PV thrombosis, refractory variceal bleeding.
   → Sugiura procedure:
   - Extensive devascularization of stomach and distal esophagus
   - Transection of esophagus
   - Splenectomy

- Truncal vagotomy
- Pyloroplasty

Liver Transplantation
- 1 year, SR is 86%.

- **Kings College criteria for liver TPx:**
  - Acetaminophen-induced
    - Arterial pH <7.3
    - Lactate > 3mmol/L
    - The 3 following criteria:
      o Hepatic encephalopathy > grad 3
      o Serum creatinine > 3.4
      o INR > 6.5
  - Non-acetaminophen-induced
    - INR > 6.5
    - 3 out of 5 following criteria:
      o Indeterminate etiology
      o INR > 3.5
      o Bilirubin > 17.6 mg/dl
      o Age ≤ 10 or > 40
      o Interval jaundice encephalopathy
  - These criteria are only for fulminant liver failure.

Liver TPx Technique
- Bicaval anastomosis
- Piggyback technique
- Modified piggyback
- Vascular reconstruction
- Arterial reconstruction
- Biliary anastomosis

Complications Following LTPx
- Arterial
  - Interruption or reduction → bile duct necrosis, liver abscess, graft dysfunction, but can survive because of PV.
    → Hepatic artery thrombosis, 2%–5% → thrombectomy or reconstruction of artery
      → Hepatic artery stenosis, 2%–10% → surgical revision or percutaneous angioplasty

- Biliary tree depends on arterial blood supply.

- Venous
  - PV thrombosis, PV stenosis.
    - → if early → surgery
    - → if late → percutaneous (balloon) removal.

- Biliary
  - Duct to duct anastomosis is better than duct to bowel.
  - Bile leak, 20% → ERCP and stent, 85% success rate.
  - Bile duct stricture, 15% → MRCP → dilation and stent and replacement of large stent after 3 months.
    - → If non-anastomotic stricture → stent.
    - → If failed → Roux-en-Y hepaticojejunostomy.

Prevention of Variceal Bleeding

- Nonselective β-blocker: ↓ COP → VC of splanchnic → ↓ PV pressure.
- It decreases mortality by 50%, decreases bleeding by 45% (20% will not respond and 20% will not tolerate side effects).
- Prophylaxis endoscopy surveillance → variceal band ligation is recommended in medium and large size of varices.
- Perform 1–2 weeks until obliteration, followed by 1–3 months follow-up, and Q6M EGD surveillance.

Other complication of Portal HTN

Hepatic Hydrothorax

- Treatment: TIPS.
- Pleural effusion in patient with cirrhosis and PHTN without cardiopulmonary disease.
- 10% in patient with ascites.
- Common in right but can be bilateral, accumulation of 500 cc.
- Trans-diaphragmatic migration of ascites fluid via lymph and diaphragmatic defect but can be without ascites.
  - → Thoracentesis and analysis.
  - → Definitive diagnosis by technetium sulfur colloid study → passage of radioactive to chest cavity confirms diagnosis.
- Can be infected → SBEM.

Treatment

- Na$^+$ restriction and diuresis.
- In refractory cases → therapeutic thoracentesis, TIPS, PV shunt.
- Tube thoracostomy with injection of sclerosing agent can be for long term.
- In patient with SBEM → ceftriaxone, 1 g IV OD × 10 days.
- Hepatic hydrothorax: serious late complication → liver TPx.

Hepatorenal Syndrome

- Alteration in vasoactive hormones → splanchnic VD, renal artery VC → ↓renal hypoperfusion.
- Types:

    I   Progressive, rapid decline in renal function

    II Slow, gradual decrease in renal function

- Tx: TIPS, especially type II.

Hepatopulmonary Syndrome

- Intrapulmonary VD.
- Right to left shunt → ↓ ventilation.
- TIPS bridging to surgery (LTPx).

Portal Hypertensive Gastropathy

- Inflamed fragile mucosa of stomach → treatment: mucosal protection → TIPS.

Management of Refractory Ascites

- Ascites: abnormal accumulation of fluid in peritoneal cavity.
- Results from PHTN, impaired renal function, ↓ plasma oncotic pressure.
- Liver causes 80% of ascites.
- Others: peritoneal carcinomatosis, abdominal TB, CHF, nephrotic syndrome, Budd-Chiari syndrome, pancreatic disease, alcoholic hepatitis.

Pathophysiology

- Peripheral arterial VD.

    PHTN → nitric oxide → VD → splanchnic artery VD.

Refractory Ascites
1. Resistance
2. Intractable

- Resistance: does not respond to diuresis (spironolactone, 400 mg, or Lasix, 160 mg/day).
- Intractable when patient cannot tolerate diuresis because of low Na^+, encephalopathy, azotemia.
- Refractory happened in less than 10%.

Diagnosis of Ascites
- All patients (new or known) should go for paracentesis as 10%–25% risk of spontaneous bacterial peritonitis.
  - → Analysis of ascites
    Cell count, gram stain, C/S, albumin, total protein, glucose, LDH (TG added if suspected chylous ascites).
  - → Cytology if suspected malignancy.
  - → Serum albumin, protein, LDH to compare it with ascites.
- To determine the cause of ascites → calculate serum-ascites albumin gradient (SAAG).
  SAAG = serum albumin − ascetic albumin

Causes of ascites according to SAAG

SAAG ≥ 1.1 g/dL with PHTN	SAAG ≥ 1.1 g/dL: No PHTN
Cirrhosis	Peritoneal CA
Alcoholic hepatitis	Nephrotic syndrome
Vascular obstruction (Budd Chiari syndrome, PV thrombosis)	Pancreatitis
CHF, Myxedema	Peritoneal TB
Metastasis to liver, Fatty liver	Serositis

Paracentesis
- Mostly cirrhotic and have prolonged PT and low platelet.
- INR is not accurate.
- Routine platelet, FFP transfusion is not recommended.

- Major contraindication to paracentesis is DIC.
- Needle introduced in 3 cm medial and superior to ASIS on LLQ because right → cecum is distended, most patients taking lactulose.
- Angular technique (oblique) or Z-track technique (straight then to peritoneum).

Treatment of Ascites
- Decrease Na^+ intake and increase Na^+ excretion.

Non-pharmacologic Treatment
- Dietary sodium restriction
  - Typical dietary Na^+ content = 4–6 g/day.
  - Daily Na^+ restriction is 1.5–2 g (recommended).
  - 1 teaspoon contains 2,300 mg Na^+.
  - Processed food has higher Na^+.
  - Measure Na^+ urine for 24 hrs.
  - 15%–20% can achieve −ve Na^+ balance by restriction.
- Fluid restriction
  - Not necessary except if Na^+ is 125 mg/dL.

Pharmacological Treatment
- Diuretics
  - Most commonly used is K^+ sparing, spironolactone and Lasix.
  - Dose:
    - → spironolactone 100 mg and maximum 400 mg
    - → Lasix 40 mg and maximum 160 mg
  - Thiazide is not recommended → ↓ K^+ and ↑ ammonia → encephalopathy.
- Albumin
- VC: in management of hepatorenal syndrome (HRS).
  - Improve renal function, ↓ ascites.
  - Octreotide → splanchnic vasoconstriction → ↓ ascites.
- Drug to avoid
  - NSAIDs → nephropathy.

Intervention Therapy
- Large volume paracentesis (LVP)
  - 4–5 L removed.
  - Albumin infusion doesn't improve mortality and morbidity but improves electrolyte imbalance.
  - Need albumin if large ascitic fluid is drained, 6–8 L.
- TIPS
- Peritoneovenous shunt (PVS)
- Currently not used → not safe → TIPS is better.
  - 40% failure of shunt in first year.
  - Complications: DIC, coagulopathy, pulmonary edema, ↑ variceal bleeding, encephalopathy.

Spontaneous Bacterial Peritonitis (SBP)
- 30% of cirrhotic liver with ascites will develop SBP.
- Mortality rate is 20%.
- All hospitalized patients → ascites fluid analysis.
- Normal patient who developed abdominal pain, fever, encephalopathy, leukocytosis, or renal failure → repeat paracentesis.
- Treatment: SBP with empiric antibiotic is not recommended without definitive C/S.

Treatment
- Ascites fluid with absolute neutrophil count more than 250 cell/m^3 is diagnostic → empiric antibiotic should be given, then C/S → antibiotic should narrow down accordingly.

- Empiric Antibiotic
  First line
  - Cefotaxime   2 g IV Q8H
  - Ofloxacin   400 mg PO Q12H

  Second line
  - Ceftriaxone   1 g IV Q12H
  - Ciprofloxacin   400 mg IV Q12H
  - Tazocin   3.375 mg IV Q6H
  - Ertapenem   1 g IV Q24H for resistance
  - Cefepime   1–2 g IV Q18H for resistance

- Prophylactic Antibiotic
  First line with GI bleeding
  - Ceftriaxone, 1 g IV daily for 7 days.
  - Weekly prophylaxis: ciprofloxacin, 750 mg PO.
  - Decreases mortality and morbidity if you give albumin + antibiotic.
    - → Albumin 1.5 g/kg within 6 hrs, then 1 g/kg at day 3.
  - Patient with ascites can have secondary bacterial peritonitis → bowel perforation, abscess.
  - Need to distinguish between primary and secondary, although SBP comes with mild symptom.
  - Peritoneal analysis (fluid).
  - X-ray or CT for perforation or abscess.

Prophylaxis
- oral ciprofloxacin, 750 mg/ week.
- Trimethoprim, sulfamethoxazole recommended after first episode of SBP.
- Primary prophylaxis is controversial.
- Current recommendation:
  Give primary prophylaxis with oral ciprofloxacin to patient with protein
    < 1.5 gl/dL with one of the following:
      Creatinine > 1.2 mg/dL
      Urea > 25 mg/dL
      $Na^+ < 130$ mEq/L
      Child score > 9 and bilirubin > 3 mg/dL
- Patient with prior SBP and now has UGI bleeding → ciprofloxacin IV for 7 days is recommended.

Hepatic Encephalopathy
- Treatment:
  - ICU, intubation as GCS.
  - Determine the cause, e.g., cirrhosis, acetaminophen ingestion.
  - Determine its child class A, B, C.
  - If child A, call tertiary center for liver TPx.
  - If B and C → TIPS.

- No protein restriction, use branched chain amino acid, as those patients are already malnourished.
- Lactulose enema to ↓ ammonia.
- Neomycin orally.
- Others: probiotics.

Budd-Chiari Syndrome (BCS)
- Congestive hepatopathy.
- Thrombosis or obstruction of hepatic vein.
- Incidence: 1 in 100,000.
- Symptom mimics to liver failure.
- Types:
  o Primary: when thrombosis is intraluminal.
  o Secondary: when compression by any lesion.
- Primary, 75%–90%.
- Causes: thrombocytopenia, polycythemia rubra, 35%–50%.
- All coagulopathy disease can cause BCS.
- When obstruction of two or more of HV → low perfusion.
- Biopsy: non-inflammatory centrilobular necrosis.
- Can cause PHTN.
- Caudate lobe hypertrophy, 50% → further obstruction IVC.
- US, initial tool → absence of hepatic vein flow, spiderweb hepatic vein.
- CT → thrombosis.
- Best and definitive → hepatic venography.
- Treatment:
  - Initial treatment of underlying cause and prevention of further thrombosis by anticoagulant.
  - Management of ascites.
  - Percutaneous angioplasty and TIPS + thrombolytic therapy.
  - Thrombolytic alone in acute phase.
  - Portacaval shunt if all measures fails.
  - If progressive and ESLD → liver TPx.

Evaluation of Liver Mass

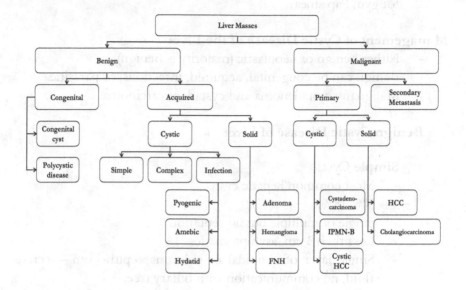

- History and physical examination
  - Abdominal pain, early satiety, weight loss
  - Liver disease, cirrhosis, alcohol
  - Hepatitis, blood transfusion, tattoo
  - OCP, CA history
  - Jaundice
  - Palpable mass, splenomegaly, stigmata of PHTN

- Laboratory
  - CBC
  - U&E
  - LFT, albumin, ammonia
  - PTT, PT, INR.
  - Hepatitis screening
  - Tumor marker (CEA, AFP, CA 19)

- Imaging
  - US
  - CT, MRI (contrast pattern)
  - Nuclear medicine (PET)
  - Angiography

- Occult Primary: EGD, colonoscopy, mammogram, US neck, and for gyn, Pap smear.

Management of Cystic Disease of the Liver
- Either benign or neoplastic (majority is benign).
- Benign can be congenital, acquired, infectious, or parasitic.
- Malignant: cystadenoma and cystadenocarcinoma.

Benign Cystic Disease of Liver

- **Simple Cyst**
  - Most common hepatic cyst.
  - 5%–18%.
  - Single or multiple but no septation.
  - Less than 3 cm, asymptomatic.
  - Single layer of cuboidal or columnar epithelium—secrete fluid, no communication with biliary tree.

  - **Pathogenesis**
  - Aberrant intrahepatic bile duct lost communication to biliary tree.
  - Size: few mm to 20 cm.
  - Serous, brown if previous hemorrhage.

  - **Indication for Intervention**
  - Usually asymptomatic → none.
  - No follow-up if diagnosis established as simple cyst
  - Symptom is rare if < 5 cm.
  - Symptom: vague discomfort, fullness, early satiety.
  - US: round, oval, sharp edge, serous fluid, no septation (if +ve → 2 cysts adjacent).
  - CT: location, vasculature nearby, well circumscribed, no enhancement with contrast.
  - MRI: T1 Hypointense, T2 Hyperintense

  - **Intervention**
  - Aspiration, 100% recurrence.
  - Sclerotherapy is mainstay; US-guided, makes sure no biliary communication.

→ Aspiration → instilled 95% ethanol and not exceeding 120 mL to avoid intoxication.

→ Then reaspiration after 2–4 hrs.

- Sedation is required → because of pain.
- Repeat procedure if necessary.
- Follow up after 6 months for symptom relief.
- Recurrence, 5%.

• **Surgical**
- Treatment of choice.
- Isolated → fenestration.
- Laparoscopic resection.
- Puncture and remove anterior wall and send histopathology.
- Cyst cavity fulgurated with organ beam coagulation.
- Bile leak is the most common complication.
- 5% require open conversion.

■ **Polycystic Liver Disease**
- Staged by Gigot classification:

Type I	Limited number < 10, of large cyst > 10 cm
Type II	Diffuse involvement of parenchyma by medium-sized cyst with large area uninvolved
Type III	Massive diffuse by small and medium cysts with little spared liver parenchyma

• **Pathogenesis**
- commonly associated with Polycystic kidney disease.
- Autosomal dominant.
- Genetic mutation: PRKCSH chromosome 19 or SEC63 chromosome 6, both 90%.
- 10%–20% isolated PLD.
- Liver cyst develops later than renal.
- Other extrarenal manifestation: cerebral aneurysm → brain image.
- Similar to gross and microscope to simple cyst.
- Overgrowth → cells secrete fluid → biliary micro hamartoma.

- **Indication for Intervention**
- Minority needs intervention → Unless symptom occurs or when cyst: parenchyma ratio > 1
  - → Compressed IVC, stomach, lower limb dema, early satiety.
- Normal LFT, high ALP and GGT.
- Cyst may get infected or hemorrhage.
- Serious complications: biliary compression, PHTN, ascites (refractory), and/or pleural effusion.
- Malignant transformation may occur (rare).

- **Medical Therapy**
- Somatostatin may ↓ liver volume, but no cyst regression.
- mTOR for small cyst (may regress).

- **Intervention Therapy**
- Transcatheter arterial embolization.
- Aspiration: no benefit unless infected.

- **Surgical Therapy**
- Open cyst fenestration, superficial to deep.
  - → Laparoscopy not recommended.
  - → Debulk liver as much as possible.
- Take care for vessels and biliary duct.
- Mortality rate is 4% and morbidity is 30% for fenestration, 65% for resection.
- Complication: ascites.

- **Transplantation (TPx)**
- Single most definitive treatment.
- Pre-operative MELD score.
- SR is 5 years of PLD and PKD, 80%–85%.

- **Ciliated Hepatic Foregut Cyst**
  - Any region of foregut including liver and gallbladder.
  - Four layers.
  - Subcapsular close to insertion of falciform ligament IV.
  - Appearance of atypical solid tumor.

- CA 19-9 may be high, difficult to distinguish from cystadenoma and cystadenocarcinoma.
- FNA is helpful.
- Malignant transformation may occurs.
- Resection if > 4 cm.

- **Traumatic Cyst**
    - Liver hematoma can occur after trauma but may also be rupture adenoma.
    - Symptoms: pain due to peritonitis, hypovolemic shock.
    - Conservative unless rupture, bile leak, compression.

- **Caroli Disease**
    - Congenital duct malformation (intrahepatic).
    - Segmental cystic dilation of intrahepatic radicles.
    - ↑ biliary lithiasis, cholangitis, biliary abscess.
    - Occurs in absence of liver cirrhosis.
    - Mostly present symptom → fever, chills, abdominal pain.
    - In aged 30.
    - Rarely present with PHTN.
    - 33% → biliary lithiasis.
    - 7% → cholangiocarcinoma.
    - Investigation: MRCP, ERCP.
    - Treatment: ERCP, PTC drainage.
        - → If single lobe → resection.
        - → Liver TRx for recurrent cholangitis decompensation.

Cystic Lesion	Clinical Picture	Radiological	Management
Simple cyst	Asymptomatic, may have symptom with pregnancy	Well-defined Unilocular Round/oval Low fluid density	None unless with symptom Alcohol Sclerotherapy Laparotomy fenestration
Ciliated foregut cyst	Painful if 5 cm	Unilocular Subcapsular Near falciform (segment IV) Four layers in US	Resection if > 4 cm
Polycystic	Family history of PLD or PKD	Multiple cystic Liver ± kidney Hepatic Enlargement	Open fenestration Liver resection Liver TPx
Amebic abscess	Travel to endemic region	Complex cyst Double target appearance	Metronidazole
Pyogenic liver abscess	Clinical finding of infection	Complex cyst with rim enhancement	Percutuaneous drainage + antibiotic Surgery if refractory
Hydatid cyst	Travel to endemic	Complex cyst with peripheral daughter cyst	Excision of cyst or pericystectomy
Traumatic cyst	History of trauma	Cystic liver lesion with variable density	None unless with symptom or complication

Neoplastic Liver Disease

- **Hepatic Cystadenoma**
  - In right lobe (mostly), slow-growing benign lesion, but it can transform to malignant.
  - Similar to mucinous cystic pancreatic neoplasm and IPMN.

- **Pathogenesis**
  - Mostly intrahepatic and may arise from biliary structure.
  - Solitary lesion is 1–40 cm.
  - Lobulated, multiloculated.
  - Content is serous to mucinous.
  - Three layers: inner epithelium, middle mesenchymal stroma, and outer collagen or pseudocapsule.
  - Luminal dysplasia, metaplasia, high risk of malignancy transformation.
  - 85% with ovarian-like stroma occur only in female; in male, usually with biliary communication.

- **Indication for Intervention**
  - Incidence: 40s–50s in female.
  - Can cause symptoms and complications.
  - Mildly high ALP.
  - US: septation, papillary projection.
  - CT: hypodense, multiloculated, well-definitive border. The septation → fine calcification and contrast enchancement.
  - MRI: reveals septation:

    | T1 | Hypointense or isointense |
    | T2 | Hyperintense |

  - Rarely multiple.
  - Cytology: not specific, chronic inflammation.
  - High CEA, high CA 19-9 (not diagnostic).
  - Because of potential malignancy → remove.

- **Technique**
  - Surgical therapy is mainstay.
  - Fenestration with fulguration is not recommended.
  - So either enucleation or partial hepatectomy.
    - → Careful in segment 4 (biliary bifurcation).
    - → IOC is recommended if communication.
    - → Frozen section to exclude IPMN-B.
  - Extrahepatic often requires bile duct resection and biliary-enteric reconstruction.

- **Cystic intra-ductal papillary mucinous neoplasm – biliary (IPMN-B)**
  - Similar to pancreatic IPMN and hepatic cystadenoma.
  - Can have communication with biliary duct.

  - **Pathogenesis**
    - Produce mucin.
    - Found in intrahepatic bile duct.
    - similar to side branch of pancreatic IPMN.
    - Mimic cystadenoma and CA → cystic and solid component.
    - Multiloculated and hemorrhagic.
    - High malignancy potential.
      - → Incidence of invasive adenocarcinoma, 60% of cystic IPMN-B.

  - **Indication for Intervention**
    - Difficult to distinguish from cystadenoma and CA.
    - Large mural duct nodule with distal dilatation.
    - ERCP or IOC (but not MRCP) demonstrates biliary communication.

  - **Technique**
    - Because of high risk of malignancy → intervention.
    - IOC should be performed.
    - Superfacial spread along biliary duct.
      - → Formal hepatectomy is the preferred approach.
      - → Extrahepatic biliary resection and/or partial LNs dissection.
    - Outcome is better than cholangiocarcinoma.
    - 5 years, SR is 60%–80%.

- **Hepatic Cystadenocarcinoma**
  - Malignant transformation from cystadenoma.
  - Mostly intrahepatic, no biliary communication.
  - If communication → IPMN-B or cystic cholangiocarcinoma.

  - **Pathogenesis**
    - With or without ovarian-like stroma.
    - Solitary, can be distinguished from liver metastasis.

- Pain, jaundice (20%), rupture is not uncommon.

- **Indication for Intervention**
  - Size: 2–40 cm.
  - Mild elevation of CA 19-9.
  - Cystic fluid analysis is helpful in DDx.
  - No aspiration → peritoneal seeding.
  - Nodularity and septation.

- **Technique**
  - Surgical resection.
  - IOC is recommended to exclude biliary communication and to distinguish from IPMN-B.
  - Tumor extension may exceed → formal hepatic resection or wedge resection.
  - Extrahepatic biliary resection + reconstruction may be necessary.
  - Spillage → carcinomatosis.

- **Embryonic Hepatic Sarcoma**
  - Rare, age of presentation 2–15 years old.
  - Large poorly differentiated tumor.
  - Myxoid and necrotic content.
  - CT, MRI.

Cystic Lesion	Clinical Picture	Radiological	Management
Cystadenoma	More in female No history of infection or trauma	Complex, multilocular Septation Microcalcification Contrast enhancement of septation	Enucleation Partial hepatectomyor lobectomy
Cystadenocarcinoma	More in female No history of infection or trauma	Complex, multilocular Septation Microcalcification Contrast enhancement of septation	Partial hepatectomyor lobectomy
IPMN-B	No history of infection or trauma History of IPMN-P	Complex, multilocular Septation Microcalcification Contrast enhancement of septation Biliary communications on ERCP or IOC Bile duct dilation Distal to tumor	Partial hepatectomyor lobectomy + IOC ± extrahepatic Biliary resection and portal lymphadenectomy
Embryonal sarcoma	Adolescent	Large complex cyst on CT, MRI Solid on US	Partial hepatectomy or lobectomy + chemotherapy
Cystic HCC	History of HBV HCV, cirrhosis	Complex hypervascular with PV washout	RFA, TACE Partial hepatectomy or lobectomy LTPX
Cystic metastasis	History of malignancy	Multiple complex cysts with enhancement	Chemotherapy

Infections of the Liver
- Largest portion of reticuloendothelial system (RES) in the liver.
- Thus, nonviral infection is unusual.
- Most common visceral abscess.
- Three categories:
    1. Pyogenic: aerobic or anaerobic from GIT
    2. Amoebic: Entamoeba histolytica
    3. Fungal (candida), parasitic (Echinococcus granuloses)

Pyogenic Liver Abscess
- Single or multiple, more frequently in right lobe.
- If multiple, variable in size and may have a honeycomb appearance.
- 40% monomicrobial, 40% ploymicobial, 20% culture −ve.
- Common organism: E. coli, then streptococcus faecalis, klebsiella, bacteroides.
- In patient with endocarditis, most common cause is infected catheter→ staph and streptococcus.
- In the past, caused by acute appendicitis, diverticulitis.
- Now, commonly caused by instrumentation of biliary system, subacute bacterial endocarditis, infected catheter, direct extension (cholecystitis), injury from trauma, hepatic artery from septicemia, and cryptogenic process.
- In immunocompromised, HIV, chemotherapy, transplanted patient.
- Symptoms: RUQ pain, jaundice, ⅓ with constitutional symptom, leukocytosis, high ESR, high alkaline phosphatase.
- Blood C/S → 50% will identify caustic organism.
- X-ray: Elevated right hemidiaphragm
            Right pleural effusion
            Lower-right atelectasis
            Gas in RUQ
            Portal gas if pylephlebitis
- US → round or oval hypoechoic lesion with well defined wall.
- CT localization, hypodense, and peripheral enhancement may contain air fluid level (gas-forming organism).
- MRI not superior to CT.

Treatment

- Treatment of abscess and underlying cause and mostly with IV antibiotics + drainage.

- • Antibiotics
  - First, blood culture.
  - IV antibiotic (empiric) then modified as C/S → bacteria can identify the source.
  - If colonic, ciprofloxacin or third generation cephalocporin + metronidazole.
  - If biliary source, broad-spectrum (tazocin).
  - If patient is severely ill and has recurrent cholangitis → meropenem to treat drug resistance for gram −ve + linezolid to treat VRE.
  - If endocarditis → vancomycin to treat MRSA, also antibiotic for 4–6 weeks.
        → Shorter if drainage is achieved.

- • Drainage
  - Either percutaneous, closed aspiration, or surgery.
  - Catheter placement vs. percutaneous aspiration → catheter placement is superior, 100% vs. 60%.
  - Small abscess with no biliary obstruction → IV antibiotic only
  - All abscesses, C/S + biopsy for malignancy.
  - Hepatic resection in some circumstances:
    1. Patient with inflammatory mass.
    2. Chronic biliary obstruction (multiple biliary drainages)

Amebic Liver Abscess

- Causative organism: Entamoeba histolytica.
- Worldwide, 10% are infected by E. histolytica.
- Entamoeba histolytica enters GIT by ingestion of mature cyst in fecal-contaminated vegetable → goes to stomach and small bowel and (colon → transferred to trophozoite) invades mucosa → ulcer → to Portal V to liver or lung or brain.
- Single or multiple (right lobe commonly).
- Contains central necrosis, thick reddish pus, like anchovy paste or chocolate sauce.

- Considered in patient who travelled to endemic area.
- Symptoms: RUQ pain, fever, and diarrhea (unusual).
- Leukocytosis, hepatomegaly, high LFT, and jaundice are unusual, but alkaline phosphatase is high.
- Patient has +ve fluorescent antibody test (most).
- CT: well-defined, low-density round lesion with enhanced wall, peripheral zone edema, and can have septation.

Treatment
- Flagyl, 750 mg IV Q8H for 7–10 days, successful in 95%.
- US or CT as follow-up.
- Aspiration is rarely needed.
- Abscess in left lobe → risk of rupture → pericarditis, so should be treated with aspiration.

Drainage
- Aspiration did not improve outcomes.
- Used for the following:
    1. No clinical response within 5–7 days of antibiotic.
    2. High risk of rupture.
- Surgery if hemorrhage, rupture, and erosion to adjacent or sepsis.

Outcomes
- Majority responds within 3 days.
- Factors predicting mortality:
    1. High bilirubin, 3.5
    2. Encephalopathy
    3. Large volume > 500 mL
    4. Albumin less than 2
    5. Multiple abscesses
- Radiological resolution takes 9 months.
- Follow-up imaging is advisable.

Fungal Liver Abscess
- High in immunocompromised, liver TPx, bone marrow TPx.
- Treatment: same principle of pyogenic abscess.
- Most common organism is candida.
- Treatment: Historically, amphotericin B, Now, caspofungin.

- Outcome: MR is 50%.

Hydatid Disease

- **Echinococcus Granulosus**
    - Infected by eating the viscera of sheep that contains hydatid cyst → scolices in the cyst adhere to small bowel of dogs and become adult taenia then shed 500 ova into the bowel → feces → to the grass and contaminate it, then grass with ova is ingested by intermediate host (sheep, cattle, pigs, human).
    - The ova has envelope dissolved by gastric juice → small bowel → portal vein → liver → adult cyst.
    - Few of the ova pass through liver → lung, spleen, brain, bone.
    - The disease is common in area with sheep where dogs have an access.
    - Mainly in right lobe.
    - It could be silent and found in autopsy.

Pathogenesis and Subtypes

- Types: cystic and alveolar
- Cystic is the most common (E. granulosis)
- Liver, 80%; lung, 20%.
- Pericyst, exocyst, endocyst, daughter cyst containing protoscolices.

Clinical Picture and Diagnosis

- 50% are asymptomatic.
- RUQ pain, fever, jaundice, PHTN, Budd-Chiari syndrome, secondary cyst infection.
- May rupture to biliary tree or peritoneum → biliary obstruction and anaphylaxis.
- E. multilocularis—no rupture nor anaphylaxis.
- CBC → eosinophilia.
- LFT, serum Ag test (previous gold standard).

Diagnosis
Laboratory

- ELISA for echinococcal antigen → +ve 85% of patient (immunoassay).

- If −ve, i.e., cyst, not leaked or no scolices or parasite, it is not viable.
- Alveolar disease → Em2Ag, 99% sensitivity.
- Eosinophilia in 30%.

Imaging

- Modified Gharbi classification (CE).
- CL: lesion is parasitic.
- CE1, CE2: active cyst.
- CE3: transitional zone.
- CE4, CE5: inactive cyst.
- Inactive → no treatment required; whereas active or transition, cyst should be treated.
- CT, MRI preferred.
- MRCP if cyst-biliary communication.

WHO-IWGE Classification	CL	CE1	CE2	CE3	CE4	CE5
US feature	Unilocular, round Cyst wall not visible	Unilocular Cyst wall visible Hydatid sand	Septated Honey-comb Rosette	Detached, floating Water lily sign	No daughter cyst Ball of wall	Thick, calcified Cone-shaped shadow
Medical treatment	Need diagnosis for treatment	Snowflake Yes	Yes	Yes	No	No
PAIR	-	Yes	Yes	Yes	No	No
Surgery	-	No	Yes	Yes	No	No

Treatment

- Treatment: prevent progression, complication and eradicate parasite.
- WHO-IWEG recommendation depends on image feature.

Medical Treatment

- Albendazole 10–15 mg/kg/day divided to 2 doses/day (best).
- Mebendazole, praziquantel can be used also.
- Benzimidazole is teratogenic, so contraindicated in pregnancy.

- Contraindicated in CLD, bone marrow suppression → hepatotoxicity, leukopenia, thrombocytopenia.
- Albendazole + praziquantel, 40 mg/kg/day, more effective than albendazole alone.
- Patient with < 5 cm, uncomplicated (CE1, CE3) → responds well to medical treatment.
- For large or complicated cyst, success rate is 30% → medical + percutaneous or operative.

Percutaneous Approach

- puncture, aspiration, injection, re-aspiration (PAIR)
- US-guided, transhepatic: puncture of cyst and avoid intraperitoneal spillage → aspiration → injection of scolicidal (20% hypertonic saline or 95% ethanol for 10–15 min) then reaspiration.
- Indication:
  - → Small (< 5 cm) unilocular CE1, CE3, accessible, inoperable (not fit for surgery), pregnant.
- Contraindication:
  - Complicated cyst with infection, rupture, biliary communication, or pulmonary.
  - → WHO recommends albendazole 4 hrs before PAIR and continue for 1 month after.
- Percutaneous drainage for large cyst > 10 cm left in place till output < 10 mL/day.
- Advantage: minimally invasive, low cost.
  Note: if biliary communication → post procedure fistula → sclerosing cholangitis.
- PAIR + medical treatment superior to surgery.

Surgical Treatment

- WHO guideline:
  For large complicated (infection), communication with biliary tree, superficial, multiple daughter cysts.
- Conservative and radical treatment.
- Conservative: partial or subtotal resection of cyst (pericyst) left behind, marsupialization.

- Radical: entire cyst with pericyst.
- Pericystectomy, segment or lobe resection.
- Both can be done laparoscopy or open.
- Albendazole 1 day preoperative and 1 month post-op.

- **Laparoscopy**
    - For easy access such as segment 3, 4b, 5, 6 → place sponge (soaked) with scolicidal → puncture + aspiration, then resection → fill space with omentum + drain.
    - Disadvantage: no access for deep cyst such posterosuperior segment.
    - Meta-analysis → partial cystectomy or complete pericystectomy or segment resection → recurrence, 1%.

- **Open**
    - Recommended for large multiloculated, complicated, posterosuperior segment, biliary fistula.
    - Need pre-operative: MRCP.
    - Intra-operative: H_2O_2 in cavity is helpful in identifying biliary communication.
    - If it is closed primarily, if large bilioenteric anastomosis (rare) or if bile leak post-operative → ERCP → pericystectomy or liver resection.
    - Liver resection can range from wedge to formal resection → if patient fails medical or percutaneous, conservative surgery → radical resection.
    - Liver TPx if concomitant liver disease or with complications such as Budd-Chiari syndrome or PHTN.

- **Outcomes**
    - PAIR: Mortality, 8%–13% Morbidity, 0.1% Surgery: Mortality, 1%–4% Morbidity, 25%–66%

- Recurrence   2% with radial resection

                        10% with percutaneous and conservative surgery
- Follow-up WHO guidelines:

        CBC, LFT every 3–6 months.

- **Echinococcus Multilocularis (Alveolar)**
  - Same mode of infection.
  - Infection to lung is common (alveolar), i.e., alveolar echinococcosis (AE).
  - CT: hypoechogenicity and hyperechogenicity, irregular border, and central necrosis.
  - For AE, PCR is needed to identify E. multilocularis.
  - More aggressive, infiltrative → biliary → Budd-Shiari syndrome, liver failure.
    → PNM stage:

P	Extension of parasite
N	Involvement of adjacent organ
M	Metastasis (extrahepatic)

  - Percutaneous is not an option, and surgery is mandatory → surgical resection.
  - Albendazole for 2 years post-operative.
  - Treatment: albendazole.
  - This procedure is a more generalized reaction → so it requires surgery.
  - CT, MRI is recommended every 1–2 years.

Ascariasis

- Far East, India, South Africa.
- Lodge in CBD → bile duct obstruction → cholangitis, also stone formation.
- US, ERCP, filling defect (linear).
- Occasionally from duodenum to biliary.
- Treatment piperazine citrate, albendazole + endoscopic extraction of worm.
- Surgery if worm is not removed by ERCP.

Schistosomiasis

- 200 million in 74 countries.

- Ova goes from bowel to liver.
- Enters skin during contact with infected water.
- Portal fibrosis.
- Three stages of symptom:
    1. Itching in skin
    2. Fever, urticaria, eosinophilia
    3. Hepatic fibrosis and Portal HTH → hepatic shrinkage and splenomegaly
- Serology → postexposure.
- AST, ALT, AP, and low albumin.
- Treatment: praziquantel, 40–75 mg/kg single dose.
- GI bleeding by endoscopy, if refractory with portal HTN → distal splenorenal shunt or gastric devascularization and splenectomy.

Viral Hepatitis
Hepatitis A, B, C, E
- Hepatitis A
    - RNA virus.
    - Self-limited, rarely → fulminant hepatic failure.
    - RUQ pain, nausea and vomiting, anorexia, malaise, jaundice, and hepatomegaly.
    - Treatment: suppression, but if → fulminant hepatic failure → liver TPx.

- Hepatitis B
    - DNA virus.
    - Complication: chronic liver disease, cirrhosis; in USA, 0. 27% of HCC, but in third world, 30%–55% of HCC.
    - If chronic HBV, treatment → viral suppression to prevent complication, antiviral interferon, tenofovir, nucleoside (well tolerated).

- Hepatitis C
    - Acute 2–26 weeks after exposure (icteric phase).
    - Diagnosis: presence of HCV RNA and anti-HCV antibody.
    - PCR can detect it after days/weeks expose, while antibody will appear 2–6 months.
    - If not cleared in acute, 1 dose of interferon.

- Chronic → cirrhosis, HCE.
- Need TPx.
- Treatment: triple therapy—interferon, ribavirin, and protease.

▪ Hepatitis E

Benign Liver Lesion
Hemangioma
- Most common benign tumor of liver.
- 2%–20% of population.
- Four times more in female.
- In ages 30s–50s.
- 50% have multifocal lesion.
- Well-defined, soft dark lesion, ranging from 1 cm to large, if > 5 cm → giant → indication for resection.
- Microscopic: single layer of endothelium lining with dilated cavernous vascular channel surrounded by thin connective tissue, calcification, and fibrosis.

- **Etiology**
  - Congenital or acquired.
  - Tumor regression after treatment with anti-VEGF antibody.
  - Hormonal predisposition → four time more in female → also estrogen receptor seen in hemangioma surface and ↑ rate of growth while on steroid or OCP.

- **Clinical Picture**
  - 50%–90% are asymptomatic, incidentally during US or CT.
  - Pain is secondary to hemangioma because of thrombosis or stretching of Glisson's capsule.
  - RUQ pain, nausea, early satiety → also right shoulder pain → irritation of diaphragm.
  - Compression: gastric outlet obstructive jaundice.
  - Large hemangioma → AV shunt → CHF.
  - Rupture is less than 5% but life-threatening → ⅓ death.
  - DIC, thrombocytopenia → trapped platelet and trigger by small procedure → mortality, 30%.

- **Diagnosis**
  - US, CT, MRI.
  - US → well-defined, hyperechoic, homogenous mass.
  - CT: triphasic contrast, sensitivity is 90% → peripheral enhancement on arterial phase, central filling on portal (venous) phase, and retention of contrast on delayed phase.
    - → Thrombosed hemangioma may mimic malignancy NET with liver metastasis
    - → so further MRI imaging; sensitivity is 90% and specificity is 95% → light bubble sign can be differentiated from metastasis.
  - Percutaneous biopsy is contraindicated.
  - If diagnosis is still unclear → angiography or CT with technetium-labeled RBCs.
  - CBC is normal except in Kasabach-Merritt syndrome → fibrinolysis → low platelet and coagulopathy.
  - Obstruction of biliary, ALP, and bilirubin.
  - Tumor marker CA 19-9, CEA, αFP, unusually mild elevation.

- **Management**
  - Most lesions remain stable, 10%–15% regression.
  - Retrospective study: operative vs. conservative = equal.
  - Size is not one of the criteria for resection even if pregnant or on OCP as long as asymptomatic.
  - Most common indication of resection·is symptomatic hemangioma after exclusion of other cause of pain.
  - Complication is an indication of an intervention, e.g., rupture → resuscitation and angiography then interval resection.
  - If failed angiography → emergent resection.
  - Kasabach-Merritt syndrome warrants emergent surgical resection if failed medical treatment (interferon), embolization is an option also.
  - Rapidly enlarged hemangioma, ↑ malignancy risk → laparoscopic or open resection.

Non-operative Therapy

- For patient with spontaneous or traumatic rupture or patient refuses surgery.
  - → Embolization, RFA, ethanol ablation, and hepatic radiotherapy.
- Elective embolization in symptomatic patient can be a transient response, but recurrence of symptom is usually common.
- Non-operative is also used in pediatrics, 10% of liver lesion in pediatrics.
  - → Symptom of pediatric hemangioma → mortality, 70%.
  - → First line is medical treatment with prednisolone or b-blockers (propranolol).
  - → Embolization.
  - → Surgery for severe symptom or rupture.

Surgical Approach and Technique

- Enucleation or resection or liver resection (anatomic and nonanatomic).
  - → Enucleation is the most common used approach, as well as ↑ success rate.
- Blood supply of hemangioma comes from hepatic artery.
  - → Large lesion may require ligation of ipsilateral lateral hepatic artery.
  - → Pringle maneuver, clamp for less than 30 mintues and unclamping 5 min with gentle pressure on hemangioma during 5 mintues.
- Dissection by incision of Glisson's capsule and identification of pseudocapsule → IOUS may be useful.
- Dissection by ultrasonic, blunt, energy device, stapler.
- Non-anatomic resection for small peripheral location → especially in segment II, III.
- For deeper → standard liver resection.
- Laparoscopy can be used to all situations.
- Tumor in the right side is adjacent to major intrahepatic vessels.
- TPx for Kasabach-Merritt syndrome (rare).

- **Prognosis**
  - MRI to reduce radiation exposure.
  - MRI 3 months after diagnosis with repeat MRI in 3–6 months if lesion is atypical or suspected malignancy.

→ If the lesion is stable in first imaging in follow-up →
annual imaging is recommended with more interval
follow-up if unchanged.

- In general, treating a patient with hemangioma with
surgery → improves quality of life and satisfaction.

Adenoma

- Benign, solid, commonly in premenopausal patients older than
30, solitary can be multiple.
- OCP is a risk factor.
- Grossly: well-circumscribed, soft tan (light brown) lesion with or
without capsule.
- Microscopic: sheet of hepatocyte containing glycogen and lipid
with no Kupffer cells and bile ductule.
- Risk of rupture and intraperitoneal bleeding.
- Risk of malignancy transformation to HCC, so surgical resection
is recommended.
- Anywhere but common in right side.
- only 4.2% is > 5 cm.
- AFP is helpful to distinguish from HCC.
- Divided to four subtypes.
  Hepatocyte nuclear factor-1α is the commonest and characterized
  by noninflammatory infiltrate.

- **Presentation**
  - Young female, 20s–40s.
  - ↑ by use of OCP.
  - RUQ pain or epigastric related to rupture and
  hemorrhage and rarely causes hypovolemic shock.

- **Image**
  - CT: sharply defined border can be confused with metastasis.
    Arterial phase: hypervascular enhancement.
    Venous phase: hypodense or isodense.
  - MRI: hypertense on T1.

- **Management**
  - Initially if < 5 cm → stop OCP and anabolic steroid →
  regress.

- For patient with no history of OCP → and > 5 cm or symptomatic → surgical resection (risk of bleeding from rupture and malignancy).
- Resection should be with −ve margin.
- Formal resection vs. parenchymal sparing, depending on suspected malignancy.
- Intraoperative ultrasound (IOUS) is useful.
- Laparoscopy may be possible.
- RFA for small or multiple adenomas.
- If life-threatening hemorrhage → angioembolization; if not possible, i.e., unstable or not available → laparotomy (laparoscopy is not recommended here).
- Mortality rate from hemorrhage is 5%–10%.
- Pringle maneuver, hemostatic agent, if cannot be controlled → formal resection.

Focal Nodular Hyperplasia (FNH)
- **Pathogenesis**
  - Second most common after hemangioma.
  - Common with female of childbearing age and usually not related to OCP.
  - No risk of malignancy or hemorrhage or rupture.
  - Histopathology: fibrous scar of vessels found in center.
  - 20% atypical (absence of central scarring).
  - Single, mostly < 5 cm.

- **Presentation**
  - Female, 20s–50s.
  - Incidental.

- **Imaging**
  - CT biphasic, circumscribed with central scar, homogenous enhancement with hyperintense on arterial phase. Isointense on venous phase, well-circumscribed with central scar.
  - Fibrous septation extending from central scar.
  - MRI hypointense T1 and hyperintense in T2.

- **Management**
    - Conservative, never perform surgery.
    - Reassurance, observation.
    - If atypical and symptomatic → follow up, surgery is not recommended; with pain or (atypical central scar) → should be distinguished from fibrolamellar HCC (central scar on CT).
    - No risk of bleeding or malignancy.
    - Open or laparoscopic resection.
    - Formal resection may be needed with suspicious lesions.

Bile Duct Hamartomas
- Small white lesions of 2–4 mm (incidental).
- Visualized during laparotomy.
- Firm, smooth, white yellow.
- Cannot be distinguished from malignancy → biopsy.

Type	US	CT	MRI
Hemangioma	Well demarcated Hyperechoic	Asymmetric peripheral enhancement, gradual central on delayed phase	T1: hypo T2: hyper
Adenoma	Well demarcated Hypo- or hyperechoic mass	Well encapsulated Iso or hypo in noncontrast Heterogeneity because of hemorrhage or necrosis	T1 and T2 Iso, hypointense
FNH	Hypo, hyper, iso Central scar	Well circumscribed Hyperintense or arterial iso on venous Central scar on venous phase	T1: iso or hypo T1: hyper with central scar Hyperintense

Malignant Liver Tumor

- Primary or secondary (metastasis) → 2 ry is the most common than 1 ry.
- Primary originates from hepatocytes (HCC), if arising from bile duct → cholangiocarcinoma.
- 60% of colorectal cancer will develop liver metastasis.
- In one study, HCC, 47%; CRC metastasis, 17%; cholangiocarcinoma, 11%; NET, 7%; others, 18%.
- Surgical resection is mainstay of treatment.
- Lesion is considered resectable for the following conditions:
    1. −ve margin can be obtained.
    2. Leaving adequate amount of functioning liver.
    3. Intact hepatic artery and venous (PV).
    4. Biliary drainage.
- If unresectable → Ablation by → alcohol, thermal, RFA, cryoablation, microwave embolization and EBR.
- RFA and microwave are the most successful methods.
- Irreversible electroporation: thermal ablation for tumor adjacent to vascular structure (no effect on vascular).
- Embolization: TAE, TACE, or radioembolization.

Hepatocellular Carcinoma (HCC)

- Fifth most common tumor.
- Third most common cause of death.
- Most common primary tumor.
- Risk factor: hepatitis B or C, alcoholic cirrhosis, hemochromatosis, and NASH.
- In cirrhotic patient, annually risk of HCC transformation is 2%–6%.
- In hepatitis C, HCC developed after cirrhosis while hepatitis B, HCC developed before cirrhosis.
- Variants of HCC: clear type HCC, fibrolamellar HCC, combined hepatocellular cholangiocarcinoma, sclerosing HCC.
- CT finding: arterial phase → hypervascular and hypodense in delayed phase.
- MRI is variable on T1 but hyperintense on T2.
- Usually, HCC invades PV → thrombosis is diagnostic.

Treatment

- Most widely used treatment is resection, TACE, ablation.
- If HCC, no cirrhosis → resection (Tx of choice).

- Milan criteria for liver TPx with HCC:
  o One lesion smaller than 5 cm; *alternatively*, up to 3 lesions, each smaller than 3 cm.
  o No extrahepatic manifestations.
  o No evidence of gross vascular invasion.
- Usually, major resection is reserved to patient with good liver reserve or child A with no evidence of PHTN.
- Tumor size is not a predictor for survival, as well as solitary lesion.
- Recent randomized trial: ↑ SR in 2 cm −ve margin vs. 1 cm.
- Anatomic resection increases SR.
- Thermal ablation for < 3 cm lesion = surgery resection.
- Ablation to tumor adjacent to major vascular structure > 4 cm should be avoided.
- Cirrhotic patient → Liver TPx → can address both HCC and CLD → but it's limited.
- If child A has cirrhosis with preserved liver function → resection, and if resection is not possible (poor function) → liver TPx.
- Combination of TACE + RFA ↑ SR vs. TACE alone.
- Responds to TACE as high as 80% but should repeat it within 3–6 months.
  → Total bilirubin > 3 mg/dL is contraindicated to this treatment.
  → PV thrombosis is relatively contraindicated. These patients can be treated with radioembolization or EBR.
- Surgical resection and Liver TPx are contraindicated when extrahepatic disease is present.
- MR is 5%, and SR is 30%–60%, 5 years.
- Recurrence is 30% and usually with patient with cirrhosis.
- Barcelona—clinical liver CA ground refined HCC management, see algorithm:

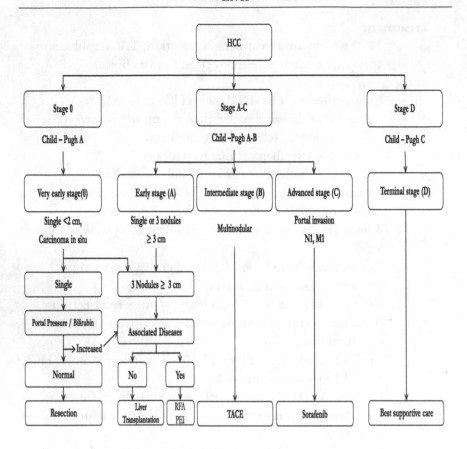

Cholangiocarcinoma

- Second most common primary tumor of the liver
- It is adenocarcinoma.
- classified into the following:
    1. Peripheral (intrahepatic) liver mass.
    2. Central (extrahepatic), subclassified into:
        - Distal.
        - Proximal (hilar), i.e., Klatskin tumor—originated from duct wall at hepatic duct confluence → presented with obstructive jaundice.

- Risk factors: Sclerosing cholangitis, 8%–20%
                    Choledochal cyst, 3%–28%
                    And cirrhosis.

- ## Intrahepatic Cholangiocarcinoma (ICC)(Peripheral)

  ### Presentation and Pre-operative Evaluation
  - Often incidentally during image.
  - Types:
    1. Mass forming
    2. Periductal infiltrate (worst prognosis)
    3. Intraductal
  - Nonspecific symptoms: abdominal pain, fatigue, weight loss.
  - Physical examination: unremarkable, jaundice in advanced disease.
  - Laboratory: often mildly high AFP, CEA, CA 19-9, chromogranin A.
  - CT: low attenuation, peripheral enhancement, better liver protocol MRI.
  - Diagnosis by biopsy, if no source, work up for primary tumor with mammogram, upper & lower scope or PET.
  - Liver biopsy for patient, not going for surgery, to guide chemotherapy.
  - FLR estimated by CT volumetry at least 25%, if cirrhotic patient, 40%–50%.
  - Child score, MELD can be used.

  - Criteria for unresectability:
    1. Locally advanced, involve in-out flow bilaterally.
    2. Multiple bilateral
    3. Distant metastasis
    4. Perihepatic LNs, PHTN → non-operative.

  ### Staging
T1s	CA in situ (intraductal)
T1	Solitary tumor with no vascular invasion
T2a	Solitary tumor with vascular invasion
T2b	Multiple tumors with or without vascular invasion
T3	Tumor perforating visceral peritoneum
T4	Tumor with periductal invasion
N0	No LNs
N1	Regional LNs present
M	Metastasis

Management
- **Resection**
  - Surgical resection is the only curable option.
  - Range from wedge resection for small lesion to formal anatomic resection, e.g., extended hepatectomy.
  - ICC can associated with carcinomatosis → should start with diagnostic laparoscopy.
  - If FLR is small → PV embolization at the side of the tumor → contralateral hyperplasia, to increase FLR.
  - With major liver resection, combined PV, IVC resection, and reconstruction.
  - Hilar LNs should be dissected → because 30% is +ve.
  - 5 years, SR is 40%–60%.
  - +ve margin → worst prognosis → adjuvant chemoradiotherapy.
  - Because of high incidence of locoregional metastasis (LNs) → neo-adjuvant chemoradiation is given.
  - Steps:
    - → Open or MIS.
    - → division of the triangular ligament to mobilize the liver.
    - → IOUS to assess the liver, removed gallbladder.
    - → Inflow controlled in the hilar of liver.
    - → HV outflow controlled.
    - → Ramel clamp using for Pringle maneuver, 15 min/5 min off.
    - → Parenchyma divided high-energy technique, stapler, or other techniques.

- **Other Treatment**
  - Adjuvant chemotherapy in R0 and high risk.
  - If R1 (+ve microscopic) or +ve LNs → chemoradiation.
  - Usually, dismal result and mandate liver TPx.
  - 5 years SR in patient who underwent autologous liver TPx is 70%.
  - Presence of extrahepatic disease including LNs and porta hepatis is contraindicated for resection.
  - R2 (macroscopic) → managed as unresectable disease.

- Unresectable disease → EBR, TACE, TARE or ablation (RFA, microwave), embolization.
  - PDT photodynamic therapy can be used.

- **Central Cholangiocarcinoma**
  - Distal + proximal: to be discussed in biliry chapter.

  Metastatic Colorectal CA
  - CRC third most common of liver lesion.
  - 50%–60% with colon CA will develop liver metastasis during lifetime.
  - Predictor of poor outcome:
    1. +ve LNS
    2. Disease-free interval < 12 months
    3. More than 1 tumor
    4. Tumor > 5 cm
    5. CEA > 200 ng/mL
  - Liver resection of metastasis fewer than 4 nodules, should consider future liver remnant (FLR).
  - 10 years, SR with metastasis > 4 nodules is 29%, and if solitary nodules, 32%.
  - Aggressive strategy, chemotherapy (HIPEC), improve outcome.
  - Approach is neo-adjuvant chemotherapy, portal vein embolization, two-stage hepatectomy.
  - Surgical resection is the mainstay.
  - Width of −ve margin does not ‾ recurrence.
  - In patient with CRC with single live metastasis → resection of the primary tumor + liver metastasis can be resected at the same time.
  - Major liver resection with complex procedure such pelvic exenteration, can address liver lesion first or after CRC resection (staged)
    - → Liver first is an attractive option, but most prefer primary tumor resection first.
  - Pre-operative chemotherapy is administered to assess response.
    - → Irinotecan steatohepatitis

> → Oxaliplatin sinusoidal congestion, usually small lesion < 2 cm disappears with chemotherapy → but if not resected surgically → recurrence is 80%.

- Need multidisciplinary approach (tumor board).
- Prognostic factor: size of tumor, extrahepatic disease, and nodal status of primary tumor.

Neuroendocrine Tumors

- Hepatic metastasis.
- Many advocate debulking and aggressive surgery to control symptom.
- SR 5, 10 years after resection is 61%, 35% respectively.
- Major hepatectomy → recurrence is 84% at 5 years.
- There is staged resection for left hepatectomy:
- First, left PV embolization, after 8 weeks → i.e., hypertrophy of right side → left hepatectomy → SR is 94%, 79%, and disease-free, 50%–85%.
- Systemic therapy is not effective, so use any modality RFA, microwave ablation, intra-arterial chemoembolization, or radioembolization.
- Some center performed outologus liver TPx.

Pre-operative Assessment

- Child-Turcotte-Pugh scoring.
- MR is 5%, 30%, 80% in Child A, B, C, respectively.
- Total bilirubin, albumin, prothrombin time (INR), ascites, and encephalopathy.
- PHTN: thrombocytopenia, splenomegaly, and esophageal varices.
- CT, MRI to look for location, relation to vasculature and biliary tree.
- FLR is estimated to decrease post-operative liver failure.
  - → For healthy patient, FLR must be > 20%.
  - → Patient on chemotherapy, > 30%.
  - → Cirrhosis, > 40%.
- Volumetry is calculated with 3D CT-MRI.
  - → Alternately calculated with body weight or body surface area, i.e., total liver volume in cm^3 = (794.41 + 1,267.28 × body surface are in m^2).

- Patient with insufficient FLR volume should undergo PV embolization of the branch planned for resection to induce growth to contralateral side → repeat volumetry after 4 weeks of PV embolization.

- **Hepatic Malignancy Resection vs. TPx**
    - Only 20%–30% are candidates for surgical therapy.
    - Multidisciplinary approach.
    - Assessment, history, physical examination, CBC, serology.
    - CTP or MELD.
    - CTP is better to predict postoperative mortality.
    - MELD > 9 benefits from TPx, not resection.
    - Use Barcelona and Milan criteria for appropriate management.
    - HCV, 1.5% chance to have CA.
    - HBV, 0.2% chance to have CA.
    - Primary biliary cirrhosis, hemochromatosis.

- **Screening**
    - AFP and US → no longer used, but AFP remains an important tool in tending response to treatment and surveillance.
    - Prothrombin induced by vitamin K absence-II (PIVKA-II). → Most importantly, sensitivity and specificity is 100%
    - AFP: sensitivity and specificity is 44%, 73%
    - CT: sensitivity and specificity is 81%–93%
    - MRI: sensitivity and specificity is 91%–95%

    Treatment Option for Liver CA
    1. Hepatic resection
    2. Liver transplant
    3. Ablation RFA, ethanol, cryoablation, microwave.
    4. Regional liver therapies: chemoembolization, arterial embolization, internal radiation
    5. External beam radiation: stereotactic radiosurgery
    6. Systemic chemotherapy
    7. Combined multimodality
    - Need multidisciplinary approach (tumor board).
    - CT, MRI Q3–4M in first year after diagnosis to observe response, progression, recurrence.

- **Radiofrequency Ablation (RFA)**
  - No pain or CNS excitation.
  - Recurrence is four times than resection.
  - No difference between RFA with resection and resection alone.

- **Ethanol Ablation and Cryosurgery, Microwave Ablation**
  - Ethanol is effective in small HCC (percutaneous) bridge to OLTPx.
  - Microwave: unresctable tumor to produce coagulation necrosis.
  - Local recurrence after ablation is 2.7% and locoregional, 43%.

- **Chemoembolization**
  - Hepatic artery pump chemoperfusion.
  - Chemotherapy + embolization through hepatic artery.
  - SR is 57.26%, 1–3 years.
  - Complications of TACE → liver dysfunction, liver failure.

Hepatic Resection Surgical Technique
- **Technique and Device for Dividing Liver Parenchyma**
  - Blunt fracture and clip.
  - Monopolar cautery (Bovie).
  - Bipolar.
  - Argan beam coagulation.
  - CUSA ultrasonic dissector.
  - Hydro-jet, water-jet dissector.
  - Harmonic scalpel.
  - Ligasure.

- **Steps Common to All Open Major Hepatic Resections**
  - Make the skin incision—right subcostal with or without a partial or complete left subcostal extension.
  - Open and explore the abdomen, and place a fixed table retractor (e.g., Thompson or Bookwalter).
  - Examine the liver, perform liver ultrasound.
  - Take down the round and falciform ligaments, and expose the anterior surface of the hepatic veins.
  - For a left hepatectomy, divide the left triangular ligament; for a right hepatectomy, mobilize the right lobe from the right coronary and triangular ligaments.
  - Open the gastrohepatic ligament, palpate the porta hepatis.
  - Perform a cholecystectomy.

Right Hepatic Lobectomy (Right Hepatectomy or Hemihepatectomy)
- Mobilize the liver from the anterior aspect of the IVC in "piggyback" fashion.
- ligate the short hepatic veins up to the right hepatic vein.
- ligate and divide the right hepatic artery.
- Expose the portal vein, identifying its right and left branches.
- Divide the right portal vein.
- Repeat ultrasound and confirm the transection plane.
- Cauterize approximately 1 cm into the liver parenchyma, then switch to a hydro-jet dissection device in combination with Bovie electrocautery and suture ligation.
- During division, identification, control, ligation, and transection of the right hepatic ducts.
- place a figure-of-eight ligating vascular suture if bleeding is encountered.
- Ensure hemostasis of the transected liver edge with an argon beam coagulator and suture ligation.
- Inspect the transection surface for bile leaks. These should be clipped or suture ligated.
- Inspect the IVC and right retroperitoneal space for hemostasis.
- Jackson-Pratt drain in the right subphrenic space and close the abdomen.

Pringle and Ischemic Pre-condition
- Pringle described clamping of portal triad to cease and minimize the bleeding in trauma.
- Liver can tolerate 1 hr of warm ischemia.
- But Pringle maneuver occlusion, 15 min and 5 min off.
- Ischemic precondition: brief interruption of blood flow to organ followed by short reperfusion.

Preoperative PV Embolization
- PV embolization induces → thrombosis of tumor and ipsilat atrophy and hypertrophy of centra lateral lobe.
- PVE: compensatory hypertrophy.
- Normally, 25%–30% is adequate.

Gallbladder and Biliary System

Anatomy

- Pear-shaped sac, 7–10 cm long, capacity is 30–50 mL, when distended, increase to 300 mL.
- Located in gallbladder fossa, a line from it and IVC—divides the liver to right and left lobe.
- Composed of fundus, body, infundibulum (Hartmann's pouch), and neck.
- Usually covered with peritoneum and rarely embedded in liver.
- Lined by single folded tall columnar epithelium containing fat and cholesterol.
- Mucus secreted from tubulo-alveolar gland in neck and infundibulum.
- Layers: mucosa, muscolusa (longitudinal circular and oblique fibrous), serosa.
- No muscularis mucosa nor submucosa.
- Perimuscular layer contains serosa: connective tissue, Nerves, V, LNs.
- Blood supply: cystic artery from hepatic artery, 90%.
- Calot's Δ: cystic artery runs through it, bonded by cyst duct, CHD, and liver margin. When artery reaches neck → divided to anterior and posterior.
- Venous return to small veins in liver and rarely cystic vein to portal vein.
- LNs is in the neck of gallbladder (laund, Calot) overlies insertion of cystic artery.
- NS: vague and sympathetic through celiac plexus (T8, T9).

Bile Duct

- Extrahepatic bile ducts consist of right, left hepatic ducts joins to form CHD, when cystic duct join CHD → CBD.
- Enter 2nd part of the Duodenum through muscular structure (sphincter of Oddi).
- Left hepatic duct is longer and more distendable.
- CHD is 1–4 cm in length and 4 mm in diameter, lies in front of Portal vein and to the right of hepatic artery.

- Cystic duct is variable: short, long or absent → near to neck → spiral valve of Heister → no valvular function but makes cannulation difficult.
- CBD is 7–10 cm and 5–10 mm in diameter.
- Upper ⅓ (supraduodenal) passes in hepatoduodenal ligament to the right of hepatic artery and anterior to PV.
- Middle ⅓ (retroduodenal) curves behind of D1 lateral to PV and hepatic artery.
- Lower ⅓ (pancreatic portion) curves behind head of pancreas in groove and enters D2, before that, it joins pancreatic duct 1–2 cm before opening of ampulla of Vater.
- 10 cm distal to the pylorus, 70% join outside of duodenum, 20% join within duodenum, 10% separate opening.
- Sphincter of Oddi is a thick, smooth circular muscle.
- Extrahepatic ducts lined by columnar mucosa then smooth muscle cells → no distinct muscle layer.
- Arterial supply: GDA and right hepatic artery.

Anomalies
- Classic description in ⅓ of patient.
- Abnormal position, e.g., intrahepatic (embedded).
- Absence is rare, 0.03%.
- Duplication with two separate cavities is 1:4,000, either separate duct or merge together.
- Intrahepatic gallbladder increases incidence of gallbladder stone.
- Small ducts of Luschka drain directly from liver to body of gallbladder → bile leak (biloma).
- Accessory right hepatic duct, 5%.
- Anomaly of right hepatic duct and cystic artery, 50%.
- Two right hepatic—one from hepatic artery and the other from SMA.
- Cystic artery from left hepatic, 90%.
- → 20% right hepatic from SMA.
- → 10% from left hepatic, common hepatic GDA, SMA.

467

Physiology

- Bile: 500–1,000 mL/day.
- Neurohormonal, chemical stimuli to increase or decrease the bile flow such Vagus increases bile flow whereas splanchnic nerves lowers it.
- HCl and fatty acid increase it.
- Bile composition and metabolism (see liver).
- The pH of hepatic bile is neutral or slightly alkaline; diet like protein makes it more acidic.
- Bile salt synthesized in liver from cholesterol → conjugated there with taurin and glycin → bile acid.
- 95% of bile acid reabsorbed and return to Portal vein (enteropehatic circulation), 5% in stool and urine.
- Cholesterol and phospholipid synthesized in liver.
- The color of bile because bile pigment which is breakdown of Hb, present in bile ten times than serum.

Gallbladder Function

- Absorption and Secretion
  - In fasting → storage of bile → mucosa absorbs Na, Cl, and water and concentrate it ten times.
  - Gradual relaxation to lower the pressure.
  - Epithelial cells secrete glycoprotein and H^+ ions.
  - Mucosal glands in infundibulum and neck secrete mucus to protect mucosa from bile, this mucus makes white bile in obstructive condition.
  - H^+ acidification → lower pH of gallbladder bile → prevents precipitation as Ca^{++} salt.

- Motor Activity
  - Gallbladder filling by tonic contraction of sphincter of Oddi (pressure gradient).
  - During fasting → phase II interdigestive MMC and empty in small volume. This process is mediated by motilin.
  - In response to meal, CCK released from duodenal mucosa, relaxation of sphincter of Oddi and contraction of gallbladder.
  - With eating, emptying 50%–70% within 30–40 min, then 60–90 min to refill.

- Defect in motor activity plays a role in cholesterol nucleation and gallbladder stone formation.

- Neurohormonal Regulation
  - Atropine relaxes gallbladder (sympathomimetic) and parasympathomimetic contracts it.
  - CCK ↑ in blood in response by acid, fat, amino acid.
    - CCK half-life is 2–3 min, metabolized in liver and kidney.
    - CCK acts on smooth muscle.
    - In vagotomy the response to CCK is decreased.
  - VIP and somatostatin ↓ contraction, i.e., gallbladder stasis.

Sphincter of Oddi

- Regulates bile and pancreatic secretion and prevents regurgitation of duodenal content.
- 4–6 mm in length.
- Resting pressure is 13 mmHg.
- Four contractions/min in manometry, 12–140 mmHg.
- Regulated by interstitial cells of Cajal.

Diagnostic Study

- Blood Test
  - CBC.
  - LFT, bilirubin (indirect, direct), ALP, GGT.

- US
  - Initial investigation.
  - Sensitivity and specificity > 90%.
  - Stone showed with acoustic shadow.
  - Polyps, calcification and reflect shadows.
  - Thickness gallbladder wall.
  - Visualization of biliary tree.
  - Periampullary region is difficult to be assessed.

- Oral Cholecystography
  - Previously was the procedure of choice.
  - Now, replaced by US.

- Admistration of oral radiopaque and excreted by liver into biliary tree.
- No value if malabsortption, vomiting, obstructive jaundice, and liver faliure

- HIDA Scan
  - Biliary scintigraphy, technetium-99m injected IV → cleared by Kupffer cells in liver to the bile.
  - Uptake in 10 min and seen in gallbladder, duodenum within 60 min.
  - Primary use → acute cholecystitis appears as non-visualizing gallbladder and fills biliary and duodenum.
  - Sensitivity and specificity is 95%.
  - False +ve in stasis, critically ill, TPN.
  - Filling of gallbladder and CBD with delayed or absent duodenal filling → obstruction at ampulla.
  - Localize the are of leak post-operatively.
  - Also used to diagnose biliary dyskinesia (chronic cholecystitis).

- CT
  - Inferior to US for gallbladder stone.
  - Test of choice to evaluate gallbladder CA and nearby structure.
  - Staging and vascular involvement.

- Percutaneous Transhepatic Cholangiography (PTC) and Percutaneous Biliary Drainage (PBD)
  - Intrahepatic duct accessed percutaneousely.
  - Catherization and wire cholangiography → intervention.
  - Identify bile duct stricture and tumor.
  - Complications: bleeding, cholangitis, bile leak.
  - Can keep catheter for drainage.

- MRI
  - T2 with or without contrast.
  - Sensitivity, 95%; specificity, 89%.
  - MRCP: diagnose biliary and pancreatic pathology.
  - Reserved ERCP for therapeutic purposes.

- ERCP
  - CBD cannulation: cholangiogram by fluoroscopy.
  - Required IV sedation.
  - Diagnostic and therapeutic.
  - Once showed ductal stone → sphincterotomy and stone extraction +/− stent.
  - Success rate is 90%.
  - Complications: pancreatitis, cholangitis (5%).

- EUS
  - Noninvasive.
  - Evaluation of tumor and resectability.
  - There is channel for biopsy.
  - Less sensitive than ERCP.
  - Cannulation of sphincter is not necessary.

Pathology
Gallstone Disease
Prevalence
  - In autopsy, 11%–36%.
  - Differ for age, gender, and ethnicity.
  - Etiology: obesity, pregnancy, dietary factor, CD, terminal ileum resection, gastric surgery, bariatric surgery, hereditary spherocytosis, SCD, thalassemia, OCP, TPN.
  - Women: Men = 3:1.
  - First-degree relative, ↑ twofold greater prevalence.

Natural History
  - Mostly asymptomatic.
  - Symptoms: biliary colic and complications.
  - Complications: acute cholecystitis, mucocele, empyema, CBD stone, ± cholangitis, gallstone pancreatitis, fistula to CBD, duodenum and small bowel, gallstone ileus, gallbladder CA.
  - Diagnosis: incidentally by US.
  - 3% of asymptomatic → become symptomatic per year.
  - 20% of gallstone is symptomatic, 1%–4% biliary complication.

- Gallstone size < 5 mm → biliary pancreatitis.
  > 3 cm → acute cholecystitis, CA
- Once symptomatic → recurrent attack.
- Complication: 3%–5% of symptomatic gall stone/year.
- Over 20 years, ⅔ of asymptomatic remain symptom-free.

Gallstone Formation
- It's either 80% cholesterol or 15%–20% pigmented (black and brown).

- Cholesterol Stone
  - Pure cholesterol, uncommon < 10%, usually a single large stone.
  - Most other cholesterol stones contain bile pigment and Ca^{++} but always cholesterol > 70% of weight.
  - Multiple, maybe hard and faceted, or irregular mulberry shape and soft.
  - Color is from white yellowish to brown.
  - Primary event of formation → oversaturation of bile with cholesterol.
  - Cholesterol solubility depends on concentration of bile salt, lecithin.
  - Cholesterol secreted in the bile as cholesterol phospholipid vesicles.
  - Vesicles will be enriched with cholesterol → nucleated cholesterol crystal.

- Pigment Stone
  - Contain < 20% cholesterol and are dark because of presence of Ca^{++} bilirubinate.
  - Black or brown pigment stones have little in common and should be considered as separate entities.
    - A. Black pigment is small, brittle, black, speculated to be supersaturated of calcium bilirubinate.

Mostly from hemolytic anemia and cirrhosis and from unconjugated bilirubin and found in gallbladder like cholesterol type.

A. Brown stone < 1 cm, brownish yellow, soft, mushy, found in gallbladder and ducts.

Usually secondary to bacterial infection.

Bacteria such as E. coli secretes β-glucuronidase that clears bilirubin glucuronide to produce insoluble unconjugated bilirubin. Participitate with Ca^{++} and bacterial dead body → stone → typically found in biliary tree.

Indication of Prophylactic Cholecystectomy

1. Old age with DM.
2. For the one who will be isolated from medical care.
3. Patient with gallbladder CA.
4. Calcification and porcelain gallbladder.
5. Polyps more than 2–3.
6. Women in childbearing age.
7. SCD.
8. Patient will perform bariatric surgery.
9. Ileal resection and spinal cord injury.
10. Transplantation.

Polyps and Gallstones

- Polyps > 1 cm + radiovascular stalk or more than 2–3 polyps → cholecystectomy.
- Serial US is recommended for patient with polyps and gallstone → prophylactic laparoscopic cholecystectomy is recommended.

Gallbladder Wall Calcification

1. Selective mucosal calcification (focal Ca^{++} deposit).
2. Diffuse intramural calcification (porcelain gallbladder).
   - Previously, porcelain gallbladder is considered premalignant, now can be observe → follow-up.

- But selective mucosal calcification → is premalignant in 60% compared with diffuse calcification, 1%.
- Incidence of CA with selective vs. diffuse, 35% vs. 16% respectively.

Gastric CA

- Gastrectomy + denervation of parasympathetic and sympathetic with extensive lymphadenectomy.
- Duodenal exclusion → ↑ risk.
- So prophylactic cholecystectomy is advisable to avoid acute acalculous cholecystitis, ERCP, CBD exploration in presence of Roux-en-Y.

Small Bowel Resection

1. Short Gut Syndrome
   - Alter enterohepatic circulation of bile salt from ileal resection.
   - Prolonged TPN.
   - Cholecystectomy with extended bowel resection can prevent complication and can prevent need for reopening hostile abdomen and decrease risk of bowel injury.

2. Intestinal carcinoid will require long-term somatostatin → ↓ CCK → ↓ gallbladder motility.
   - 65% of patient on somatostatin → gallstone → 17% require cholecystectomy within 5 years.

Hemoglubinopathy

- SCD, 70% will have gallstone at the age of 30; in children, 40%.
- 50% will have complication within 5 years.
- It's hard to distinguish biliary colic from VOC.
- ↑ risk of CBD stone and ↑ IOC use.
- Strongly advisable.
- Patient at age 50 → mostly need splenectomy and cholecystectomy.

- Limited role of cholecystectomy and silent gallstone in thalassemia.

Transplant

- ↑ gallstone.
- Kidney and pancreatic TPx can benefit from prophylactic cholecystectomy.
- Heart TPx is a must to do prophylactic cholecystectomy.

Spinal Cord Injury

- 30% will have gallstone.
- Complication is 2.2%
- Difficult to diagnose in high spinal cord injury.

Bariatric Surgery

- Roux-en-Y bypass and sleeve gastrectomy.
- 30% will develop symptom.
- Rarely severe complication, 1%.
- Ursodeoxycholic acid used as prophylaxis to prevent gallstone formation in the first 6 months of post-bariatric surgery.
- Meta-analysis: 8.8% with ursodeoxycholic developed gallstone whereas 27.7% with placebo developed gallstone.
- With sleeve gastrectomy, gall stone formation is 7%–15%; whereas the bypass surgery, > 30%.

Symptomatic Gallstone

Chronic Cholecystitis (Biliary Colic)

- The pain developed when stone obstruct cystic duct, ↑ tension on the wall.
- Mucosa is initially normal or hypertrophied but late atrophied → epithelium protrusions into muscle → Rokitansky-Aschoff sinus.

- **Clinical Presentation**
  - Pain is constant and ↑ in severity over the first ½ hr and lasts for 1–5 hrs.

- Located in epigastrium, or RUQ radiate to upper-right back or between scapula.
- Typically in the night or after fatty meal.
- Often associated with nausea, vomiting (sometimes).
- On and off, i.e., episodic.
- On physical examination → mild right hypochondrial tenderness during episode → between attack, no pain, no tenderness.
- Atypical symptoms: pain primarily in the back, bloating, blenching.
- If atypical symptoms, you should rule out PUD, GERD, hernias, IBD, diverticular disease, liver disease, renal stone, pleuritic chest pain, and MI.
- When pain is persisting and lasts > 24 hrs → impacted stone or acute cholecystitis.
- When impaction → hydrops of gallbladder → bile absorbs and continuously secretes mucus → mucocele.
- Usually palpable gallbladder but not tender → hydrops → inflammation, infection, perforation → early cholecystectomy to avoid complication.

- **Diagnosis**
  - Laboratory: WBCs, LFT → normal.
  - US is the gold standard.
  - If the patient has typical pain in two or more occasions → cholecystectomy.
  - Sludge, stone, adenomyomatosis → causes typical biliary symptom and detected on US.
  - Cholesterolosis is caused by accumulation of cholesterol and macrophage in gallbladder mucosa either locally or polyps → produces "strawberry gallbladder."
  - Adenomyomatosis: glandular proliferation and hypertrophy of smooth muscle.
  - Granulomatous polyps developed in lumen → cholecystectomy.

- **Management**
  - If symptomatic → elective laparoscopic cholecystectomy.
  - If waiting for surgery or postponed → patient advised to avoid fatty meal.
  - DM patient with symptoms → cholecystectomy directly as they are more prone to develop acute cholecystitis that is often severe.
  - Pregnant with symptom → low fat diet until secondary trimester → laparoscopic cholecystectomy.

Acute Cholecystitis

- **Pathogenesis**
  - Secondary to gallstone, 90%–95%.
  - 1% is tumor obstructing cystic duct.
  - Obstruction of cystic duct are initial event that lead to distension, inflammation, and edema.
  - Inflammatory process is thought to be long irritation of lecithin → prostaglandin → secondary bacterial contamination, 15%–30%.
  - Gallbladder becomes thick, reddish with subserosal hemorrhage → mucosa is hyperemic with patchy necrosis.
  - Mostly, gallbladder stone will dislodge and inflammation subside.
  - When it remains obstructive + bacterial infection → acute gangrenous cholecystitis and abscess or empyema.
  - Perforation is rare.
  - When gas-forming organism → gas seen in the wall and lumen of gallbladder → emphysematous gallbladder.

- **Clinical Manifestation**
  - 80% will give history of chronic cholecystitis.
  - Begins like biliary colic but persists, i.e., pain does not subside for several days.
  - In RUQ or epigastrium radiating to right scapula and back.
  - Fever, anorexia, nausea and vomiting.
  - On examination: focal tenderness and guarding in RUQ, mass can be palpable.

- Murphy's signs: inspiratory arrest with deep palpation in right subcostal area.
- Severe jaundice → CBD stone or obstruction of bile duct by severe pericholecystic fluid inflammation secondary to stone in infundibulum (Mirizzi syndrome).
- Patient with DM has usually delayed presentation with complication tenfold.
- DDx: PUD, pancreatitis, appendicitis, hepatic pneumonia (Fitz-Hugh-Curtis syndrome), MI, pneumonia, herpes zoster.

- **Diagnosis**
  Laboratory
  - Leukocytosis is 12–15,000, but can be normal.
  - if > 20,000 → complicated or cholangitis.
  - LFT is normal or slightly high, but bilirubin may be slightly high as well as ALP and amylase.

  Radiological
  - US: stone, pericholecystic fluid, ticked wall + sonographic Murphy's sign.
  - Typical history of acute cholecystitis → US is cheap, no radiation.
  - Sensitivity is 90% to detect gallstone but 60%–70% to detect acute cholecystitis.
  - Picture of acute cholecystitis → US → gallstone → cholecystectomy → shall we proceed to CT? → never.
  - CT is more sensitive in acute cholecystitis.
  - If the patient with picture of acute cholecystitis → US reveals only gallstone, but significant concern of other intra-abdominal pathology → CT with IV contrast (e.g., LLQ → diverticulitis).
  - HIDA scan if suspicion of acute cholecystitis (unclear) and US −ve → HIDA is better than US and CT.
  - normal HIDA excludes acute cholecystitis.

- **Management**
  - IVF, IV antibiotic (gram −ve and anerobe), third generation of cephalosporin + Metronidazole.
  - For patient with allergy to cephalosporins → aminoglycosides + Metronidazole.
  - More than ½ has +ve bacteria in C/S.
  - 85% will respond to conservative treatment.
  - If patient did not improve within 72 hrs → percutaneous cholecystostomy or surgery.
  - Most patients will recur biliary event within 1–3 years.
  - Analgesia: Adol, NSAIDs, opiate.
  - Minimal comorbidity → laparoscopic cholecystectomy.

- **Cholecystectomy**
  - Laparoscopic cholecystectomy is the procedure of choice.
  - Within 72 hrs, the sooner the better.
  - Should be familiar with open cholecystectomy.
  - Should know bailout option.
  - Conversion rate is 10%–15%.
  - When patient is late or unfit → delay 2 months and treat with antibiotics.
  - 20% failure rate of medical treatment.
  - For patients unfit for OR → percutaneous cholecystostomy or open cholecystectomy under local anesthesia → failure of improvement after cholecystostomy, i.e., perforation or gangrene → surgery.
  - If patient improved after cholecystostomy → cholangiography should show patent ductus cysticus → then remove cholecystostomy tube → schedule for surgery in the near future.
  - If patient cannot tolerate surgery → remove stone via cholecystostomy tube before removal.

- **Bailout Option**
  - If gallbladder is fused in liver (abut) → back wall of gallbladder left and cauterize the mucosa to decrease mucocele.

- If cystic duct is difficult to identify → subtotal cholecystectomy (remove all stones and oversewn a small remaining cuff → close suction drain.

- **Complication and posto-perative Care**
  - Most leak is from cystic duct stump or small subvesical duct (duct of Luschka)→ drain and remove it the next day when no sign of leak.
  - If still high output, leave the drain.
  - Biloma → percutaneous drainage → ERCP sphincterotomy ± stent to define anatomy and decompress biliary system.

- **Bile gallstone spillage** → irrigation and aspirate and remove stone as much as you can → large stone → abscess → drain → antibiotic if SIRS or sepsis.

- **Pneumonia** → after open cholecystectomy → regional anesthesia with transverse abdominal plane block, paravertebral block, epidural.

- **Percutaneous Drainage**
  - Used in patient who fail in medical treatment and have contraindication or high risk of GA or have prolonged Symptom 3–4 days.
  - 90% effective.
  - Under LA.
  - 15% dislodge or blockage.
  - Contrast injection in 4–6 weeks → if cystic duct in patent → remove.

- **Endoscopic Therapy**
  - Transpapillary: ERCP and stent into gallbladder via cystic duct: 90% effective.
    Transmural: puncturing of gallbladder under EUS → dilation of tract → stent.

Special Situation (Pregnancy)
- DDx: HELLP syndrome, acute fatty liver with pregnancy.
- Previously, avoid laparoscopic cholecystectomy in first and third trimester.
- Now it's safe in all trimesters to perfrom the surgery but most centers will do:
  - First trimester → medical treatment, if failed → percutaneous drainage → bridging to laparoscopic cholecystectomy at second trimester.
  - Second trimester → laparoscopic cholecystectomy.
  - Third trimester → postpone till postpartum.

Acalculous Cholecystitis
- In critically ill patient, TPN, burn, sepsis, major operation, multiple traumas, prolonged illness, stasis, ischemia.
- The cause is unknown but gallbladder is distended with bile stasis and ischemia is cofactor.
- Histopathology: edema to the wall with patchy thrombosis of arterioles and venules.
- Symptom: same as acute cholecystitis.
- If unconscious, ↑ WBC, high ALP and LFT.
- US: diagnostic tool of choice.
- CT: to rule out other cause of sepsis.
- HIDA: nonvisualization of gallbladder but less sensitive when patient is fasting or on TPN.
- CT-guided cholecystostomy is the treatment of choice.
- As usually patient is unfit for surgery, 90% impairment.
- If patient did not improve → open cholecystostomy or open cholecystectomy.

Laparoscopic Cholecystectomy
- After induction of anesthesia, time-out performed, the patient is positioned in reverse Trendelenburg.
- The entire abdomen is prepped and draped in standard sterile fashion.
- Access is gained by either the Veress needle technique (closed technique) or open technique (Hasson).
- CO_2 insufflation is initiated to a pressure of 15 mmHg.

- The first trocar sized 10 mm is placed at or around the umbilicus.
- Better to use angled camera (30 degrees).
- Then three trocars sized 5 mm are introduced in epigastrium, right subcostal in midclavicular line, and the last one in right subcostal anterior axillary line.
- The fundus of the gallbladder is grasped with an instrument.
- the tip of the gallbladder is retracted cephalad toward the right axilla, and the infundibulum of the gallbladder is retracted laterally.
- A Maryland dissector is used to clear the peritoneum over the infundibulum and cystic duct.
- Sharp dissection to the peritoneal fold around the gall, making a V-shaped dissection by L-hook.
- The cystic duct is cleared of the attachments circumferentially, i.e., skeletonize the duct and artery.
- Obtain critical view of safety.
- Cystic duct is clipped by endoclips as well cystic artery.
- The gallbladder is dissected from liver bed by L-hook, placed into a specimen retrieval bag, and removed through either the subxiphoid or the umbilical port.
- Use irrigation and suction if needed.
- Close the wounds and place the dressing.

Choledocholithiasis (CBD) Stone
- Small or large, single or multiple.
- CBD stone, 5% of gallstone require surgery, increases with age.
- 20%–25% above 60 of age will have CBD stone.
- Vast majority is secondary stone, i.e., from gallbladder, whereas primary is brown pigment → stasis + infection (Asia).

- **Clinical Picture**
  - May be silent and discovered incidentally.
  - May cause obstruction → obstructive jaundice or biliary pancreatitis.
  - The pain with CBD stone is similar to biliary colic.
  - Nausea and vomiting, dark urine, pale stool.
  - Signs: may be normal or may experience epigastric pain or RUQ tenderness, icterus is common.

- May present with complete obstruction → ALP, bilirubin is shooting high.

- **Diagnosis**
  - Lab: ↑ bilirubin (mainly direct), ↑ ALP, normal or slight increase in amylase.
  - First test is US for decimating of gallbladder stone.
  - The stone may be more distal.
  - CBD dilation > 8 mm suggests obstruction.
  - MRCP sensitivity and specificity is 89%–95%, can detect > 5 mm stone.
  - ERCP is the gold standard for diagnosis; it provides therapeutic option.
  - EUS is as good as ERCP sensitivity and specificity, 91%, 100%, but lack therapeutic option.
  - PTC rarely needed in secondary CBD stone.

- **Management of CBD stone**
  - Patient with gallstone and suspected CBD stone, either preoperative ERCP or intra-operative cholangiogram (IOC).
  - If ERCP → sphincterotomy and ductal clearance +/- stent followed by laparoscopic cholecystectomy.
  - Vast majority treated by ERCP.
  - The classic open CBD exploration is rarely done.
  - Now laparoscopic CBD exploration (LCBDE) gain popularity.
  - LCBDE at the time of laparoscopic cholecystectomy vs. laparoscopic cholecystectomy with pre- or postoperative ERCP is almost the same → but ↓ stay and cost with LCBDE.
  - Post-operative ERCP failure is 4%–10%, which requires return to the theater for open CBD exploration.
  - LCBDE: ↑ time, need expert surgeon and sufficient instrument.

Patient Selection
  - If suspicion of CBD stone → laparoscopic cholecystectomy + IOC ± LCBDE.
    → if history or coexisting of the following finding:
      o Jaundice

o Dark urine, acholic stools
o Gallstone pancreatitis
o High LFT
o Dilated CBD
- Incidence of CBD stone during laparoscopic cholecystectomy is 15%–20%.
- CBD stone may persist despite ERCP, and stone may enter the duct after ERCP → so IOC after ERCP.
- Patient should be counseled for LCBDE, OCBDE, or post-operative ERCP.

Surgical Planning for LCBD
- Confirm CBD stone by image or post-ERCP with residual stone.
- Prepare instrument, e.g., C-arm and instruments.
- Trocar-like laparoscopic cholecystectomy.
- IOC or US → 99% specificity and sensitivity.

Transcystic Laparoscopic CBD Exploration (LCBDE)
- Transcystic approach → contrast → define anatomy → flush with normal saline → glucagon to relax sphincter of Oddi (should be avoided if patient is taking β-blocker) or nitroglycerin.
    - Advantage: incision of CBD is avoided.
    - Disadvantage: proximal stone is not possible to reach.
    - **NB**: should not be done if CBD < 3 mm.

- Cystic Ductotomy
    - If large and tortuous → incision in the neck of gallbladder, proximal to CD and HD junction.
    - If too small → incision near CBD.

- Wire Access
    - Cholangiogram catheter is 0.035 inch; guidewire passes through catheter under fluoroscopy till it reaches duodenum.
    - Oslen clamp over wire.
    - Access passes over the wire.

- Balloon Dilation
  - Routine balloon dilation is recommended to traverse valve of Heister in cystic duct.
  - Balloon should cross CD and CBD junction under fluoroscopy.

- Stone Clearance
  - Wire basket passes through CD to CBD.
  - Fogarty biliary balloon may be used to dislodge stone or pull them retrogradely but can migrate stone to HD.
  - Use of flexible scope with dormia basket is the most direct way to ensure clearance.
  - Choledochoscope is connected with normal saline irrigation.
  - Can be directed toward HD.
  - Once wire basket advances beyond the stone, the basket is opened and pulled back to remove stone from cystic duct.
  - After clearance, advance scope till ampulla until mucosa of duodenum is visualized.
  - If stone is too large → laser lithotripsy.

- Duct Closure
  - Closing cholangiogram should be performed to check residual stone and rule out duct injury.
  - Preferable to use loop for ligation rather than clip (because of cystic duct manipulation).
  - Drain: not routinely.

Transcholedochal Laparoscopic CBD Exploration (LCBDE)
- If transcystic approach failed → TCLCBDE.
- Alternative procedure: post-operative ERCP or conversion to open.
- Should be reserved for CBD ≥ 7 mm, not performed if there's inflammation in porta hepatis.
- Transcholedochal approach:
  - Incision in CBD is just distal to cystic duct and CHD junction.

- Suture of CBD if stone is extracted.
- Disadvantage: bile leak, stricture.

- Exposure and Ductotomy
  - Expose anterior supraduodenal CBD.
  - Lateral and upward traction.
  - Longitudinal incision at anterior aspect of CBD.
  - Avoid arterial supply of CBD typically at 3 and 9 o'clock.
  - Length is 1–2 cm.
  - Stay suture may be placed.

- Stone Clearance
  - Flush out or capture with choledochoscope as in transcystic approach.

- Duct Closure
  - Fine 4-0 absorbable monofilaments (PDS) to prevent stone formation.
  - Suture over T tube, typically (14F) to decompress biliary, protect closure, and prevent stricture formation.
    → May be used postoperatively for cholangiogram.
  - Removal is usually 3 weeks post-operative.
  - T-tube is controversial because of discomfort, fistula after removal, dislodgement.
  - Close by primary closure.
  - Adjacent to primary closure → ampullary stent.
  - Stent complications: dislodgment and migration, occlusion, cholangitis, pancreatitis, erosion of duct and duodenum.
  - After closure → cholangiogram via T-tube or cystic duct stump.

- Result of LCBDE
  - Transcystic success rate is 70%.
  - Transcholedochal success rate is 95%–98%.
  - Bile leak is more with transcholedochal.
  - LCBDE vs. OCBDE (gold standard):

→ OCBDE—success rate 98%

→ LCBDE—lower infection.

- One stage, ↓ stay and cost.

Open CBD Exploration

- Failure of the other technique.
- Major principles of OCBDE:
  - Bile duct ≤ 5 mm is relative contraindication; if ≤ 3 mm, absolute contraindication.
  - Stone ≤ 3 mm will pass spontaneously.
  - Avoid forceful manipulation → false passage.
  - Cholangiogram before exploration (position and number) of stone and duct anatomy.
  - Procedure: right subcostal or upper midline.
  - Extensive Kocher maneuver for retroduodenal and intrapancreatic biliary duct.
  - From left side is easier.
  - Incised overlaying peritoneum.
  - Place two stay sutures in th bile duct.
  - Avoid arterial supply of CBD typically at 3 and 9 o'clock
  - Incise duct longitudinally by 15 blades at the level of cystic duct entry, 1.5 cm.
  - Obvious stone is extracted.
  - Stone palpation and milking up and down.
  - Duct explored by Randall stone forceps.
  - Flush the duct.
  - Choledochoscope may be used, as well as Fogarty biliary catheter.
  - Ampullary potency → Bakes dilator and gradual dilation by big size one by one.
  - Use of Fogarty catheter is a superior way to ensure patency, flexible, if passed duodenum inflation of balloon and pull back.
  - Steel sign: seeing tip of sound in duodenum.
  - Choledochoscope is performed.
  - If stuck → electrohydraulic lithotripsy via choledochoscope.
  - If failed lithotripsy → T-tube and terminate OR.

- In the past, transduodenal sphincteroplasty, duodenum is incised transversally and sphincter is incised at 11 o'clock to avoid pancreatic duct injury, then sphincteroplasty.
  → It's abundant nowadays.
- After choledochoscope is completed → T-tube (14F) oversewn into place (should fit to the duct).
- Closure by absorbable 3-0, e.g., chromic.
- Bite 1–2 mm in depth and 2 mm apart.
- Last bite should be watertight to test tube.
- Cholangiogram is obtained.

Special Concern

- Retained stone post operatively or recurrence after months or years following laparoscopic cholecystectomy → ERCP.
- T-tube: a gutter is cut out of the cross arm to lower resistance during removal, thus to reduce risk of fistulous tract disruption.
- If CBD exploration done with T-tube → cholangiogram before removal.
- Retained stone can be retrieved by endoscopy or via T-tube once tract has matured 2–4 weeks.
  → T-tube removed → catheter passes to tract under fluoroscopy.
  → Removal of stone by basket or balloon.
- Recurrent stone → generous sphincterotomy.
- Bile duct drainage procedure:
  → Rare when stone cannot be cleaned and/or bile duct is very dilated > 1.5 cm:
    - choleduocoduodenotomy by mobilization of second part of duodenum (Kocher maneuver).
    - Choledochojejunostomy by 45 cm Roux-en-Y and end-to-side anastomosis.
    - Hepaticojejunostomy for bile duct stricture or palliative procedure of malignant periampullary neoplasm.

Management of Gallstone Ileus

- Rare, 0.3%–0.5%, from complication of gallstone.
- Bilioenteric fistula by inflammation.
- Similar pathophysiology with Mirizzi syndrome in which large stone in infundibulum erodes through gallbladder to CBD.
  - → Another Bouveret's syndrome in which gallstone erodes gallbladder into stomach and is impacted in pylorus, resulting in gastric outlet obstruction.
- Location of fistula is mostly in duodenum, followed by small bowel (mid-end).
- Cholecystocolic is rare.
- Stone usually > 3 cm.
- 3.7% of bowel obstruction.

Diagnosis
Clinical
- Bowel obstruction.
- Classically, biliary colic before 1–2 days.

Radiological
- Rigler's triad: bowel obstruction, pneumobilia, aberrant stone in GI tract, 20%–50%.
- CT is diagnostic, 93%.

Management
- Resuscitation, NGT, Foley catheter.
- Laparotomy: palpate manually from ligament of Treitz and distally to obstruction.
- Most often in terminal ileum or at ileocecal valve.
- Enterotomy is made in healthy small bowel part 30 cm proximal to obstruction → longitudinally in antimesenteric border.
- Stone is milked out.
- Enterotomy is closed in a transverse fashion.
- Repair of fistula is controversial.
  - → Single stage is better but ↑ mortality and morbidity, 16% vs. 11% with enterotomy alone.

- only 10% required to re-open, i.e., interval cholecystectomy.
- Laparoscopy should be avoided because of the following:
    1. Dilated bowel.
    2. Patient is hypovolemic $\rightarrow$ pneumoperitoneum $\rightarrow$ low VR, low COP.
    3. Evaluation of bowel is limited.

Discussion

- The recommended approach in acute surgical intervention is enterolithotomy alone.
- Complex surgery $\rightarrow$ $\uparrow$ mortality and morbidity.

Management of Acute Cholangitis
Etiology

- 70% caused by secondary gallstone.
- Non-iatrogenic:
    - Benign: gallstone (primary, secondary), pancreatitis (acute, chronic), Mirizzi, choledochal cyst, biliary stricture, PSC.
    - Malignant: pancreatic CA, cholangiocarcinoma, periampullary CA, tumor compressing CBD.
- Iatrogenic:
    - Post-ERCP, direct trauma, ischemia-induced stricture, anastomotic stricture.
    - Most common location of obstruction is distally.

Pathogenesis

- Continuous flow of bile is preventive mechanism + bile salts that are inherently bacteriostatic and contain IgA.
- Bacteria can enter the biliary system via duodenum, typically prevented by the sphincter of Oddi.
- Hematogenous spread from the portal vein rarely occurs.
- ERCP represents 0.5%–1.7% of ascending cholangitis.
- Polymicrobial: E. coli, 25%–50%; klebsiella, 15%–20% (−ve).
- Most common gram +ve organism is enterococcus, 10%–20%.

Presentation

- Charcot's triad: fever, RUQ pain, jaundice → 75%.
- Reynolds pentad: Charcot's triad + hypotension, confusion, i.e., sepsis.

Decision-Making

- Tokyo guideline:
    - A. Clinical manifestation
        - (1) History of biliary disease and (2) fever
        - (3) jaundice (4)abdominal pain
    - B. Laboratory
        - (1)↑ WBC and (2) abnormal LFT
    - C. Image finding, i.e., dilatation
    - D. Suspected diagnosis: 2 or more item in A
    - E. Definite diagnosis: charcot triad + both item B + item C.

Diagnosis

- CBC: high WBCs.
- Chemistry: high LFT, ALP, rarely ↑ amylase and lipase → could be gallstone pancreatitis.
- C/S from blood, bile.
- US is the first tool.
- HIDA: identify cystic duct obstruction.
- EUS, CT.
- MRCP: great sensitivity to gallstone.
- ERCP: the diagnostic of choice.
- → Remove the stent if it is there.
- PTC and PBD: to locate, drain, C/S, Bx.

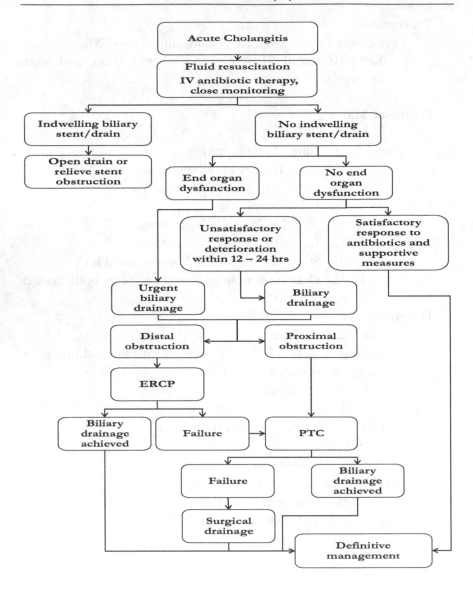

Treatment

- ICU, resuscitation, correction of electrolyte, coagulopathy.
- Antibiotic for 7–14 days and send C/S; if C/S came → tailored accordingly.
- Second- or third-generation cephalosporin is not recommended, no coverage to enterococcus.
- Tazocin is the best (can stand alone) with good penetration into bile.

- Severity assessment → Tokyo guideline.
  - → Mild: patient responds to medical treatment.
  - → Moderate: patient does not respond but no MOF.
  - → Severe: patient does not respond with MOF, i.e., one of the following:
    1. CVS: hypotension.
    2. CNS: disturb level of consciousness.
    3. Respiratory: $PaO_2/FiO_2 < 300$.
    4. Renal: creatinine > 2.
    5. Liver: INR > 1.5.
    6. Hematology: platelet < 100,000.
- Biliary drainage is not required if stone is passed.
- If patient improved clinically but not in laboratory → MRCP.
- ERCP is the gold standard, 90%–98% effective → sphincterotomy + stent.
- If PSC → avoid instrumentation.
- ERCP complication: 7%–15%.
- PTC if IHBD without extrahepatic dilatation, i.e., proximal or hilar pathology.
- Percutaneous cholecystostomy is not advisable unless cholecystitis.
- Surgery is rare, and usually the last option, but ↑ mortality and morbidity, 40%.
- If all failed or if previous Roux-en-Y with inadequate PTC → surgery.
- Surgery → choledochotomy with limited CBD exploration and T-tube, removed 10 days to 6 weeks.
- These procedures should be avoided in ascending cholangitis: formal CBD exploration, transduodenal sphincteroplasty, biliary enteric bypass.
- Definitive surgical intervention should be deferred till infection subsided.
- Cholecystectomy can be performed at the same admission, if no MOF.

Prognosis

- Most cases are mild; 85% respond to conservative treatment without biliary drainage.

- Mortality rate is 2.8%–10%.
- The poorest prognosis with MOF.

Cholangiohepatitis
- Recurrent pyogenic cholangitis, 30%–40%.
- Caused by bacterial (E. coli, strep, enterococcus) contamination or parasite.
- Bacterial enzyme causes deconjugation of bilirubin → bile sludge → brown pigment stone.
- The nucleus may contain worm, ovum.
- Repeated cholangitis → stricture → obstruction → stone → infection, liver abscess, and liver failure (secondary biliary cirrhosis).
- Classic Charcot's triad.
- US → stone in CBD and pneumobilia from gas-forming organism.
- MRCP and PTC → for imaging.
- Emergent decompression of biliary tree in septic patient
- Removal of stone and debris.
- Long-term therapy: Roux-en-Y hepaticojejunostomy.
- Resection of involved liver.

Mirizzi Syndrome
- Mirizzi syndrome is defined as a common hepatic duct obstruction caused by extrinsic compression from an impacted stone in the cystic duct or infundibulum of the gallbladder.
- Patients with Mirizzi syndrome can present with jaundice, fever, and upper-right quadrant pain.
- Mirizzi syndrome is often not recognized preoperatively in patients undergoing cholecystectomy and can lead to significant morbidity and biliary injury.

Epidemiology
- 0.05%–4% of patients undergoing surgery for cholelithiasis.
- 50%–77% of patients with Mirizzi syndrome are women, which may in part be due to a higher incidence of gallstones in women.
- Can be associated with gallbladder cancer.

- It has been hypothesized that recurrent inflammation and biliary stasis may predispose to both conditions.

Pathophysiology

- Large gallstones can become impacted in the cystic duct or the infundibulum; these stones can produce common hepatic duct obstruction because of the proximity of the cystic duct and the common hepatic duct + secondary inflammation.
- In rare cases, chronic inflammation may result in bile duct wall necrosis and erosion of the anterior or lateral wall of the common bile duct by impacted stones, leading to cholecystobiliary (cholecystohepatic or cholecystocholedochal) fistula.

Classification

- Mirizzi syndrome has been classified based on the presence and extent of a cholecystobiliary fistula.

  - Type I (11%): external compression of the common hepatic duct due to a stone impacted at the neck/infundibulum of the gallbladder or at the cystic duct.
  - Type II (41%): the fistula involves less than one-third of the circumference of the common bile duct.
  - Type III (44%): involvement of between one-third and two-thirds of the circumference of the common bile duct.
  - Type IV (4%): destruction of the entire wall of the common bile duct.

Clinical Manifestations

- Jaundice, fever, and upper-right quadrant pain. However, all three symptoms are only present in 44%–71%.
- Pain is the most common presenting feature (54%–100%), followed by jaundice (24%–100%) and cholangitis (6%–35%).
- Up to one-third of patients have acute cholecystitis on presentation and, in rare cases, acute pancreatitis.

Laboratory Findings
- The major laboratory findings are elevations in the serum concentrations of alkaline phosphatase and bilirubin in over 90% of patients.
- Patients with concurrent acute cholecystitis, cholangitis, or pancreatitis may have leukocytosis.

Diagnosis
- Should be suspected in any patients with upper-right quadrant pain, jaundice, and fever.

Diagnostic Imaging
- **US**
  - Dilatation of the biliary system above the level of the gallbladder neck.
  - The presence of a stone impacted in the gallbladder neck.
  - An abrupt change to a normal width of the common duct below the level of the stone.
  - The sensitivity of abdominal ultrasound in the diagnosis of Mirizzi syndrome is 23%–46%.

- **CT scan**
  - does not significantly add to the diagnostic yield of abdominal ultrasound in identifying the cause of biliary obstruction.

- **Magnetic resonance cholangiopancreatogram (MRCP)**
  - Dilatation of the biliary system above the level of the gallbladder neck, an abrupt change to a normal diameter of the common duct below the level of the stone

- **ERCP**
  - confirm the diagnosis of Mirizzi syndrome and determine if a cholecystobiliary fistula is present. Sphincterotomy allows for biliary decompression by internal stenting in patients with obstructive jaundice or cholangitis.

- **PTC**
  - is typically reserved for patients who are not candidates for ERCP, who have failed ERCP, or who have surgically altered anatomy, preventing endoscopic access to the biliary tree.

Differential diagnosis
- **Choledocholithiasis**
- **Acute cholecystitis**
- Biliary leaks
- Pancreatitis
- Liver abscess
- Infected choledochal cysts
- Recurrent pyogenic cholangitis

Management
- Type I: partial or total cholecystectomy, either laparoscopic or open. Common bile duct exploration is typically not required.
- Type II: cholecystectomy + closure of the fistula, either by suture repair with absorbable material, T tube placement, or choledochoplasty with the remnant gallbladder.
- Type III: choledochoplasty or bilioenteric anastomosis (choledochoduodenostomy, cholecystoduodenostomy, or choledochojejunostomy), depending on the size of the fistula. Suture of the fistula is not indicated.
- Type IV: bilioenteric anastomosis, typically choledochojejunostomy, is preferred because the entire wall of the common bile duct has been destroyed.

Management of Biliary Injury and Stricture
- Complications of injury and obstruction: sepsis, cholangitis, secondary biliary cirrhosis, PHTN.
- It costs 50,000 USD.
- ↑ mortality by ninefold.
- Affects the quality of life.

- Causes:
  - Non-iatrogenic: chronic pancreatitis, autoimmune hepatitis, PSC, pyogenic cholangitis.

- Iatrogenic injury to bile duct.
  - 0.2% with open cholecystectomy.
  - 0.4% with laparoscopy.
  - ⅓ of surgeons will create injury in their life career.

Mechanism of Bile Duct Injury

- Most common cause: excessive cephalad retraction of gallbladder fundus.
- Insufficient lateral traction → alignment of CD and CBD, excessive diathermy.
- Aberrant biliary anatomy → right hepatic duct may run aberrantly crossing Calot's Δ.
  - → Bile duct is very narrow that it's mistaken as cystic.
  - → Cystic duct runs along CBD.
- Most common vascular injury is right hepatic artery → complications are pseudoaneurysm, bile duct necrosis, stenosis, cholangitis, liver atrophy, necrosis.
- Single-incision technique → ↑ chance of injury.

Preventing Bile Duct Injury

1. Optimal timing.
2. Use angled camera, e.g., 10°, 30°.
3. Obtain critical view of safety.
4. Always dissect above sulcus of Rouviere.
5. Use intra-operative cholangiogram (IOC)
6. Call senior surgeon when in doubt.
7. Convert to open, not a shame.

Classification of Injury

- Many classifications: Bismuth, Strasberg, Amsterdam, Neuhaus.
- Most widely used is Bismuth, which respects HD bifurcation.
- **Strasberg classification**:
  - A. Cystic duct leak or leak from small duct in liver bed.
  - B. Occlusion of part of biliary tree → typically clipped and divided of right hepatic duct.
  - C. Transection (but not ligation) of aberrant right HD.
  - D. Lateral injury of major BD.
  - E. E1 (Bismuth type 1): CHD division > 2 cm from bifurcation.

E2 (Bismuth type 2): CHD division < 2 cm from bifurcation.

E3 (Bismuth type 3): CHD at bifurcation.

E4 (Bismuth type 4): destruction of biliary confluence.

E5 (Bismuth type 5): involvement of aberrant right HD alone or with concomitant stricture of CHD.

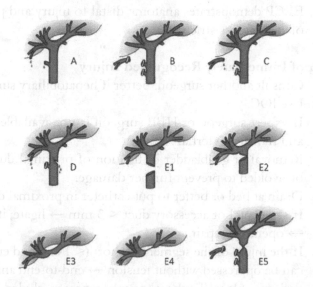

Clinical Presentation
- < 40% recognized during procedure.
- Finding includes the following:
    1. Evidence that clip size 10 is not sufficient to clip.
    2. Persistent biliary leak.
    3. Identification of second ductal structure.
    4. Extrasoft tissue adjacent to porta hepatis.
    5. Presence of larger artery.
    6. Sustain bleeding from right to gallbladder.
    7. Excessive number of clips.
    8. Inability to identify regional anatomic structure.
- Abdominal discomfort, nausea, anorexia, vomiting, malaise.

- Bile leak, biloma or free in peritoneum → if partially clipped.
- If completely clipped → jaundice, cholangitis.
- Chemistry: high LFT, AP, ↑ bilirubin.
- US: biloma, biliary dilatation.
- MRCP.
- HIDA scan to identify the site of leak (initial).
- PTC outlines anatomy and decompression with catheter or stent (PBD).
- ERCP demonstrates anatomy distal to injury and placement of stent across stricture.

Repair of Immediately Recognized Injury

- Consult another surgeon, better if hepatobiliary surgeon.
- Use IOC.
- If expert surgeon or HBP surgeon is not available → drain and transfer to tertiary center.
- Removal of gallbladder or ligation of proximal duct should be avoided to prevent further damage.
- Drain at bed or better to put catheter in proximal duct.
- If segmental or accessory duct < 3 mm → ligate; if > 4 mm → operative repair.
- If the injury of the segment is short (< 1 cm) and end-to-end can be oppressed without tension → end-to-end anastomosis and can place T-tube through separate choledochotomy either above or below anastomosis.
- Generous kocherization of duodenal is helpful → primary repair should be avoided if it's near hepatic bifurcation, ↑ stricture.
- If proximal injury *or* injured bile duct > 1 cm → end-to-end should be avoided → distal duct oversewn + proximal duct debridement and anastomosis with jejunal loop = end-to-side Roux-en-Y hepaticojejunostomy, which is better than choledochoduodenostomy → less stricture, less leak.
- Repair by primary surgeon has 20% success rate.
- Generally, in residency, 112 laparoscopic cholecystectomies are performed, 0.9 CBD exploration, 1.6 choledochal anastomosis.

- Biliary tree should be drained via retrograde catheter to facilitate cholangiogram.

Initial Management after Delayed Recognition in Post-operative

- If early, < 72 hrs → biloma, ascites, peritonitis.
    - → Control leak, control sepsis, IV antibiotic.
    - → Operation by hepatobiliary surgeon.
- PTC, ERCP, MRCP.
- also CTA, MRA to rule out right hepatic artery injury.
- If late, after 72 hrs → percutaneous drain + PTC; when acute inflammation subsided within 6–8 weeks → operative repair.

Definitive Management of Bile Duct Stricture

- Type A   → ERCP and stent
- Type B & C → No intervention or right posterior sectionectomy
- Type D   → Endoscopic or interventional radiology Stent
                      → If side-to-side anastomosis → failed (⅔)
                      → Roux-en-Y hepatico- jejunostomy is preferred (the procedure of choice)
- Type E   → Biliary enteric anastomosis, almost to all case → Roux-en-Y hepaticojejunostomy
- Finally, if all failed → ESLD → liver TPx.

Outcomes and Long-Term Surgical Reconstruction

- Best result if recognized during cholecystectomy and repair immediately by expert hepatobiliary surgeon.
- The more proximal, the more worse.
- Operative mortality rate is 5%–30%.
- Complications: cholangitis, exterior biliary, and hematic biliary.
- 70% stricture within 2 years, 90% within 7 years.
- Factor ↓ risk of stricture → Roux-en-Y anastomosis, no liver fibrosis, no infection, and use of transhepatic stent.
- Four factors to predict outcome:
    1. Performing complete cholangiogram
    2. Choice of repair
    3. Operative repair
    4. Experience of the surgeon

Effect of Repair to Quality of Life
- Psychological is the most important.
- Intestinal adhesion, internal hernia.
- Roux syndrome.

Management of Cystic Disorder of Bile Duct
- Rare, congenital disorder.
- Affects intra - and extrahepatic biliary tract.
- Weakness of bile duct wall and ↑ pressure.
- 1:100,000.
- Diagnosed in childhood but ½ diagnosed in adulthood.
- Male: Female = 1:4.
- 90% in pancreaticobiliary junction > 1 cm proximal to ampulla → reflux of pancreatic juice to biliary.
- ↑ risk of cholangitis, pancreatitis, malignancy transformation.

Etiology and Classification
- Anomaly in pancreaticobiliary duct junction, 15 mm proximal to ampulla → reflux of pancreatic secretin → formation of the cyst by change in BD epithelium.
- Classification by Alonso-Lej and modified by Todani.
- Types:

Type I		Dilation of extrahepatic biliary tract (most common 80%–90%).
	Ia	Cystic.
	Ib	Focal.
	Ic	Fusiform.
Type II		Saccular diverticulum of extrahepatic biliary tract.
Type III		Bile duct dilatation within duodenal wall (choledococele).
Type IV		Cystic dilatation of extra- and intrahepatic duct (second most, 15%–20%).
Type V		Caroli disease, intrahepatic cysts (less common).

Clinical Presentation
- Δ: RUQ pain, jaundice, abdominal mass (10%).
- In pediatrics: jaundice and mass.
- In adults: pain, 87%; jaundice, 42%; nausea, 29%; cholangitis, 26%; pancreatitis, 23%; mass, 13%.

Diagnosis
- Mildly elevation of LFT, 60%.
- By US or CT: CBD > 1 cm.
- Cholangiography (endoscopic, transhepatic, MRCP).
- MRCP is diagnostic of choice, most sensitive (noninvasive). .

Management
- Cholecystectomy + complete resection of the cyst to avoid the complication.

Type I	Resection of the cyst completely till inferior portion and up at the level of bifurcation of CHD.
	→ Send frozen to exclude malignancy then Roux-en-Y hepaticojejunostomy.
	→ Better than hepaticoduodenostomy → reflux, gastritis, gastric CA.
Type II	Simple diverticulectomy, no malignancy risk.
Type III	Small: ERCP and sphincterotomy.
	Large: transduodenal excision.
Type IV	Intrahepatic and extrahepatic.
	Intrahepatic: partial hepatectomy
	Extrahepatic: as Type I
Type V.	If concise to one lobe → hepatic resection.
	If bilobar, recurrent cholangitis, PHTN → liver TPx.

Prognosis
- Common surgical complications: wound infection, leak.
- Late complications (40%): stricture, cholangitis, and cholangiocarcinoma.
- All patients → surveillance of cholangiocarcinoma → serial image and CA 19-9.
- 5 years, SR with resection and reconstruction > 90%.

- Risk of cholangiocarcinoma is high → so long-term surveillance.

Sclerosing Cholangitis
- Uncommon disease → inflammatory stricture, intra- and extrabiliary system.
- Progressive disease resulting in secondary stricture.
- There are two types:
    - Primary sclerosing cholangitis
      Unknown cause, associated with IBD (UC, CD) 80% and Riedel thyroiditis, retroperitoneal fibrosis, i.e., autoimmune disease.
    - Secondary sclerosing cholangitis: bile duct stone, cholangitis, previous biliary surgery, or toxin.
- Patients with sclerosing cholangitis are at risk to develop cholangiocarcinoma.
- ⅔ female in their 40s.
- SR 12–18 years.
- 75% involve both intrahepatic and extrahepatic—15% isolated intrahepatic, 10% is extrahepatic.
- Symptoms: intermittent jaundice, fatigue, weight loss, pancreatitis, abdominal pain (½ of the patients).
- Colectomy to UC will not improve of PSC.
- Malignancy in 15% of PSC.
- SR 10–12 years after diagnosis.
- Mostly die from liver failure.

Associated Disease
- 70%–80% → IBD.
- Risk of colon CA is high after LTPx → colonoscopy surveillance.
- Other diseases: thyroiditis, DMI, ankylosing spontaneous, celiac disease.
- Gallstone develops in 25% of PSC; polyps, 5%.
- HCC, 2%–4%.
- Cholangiocarcinoma is 15% of PSC.

Clinical Presentation and Diagnosis
- May be asymptomatic.

- May have elevation LFT, bilirubin, ALP.
- RUQ pain, pruritus, fatigue.
- MRCP is the gold standard to diagnose PSC: multiple dilations and strictures (beading) of both intra and extra.
- ERCP, PTC: diagnostic and offer Bx, and stent.
- Liver biopsy for all patients to document degree of liver fibrosis.
- Colonoscopy surveillance.

Biliary Malignancy in PSC

- Risk is 15%.
- Annually, 1%–2%; incidental, 3%–9%.
- MRI, MRCP.
- CA 19-9 is relatively specific → if > 130 with no jaundice → cholangiocarcinoma.
- Histology is the gold standard for diagnosis → sensitivity of biopsy or brush FNA is 40%, but specificity is 100%.
- FISH → chromosol abnormality, 80%.
- PET has the highest specificity and sensitivity.

Medical Treatment

- Ursodeoxycholic acid, 15 mg/k/day.
- Immunosuppressant is not beneficial.
- No dramatic improvement with steroid but risk of infection.

Endoscopic

- Dominant stricture < 1.5 mm.
- Stent 6–8 weeks then remain or change.
- PTC if patient has Roux-en-Y.

Surgical Resection

- Selected patient if dominant in extrahepatic, no cirrhosis → resection of biliary tree + Roux-en-Y hepaticojejunostomy.
- Hepatic bifurcation, 80% of stricture → preoperative PTC facilitates dissection of hepatic bifurcation and provides stenting for reconstruction + cholecystectomy.
- If associated with liver cirrhosis → liver TPx.
  MR is 5%, survival rate in 1, 5 years is 90%, 70%, respectively.
  → Retransplantation within 2 years, 10%.

Stenosis of Sphincter of Oddi
- inflammation, fibrosis, muscular hypertrophy.
- Trauma (passage of stone), sphincter motility disorder, congenital anomaly.
- Episodic pain of biliary type and abnormal LFT are common presentations.
- Recurrent jaundice or pancreatitis play roles.
- Dilated CBD and difficult cannulation with delay emptying → diagnostic.
- Ampulla manometry.
- Surgical sphincteroplasty if failed endoscopic intervention.

Tumors
Carcinoma of Gallbladder
Epidemiology
- Fifth most common CA in GI.
- 2%–4%% of GI malignancy.
- Male: female = 1:2–3.
- High in 70s age-group.
- Autopsy, 0.4%, and 1% has undergone laparoscopic cholecystectomy.

Risk Factors
- Gallstone, 95%, i.e., 95% of gallbladder CA has gallbladder stone.
- Risk of CA is ↑with size of stone.
- Large stone > 3 cm, ↑ risk for gallbladder CA, tenfold.
- 20 years risk of developing gallbladder CA with gallbladder stone is 0.5%.
- Pathogenesis mostly because of chronic inflammation.
- Polypoid lesion ↑ particularly > 10 mm.
- Porcelain gallbladder, 20% incidence of gallbladder CA → gallbladder should be removed even if asymptomatic.
- Sclerosing cholangitis, especially in biliary pancreatic junction.
- Salmonella infection.
- Medication: methyldopa, isoniazid.

Pathology
- 60% of tumor originates from fundus, 30% from body, 10% from neck.
- Diffuse or nodule pattern are the most common types.
- Gallbladder lies on segment 4-B and 5.
- Tumor spreads through subserosal plane.
- 80%–90% adenocarcinoma.
  → Others: SCC, adenosquamous, oat cells, and anaplastic
- Adenocarcinoma is papillary, nodular, tubular.
- Less than 10% is papillary, it has better outcome as always is localized in gallbladder.
- Gallbladder CA spreads through lymphatic and venous drainage and directs invasion to liver.
- Lymphatic drainage first to cystic (Calot's Δ) node → pericholedochal → hilar LNs → peripancreatic and duodenal, periportal, celiac, SMA node.
- Gallbladder veins drains to liver usually to segment IV and V.
- Gallbladder lacks submucosa and muscularis mucosa → if it doesn't invade muscular layer, ↓ nodal metastasis.
- 25% localized to gallbladder, 35% reginal LNs, 40% distant metastasis.

Presentation
1. Preoperative on workup for symptoms
2. Preoperative incidental finding
3. Intraoperative
4. Postoperative by histopathology

- 50% discovered pre-operatively.
- Unfortunately, most gallbladder CA diagnosed at late stages 37% (stage IV).
- ⅓ has metastasis.

Diagnostic Evaluation
- History and physical examination are inadequate.
- CEA, CA 19-9 are not diagnostic.
  CEA is 93% specific and 50% sensitive.

CA 19-9, 79% sensitive and 69% specific, but not routinely used.
- US → any, mass, polyp > 1 cm, porcelain gallbladder → high index of suspicion.
- DDx of gallbladder masses: cholesterolosis, cholesterol polyp, adenomyomatosis.
- CT for staging but poor for nodal staging.
- PTC, ERCP for jaundiced patient.
- MRCP is the best tool to asses biliary, vascular, nodal.
- If imaging diagnosed as unresectable → biopsy to provide pathologic diagnosis.

Staging

Tis	In situ
T1a	Invade lamina propria
T1b	Invade muscular layer
T2	Perimuscular connective tissue
T3	Perforate serosa / invade liver
T4	Invade PV, HA
N1	Node for cystic duct, CBD, HA, PV
N2	Periaortic, pericaval, SMA
M	Metastatic disease

Surgical Treatment

Only surgery is curative.

I	T1a	→	Cholecystectomy
	T1b	→	Radical, i.e., cholecystectomy + segment 4b, 5 ± lymphadenopathy
II	Like Tb		
III	Diagnostic staging laparoscopy if no LNs →T1b		
IVa	Like T1b + adjuvant chemoradiation		
IVb	Palliative therapy		

- If cholecystectomy has been done → histopathology → Tis or T1a → nothing to do.
- T1b → radical surgery showed improve overall survival.

T1a

- LNs metastasis is 1.1%, but simple cholecystectomy is enough.
- Should obtain −ve margin.
- If cystic duct ivolve → cystic and bile duct resection + reconstructions, Roux-en-Y hepaticojejunostomy.

T1b

- Recent data showed aggressive resection → improves survival.
- LNs metastasis is 10%.
- Complete staging with CT CAP.
- Radical cholecystectomy + portal LNs dissection is recommended.

Liver Resection

- Range from resection of segment 4b and 5 to extended right hepatectomy → R0 should be achieved.
- Frozen section is helpful.

Portal Lymphadenectomy

- T2–T4 has +ve LNs by 50%.
- Minimum 6 LNs must be removed.

Extrahepatic bile duct Resection

- If +ve cystic duct margin.
- If extensive lymphadenopathy → risk of biliary ischemia.
- Resection then Roux-en-Y hepaticojejunostomy.

Excision of Port Site

- Not recommended by NCCN.
- Because if +ve, that means → peritoneal dissemination.

Re-operation for Incidentally Discovered Gallbladder CA

- No different in outcomes between one operation and two operations, i.e., reopen.
  → No difference in SR as well.
- John Hopkins → no difference between conversion to open and laparoscopic cholecystectomy then reopen.
- Biopsy is not recommended as peritoneal dissemination.

Advanced Disease

- Stage III: aggressive surgery management, i.e., R0 may improve survival.
- Laparoscopy staging is not routinely recommended.

Adjuvant Therapy

- ↑ resectability by 50% unresectable.
- Usually, 30% present with metastatic disease.
- Thus, chemotherapy is mainstay of gallbladder CA.

Management of Unresectable Metastatic Disease

- As mentioned previously, mainstay is chemotherapy.
- For jaundiced patient → ERCP (preferred) or PTC.

Biology and Future Direction

- In the past, Mutation in TP53 and K-RAS was discovered
  → Now
  - o PBRM1   53%
  - o TP53   4%–41%
  - o ERBB2   15%–16%
  - o P1KCA   12%–14%
  - o K-RAS   4%–11%
  - o APC   4%
  - o BRAF   1%

Prognosis

- Most common unresectable tumor → 5 years, SR is 5%, with median survival of 6 months.
- T1 with laparoscopic cholecystectomy only, SR is 80%–100%, 5 years.
- T2 with 5 years SR, simple cholecystectomy vs. radical cholecystectomy and lymphadenectomy, 25%–40% vs. 70%.
- Patient with advanced but resectable tumor, 5 years, SR is 20%–50%; with median, SR is 1–3 months.
- Recurrence after resection is common in liver, retroperitoneal LNs.
- Prognosis of recurrent disease is poor.

Management of Bile Duct CA (Cholangiocarcinoma)

- From biliary epithelial, anywhere is biliary tree.
- 3% of GI malignancy.
- Many patients have advanced disease when diagnosis.
- Most with unresectable die within 1 year.

Incidence

- Autopsy, 0.3%.
- 1:100,000 per year.
- Male: Female = 1.3:1.
- 50s–70s age-group.

Etiology

- PSC, choledochal cyst, hepatolithiasis, biliary enteric anastomosis, typhoid infection.
- Others: liver flukes, dietary nitrosamines and exposure to dioxin, hepatitis B and C, alcohol, obesity, UC.

Pathology

- 95% is adenocarcinoma.
- Divided into sclerosing (most common) and arises in the hilar region, papillary and nodular is the most favorable prognosis.
- Anatomically: divided into proximal (intrahepatic), 5%–10%; hilar (Klastskin), 60%–70%; and distal, 20%–30%.
- Intrahepatic cholangiocarcinoma is treated like HCC.

Clinical Manifestation and Diagnosis
- Painless jaundice is the most common presentation.
- Pruritus, mild RUQ pain, anorexia, fatigue, weight loss.
- ↑ bilirubin, ↑ALP, ↑ GGT.
- Most common diagnosing marker is CA 19-9 → sensitivity and specificity, 79%–98%.
- High CA 125, high CEA.

NB
- CA 19-9, mild elevation in cholangitis.
- US, CT is the initial tool.
- MRCP for tumor, LNs, vasculature.
- Biliary anatomy identified by PTC (mainly proximal).
- ERCP mainly for distal tumor.
- For vascular involvement → celiac angiography.
- Biopsy by percutaneous FNA, biliary brush or scrape biopsy and cytology.
- Patient with resectable tumor → offer surgery based on radiologic finding and clinical suspicion.

Management
- Resistant to chemoradiation and surgery is the mainstay.
- Surgical exploration if resectable and no metastasis.
- ½ of patient who explored have peritoneal implants, nodal or hepatic metastasis, or locally advanced disease → surgical bypass for decompression and cholecystectomy to prevent cholecystitis.

Intra-hepatic Cholangiocarcinoma (Proximal)
See liver.

Hilar Cholangiocarcinoma (CCA)
- Painless, jaundice, other nonspecific constitutional symptoms.
- US → dilation of IHBD with no dilation in CBD.
- Diagnosis by liver or pancreatic protocol CT or MRI before stent because of artifact.
- ERCP, PTC may add benefit → biopsy or drainage.
- Bx is difficult, so proceed for surgery if resectable.

- Pre-operative drainage, ↑ risk of post-operative infection, but normalized bilirubin before surgery is better. The goal is < 6–7 mg/dL.

Staging
- Perihilar (Klatskin tumor) and classified as Bismuth-Corlette classification:

Type I	Confined to common hepatic duct
Type II	Involve bifurcation without intrahepatic Ducts (most common 60-80%)
Type IIIa	Tumor extended to right HD.
IIIb	Tumor extended to Left HD.
Type IV	Involve both right and left HD

- TNM classification:

T1	Tumor confined to BD
T2a	Tumor invaded beyond wall of BD
T2b	Tumor invaded liver parenchyma
T3	Tumor invaded unilateral of PV or HA
T4	Tumor invaded PV, HA
N1	Regional LNs
N2	Periaortic LNs, pericaval
M	Metastatic disease

Management
- **Resection**

Exploration before resection preferred by laparoscopy.
→ Dissect hepatoduodenal ligament.
→ Transect CBD early and send distal end for frozen to achieve −ve margin.
  If +ve → Whipple.
→ Bile duct reflected upward with all LNs → till HD confluence.
→ Exposed left duct and divided and send for frozen.
  If −ve → extended right hepatectomy.
  If +ve → divided right hepatic duct with −ve margin + extended left hepatectomy

(because left duct is taller than right) + caudate lobe resection.
→ Reconstructions via Roux-en-Y hepaticojejunostomy.

- **Other Treatment**
  - Chemotherapy resistant but adjuvant chemotherapy given for +ve margin and +ve LNs.
  - If unresectable → biliary stent with chemotherapy or chemoradiation.
  - If disease found to be unresectable at the time of laparoscopy → operative bypass to segment 3 or 4, hepaticojejunostomy.
  - Sometimes needs liver TPx after neoadjuvant.

Distal CBD Cholangiocarcinoma
- Presentation similar to periampullary tumor.
- Painless jaundice ± nonspecific constitutional symptom.
- High liver enzyme, alkaline phosphatase, bilirubin > 8–10 mg/dL, suggest malignant process rather than benign.
- Initially US → shows intra- and extra-hepatic ducts dilation.
- Pancreatic protocol CT is very useful for lesion, LNs, metastasis.
- ± secondary pancreatic sign of periampullary malignancy such as atrophy and duct dilatation.
- ERCP can be used, but stent is not recommended → ↑ colonized bacteria in biliary tree and ↑ post of infection after Whipple procedure.
- Distal CBD cholangiocarcinoma never requires hepatectomy.
- EUS detailed image, biopsy (no risk of colonization).

Staging
- Like hilar CA.

Management
- **Resection**
  - Require Whipple procedure.
  - Criteria of resectability: absence of metastasis and locally advanced disease.

- Open approach mostly used but laparoscopy and robotic are used in some centers.
- Upper midline provides good exposure.
- Intraoperative US to assess liver for metastasis.
- Steps:
  - Right colon and hepatic flexure mobilized.
  - Extensive Kocher maneuver.
  - Tunnel-created cephalad along anterior surface of SMV and under the neck of pancreas.
  - Full right medial visceral rotation to help exposure of SMV.
  - Remove gallbladder.
  - Hepatoduodenal ligament skeletonized.
  - GDA identified and ligated.
  - Another tunnel is made under the neck of pancreas.
  - Two tunnels meet → Penrose drain passed.
  - CBD divided.
  - Distal stomach or proximal duodenum divided.
  - Neck of pancreas divided on Penrose drain to protect the vein below.
  - Frozen section for CBD to confirm −ve margin.
  - Divide proximal jejunum and bring it under SMV and SMA.
  - Reconstruction: gastrojejunostomy, choleduchojejunostomy and pancreaticojejunostomy.

- **Other Management**
  - Distal CBD is chemotherapy resistant.
  - But adjuvant chemoradiation may be used in case of +ve margin or LNS.
  - Unresectable tumor → durable stent + chemotherapy, radiation.

Patient with Unresectable Disease
- Patient with unresectable disease → 5FU alone or in combination of mitomycin C, ↑ response, 10%–30%.
  - → Combination of chemotherapy and radiation is more effective.
- Chemotherapy, ↓ immunity, ↑ risk of cholangitis.

- External beam radiation is not effective.
- Intraoperative radiation via stent.

Prognosis
- Perihilar presents with advanced unresectable disease, the median SR is 5–8 months.
- 5 years, SR of resectable tumor is 10%–30%, but patient with −ve margin ↑ SR (40%).
- Operative mortality rate is 5%–8%.
- Distal cholangiocarcinoma, 5 years, SR is 30%–50% and median survival is 32–38 months.
- Greater risk with +ve margin +ve LNs.
- Therapy for recurrent disease → palliative, and surgery is not recommended.

Ampullary and Periampullary Neoplasm
- Four most common malignant neoplasm:
  1. Pancreatic ductal adenocarcinoma
  2. Distal cholangiocarcinoma
  3. Ampullary adenoma or carcinoma
  4. Duodenal adenocarcinoma
- Mostly PD adenocarcinoma, which is 75%–85%, followed by distal cholangiocarcinoma and ampullary lesions then duodenal adenocarcinoma.
- other rare lesions: NET, pancreatic cystic neoplasm, GIST, sarcoma, lymphoma.
- Pancreaticoduodenectomy mortality is > 2%.

- **Pancreatic Ductal Adenocarcinoma**
  - See pancreas.

- **Distal Cholangiocarcinoma**
  - See before.

- **Ampullary Adenoma and Carcinoma**
  Ampullary Adenoma
  - Diagnosed by EGD and biopsy false −ve, 25%–50%.

- Benign villous adenoma excised locally and transduodenal excision for < 2 cm.
- EUS may be helpful.
- Preoperative → CA → not transduodenal excision but pancreaticoduodenectomy.
- Patient with FAP and periampullary adenoma → high incidence of CA.
- Whipple (not pylorus sparing) is the standard procedure of choice in FAP with periampullary lesion.

Ampullary Adenocarcinoma
- Accounts 0.2%–0.5% of GI malignancy.
- Third most common in periampullary, 6%–8%.
- Present with obstruction, symptom → early pickup → resectable is 80%.
  - → More favorable than pancreatic duct carcinoma.
- 5 years, SR is 34%–68%.
- Two pathology subtypes: intestinal and pancreaticobiliary.
- Intestinal is more favorable than pancreaticobiliary.

• **Duodenal Adenocarcinoma**
- Least of periampullary, 4%–7%.
- 0.4% of GI malignancy.
- Despite its rarity, it's the most common site of small bowel malignancy, accounting for 56%.
- Arises from duodenal polyps.
- Majority are sporadic, but patient with FAP carries 100%–200% high risk of CA as they have duodenal adenoma.
- More favorable.
- 5 years, SR is 45%–71%.

Pancreas

Anatomy

- Weight is 75–100 g; length is 15–20 cm.
- Divided into head, neck, body, tail.
- Relation:
    - Anteriorly: transverse mesocolon.
    - Posteriorly: IVC, right renal artery and vein.
- At inferior border of the neck of pancreas, SMV + splenic vein → portal v.
- Variations of PV:
    - (SMV + IMV) + splenic vein
    - Trifurcation
    - SMV + (IMV + splenic vein)
- SMA parallel to vein and just left to it.
- Head and uncinate process wrap right side of Portal vein and posteriorly.
- Venous drainage → portal vein (right lateral and posterior of PV).
- CBD runs in deep groove posterior to pancreas then passes through parenchyma to join main pancreatic duct.
- Body and tail lie anterior to splenic artery and vein.
- The splenic vein lies behind pancreas and artery at superior border and gives branches to pancreas, must be divided to perform spleen sparing distal pancreatectomy.
- Once divided, gastrocolic ligament (omentum) → lesser sac, pancreatic pseudocyst develops in this area.
- The transverse mesocolon attaches to inferior margin of body and tail of pancreas.
- The body of pancreas is anterior to aorta and the origin of SMA.
- The pancreatic neck is anterior to L1 and L2.
- The tail is anterior to left kidney and nestled spleen and splenic flexure of colon (avoid injury of pancreas during splenectomy and left colectomy).

Pancreatic Duct Anatomy

- Ventral (major) Wirsung duct.
- Dorsal (minor) Santorini duct.

- In ⅓ of patients, the pancreatic duct and bile duct are distinct.
- ⅓ emerge in two ducts and ⅓ has common channel.
- 30% of patients have blind Santorini duct.
- 10% of patients, the two ducts fail to fuse together (separate) Santorini duct drain into minor papilla and Wirsung duct drain into major papilla → pancreatic divisum.
    - → Majority of drainage of pancreas is through minor duct and is incapable to handle it → stasis and obstruction → repeated attacks of acute pancreatitis.
- Main pancreatic duct is 2–3 mm in diameter.
- Pressure inside pancreatic duct is twice than bile duct → prevents bile reflux to pancreatic duct.
- Pancreatic duct join bile duct to empty in ampulla of Vater (sphincter of Oddi) located in medial aspect in second part of the duodenum.
- Muscle fiber around the ampulla is contracted and relaxes by neural and endocrine (hormonal) factor.

Vascular and Lymphatic Anatomy

- Arterial supply:
    - Celiac → common hepatic → gastroduodenal artery (GDA)→ Superior pancreaticoduodenal arteries (anterior and posterior).
    - SMA → behind neck of pancreas → inferior pancreaticoduodenal (anterior and posterior).

    - You cannot resect head of pancreas without devascularizing the duodenum.
    - Variation of 15%–20% replaced right hepatic, common, GDA arise from SMA.
    - Body and tail supplied by branches of splenic artery.

- Venous drainage:
    - Superior veins → portal vein.
    - Posterior and inferior veins → inferior mesenteric vein.

- Lymphatic:
    - The head: pyloric, pancreatic duodenal LNs.

- The neck: superior mesenteric and aortic LNs.
- The body: superior and inferior pancreatic LNs.
- The tail: splenic LNs.

- Neuroanatomy
  - Sympathetic and parasympathetic.
  - Acinar cells (exocrine).
  - Islet cells (endocrine).
  - Parasympathetic stimulates exocrine and endocrine, while sympathetic inhibits them.
  - Pancreas is innervated by neuron that secretes somatostatin, VIP, CGRP (both exocrine and endocrine).
  - Rich of afferent sensory fibers in advanced pancreatic tumor, somatic travel to celiac ganglia.

Histology and Physiology

- Exocrine, 85%.
- Extracellular matrix, 10%.
- Bloog vessels and ducts, 4%.
- Endocrine, 2%.
- Can live without pancreas with insulin and digestive enzyme.
- 20% of pancreatic volume required to prevent insufficiency.

Exocrine Pancreas

- Ouput 500–800 mL/day, colorless, odorless, alkaline iso-osmotic juice.

- Acinar cells (amylase, protease, lipase), pyramidal in shape → secrete all types of enzyme.
  - Amylase → salivary and pancreatic → hydrolyzed starch to glucose and glycogen.
  - Gastric protein hydrolysis → stimulates intestine to secrete CCK and secretin.
  - Proteolytic—trypsinogen → trypsin positive enterokinase (duodenal mucosa). Trypsinogen is activated in pancreas and inhibited by enzyme secreted in acinar cells → failure to express normal trypsinogen inhibitor, PSTI, SPINK1 → familial

pancreatitis, i.e., mutation of cationic trypsinogen or PRSS1.
- Lipase secretes in active form.
- Phospholipase A2, as with all lipase, requires bile salt for its action.

- Centroacinar cells and intercalated duct → secrete water and electrolyte in pancreatic juice.
    - 40 acinar cells → spherical units = acinous.
    - Centroacinar cells contain carbonic anhydrase needed to secrete bicarbonate.
    - Secretin is a major stimulation of bicarbonate secretion, as well as CCK, gastrin, and acetylcholine but much less than secretin.
    - In vagotomy, ‾ bicarbonate and fluid juice.
    - Endocrine inhibits exocrine secretion.
    - Pancreatic juice → intercalated duct → interlobular duct (concentration) → 20 secondary intralobular ducts → drain in main duct.

Endocrine Pancreas
- 1 million islets of Langerhans, 40–900 mm.
- Most islets contain 3,000–4,000 cells of five major types:
    1. α (alpha) cells secrete glucagon.
    2. β (beta) cells secrete insulin.
    3. δ (delta) cells secrete somatostatin.
    4. ε (epsilon) cells secrete ghrelin.
    5. PP cells secrete pancreatic polypeptide.

- Insulin
    - Stimulated by glucose, protein, fat, glucagon, and CCK.
    - Inhibited by somatostatin, amylin.
    - Inhibits endogenous liver glucose to release and facilitate glucose transport into cells → ↓ plasma glucose and inhibits glycogenolysis, fatty acid breakdown, and ketone formation and stimulates protein synthesis.

- Up to 80% of pancreas can be resected without being diabetic.
- Type I: overexpression of insulin receptor → ↑ sensitivity to insulin in muscle and SC → ↓ hypoglycemia.
- Type II: downregulation of insulin receptor → insulin resistance.
- Type III: impairment of hepatic or peripheral insulin receptor.

- Glucagon
    - ↑ hepatic glycogenolysis and gluconeogenesis.
    - . ↑ glucose → ↓ glucagon.
    - Release in hypoglycemia.

- Somatostatin
    - Two bioactive products: somatostatin 14, 28 → inhibit endocrine and exocrine, ↓ GI mortality, intestinal absorption, vascular tone.
    - There are five different types of somatostatin receptor (SSTR).
    - All are G proteins.
    - Somatostatin 28 is a selective type of SSTR.
    - Hexapeptide and octapeptide such as octreotide bind only SSTR 2, 3, 5 → large H2 inhibitor, only endocrine and exocrine.
    - Major stimulant is fat (intraluminal).
    - Acetylcholine ↓ somatostatin and exocrine.

- Pancreatic Polypeptide (PP)
    - Protein is the most stimulant then fat and glucose.
    - Hypoglycemia → stimulate PP.
    - Insulin and somatostatin lower it, also glucagon.
    - Pancreatic polypeptide ↓ biliary contraction.

- Ghrelin
    - Found in pancreas and fundus of stomach.
    - Blocks insulin effect on liver.
    - In addition to the five above, there is amylin, VIP, and serotonin.

Islet Distribution
- β cells are located in the center, it represents 70% of islet mass.
- The others in periphery are: α cells, 10%, and PP cells, 15%, and the least is d cells, 5%.
- More than twenty hormones are secreted by the islet.
- Head and uncinate are high in PP, low in α.
- But body and tail are high in α, low PP, i.e., Whipple removes PP cells by 95% → glucose intolerance compared to distal pancreatectomy.
- Chronic pancreatitis → affects the head → pancreatogenic diabetes.
- Distal pancrease rich in α → glucagonoma.

Pathology
Acute Pancreatitis (AP)
- Acute inflammation with little or no fibrosis.
- Range from self-limiting to critical disease, infected pancreatic necrosis, and MOF.
- Most common GI disease in the US.
- Fourteenth most fatal illness.
- Ninth most common noncancer GI disease leading to death.

Etiology
- Gallstone is 80% of the causes, mostly in female.
- Alcohol, mostly in male.
- Hyperlipidemia.
- Hereditary.
- Trauma: external, surgery, ERCP.
- Hypercalcemia.
- Ischemia: low perfusion, thromboembolic, vasculitis.
- Obstruction: neoplasm, divisum.
- Others: infection, venom, drug, and idiopathic.

Gallstone
- Hypothesis:
    1. Transient lodged distally.
    2. Transient incompetence of sphincter of Oddi → duodenal fluid reflux.

3. Obstructive pancreatic duct → duct hypertension → minor duct disruption → extravasation of pancreatic juice.

Alcohol
-   Recurrent attacks of acute pancreatitis → chronic.
-   Consumption of 100–150 g/day ↑ the risk.
-   Mechanism:
    1. Ethanol ↓ bicarbonate, ↓ trypsin inhibitor.
    2. By ethanol metabolic toxins.
    3. Spasm of sphincter of Oddi.
    4. Ethanol increase duct permeability → prematurely activated enzyme → damage.
    5. Ethanol increases protein in pancreatic juice → obstruction.

Iatrogenic
-   Pancreatic biopsy, exploration of biliary tree, distal gastrectomy, cardiopulmonary bypass, and ERCP.

Hereditary Pancreatitis
-   Autosomal dominant → mutation of cationic trypsinogen gene (PRSS1).

    → Activation of trypsinogen to trypsin → abnormal duct secretion → pancreatitis.
-   Mutation of SPINK1 also referred as pancreatic secretory trypsin inhibitor (PSTI)→ blocks active-binding site of trypsin, so mutant enzyme → activate acinar cells → destructs first line of defense, trypsin inhibitor → proteolytic.

Tumor
-   Pancreatic or periampullary tumor.
-   1%–2% with acute pancreatitis → have underlying tumor.

Hyperlipidemia
-   Type I and V hyperlipoproteinemia → abdominal pain associated with marked hypertriglyceridemia.

- Lipase liberates toxic fatty acid into pancreatic microcirculation → impairment and ischemia.
- Managed by dietary modification to restrict triglycerides, clofibrate.

Drug and Miscellaneous Causes
- Many drugs produced hyperamylasemia and/or abdominal pain: thiazide, furosemide, estrogen, mercaptopurine, methyldopa, valproic acid, acetylcholinesterase inhibitor, lipid base IV, propofol.
- High Ca^{++} such as HPT → formation of calcified stone intraductally.
- Infestation, ascaris → cholangitis.
- Azotemia, vasculitis.
- Scorpion venom.
- Idiopathic.

Pathophysiology
- Activation of digestive enzyme inside acinar cells → acinar cells injury → inflammatory cells activation → release of cytokines and chemical mediator.

Precipitating Initial Events
- Acinar Cell Events
  Key roles of trypsin activation (protective mechanism):
  1. Enzyme synthesis in inactive precursor called zymogen.
     → Transported and secreted outside the gland → normally activation in duodenum (enterokinase).
  2. Digestive enzyme surrounded by cytoplasm (zymogen granules).
  3. Trypsin inhibitor.
     - Inhibitor of acinar secretion → activation of trypsinogen → zymogene is not secreted outside → cytoplasm contains vacuoles (lysosomal enzymes) such as cathepsin B → activation of trypsinogen → ↑ cytosolic Ca^{++}.

- Pre-ERCP infusion of Mg^{++} → natural antagonist of Ca^{++}, lower risk of ERCP pancreatitis.
- Cathepsin → cytochrome C → cell death (apoptosis).

- Intrapancreatic Events
  - Activate neutrophils and proteolytic enzymes (cathepsin, elastase).
  - Macrophage release (TNF-α, IL-1, IL-6, IL-8) → local and systemic inflammatory response.
    - → ↑ vascular permeability → edema, hemorrhage, microthrombi, fluid around pancreas.
  - Failure of microcirculation (severe acute pain) → hypoperfusion and necrosis.
  - Without necrosis → interstitial edematous pancreatitis.

- Systemic Events
  - Systemic inflammation and multiple organ failures (MOF).
  - Pro-inflammatory mediators increase, such as TNF-α, IL-1, IL-2, IL-6, and chemokines, as well as anti-inflammatory.
  - MOF with overwhelming pro-inflammatory response.
  - ↓ suppression immunity in response to inflammatory response → infected pancreatic necrosis → third to fourth week.
  - SIRS, MOF.
  - Organ failure score using Marshall or SOFA → mostly CVS, respiratory, renal.
  - MOF is defined as two or more points on score system.

Clinical Picture
- General consideration
- Incidence, 13–45:100,000.
- Mild, moderate, severe, or critical.

- Needs hospitalization.
- The recovery for mild is less than a week.
- Severe—weeks to months of intensive treatment.
- MR of mild is 1%, moderate, 10%; severe, 20%–40%; critical, 50%.
- Recurrence, 20%–30%.
- Chronic pancreatitis, 10%.
- Scoring system: Ranson, modified Glasgow criteria, modified Marshall, APACHE II, and BISAP.

Diagnosis
- 2–3 criteria to diagnose.
  - → Clinical: upper abdominal pain (acute onset), epigastrium radiates to mid back.
  - → Laboratory: amylase > 3 times.
  - → Radiology: US, CT, MRI.
- Amylase increases after several hours and remains for 3–5 days.
  Causes of hyperamylasemia are acute pancreatitis (AP), small bowel obstruction, perforated duodenal ulcer, fractures, intra-abdominal inflammation, i.e., not specific.
- Urinary clearance is higher during AP → so do urine amylase diagnostic and remain several days after normalized serum amylase.
- Severe disease → intravascular fluid loss → sequestration in retroperitoneum → hematocrit.
- 1% bleeding from necrotizing pancreatitis → bluish discoloration of the umbilicus (Cullen's sign) or flank Grey-Turner sign.
- Fluid loss → prerenal azotemia, BUN, creatinine.
- Hypoalbuminemia, low Ca^{++}, hyperglycemia.
- Routinely and early CT should be avoided unless uncertain diagnosis → indicated if same abdominal pain when hollow viscus perforation is suspected.
- Optimal initial CT between 72–96 hrs as the extent of pancreatic and peripancreatic necrosis become apparent at 72 hrs.
- Follow-up CT if clinical deterioration or failure of treatment, but no routine follow-up.

Stratification and Scoring

- Ranson, modified Glasgow criteria, APACHE II, or BISAP → most recent.
- Ranson and Glasgow for the first 48 hrs, 3 pts or more → severe.
- APACHE, 8 pts or more or CRP > 150 mg/dL for the first 24 hrs.
- BISAP: BUN > 25, GCS < 15, SIRS, age > 60, and pleural effusion for the first 24 hrs.
- Accuracy of these scales is 70%.

- **Ranson Scoring**

Ranson (alcoholic or other)	Ranson (biliary)
At admission	At admission
Age > 55 Y	Age > 70
GB > 16000/mm3	GB > 18000/mm3
LDH >350	LDH > 250
AST< 250	AST > 250
Glycaemia < 200 mg /dl	Glycaemia > 220 mg /dl
In 48 h	In 48 h
Drop in hematocrit > 10 %	Drop in hematocrit > 10%
BUN increase > 5 mg /dl	BUN increase > 2 mg /dl
Calcium > mg /dl 8	Calcium > mg /dl 8
PO2 < 60 mmHg	PO2< 60 mmHg
Bases deficit > 4 mEq/L	Bases deficit > 5 mEq\L
Fluid lose > 6 L	Fluid lose > 4 L
Each item worth 1 point (0-11 point)	

- **Atlanta Classification (According to 2012 Revision)**
  - Mild: no MOF, no local or systemic complications.
  - Moderate: MOF resolved within 48 hrs or local and systemic complication without persistent MOF.
  - Severe: persistent MOF > 48 hrs, single intervention.

- **Modified Marshall Scoring System**
  - Elements: PaO_2, FiO_2, creatinine, SBP.

- **Balthazar (CT scan) Severity Index**
  Grade
  A   Normal
  B   Pancreatic enlargement (edema)
  C   Pancreatic inflammation, peripancreatic fat
  D   Single fluid collection
  E   Two or more fluid collection or retroperitoneal air

Determining of etiology
- Alcohol ingestion (blood ethanol level).
- Gallbladder stone (US), ALP, ALT, amylase.
- If all are absent → drug, trauma, ERCP, infection, serum TG and Ca^{++}.

Initial Management
- **Resuscitation**
  - Initial aggressive resuscitation is required → because of hypovolemia from vomiting, poor oral intake, high respiratory losses, diaphoresis, edema.
  - 10–20 mL/kg/hr for the first 24–48 hrs, continuous infusion.
  - But if overload → pulmonary edema, ARDS, ACS.
  - RL is the fluid of choice.
  - If patient is in shock → fluid + vasopressor.
  - Pancreatitis: pancreatic edema and microangiopathy ↓ blood flow → cellular death → release of enzyme → ↑ inflammation, ↑ vascular permeability edema.
  - Marker from resuscitation: hct, BUN, creatinine.
  - Therapy directed: CVP, PAWP, SvO_2, lactate, hourly UOP.
    → As per surviving sepsis campaign: SvO_2 above 65% correlates with adequate tissue perfusion.

- **Antibiotic**
  - No role for antibiotic in acute pancreatitis or necrotic pancreatitis to prevent infection, i.e., no prophylactic antibiotic.
  - If pancreatitis + active infection → such as cholangitis, UTI, pneumonia or infected pancreatic necrosis → broad spectrum antibiotics + antifungal and C/S.

- **Pain management:**
  - Better if IV paracetamol, NSAIDs, meperidine.
  - Morphine is avoided as S/E will produce sphincter of Oddi spasms while glucagon will relax sphincter of Oddi.

- **Nutrition**
  - Mild pancreatitis → enteral feeding should be initiated → fat-free.
  - Severe → controversy on the time of initiation, but it should be before TPN → TPN increases morbidity and mortality, but enteral feeding prevents bowel mucosa atrophy and bacterial translocation.
  - NGT or NJT feeding is considered if not tolerated orally.

- **ERCP**
  - ERCP should be avoided unless biliary obstruction.
  - If symptomatic and biochemical abnormality → MRCP.
  - If cholangitis or gallstone → ERCP within 24 hrs from admission.
  - If bleeding → CT angiography or CT with arterial phase.

- **Surgical Management**
  - Historically, pancreatic necrosectomy for necrotizing pancreas.
  - Now, surgery is reserved for infected pancreatic necrosis or gastric outlet obstruction, bile duct obstruction.
  - Infected necrosis can be diagnosed by FNA at the time of planned procedure i.e. no routine FNA.
    → or by CT: gas pocket around the pancreas.
  - Antibiotic with good pancreatic penetration → carbapenem.
  - If antibiotic fails to resolve symptom, such intra-abdominal pathology, abdominal compartment syndrome or clinical instability → (step-up approach) → percutaneous drainage for exchange irrigation or endoscopic transluminal drainage or video-assisted retroperitoneal debridement through flank incision.
  - Laparoscopic or open necrosectomy if previous modality failed.

Management of Pancreatic Necrosis
- Usually, pancreatic necrosis is self-limited.
- 20% with complication.
- 5%–10% peripancreatic necrosis, and mortality rate is 15%.
- ⅓ of necrosis → infection.
- Traditionally, infected pancreatic necrosis → urgent OR, but it has been abandoned and replaced by minimally invasive.
- Sequelae of acute pancreatitis.
  - o Interstitial edematous pancreatitis.
  - o Acute peripancreatic fluid collection (APFC) < 4 weeks.
  - o Pancreatic pseudocyst (PP) > 4 weeks.
  - o Necrotizing pancreatitis.
  - o Acute necrotic collection (ANC) if gas, indicates infection.
  - o Walled-off pancreatic necrosis (WOPN) if gas indicates infection.

Initial Treatment and Role of Antibiotic
- Necrotizing pancreatitis has ↑ mortality because of MOF and infection.
- ↓ SIRS by ↑ fluid resuscitation in first 24 hrs.
- Enteral nutrition within 48 hrs → decreased infection.
- Routine prophylaxis antibiotic for severe acute pancreatitis or sterile necrosis is not recommended → ↑ resistance of bacteria and fungi.
- Selective gut decontamination showing ↑ outcome in animal.
- use of probiotics is prohibited as no effect to infection → not recommended.

Therapeutic Intervention
- Early intervention in first 2 weeks, ↑ mortality.
- Open necrosectomy in the first 1–2 weeks, 75% mortality vs. 45% if intervention done at 14–29 days.
- Delayed intervention (operative) beyond 4 weeks, ↓ mortality.
- In 2010, Dutch RCT → compare open necrosectomy vs. step-up approach starting with percuatanous drainage catheter, followed by VARD, laparoscopic or open necrosectomy as needed → avoid surgery by 35% and mortality rate is 19%.
- Time of intervention, ideally 4–6 weeks.

- Indication for radiological, endoscopic or surgical intervention if documented infected necrotic pancreatitis + clinical deterioration.
- Asymptomatic WON is not an indication for intervention.
- If patient with infected necrotizing pancreatitis → with stable vital signs → only antibiotic is recommended.

Choices of Therapeutic Intervention in Necrotizing Pancreatitis
- Initial image-guided percutaneous catheter drainage or endoscopic transluminal drainage followed by endoscopic, laparoscopic or open surgical intervention if needed.

- **Percutaneous Drainage**
    - If liquefied necrosis.
    - Temporization in early phase of infected necrosis till definitive approach.
    - Feasible in 95% of patients.
    - The need of surgery, 23%–50%.
    - If failed → endoscopic, MIS or open intervention.

- **Endoscopic Drainage and Debridement**
    - Identify bulging in posterior stomach or duodenum.
    - EUS is recommended to be used.
    - Can use nasocystic tube for irrigation.
    - Place large bore pigtail.
    - Combined percutaneous and endoscopy ↓ fistula and surgical need.

- **Laparoscopy and VARD**
    - Laparoscopy ↓ systemic complication and MOF.

- **Open Pancreatic Necrosectomy**
    - High morbidity, 34%–95%, and mortality, 6%–25%.
    - Laparotomy or retroperitoneal flank incision.
    - Open approach if clinical deterioration and failure of minimal invasive procedure or if another pathology → such as perforation, hemorrhage.
    - After open necrosectomy:
        1. Open packing

2. Closed packing
3. Postoperative continuous lavage

Complications of Acute Pancreatitis
I. Local
    - Pancreatic
            Phlegmon, abscess, pseudocyst, ascites, infected necrosis, chronic pancreatitis.
II. Systemic
    - Pulmonary
            Pneumonia, atelectasis, ARDS, pleural effusion
    - CVS
            Hypotension, hypovolemia, sudden death, ST wave changes, pericardial effusion
    - Hematological
            Hemoconcentration, DIC
    - Gastrointestinal
            Hemorrhage, peptic ulcer, erosive gastritis, portal or splenic vein thrombosis
    - Renal
            Oliguria, azotemia, renal A/V thrombosis
    - Metabolic
            Hyperglycemia, ↓ Ca^{++}, high TG, encephalopathy, sudden blindness (Purtscher retinopathy)
    - CNS
            Psychosis, fat embolism, alcohol withdrawal
    - Fat necrosis
            Intra-abdominal saponification, subcutaneous tissue necrosis

Pancreatic Pseudocyst (PP)
- Chronic collection of pancreatic juice surrounded by nonepithelial wall of granulation tissue and fibrosis.
- Pancreatic duct leak → 3–4 weeks → sealed by an inflammatory reaction leading to development of wall of granulation and fibrosis → (acute pseudocyst) may resolve in 50% spontaneously.
- Occur in 10% of acute and 20%–38% of chronic pancreatitis.
- Most common complications are fluid collection and infection.
- Once fluid collection persists > 4 weeks → PP.

- If pseudocyst > 6 cm → will not resolve spontaneously.
- If post-necrotic peripancreatic fluid collection (PNFC) persists > 4 weeks → WOPN.
- 20%–30% drainage by IR is not sufficient.
- Difficult to distinguish PP from cystic neoplasm such as IPMN → 40% present with acute pancreatitis is later diagnosed with malignancy.
- Chronic pseudocyst lasts for > 6 weeks.
- Can be multiple in 17% or multilobulated.
- If incidentally → aspiration for cytology and C/S.

Pathophysiology
- PP and WOPN is composed of pancreatic juice with pancreatic debris and inflammatory cells such as cytokines and fibroblast.
- Most of PP and WOPN have communication between ductal system
  → Need ERCP, MRCP
- Pancreas over spine (watershed) → the duct disruption happened here.
- WOPN is a thicker wall than peripancreatic and grows out of initial necrotic material.
- Location: lesser sac pleural space, over kidneys, subhepatic in spleen.

Presentation
- Either after acute pancreatitis (AP) or trauma.
- 50% will increase amylase.
- Sign of fullness, gastric or intestinal obstruction.
- Early satiety or even not tolerated orally.
- Complications: obstruction, inferior rupture, hemorrhage, fistula.
- Pancreatic ascites from peripancreatic rupture.
- Infected peripancreatic → pancreatic abscess → higher mortality and morbidity require urgent intervention.
- Can cause compression and obstruction to adjacent organ → SMV, PV, SP thrombosis, and pseudoaneurysm.
- If perforated → peritonitis → urgent intervention.
- Hemorrhage → embolization (splenic artery).

Diagnostic Evaluation

- Amylase is high in 50%.
- Cystic neoplasm must be excluded.
- If patient is admitted actively as AP and CT shows → fully mature cyst → IPMN rather than peripancreatic fluid.
- CT: peripancreatic is rounded; debris is rare.
- No need to repeat CT sooner than 4 weeks, but if WOPN → repeat sooner.
- If clinical deterioration → CT-guided drainage of necrosis and C/S.
- If renal impairment → MRCS, EUS.
- Some advocate ERCP, and main pancreatic duct (MPD) stent may serve as a definitive management of PP.
- EUS → if mural nodules → IPMN → CEA is higher and mucicarmine stain is +ve.
- Regarding main pancreatic duct → MRCP to assess duct and can infuse secretin to increase pancreatic juice → dilation of duct.

Complications

o infection, rupture, bleeding.

Management

- Majority will resolve spontaneously.
- Intervention can be considered in 4–6 weeks.
- Defect on MPD disruption:

  Type I   Normal duct
  Type II   Stricture
  Type III   Complete disruption
  Type IV   Chronic pancreatitis

- PP type I

  → No intervention, all non-surgical intervention.

- PP type II

  - None surgical followed by surgical if failed (failure rate is 25%).
  - ERCP → transpapillary stent can be directed to fistula site.

- Percutaneous or endoscopy transluminal (gastric or duodenal) → cystogastrostomy or cystoduodenostomy.
- Cystogastrostomy has higher complication (hemorrhage) than cystojejunostomy.

- PP type III
    - Usually requires surgical intervention.
    - Mid-body disruption is the most common site.
    - Starts with percutaneous drain.
    - Three strategies:
        1. Roux-en-Y cystenterostomy
        2. Roux-en-Y Lateral Pancreaticojejunostomy.
        3. Distal pancreatectomy + splenectomy
    - Distal pancreatectomy + splenectomy is the worst and considered if recurrent, septic patient.
    - As β cell in tail of pancreas → insulin dependence is 50%.
    - Roux-en-Y cystenterostomy → recurrent AP + pain not resolved → not recommended.
    - Roux-en-Y LPJ is the best.
        → Palpate duct (often dilated) → Puestow procedure (absorbable monofilament).

- PP with chronic pancreatitis
    - Cystojejunostomy + Puestow procedure.

- WOPN
    - Avoid drainage to stomach.
    - Reoperation for debridement, 10%.
    - Always start with percutaneous drain and leave for 7 days to mature tract → grid wire to access pathology.

Management of Gallstone Pancreatitis
Clinical Presentation
- Abdominal pain (midepigastric) radiating to back, nausea and vomiting, decrease oral intake.
- Fever, jaundice, alcholic stool, dark urine → CBD stone and/or acute cholangitis.
- DDx: acute cholecystitis, PUD.

- Diagnosis is confirmed by amylase, lipase, ↑ threefold → serum concentration does not predict severity.
- If patient is hypotensive or has tachycardia → ICU.
- Multidisciplinary: surgeon, ICU, gastroenterologist, IR.
- Ranson or APACHE > 7 → ICU.
- 20% progress to severe → mortality rate is 30%.

Disease Severity

- Mild, moderate, severe according to pancreatic morphology ± MOF ± local and systemic complications.
- Morphology by CT:
    1. Acute edematous change in parenchyma
    2. Acute peripancreatic fluid collection (APFC).
    3. Acute necrotic collection (ANC).
- Organ failure: respiratory, renal, CVS.
- 2012 revised Atlanta classification of acute pancreatitis.
- Local complications: APFC, ANC, PP, WOPN.
- APFC: acute peripancreatic fluid collection.
- ANC: collection + necrosis.
- PP: pseudocyst, encapsulated homogeneous enzymes rich, mature at 4 weeks.
- WOPN: mature encapsulated collection of necrosis > 4 weeks.

Management

- Ranges from straightforward to complex.

- **Mild Gallstone Pancreatitis**
    - Abdominal pain, nausea and vomiting, high amylase, lipase, high bilirubin, AP, high ALT for 24–48 hrs.
    - US to confirm gallstone disease and to exclude biliary dilation > 11 mm.
    - CT is not indicated.
    - Resuscitation, maintenance targeted to UOP, HR, BP.
    - Enteral feeding within 24 hrs.
    - If symptoms include nausea and vomiting → NGT.
    - Avoid opioid → spasm of sphincter of Oddi.
    - No prophylactic antibiotic.
    - If cholangitis → ERCP + endoscopic stent.

- Laparoscopic cholecystectomy and IOC at the same admission as complication at the same admission, 5%, and with interval cholecystectomy, 17%.
- Management for CBD intraoperative:
    1. Watchful waiting
    2. Laparoscopic CBD exploration
    3. Post-operative ERCP

- **Moderate Gallstone Pancreatitis**
    - Persistent abdominal pain, fever, high WBCs, persistent high enzyme.
    - Transient MOF, high BUN, high creatinine.
    - If symptom persists more than 3 days → CT.
    - Patient with high bilirubin > 4 → biliary obstruction → MRCP.
    - Fluid resuscitation.
    - UOP, 0.5–1 mL/kg/hr → BUN can measure fluid status.
    - Usually edematous pancreas with APFC.
    - ↑ LFT → MRCP or ERCP ± sphincterotomy.
    - Most patients will have laparoscopic cholecystectomy + intraoperative cholangiogram at the same admission.
    - If sterile necrotic pancreatitis → will take time.
    - Follow-up CT is recommended.
    - Hospital stay is depending on oral intake, usually 7–10 days.

- **Severe Gallstone Pancreatitis**
    - Resuscitation is cornerstone.
    - SIRS → ICU and possible intubation.
    - One or multiple organ failure (MOF).
    - Abdominal compartment syndrome may require step up approach.
    - Renal failure → HD.
    - Critically ill because of cytokines ↑in 1–2 weeks, so the goals are as follows:
        1. O_2 delivery by MV
        2. Adequate resuscitation with RL
        3. Inotropes
        4. Maintain renal function
        5. Nutrition support (enteral), NG or NJ.

- Feeding ASAP, ↓ infection in pancreatic necrosis.
- Antibiotic if associated cholangitis, but prophylaxis for necrotic pancreatitis has not been shown to prevent the infection.
- Octreotide is controversial.
- US if gallstone and high LFT → MRCP or ERCP.
  - → If acute cholangitis → ERCP + endoscopic sphincterotomy (ES).
- Meta-analysis → early ERCP + endoscopic sphincterotomy ± stent vs. conservative → with intervention, ↓ complication rate.
- ERCP + endoscopic sphincterotomy (ES) in severe necrotic pancreatitis is not indicated.
- Unlike mild pancreatitis, in severe → cholecystectomy should be avoided.

Gallstone Pancreatitis in Pregnant Patient

- Diagnosis is similar to nonpregnancy.
- US., MRCP is better than CT or ERCP.
- Pancreatitis may lead to preterm labor. First trimester has highest chance of fetal loss.
- Cholecystectomy can be in all terms but safest in second trimester.
- ERCP is possible but with risk of radiation.
- Reasonable approach
  - First trimester: conservative treatment + laparoscopic cholecystectomy in second trimester ± ERCP.
  - Second trimester: laparoscopic cholecystectomy ± ERCP.
  - Third trimester: conservative treatment ± ERCP and laparoscopic cholecystectomy in early postpartum.
  - Maneuver such as left lateral decubitus, low pressure for insufflation, should be considered.

Pancreatic Divisum

- Recurrent pancreatitis, chronic pancreatitis associated with dominant dorsal duct anatomy → divisum results in obstructive pancreatopathy.
- Common in left-handed patient.

- Can be two separate ducts or absent of major duct (only Santorini duct is present).
- In brief, dorsal duct (Santorini) is a dominant duct with varieties: complete/incomplete.
- Acquired (with chronic and malignancy) → pseudodivisum → CT, MRCP, EUS to rule malignancy.
- Common in patient with gene mutation CFTR and SPIM1, PRSS1.

Variation of Pancreatic Divisum
1. Normal pancreas with no duct of Santorini
2. Normal pancreas with duct of Santorini
3. Pancreatic divisum with small duct of Wirsung
4. Pancreatic divisum with no duct of Wirsung

Diagnosis
- Acute recurrent pancreatitis (presentation).
- Usually epigastric pain (intractable to medical treatment) radiating to the back.
- ↑ lipase, ↑ WBCs.
- CT, MRI.
- Usually self-limiting, one-week duration.
- Helpful hypothesis recommended: endoscopic minor duct sphincterotomy to do as follows:
    1. Eliminate future episode of acute pain.
    2. ↓ frequency and severity of acute pain.
    3. Prevent development of chronic disease.
- Indication of surgery is pain → rarely biliary, duodenal splanchnic vein obstruction, and pancreatic insufficiency.
- MRI, EUS.

NB: If you cut scar tissue, you get more scar tissue. If you operate for pain, you get pain.

Endoscopic Treatment
- Generally, endoscopic therapy if duct is dilated or has recurrent acute pain.

- **Identify Minor Papilla**
  - 2–5 cm superior to major papilla but slightly lateral, sometimes under duodenal fold.
  - If blind probing → edema/ false tracts.
  - Can use dye.
  - IV secretin of 0.2 ug/kg IV to stimulate pancreatic juice.

- **Cannulation**
  - Sphincterotome, 3F or 4F.

- **Minor Endoscopic Sphincterotomy**
  - ➢ **Pancreatitis prevention**
    - In the past → use stent.
    - Rectal indomethacin (100 mg) decreases post-ERCP pancreatitis.
      - → Administer pre- or intra- or postprocedure.
      - → No need for stent.

  - ➢ **Postprocedure management**
    - Discharge after 1–2 hrs.
    - Common complications: pain, nausea.
    - 10%–15% need 1 day observation → majority will improve within 72 hrs.
    - Mortality rate is 1%–2%.

Surgical Treatment
  - Operative sphincteroplasty was mainstay before endoscopy.
  - Spare smooth muscle of surrounding duct.
  - Surgery before endoscopic intervention is the best.
  - Laparoscopic gastrotomy and endoscopy prograde sphincterotomy.
  - If patient with prior surgery (gastric bypass) → hybrid procedure.

- **Technique**
  - After ERCP or MRCP.
  - Abdomen entered through upper midline.
  - Falciform divided and retracted.

- Mobilization of colon (hepatic flexure).
- Kocherization of the duodenum to midline.
- Longitudinal duodenotomy in descending duodenum.
- Stay suture 3-0 silk.
- Major papilla identified by the squeezing of CBD manually.
- Minor papilla palpated and cannulated by lacrimal probe. If can't be done → secretin IV (↑ risk of post-operative pancreatitis) → sphincterotomy, then interrupted suture 5-0 monofilament (sphincteroplasty)

- **Drainage Procedure**
  Lateral pancreaticojejunostomy (LPJ), Puestow

- **Resection Procedure (Beger and Whipple)**
  - If patient is with pancreatic divisum fail sphincteroplasty, chronic pancreatitis and change in head of pancreatic tissue.
  - Internal and external stenting and post-operative octreotide, decrease leak and fistula.
  - Islet is more in body and tail; in the head, not much for that. Resection of head, no need for TPX.

Management Strategies of Pancreatic Divisum
- Non-familial dilated duct > 7 mm → LPJ.
- Familial dilated duct > 7 mm → total pancreatectomy+ TPx.
- Non-dilated duct and recent acute pancreatitis → endoscopic minor papillotomy.
- Non-dilated duct and endoscopic papillotomy failure → operative sphincteroplasty.
- Non-dilated duct and op. sphincteroplasty failure → pancreaticoduodenectomy.
- Pancreaticoduodenectomy failure → total pancreatectomy + TPx.

Annular pancreas
- A band of normal pancrearic tissue encircle the duodenum compeletly or partially

- Usually presented at neonatal period as duodenal obstruction (double bubble)
- Treatment: duodenojejunostomy.

Chronic Pancreatitis
Definition, Incidence, Prevalence
- Definition: progressive destruction of normal pancreatitis with loss of its endocrine and exocrine functions and healed by fibrosis, duct ectasia, acinar, atrophy.
- By autopsy, 5% of General population.
- 5–40 per 100,000.

Etiology
- Genetic mutation.
- Alcohol.
- Duct obstruction by trauma, stone.
- Metabolic: hyperlipidemia.
- Autoimmune.
- Nutrition: tropical pancreatitis → ingestion of certain starch.
- Idiopathic.

Genetic Cause
- Familial pattern of chronic non-alcoholic pancreatitis.
- Starts at childhood or adolescence by experiencing abdominal pain → chronic calcific pancreatitis → progressive pancreatic dysfunction is common.
- Symptom because of duct obstruction.
- ↑ risk of CA ≈ 40% > 50 years.
- Autosomal dominant.
- 7q35, 8 trypsinogen gene.
- Mutation position 117 of PRSS1 → ($\frac{2}{3}$, i.e., 70%).
- Additional mutation: R122H and N291 mutation of PRSS1.
- Recently, PRSS2 and SPINK (23% tropical pancreatitis) → inhibit trypsin action.
- Cystic fibrosis transmembrane receptor (CFTR) → which controls amount of chloride and bicarbonate and usually associated with classic pulmonary disease.
- CLDN2 abnormal expressed in acinar cells and may alter the secretory dynamic of enzyme.

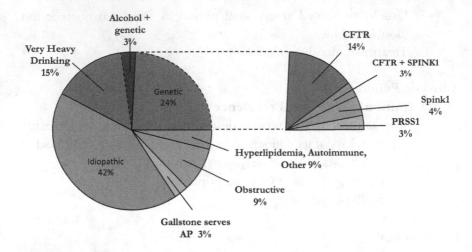

Alcohol

- Exposure to 1–20 g/day.
- CLDN2 gene.
- Higher if heavy drink, > 150 g/day, 5%–15%.
- Between 35–40 years and after 16–20 years.
- Recurrent acute pancreatitis → after 4–5 years, will convert to chronic.
- Alcohol metabolite: acetaldehyde + oxidant injury.
- Repeated severe episode → toxin → activate cascade of cytokines → collagen deposit and fibrosis.
- Interfere with intracellular transport and discharge of digestive enzyme, ↓ bicarbonate, low volume of secretion output.
- Ca^{++} complexes to protein plugs in small ductal system.
- Smoking associated with ↑ risk of chronic pancreatitis.

Hyperparathyroidism

- By ↑ Ca^{++} → ↑ calculus formation and obstruction.

Autoimmune Pancreatitis

- Treated with steroid medically.
- Appearance: mass like.
- Two types:
    1. Lymphoplasmacytic with no granulocyte epithelial lesion (GEL).
    2. Idiopathic with GEL.

- Symptoms: jaundice, pain (pancreatitis), some (minor) had constitutional symptom.
- Image: CT, ERCP, MRCP—hypoenhancing lesion involves whole pancreas, sausage-like.
- Diagnosis confirmed by serology IgG4, 70%.
- Or histologically, by EUS and FNA or US-guided Bx.
- Mayo Clinic diagnosis of AIP:
  1. Histology is characteristic.
  2. High IgG4.
  3. Responds to steroid.
- Treatment:
  - High dose of steroid, 1 mg/kg, then CA 19-9 after 2 weeks of treatment.
  - Another treatment is by Imuran.
  - if failed medical Tx → surgical inteevention

Hyperlipidemia
- Hyperlipidemia and hypertriglyceridemia predispose women to chronic pancreatitis when they receive estrogen replacement therapy.
- Fasting triglyceride levels < 300 mg/dL.

Classification
- TIGAR-O scheme for risk factor.

- Recent classification based on histopathology and etiology by Singer-Chari:
  o Chronic calcific (lithogenic)
  o Chronic obstructive
  o Chronic inflammatory
  o Chronic autoimmune inflammatory
  o Asymptomatic fibrosis

1. Chronic Calcific (Lithogenic) Pancreatitis
- Largest subgroup.
- Majority of patients have history of stone and alcohol.
- Subgroup: hereditary pancreatitis, tropical pancreatitis.

2. **Chronic Obstructive Pancreatitis**
   - Compression, obstructive in proximal duct by gallbladder stone, trauma scar, inadequate duct caliber (pancreatic divisum).
   - Obstruction of main duct (trauma or neoplasma): divisum, IPMN, ductal adenocarcinoma.
   - Fibrosis → dilation of main and secondary duct → acinar atrophy.
   - Trauma → duct leak → pseudocyst → stricture.
   - 10% of children → failure of duct of Santorini to join major (Wirsung) duct.

   Treatment
   - ➤ Temporary stent to relief symptoms.
   - ➤ Permanent surgical or endoscopy will be successful.
   - ➤ Disease high in patient with PRSS1, SPINK1, and CFTR (47%).

3. **Chronic Inflammatory Pancreatitis**
   - Diffuse fibrosis and loss of acinar element with mononuclear infiltration.
   - If diffuse infiltration by lymphocyte, plasma cells, eosinophilic cells → autoimmune pancreatitis such as Sjogren's syndrome, RA and DM I, and SLE.
   - Can present with jaundice.
   - ↑ β-globulin, IgG4.
   - Associated with CFTR.
   - DDx: lymphoma, plasmacytoma, and CA.
   - Diagnosis by biopsy.
   - Treatment: steroid.

4. **Tropical (Nutritional) Pancreatitis**
   - Common in Indonesia, India.
   - Intraductal calcifications and stone formation.
   - Protein calories malnutrition, usually due to excess starch.
   - Associated with SPINK1 mutation by 20%–55%, SFTR.

5. **Asymptomatic Pancreatic Fibrosis**
   - Elderly, tropical, alcohol.
   - Perilobar fibrosis and loss of acinar mass.
   - Cystic fibrosis.

6. **Idiopathic Pancreatitis**→ if no cause.

Pathology

- Histology
  - Early: induration nodular scarring and lobular region of fibrosis.
  - Late: loss of normal lobulation with thicker sheets of fibrosis.
  - Duct: dysplasia as cuboidal cells with hyperplastic feature + area of mononuclear cell infiltrate and area of necrosis.
  - Cystic changes may be seen.
  - In severe: broad fibrosis, ↓ islet size, small arteries appear thicker.
  - Tropical and hereditary pancreatitis are indistinguishable from alcoholic.

- Fibrosis
  - Common feature of all types.
  - Pathogenesis: activation of pancreatic stellate cells found in acini and small artery responded to pancreatic injury → loses lipid vesicles; transforms into myofibroblast →
    ↑ factors such as TGF, PDGF, and pro-inflammatory cytokines and synthesis; and secretes collagen I and II.
  - Alcohol → acute pancreatitis → ongoing exposure → fibrosis → chronicity.

- Stone Formation
  - Protein produces regular gene.
  - The protein present in all mammals (pancreas and brain).
  - Ca^{++} bicarbonate is normally present in pancreatic juice.
  - But if ↑ production → stone.
  - Lithostathine potent inhibitor of Ca^{++} carbonate and crystal formation.
  - In alcoholic, ↓ lithostathine.
  - Administer lithostathine in early stage → effective.

- Duct Distortion
  - Although calcific stone disease is a marker of advanced diagnosis, ductal calcification does not always correlate with symptom.
  - If stone developed → endoscopy or surgical removal.
  - Usually in patient with obstruction and duct hypertension.

Presentation and Natural History

- Pain is the most common in midepigastric, but it can be RUQ, LUQ, and in mid-abdomen radiation to back. Steady, boring, but not colicky for hours or days.
- Exocrine insufficiency is 40%–50% → characterized by steatorrhea and loose, fatty, malodorous stool.
- Can be exacerbated with alcohol.
- Patient typically flexes or lies on hips or lies on side in fetal position.
- Anorexia is the more common symptom, but there's also nausea and vomiting.
- The causes of pain are the following:
  1. Ductal hypertension due to stricture or stone
  2. Chronic pain related to parenchymal disease or retroperitoneal inflammation
  3. Acute increase in duct pressure
- Pain can be relieved by decompression, depending on degree of fibrosis.
- John Hopkins → 35 patients experiencing pain were treated with local resection of pancreas, head and longitudinal pancreaticojejunostomy, or Frey.
  - 80% of fibrosis → pain relieved by 100%.
  - 10% of fibrosis → pain relieved by 60%.
- So if minimal fibrosis → no decompression surgery.
- The pain of chronic pancreatic ̄ when exocrine secretion decreases (burned-out pancreatitis).
- If no intervention → narcotic addiction.
- The cause of pain → inflammation damagea perirenal layer surrounding unmyelinated pancreatic nerves and infiltration of inflammatory cells.
- Strategies to relieve pain:
  1. ↓ secretion and/or decompression.
  2. Resection of focus pathology.

3. Interrupting transmission of affected normal impulse through neural ablative procedure.

- Malabsorption and Weight Loss
  - When pancreatic exocrine is below 10% → diarrhea and steatorrhea and often weight loss.
  - Stool is bulky, foul-smelling, pale, floats on toilet (oil slick).
  - ↓ food intake and malabsorption → weight loss.
  - Lipase ↓ before trypsin deficiency.
  - Diarrhea is the first sign of pancreatic insufficiency.
  - Low bicarbonate in duct → acidification → malabsorption.

- Pancreatogenic Diabetes Mellitus (DM III)
  - Islet is 2% of pancreatic mass.
  - In chronic pain, acini is replaced by fibrosis → loss of islet.
  - 20% of chronic pain—DM and impaired glucose metabolism, 70%.
  - Alcoholic chronic pancreatitis → DM is 83% and more than ½ required insulin.
  - Ketoacidosis and nephropathy are not common with pancreatogenic DM, but retinopathy and neuropathy are common.
  - Pancreatogenic DM is common after resection. For malignancy or benign, distal pancreatectomy and Whipple have ↑ incidence than drainage procedure and the worst after subtotal or total pancreatectomy.
  - Pancreatogenic or type 3 DM is seen in cystic fibrosis and hemochromatosis.
  - Occurs in all three glucoregulatory islet cells: insulin, glucagon, polypeptide (PP).
  - Hyperglycemia in spite of insulin → due to unsuppressed hepatic glucose production or hypoglycemia due to ↑ peripheral insulin sensitivity and ↓ glucagon → brittle diabetes.
  - PP deficiency correlates with severity of chronic pain.
  - Recent study continues infusion of PP with insulin → ↓ insulin requirement.

Laboratory Test
-   Blood test (amylase, lipase).
-   PP (test meal) strongly correlates with pancreatitis (endocrine).
-   Exocrine is measured by aspiration of pancreatic juice from duodenum after nutrient (lunch test meal) (direct).
-   Indirect tests of pancreatic exocrine → measurement of metabolic by serum or urine.
    > Serum: bentiromide.
    > Urine: para-aminobenzoic acid (PABA).
-   Fecal level of chymotrypsin and elastase correlates with loss of pancreas function. These methods ↓of sensitivity in mild to moderate cases.
-   Measurement of quantification of fat in stool.

Radiology
1. Diagnosis
2. Evaluation of severity
3. Detection of complication
4. Offer treatment option

-   Historically, x-ray was the gold standard—diffuse calcification of pancreatic parenchyma, sensitivity is 30%–40%.
-   US or EUS detects small lesion < 1 cm and is the initial diagnostic tool. Sensitivity is 48%–96%. EUS can diagnose CP in early stage.
-   CT: contour, content, duct pattern calcification, calculus, cystic disease. Sensitivity is 47%- 80%; specificity is 90%.
-   Campisi study: calcification 68% with chronic pancreatitis where NET is 13.6%; IPMN, 5.8%; serous cystadenoma, 3.9%; and pancreatic CA, 3.9%.
-   MRCP sensitivity is 75%, but in early stage, 25%.
-   ERCP is the most sensitive test (gold standard), 70%–100% sensitivity and specificity.
-   Advantages: Biopsy, cytology, stent to relieve obstruction.

Cambridge classification according to main and branch duct

Grade	Main Duct	Side Branch
Normal	Normal	Normal
Equivocal	Normal	< 3, abnormal
Mid	Normal	> 3, abnormal
Moderate	Abnormal	> 3, abnormal
Severe	Abnormal	> 3, abnormal

Complication
- **Diabetes Mellitus**
- **Pancreatic Pseudocyst**
- **Pancreatic Ascites**
  - Paracentesis or thoracentesis → non-infected protein level > 25 g/L, higher amylase.
  - Serum amylase can be high, ↓ albumin.
  - Antisecretory therapy somatostatin + NPO, TPN, successful in 50%.
  - ERCP and duct stent.
  - For pleural effusion → chest tube.
  - Surgery if failed medical treatment.
  - If leak from center → Roux-en-Y.
  - If leak in tail → distal pancreatectomy.

- **Pancreatic Enteric Fistula**
  - Erosion of pancreatic pseudocyst to adjacent hollow organs.
  - Most common site is transverse colon or splenic flexure.
  - Usually present with colonic bleeding and sepsis.
  - If communicating with stomach or duodenum → close spontaneously.
  - If colon → operative intervention is usually required.

- **Head of Pancreatic Mass**
  - 30% with advanced chronic pancreatitis → inflammatory mass will develop.
  - Pain, stenosis (duodenum), PV thrombosis.

- Mutation of polymorphism of P53 is found in these patient, and ductal CA is found in 3.7%.

- **Splenic and PV Thrombosis**
    - Infrequent, 4%–8%.
    - Variceal formation (PHTN).
    - Bleeding is infrequent.
    - Mortality is 20% when gastric varices.
    - Splenectomy if you already intra operative.

Treatment
Medical Treatment

- Analgesia
    - Oral as needed.
    - Pregabalin, 300 mg PO BID.
    - Narcotic (not morphine)
    - Stopping alcohol will relieve pain by 60%–70%.

- Enzyme Therapy
    - To reserve the effect of exocrine insufficiency.
    - To prevent metabolic bone disease and prevent ↓ KEDA vitamins.
    - To decrease pain.
    - Nonenteric coated enzyme + acid suppression.

- Antisecretory Therapy
    - Somatostatin inhibits pancreatic secretion and CCK.
    - 200 ug of octreotide acetate TID SC → pain relief is 65%.
    - Some studies show octreotide + TPN decreases pain.

- Neurolytic Therapy
    - Celiac plexus neurolysis with alcohol injection especially in patient with CA.
    - Safe but last for short period.

- Endoscopic Management
  - Treatment of pancreatic duct obstruction, stone disease, pseudocyst, duct leak, and diagnosis and treatment of CA.
  - Decompression of the duct.
  - Prolonged stent should be avoided as ↑ inflammation.
  - Patient with sphincter of Oddi dyskinesia has ↑risk of post-ERCP pancreatitis after sphincterotomy.
  - Leak with 37% of complication in acute pancreatitis → decrease by stent, also post-surgery leak or post-trauma.
  - Pancreatic divisum is a mechanical obstruction of dorsal duct; stent lowers pain by to 29% after stenting.
  - Idiopathic can be treated with stent (endoscopic) and sphincterotomy.
  - ESWL can be used in pancreatic stones together with stent. 80% relief of symptom.

Surgical Therapy

- Sphincteroplasty
  - Obstruction due to sclerosing papillitis and due to scarring from pancreatitis or by stone.
  - Permanent transduodenal sphincteroplasty.

- Drainage Procedure
  - Cattell: pancreaticojejunostomy for relieving pain in unresectable pancreatic cancer.
  - DuVal and Zollinger: described caudal Roux-en-Y pancreaticojejunostomy for chronic pancreatitis.
  - Puestow and Gillesby: longitudinal decompression of the body and tail (side to side).
  - Partington and Rochelle: longitudinal Roux-en-Y pancreaticojejunostomy (universally known as Puestow procedure).
  - Puestow procedure needs pancreatic duct diameter 6 mm → decompression is 75%–85%.

- Surgical management of pancreatic stone is superior to endoscopy.

- **Resection Procedure**
  - Distal Pancreatectomy
    - For patient, focal inflammatory change localized in body and tail.
    - 40%–80% of pancreatic bulk.
    - High risk of recurrence.
    - Long-term outcome for pain relief is 60%.
    - High risk of brittle DM, hypoglycemia, and coma.

  - Proximal Pancreatectomy (Whipple Procedure)
    - pancreaticoduodenectomy (+/− pylorus).
    - Treatment of chronic → pain relief by 71%–89%.
    - MR is 1.5%–3%.
    - 25%–48% → DM.

  - Total Pancreatectomy
    - Pain relief is not better than Whipple.
    - In absence of transplantation → life-threatening, i.e., severe hypoglycemic in severe pancreatic DM.

- **Hybrid Procedure**
  - Duodenum-preserving pancreatic head resection (DPPHR) (Beger procedure).
    - Pain relief, 91%; DM, 21%; MR, 1%.
    - In comparison to Whipple in one study, pain relief is 94% whereas in Whipple, 67%.
    - Required careful dissection of GDA.

  - Local resection of pancreatic head with longitudinal pancreaticojejunostomy (LR-LPJ) (Frey).
    - Decompression for all pancreatic ducts.
    - Pain relief is 87%.

- Preserve neck of pancreas, not like Whipple or DPPHR.
- There is modification (Hamburg modification) of LR-LPJ → extensive excavation of pancreatic head.

Complication
- LR-LPJ, 16%.
- Whipple, 40%.
- DPPHR, 25%.

Comparison between the Three Procedures
Whipple, Beger, and Frey
- Beger has lower stay, higher weight gain, lower DM, lower exocrine dysfunction, and pain is equal to Whipple.
- other study showed better outcome.
- Complication: Frey ± PPPD 19% ± 53%

Total Pancreatectomy with Islet Autotransplant (TPIAT)
- 2–3 million required to achieve insulin independence, but it can be 300,000–400,000.

Cystic Neoplasm of the Pancreas
- Most are benign.
- Some undergo malignant transformation → risk vs. benefit ratio, i.e., resection vs. observation.
- Radiological features: size, growth rate, density → wall: nodular, septation, calcification, and relation to pancreatic duct.
- Usually, history and radiological features can also lead to diagnosis, but EUS-guided FNA cytology or ERCP brush for worrisome feature.
- Cystic with thick fluid with mucin, high CEA with atypical cells → potentially malignant.

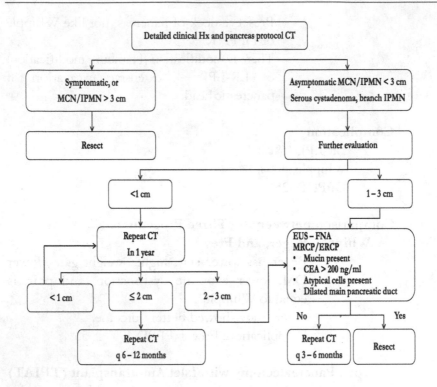

Serous Cystadenoma

- 1% of pancreatic lesion, ⅓ of cystic lesion.
- Most are asymptomatic but can cause complication such as obstruction, e.g., gastric outlet obstruction.
- Benign, true-lined epithelium, clean, glycogen-rich.
- Does not communicate with pancreatic duct.
- Thin wall capsule, thin septation.
- CT: well-circumscribed cystic mass, small septation, central scar + calcification, starburst (central scar), cluster of grapes, honeycomb appearance.
- Serous cystadenoma → benign → no risk of malignancy.
- Can show atypia, no intervention for it, but need follow up image.
- Serous cystadenocarcinoma is rare, < 1% → safe to observe.
- Rate of growth is 0.45 cm/year.
- FNA: contains serous fluid, clear → no stain with mucin and low CEA < 200.

- If conservative management is chosen → sure diagnosis → EUS-FNA, low CEA and amylase.
- If symptomatic, intervention is needed.
- Frequent in head of pancreas in male.
- Can be distinct from others as the other lesion has mucin and/or high CEA by FNA.

Mucinous Cystadenoma and Cystadenocarcinoma

- MCN spectrum ranging from benign but potentially malignant to CA with aggressive behavior.
- $2/3$ in body and tail; if in the head → mostly IPMN.
- Female: Male = 9:1.
- Common in perimenopause, usually incidentally.
- 2% of pancreatic neoplasm.
- $1/4$ of cystic neoplasm.
- Single large thick-walled, mucinous-secreting ovarian type: stroma within cyst capsule.
- 30%–50% → HGD or invasive CA.
- Never communicates with ductal system (distinguish) from IPMN.
- Symptoms: fullness, vague abdominal pain, early satiety, weight loss.
- Diagnosis by pancreatic protocol CT or MRI.
    - → Single, unilocular (more frequent), or smaller macrocytic with septation and calcification mimics chronic pseudocyst.
    - → Misdiagnosed → CT-guided drain → recurrence → so EUS + FNA is helpful, mucin-rich fluid, CEA > 200.
- The cyst lived by the tall columnar epithelium filled with viscous mucin.
- Pathology criteria to be malignant: (ovarian-like stroma) mural nodule, 5%–15% malignancy.
- Malignancy is common in large tumor and older patient (mutation of K-RAS, P53).
- The current thinking is that all MCN eventually evolve into CA if left untreated.
- Resection is the treatment of choice for most mucin-producing cystic tumor.

- Malignancy cannot be ruled out without resection or extensive sampling.
- Malignancy is 6%–36%.
- Malignant mucinous cysadenocarcinoma → deal as PD adenocarcinoma and should consider adjuvant therapy.
- Distal pancreatectomy as mostly located in body or tail.
- Small lesion → preserve spleen.
- Can use laparoscopy but do not rupture.

Intraductal Papillary Mucinous Neoplasm (IPMN)

- Duct epithelium → papillary projection and mucin production → dilation.
- 1%–3% of exocrine pancreatic neoplasm.
- 20%–50% of cystic pancreatic neoplasm.
- Diffuse or segmental involvement of main or major side branch duct.

Classification

1. Main duct (MD-IPMN)
2. Branch duct (BD-IPMN)
3. Mixed

- MD-IPMN: diffuse or segmental involvement of the main duct with dilatation of the duct > 5 mm → risk of dysplasia (CIS) is 35%–100%.
- BD-IPMN: side branch duct involvement is more common than MD-IPMN → 10:1.
  Occurs anywhere → low risk of malignancy transformation, 6%–45% or less → commonly observe.
- Mixed: like MD.

Histological Classification

- Previously classified as adenoma, borderline, CIS.
- Now mild to moderate high dysplasia.
- Four types: gastric, intestinal, pancreaticobiliary, oncocytic.
  1. Gastric: occurs in BD-IPMN and most common type overall.
     → Uncinate process, IHC: MUC5AC and 6AC.

2. Intestinal: second most common in MD-IPMN.
    → Villous growth, express MUC2–5AC.
    → 30%–50% developed invasive disease.
3. Pancreaticobiliary: main duct → 50% developed invasive disease.
4. Oncocyte: misdiagnosed with cyst cystadenocarcinoma.

Clinical Picture
-   Asymptomatic but can present nausea and vomiting, anorexia, abdominal and back pain.
-   Recurrent pancreatitis.
-   5%–10% steatorrhea, DM, weight loss → pancreatic insufficiency.

Diagnosis
-   History, physical examination, image, endoscopy.
-   CT, MRI: diffuse dilation of pancreatic duct and pancreatic parenchyma atrophy.
-   Should know if it is a main duct involvement or side branch duct.
-   ERCP: enlarged ampulla from mucin → fish-mouth sign.
-   Malignant transformation in main duct, 57%–92% → resection.
-   Branch duct found in uncinate process and malignant transformation, 6%–46%.
-   Asymptomatic, small branch lesion → annual image.
-   No ovarian stroma.
-   Can be identified early by image before invasion like adenoma in colon.
-   The lesion should be observed or resected.
    -   **High-Risk Stigmata**
        → Enhancing solid compartment.
        → Main duct is > 10 mm.
        → Obstructive jaundice.

    -   **Worrisome Feature**
        → Size > 3 cm.

559

→ Thickened enhanced cyst wall.

→ Main duct is 5–9 mm.

→ With symptom other than jaundice.

Management
- If high risk → surgery is recommended.
- If no high-risk stigmata but worrisome feature is there:
  → EUS nodule in main duct → cytology if suspicious lesion.
- If EUS is not conclusive → MRI or EUS every 3–6 months.
- Lesion < 1 cm → observation for 2–3 years, image.
- Lesion 2–3 cm → alternation with MRI, EUS every 3–6 months.
- If no internal growth and no high-risk stigmata or worrisome feature or not symptomatic → lengthen follow-up.
- If patient is fit and young and needs long surveillance → surgery should be considered.
- If patient has two or more affected first-degree relative → close surveillance → MRCP, MRI, EUS.
- If patient wants surgery rather than surveillance → do surgery.

Operation
- Enucleation, distal pancreatectomy, pancreaticoduodenectomy → if +ve margin → total pancreatectomy depending on location and pathology feature.

  - **Post-operative Care**
    - Similar to any patient with pancreatic resection.

  - **Post-operative Surveillance**
    - Depending on MD or BD and on margin or pathway grade.
    - If invasive disease,
      CT Q3M for the first year.

CT Q6M after the first year.
- If HGD,
  MRCP, CT Q3–6M.
- If moderate GD or low → depending on margin.
  If −ve → CT, MRI at 2, 5 years.
  If +ve MRCP 2 times per year.

Prognosis
- Overall survival is 36%–77%.
- Noninvasive neoplasm after resection, 5 years, SR is 70%–100%.
- Invasive Dx: 5 years, SR is 30%–60%.

Solid Pseudopapillary Neoplasm (SPN)
- Rare, young women, 27 is the mean age.
- Male: Female = 9:1.
- High tendency for cystic degeneration.
- 1%–2% of pancreatic neoplasm.
- 10% of pancreatic cystic neoplasm.
- Usually benign, but it can be aggressive and cause invasion locally and potential metastasis to liver, peritoneum → 10%–15%, rarely LNs involvement.
- Asymptomatic but can cause compression symptom.
- CT: circumscribed, heterogeneous appearance, mixed solid architecture with cystic component.
- Diagnostic by image 4C: circumscribed, cystic capsule, calcification (central).
- No FNA needed.
- Histopathology similar to NET, but no stain with chromogranin A.
- All SPN → resected surgically → −ve margin.
- Most are cured by resection.
- Excellent SR, 5 years, 90%.
- Peritoneal metastasis has been reported.

Other Cystic Neoplasm
- 5%–10% NET contain cyst.
- Von Hippel-Lindau syndrome developed pancreatic cyst, serous cystadenoma.

- Polycystic kidney, liver disease → pancreatic involvement also (cystadenoma).

Acinar Cell CA
- Mimics pancreatic adenocarcinoma, < 2% of pancreatic neoplasm, 50% in female, IHC distinguishes between them.
- More favorable than pancreatic duct adenocarcinoma (PDAC).
- Release of lipase, eosinophilia, fat necrosis, and rash (erythema nodosum) (Schmid's triad).
- Obtains CA 19-9.
- 5 years, SR is 72%.
- Localized disease, 16%.
  Regional disease, 26%.
  Distant metastasis, 50%.
- Unresectable and metastatic → palliative chemotherapy.
  Borderline → neoadjuvant chemotherapy (downstage).

Metastatic Lesion
- Renal Cell CA.
- Also melanoma, breast, lung, colon.
- Diagnosis: EUS/FNA, but not required if diagnosis is known.

Pancreatic Lymphoma
- Symptom similar to pancreatic adenocarcinoma.
  - Percutaneous or EUS biopsy; if not → laparoscopic biopsy.
  - ↑ LDH.
  - No role for resection.
  - ERCP with stent then chemotherapy.

Pancreatic Solid Neoplasm

Neoplasm of Endocrine Pancreas (Pancreatic Islet Cell Tumor) (Neuroendocrine Tumor of Pancreas)
- Uncommon—5:1,000,000.
- 2%–7% of all pancreatic tumors.
- Arising from pluripotent cells of pancreas.

- Most is sporadic but can be inherited with MEN syndrome.
- Functioning: secretes peptide products and produces symptom such as insulinoma, gastrinoma, somatostatinoma, glucagonoma, VIPoma.
  Nonfunctioning: with no symptom, identified by IHC.
- Histopathology cannot predict behavior but depends on local invasion, LNs, and hepatic metastasis.
- Confirmation by level of hormones.
- Surgery requires complete resection like insulinoma to control symptom.
- Unresectable disease in liver → chemoembolization.
- The gene mutation altered in PACU is rarely altered in PNET.
- The gene altered in PNET is mTOR, DAXX, ATRX.

Diagnosis and Prognosis

- Important factors in classification are angioinvasion, mitosis, and proliferation index by Ki-67.
- Clinical picture is dependent on functionality.
- Metastasis is 64% of gastropancreatic NET.
- Serum biomarker such as chromogranin A for diagnosis and surveillance, especially for nonfunctioning.
  - → ↑ chromogranin A associated with poor prognosis.
  - → Patient on PPI or with renal insufficiency has
    - → ↑ chromogranin A.
- CT, MRI, 22%–45%.
- Somatostatin receptor CT can detect non-insulinoma lesion by 57%–77%.
- Many of the endocrine tumors have somatostatin receptor SSTRs → detected by radio-labeled octreotide scan.
- EUS can detect tumor < 1 cm (90%), and you can obtain FNA.
- Unfortunately, mostly are malignant but more favorable than exocrine neoplasm.

Insulinoma

- Most common endocrine tumor.
- Less than 10% is malignant.
- 90% is sporadic and 10% familial with MEN I.

- Higher in female.
- Presented with Whipple triad.
    1. Symptomatic fasting hypoglycemia.
    2. Symptom relief by administering glucose.
    3. Documented serum glucose < 50 mg/dL.
- Syncopal symptoms: hypoglycemia, headache, confusion, or frequent eating.
- Symptoms: palpitation, trembling, diaphoresis, confusion, obtundation, seizure, personality change.
- Excessive catecholamines secondary to hypoglycemia.
- Low blood sugar, high serum insulin, high C-peptide.

Diagnosis

- Gold standard for diagnosis is fasting for 72 hrs and measuring C-peptide and proinsulin, insulin, and glucose level Q6H.
- Failure of insulin suppression $\rightarrow$ diagnostic $\rightarrow$ symptom is 75% within 24 hrs and 95% in 48 hrs.
- Difficult to localize as it is small, < 2 cm.
- Thin CT or MRI, 10%–40%.
- Somatostatin receptor scan is useful by 25%.
- EUS, 70%–95% (procedure of choice).
- Selective angiography + venous sampling from hepatic venous for insulin after Ca^{++} administration is rarely indicated.
- Location is ⅓ in head, ⅓ in body, ⅓ in tail.

Treatment

- Simple enucleation cure, 85%–95%.
- If located near the main duct or large (> 2 cm) $\rightarrow$ distal pancreatectomy or pancreaticoduodenectomy.
- Lymphadenectomy is warranted if malignancy is suspected.
- Intraoperative US is useful and recommended.
- Can be by laparoscopy.
- MEN I insulinoma: multifocal and higher recurrence.
- Medical treatment for metastatic disease requires small frequent meals and control of hypoglycemia.

→ Diazoxide, somatostatin analogue, and glucocorticoids in refractory cases.

- 5 years, SR is excellent, 97%.

Gastrinoma

- Zollinger-Ellison syndrome.
- ↑↑ secretion of gastrin → PUD, severe esophagitis.
- 20% have diarrhea.
- Diagnosis by serum gastric level > 1,000, but stop PPI before test for false +ve.
- Causes of high hypergastrinemia → pernicious anemia, PPI, G cell hyperplasia, atrophic gastritis, pyloric exclusion, gastric outlet obstruction.
- 70%–90% found in Passaro's triangle:
  1. Junction of cystic duct and CBD.
  2. Second, third duodenum.
  3. Neck and body of pancreas but can be found anywhere → whole body scan.
- 80% found in duodenum and 20% in pancreas.
- The test of choice SSTR (octreotide) scintigraphy + CT.
- Sensitivity is 85% and detects tumor < 1 cm.
- Octreotide scan + EUS, 90%.
- Important to rule out MEN I by checking serum Ca^{++} before surgery as rarely neutralized gastric level into patient.
- ¼ of gastrinoma associated with MEN I.
- ½ has solitary mass and ½ multiple.
- If MEN I, total parathyroidectomy + implantation in forearm.
- 50% of gastrinoma metastasized to LNs or liver → consider malignant.

Treatment

- Tumor in submucosa → full-thickness excision should be done.
- All LNs excised in Passaro's Δ.
- If tumor in pancreatic duct → enucleation.
- Pancreatic resection is justified for solitary mass with no metastasis.
- HSV (vagotomy) in unressectable tumor.
- Debulking or incomplete resection is not helpful.

- Post-operative follow-up → gastrin level, secretin stimulating test, CT scan.
- Inoperable → 5-FU, doxorubicin.
- Somatostatin analogue can control symptoms.
- 15 years, SR is 80%.
- 5 years, SR with liver metastasis is 20%–50%.
- Pancreatic tumor is bigger in size than duodenal tumor.
- Best outcome after resection of duodenal tumor.
- Large tumor outside Passaro's Δ with liver metastasis → worse prognosis.

VIPoma

- Severe intermittent watery diarrhea → dehydration and weakness from fluid and electrolyte losses, i.e., low K^+.
- VIPoma is called syndrome of watery diarrhea, dehydration, hypokalemia, achlorhydria (WDHA).
- Diarrhea, 5 L/1 day.
- ↑ VIP → ↓ gastric acid → bone reabsorption glycogenolysis, ↑ Ca^{++}, ↑ glucose and flushing.

Diagnosis

- High VIP > 200 mg/dL to thousands.
- Majority is malignant.
- 70% with metastasis.
- CT, MRI localization is 80%.
- CT localized the VIPoma, but EUS the most sensitive image.
- Somatostatin (octreotide) scintigraphy (best), 90% in localization.
- Common location in distal pancreas, tend to be metastasized.
- IVF is difficult to replace pre-operative, but it can be with octreotide.

Treatment

- Life-threatening as electrolyte disturbance.
- Resection or debulking.
- Somatostatin analogue is helpful for diarrhea.
- Hepatic artery embolization is a beneficial treatment.

Glucagonoma
- DM + dermatitis.
- DM is mild, dermatitis: necrolytic migratory erythema → cyclic migration of lesion with spreading margin and healing center in lower abdomen, perineum, perioral, feet, enlarged sensitive tongue.
- Diagnosis by serum glucagon > 500 pg/mL.
- CT, MRI.
- It's a catabolic hormone → malnutrition → low protein.
- Pre-operative preparation: DM, TPN, octreotide.
- More frequency in tail and tend to be metastasized; malignancy is 50%–90%.

Treatment
- Surgical resection or debulking.
- Normalizing glucagon either by surgery or somatostatin analogue → disappearance of dermatitis.
- 50% has metastatic disease → palliative somatostatin analogue or interference α.
- Deficiency supplement of zinc, amino acid, essential fatty acid.
- No role for chemotherapy.

Somatostatinoma
- Somatostatin inhibits pancreatic and biliary secretion.
- Gallstone formation due to stasis.
- DM due to low insulin.
- Steatorrhea due to low exocrine secretion and bile.
- Located usually in proximal pancreas in paraduodenal groove ampulla and periampullary (60%).
- Symptoms: abdominal pain, 25%; jaundice, 25%; gallstone, 19%.
- Diagnosis: high serum somatostatin > 10 mg/mL.
  → CT scan, octreotide scan.
- Malignancy, 60%–70%. If tumor > 2 cm → metastasis.
- Treatment: complete excision of the tumor and cholecystectomy (stasis)
- Resection is often not possible because of metastasis.

Non-Insulin Hyperinsulinemia Hypoglycemia Syndrome

- β cell hyperplasia (hypertrophy), islet hyperplasia, high β cell mass.
- Ectopic islet tissue, multilobulated islet, ductoinsular complex → nesidioblastosis, ↑ insulin.
- Previously, considered disease of neonate and required subtotal or total pancreatectomy.
- New cases reported post-gastric bypass after 2–5 years → hypersecretion of GIP, GLP-I.
- GLP-I is the most potent stimulant of expression of PDX-I, which normally regulates β cell development and growth.
- Treatment: conversion to gastric sleeve.
- No benefit to perfrome partial pancreatectomy without correction of bypass.

Other Functional Tumor
Ectopic ACTH
- Parathyroid hormone–related peptide.
- Curative surgery is recommended when possible pancreatic resection + lymphadenectomy.
- Somatostatin analogue alleviates symptom.

Nonfunctioning Pancreatic Endocrine Tumor
- Most endocrine tumors are not associated with high serum hormone level.
- It is considered functional if associated with clinical symptom.
- Pancreatic endocrine tumor = neuroendocrine tumor (NET), majority is malignant as ↑ growth and metastasis.
- IHC such as synaptophysin, chromogranin A are helpful in diagnosis.
- Chromogranin A can be used for recurrence or to see the response of treatment.
- Usually, NET is discovered incidentally.
- Usually enhanced by arterial phase.
- Sometimes cystic component due to central necrosis.
- Octreoscan is helpful.
- Surgical resection is recommended in fit patient with no metastasis.
- 2 cm −ve margin to achieve R0.

- Lymphadenectomy is recommended here → about 10% of patients has +ve LNs.
- Recurrent rate is 76%.
- 50% liver metastasis → give somatostatin analogue.
- Resection of primary tumor despite liver metastasis is accepted to prevent acute pancreatitis, obstruction, complication.
- Adjuvant treatment is withheld in the absence of radiological finding even if chromogranin A is high.
- Antiproliferative chemotherapy is recommended in advanced PNET (5-FU).
- Debulking for metastatic disease is controversial because of favorable SR without surgery as it's slow-growing.
- Careful selection of fit patient → pancreaticoduodenectomy + wedge resection of liver metastasis.
- It is caused by the activation of mammalian target of rapamycin (mTOR) and VEGF.
  - → Antitumor activity with everolimus → mTOR inhibitor is effecitve.

Neoplasm of Exocrine Pancreas

WHO Classification of Primary Tumor of Exocrine
Benign
1. Serous cystadenoma, 16%.
2. Mucinous cystadenoma, 45%.
3. Intraductal papillary mucinous adenoma (IPMA), 32% with no dysplasia.
4. Mature cystic teratoma.

Potential Malignant (Borderline)
1. Mature cystic teratoma with moderate dysplasia.
2. IPMN with moderate dysplasia.
3. Solid pseudopapillary neoplasm (SPN).

Malignant
1. Ductal adenocarcinoma.
2. Serous/mucinous cystadenocarcinoma.
3. Intraductal papillary mucinous neoplasm.

Pancreatic Adenocarcinoma

Epidemiology and Risk Factor

- 74% die from pancreatic CA in the first year.
- Overall, pancreatic CA is the worst prognosis of all malignancies, 5 years, SR is 6%.
- Incidence is still high, perhaps related to obesity and DM.
- Men aged 60 are affected more than women, ↑ African American.
- Risk is two- to threefold if parent has history of pancreatic CA.
- Risk factors: smoking, coffee, alcohol, high-fat diet, and low-fiber diet.
- DM 2, twofold.
   → New onset of DM or requirement of insulin →
      ↑suspicion of occult pancreatic CA.
- Chronic pancreatitis, especially familial, twentyfold.
- Mutated K-RAS oncogene, ↑ pancreatic cancer.

Gene mutation of Pancreatic CA

- K-RAS is the most common (90%) detected in serum, stool, pancreatic juice, and tissue aspiration from pancreas.
- HER2/neu and EGF are overexpressed in pancreatic CA.
- Multiple tumor suppressor genes are deleted and/or mutated P53, P16, DPCA4, and a few cases with BRCA2.
- Most pancreatic tumors have three or more from above mutation.
- 10% of pancreatic tumors are from inherited genetic predisposition.
- New modality is created to stop growth and treatment of these CA by inhibiting RGF, VEGF, but under study, combination of these drugs with standard chemotherapy → no dramatic response in overall survival.

Pathology

- Just like colon CA progresses by stages from hyperplastic polyp to invasive CA.
- Precursor lesion: pancreatic intraepithelial neoplasia.
- ⅔ of adenocarcinoma arise from head and uncinate process, 15% from body and 10% from tail.

- Tumor in body and tail is usually larger at the time of diagnosis → less commonly resectable.
- In head, diagnosed earlier because of obstructive jaundice.
- Ampullary and periampullary duodenal CA has similar fashion, but better prognosis.
- Ductal adenocarcinoma, 75% of nonendocrine CA of pancreas.
- Adenosquamous carcinoma → similar to adenocarcinoma in behavior and outcome.
- Acinar cell carcinoma, uncommon, large (> 10 cm), but prognosis is better than adenocarcinoma.

Staging
- TNM.
  o T1 tumor ≤ 2 cm is limited to pancreas.
  o T2 tumor > 2 cm is limited to pancreas.
  o T3 extends beyond pancreas but no involvement of celiac or SMA.
  o T4 lesion invdes celiac axix or SMA.
    ▪ Stage I   → T1, T2, no LNs
    ▪ Stage IIa   → T3, no LNs
    ▪ Stage IIb   → T3, one LN
    ▪ Stage III   → Locally advanced tumor T4, any LNs, no metastasis
    ▪ Stage IV→ Distant metastasis
- 8% diagnosed with confined to primary site.
- 27% spread to regional LNs.
- 53% of tumor already metastasized.
- 5 years, SR is 23% with localized disease, 9% for regional, 1.8% for metastatic disease.

Clinical presentation
- Most common presenting symptom is jaundice → pruritus, dark urine, light-colored stool, scleral icterus, and may be associated with constitutional symptom (painless jaundice).
- The pain, as pancreatitis is situated deep in the abdomen, is vague and sometimes radiating to the back.
- Weight loss.

- In advanced disease → tumor invades retroperitoneal (celiac) nerve plexus.
- Examination: jaundice.
  Abdominal examination: tender hepatomegaly, palpable nontender gallbladder in ¼ of patients (Courvoisier's sign), Sister Mary Joseph nodule, left supraclavicular lymph nodes (Virchow's node).

Laboratory

- Should perform CBC, electrolyte, and LFT. Usually high direct bilirubin and ALP.
- If prolonged biliary obstruction → coagulopathy → malabsorption of fat-soluble vitamins (K), i.e., high PT and high INR.
- Low albumin, anemia.
- High bilirubin and high ALP.
- ↑ carbohydrates antigen (CA 19-9) in 75% of patients, 10 % of patients with benign pancreatic disease, so not sensitive or specific, i.e., not effective but should be obtained as baseline.
- Some proteins are expressed in pancreatic juice.

Radiology

- Patient with jaundice → US first.
- If demonstration of gallbladder stone → ERCP.
- In the absence of gallbladder stone → CT, not ERCP.
- Diagnostic tool of choice is CT with pancreatic protocol; accuracy is 90%–95%.
- All periampullary → same degree of biliary or pancreatic duct dilation and (double duct) sign → and this is commonly associated with PDAC.
- Some lesions such distal cholangiocarcinoma, ampullary or duodenal CA cannot be visualized properly by CT or MRI → so EGD, EUS, ERCP.
- CT finding indicates tumor is unresectable if involvement of ≥ 180 degrees of SMA, celiac LNs enlargement, ascites, liver metastasis.
- SMV and PV involvement is not a contraindication as long as it's patent.

- Tumor is considered borderline resectable if there is loss of fat separation between tumor and vessels (abutment) of < 180 degrees of SMA, celiac, and hepatic artery or if short segment vein occlusion and (encasement) > 180 degrees.
- If suspicion of liver metastasis by 1 mm (small) to Bx ® consider the stage as borderline.
- PET distinguishes chronic pancreatitis from CA.
- EUS detects small lesion missed by CT, also helpful in biopsy, although tissue Bx before pancreaticoduodenectomy is not required.
- 20% of predicting resectable tumor → intra-operatively → unresectable.
- To avoid this → laparoscopic exploration with intraoperative US → higher accuracy by 98%. Multiple ports for manipulation → exploration of tissue ligament of Treitz and T colon peritoneum → gastrocolic ligament incised → lesser sac.
- US probes for liver and PV, SMA assessement.
- The percentage of patient who underwent laparoscopy to avoid laparotomy is 10%–30% in cancer head of pancreas and 50% in body and tail.
- Biliary obstruction → endoscopy with large 10F plastic stent for 3 months then replace.
- Metallic last for 5 months.

Pre-operative Stent and biopsy
- Certain circumstances call for additional workup such as tissue biopsy to guide neoadjuvent or palliative treatment for unresectable disease → EUS is the most useful invasive modality because it detects small lesion + offers FNA.
- ERCP and stent or PTC image with PBD + sampling in patient with obstructive jaundice.

Stage III (Borderline and Locally Advanced) Pancreatic CA
- Stage III is divided into two categories:
    1. Borderline resectable pancreatic CA (BRPC)
    2. Locally advanced unresectable pancreatic CA (LAPC)
- In general, BRPC refers to the technically reconstructable involvement of the portovenous axis or abutment of a major artery, whereas LAPC refers to the unreconstructable

involvement of the portovenous axis or encasement of a main artery.

- NCCN criteria for borderline resectability in pancreatic CA:
  1. No distant metastasis.
  2. Venous involvement, PV/ SMV → abutment with or without narrowing of the lumen or encasement of PV/ SMV without encasement of nearby artery, allowing for safe resection and reconstruction.
  3. GDA encasement up to hepatic artery or abutment of short segment hepatic artery or encasement without extension to celiac axis.
  4. Tumor abutment in SMA < 180.

Treatment

➤ Stage I, II: surgery + adjuvant therapy, neoadjuvant may be considered but will delay treatment.
➤ Stage III:
  o BRPD → should receive neoadjuvant chemotherapy or chemoradiation, for sterilized surgical margins and better control of micrometastatic disease.
  o LAPC → not a candidate for curative resection → so downstaging chemotherapy or chemoradiation, then re-evaluate by CT to evaluate response.
➤ Stage IV: no surgery but should offer palliative systemic therapy after Bx to guide the chemotherapy.

Surgical Treatment

- Pancreaticoduodenectomy (PD) is a method for oncological resection, for periampullary CA.
- Either standard PD or pylorus-preserving pancreatico-duodenectomy (PPPD).
- MIS, i.e., laparoscopic or robotic, is as safe and effective as open.
- Findings that are contraindications for resection:
  1. Liver metastasis (any size)
  2. Celiac LNs involvement
  3. Peritoneal implants
  4. Hepatic hilar LNs
- Findings that are not contraindications for resection:

1. Invasion to duodenum or distal stomach
2. Involvement of peripancreatic LNs
3. Involvement of LNs along porta hepatis swept down with specimen

- As before, if PV or SMV is involved, not a contraindication as long as patent.
- Venous: PV, SMV—primary repair < 3 cm; if more → interposition graft (left renal vein or IJV) → ligation of Splenic V provides more length to SMV, PV.
- Artery reconstruction, primary repair, or autologous venous graft (saphenous vein) → or left gastric artery or splenic artery.

Surgical technique

Whipple Procedure:
- After induction of anesthesia, the patient is placed in the supine position, and the abdomen is prepared for exploration.
- Incision: either extended right subcostal incision (chevron) or midline incision.
- Exploration of the entire abdomen is done.
- Place a fixed table retractor (e.g., Thompson or Bookwalter).
- In the absence of disseminated metastatic disease, begin exposure of the pancreas.
- The transverse mesocolon is retracted inferiorly, and the omentum and the stomach are retracted superiorly and anteriorly.
- The lesser sac is entered through the greater omentum.
- The middle colic vein is identified on the posterior surface of the transverse mesocolon and dissected down to its junction with SMV.
- The inferior neck of the pancreas is inspected.
- The third portion of the duodenum and the uncinate process are retracted superiorly, and the hepatic flexure and transverse mesocolon are retracted inferiorly.
- An extended Kocher maneuver is performed up to porta hepatis.
- IVC is identified.

- En bloc dissection of the retroperitoneal soft tissues is accomplished up to the level of the left renal vein.
- The gallbladder is retracted superiorly and anteriorly.
- The cystic duct is identified and dissected down to its junction with the common hepatic duct.
- A vessel loop is placed around the CBD then retracted laterally.
- Expose the takeoff of the GDA.
- The right gastric artery is identified, ligated, and divided.
- The common hepatic artery, lymph nodes are dissected circumferentially off the hepatic artery and sent for frozen section.
- If biopsies are −ve for metastatic cancer, the procedure is continued.
- The GDA is identified and ligated just distal to its origin from the common hepatic artery.
- The anterior surface of the portal vein is identified and dissected down to the superior neck of the pancreas.
- The gallbladder is dissected off the liver bed, and the cystic artery is identified, ligated, and divided.
- The common hepatic duct is divided approximately 1 cm distal to the hepatic duct bifurcation.
- Resection of the distal stomach, the greater omentum is dissected off the transverse mesocolon up to the level of the confluence of the left gastroepiploic and right gastroepiploic arteries on the greater curvature of the stomach.
- The second or third branch, the lesser omentum is dissected off the lesser curvature of the stomach, and then the stomach is divided using an 80 mm linear stapling device then oversewn with a running 3-0 polypropylene Lembert suture.
- The proximal jejunum is then divided approximately 10–15 cm distal to the ligament of Treitz.
- Dissection is carried back to the level of the SMA and uncinate process.
- The neck of the pancreas is carefully dissected off the anterior surface of the SMV and the anterior surface of the portal vein.

- The pancreas is divided with electrocautery.
- The pancreatic neck is dissected off the right lateral surface of the portal vein.
- The specimen is removed and sent to pathology for frozen sections on the bile duct margin, the uncinate process margin, and the pancreatic neck margin.
- Titanium clips are placed along the retroperitoneal margin on the lateral edge of SMA for postoperative localization by radiation oncology.
- 1 inch of the proximal body of the pancreas is mobilized for preparation of the anastomosis.
- The proximal end of the jejunum is then brought through an opening in the transverse mesocolon to the right of the middle colic vessels.
- Retrocolic or antecolic position, an end-to-side pancreatic jejunal anastomosis is done.
- The end of the pancreas is sewn to the antimesenteric border of the jejunum in two layers.
- The next anastomosis performed is the hepaticojejunostomy; this is also performed in an end-to-side fashion between the end of the common hepatic duct and the antimesenteric border of the jejunum.
- A side-to-side gastrojejunal anastomosis is then placed approximately 30–35 cm distal to the biliary anastomosis.
- Closed suction drains are placed in the upper-right quadrant.
- An inferior drain is placed posteriorly to the biliary anastomosis.
- A superior drain is placed between the pancreatic anastomosis and the incision.
- Hemostasis is secured, the abdomen closed, and dressing applied.

Post-operative Care

- Within 24 hrs → ICU, resuscitation, maintain glucose level, NGT.
- At D1, remove NG, Foley, ambulation spirometry, sips of water, then clear liquid → soft carb then progress, can use prokinetics.

- Drain left in place 4–5 days till patient can tolerate oral.
- Drain fluid, send for amylase level → if output is low and amylase is low, remove the drain.

Complications of Pancreaticoduodenectomy

- Most common causes of death are sepsis, hemorrhage, CVA event, leak, delayed gastric emptying, fistula.
- Delayed gastric emptying → diagnosed by contrast study and treated with erythromycin.
- Some of maneuvers decrease leak complication such as use of stomach or jejunum for drainage, pancreatic duct stent, use of octreotide.
- For octreotide, most studies showed decrease leak whereas some studies showed ↑ incidence of leak.
- Recent meta-analysis showed superiority of pancreaticogastrostomy over pancreaticojejunostomy.
- Optimal option:
  > If large pancreatic duct and fibrosis: duct → mucosa.
  > If small pancreatic duct: end-to-end invagination.
- Some studies showed Roux-en-Y lowers pancreatic leak, i.e., separate limb for biliary and for pancreas → no activation of pancreatic juice.
- Use of duct stent decreases leak.
- Use of nonabsorbable glue increases pancreatic atrophy and endocrine insufficiency with no decrease leak.
- Fibrin glue to limit action of pancreatic juice and occlude pancreatic duct, pancreatic stump, and anastomosis site, but no decrease in leak.
- If not combined with biliary leak → will resolve spontaneously in 95% of cases.
- Hemorrhage can occurs intra or post-operative
- Intra-operative portal vein bleeding → control by hand → divide the neck of pancreas → distal control. Graft (IJV) may be needed (interposition).
- Post-operative → hemorrhage due to digested vessels in retroperitoneum.
- Uncommon cause → GI hemorrhage, marginal ulcer → PPI.

Outcome of Pancreaticoduodenectomy

- SR according to stage of disease.
- Most patients have advanced local disease.
- Most hematogenous metastasis → liver.
- Malignant ascites with peritoneal implants and malignant pleural effusion are common.
- Medial SR after pancreaticoduodenectomy is 22 months.
- Long SR (5 years), dies from late recurrence, so palliation is mainstay.

Adjuvant Chemotherapy

- ↓ disease recurrence after resection; multiple randomized clinical trials have assessed the benefit of adjuvant chemotherapy or chemoradiotherapy.
- The CONKO-001 trial, which compared 6 months of adjuvant gemcitabine with best supportive care, demonstrated a two-month survival benefit with adjuvant chemotherapy and established the standard adjuvant therapy to be single-agent gemcitabine.
- One study showed adjuvant chemotherapy 5-FU and radiation improve outcome by 9 months.
- Three studies showed combination of 5-FU, cisplatinum, interferon α, and external beam radiation increase SR.

Neoadjuvant Treatment
Advantages
- Avoid risk of adjuvant treatment delay as complication of surgery.
- Identification of patients with aggressive tumor biology.
- Decreased tumor size.
- Increased efficacy of radiation therapy.
- Avoid patient with occult metastasis from morbidity.
- Pre-operative neoadjuvant does not increase preoperative mortality and morbidity
    → May decrease incidence of pancreatic fistula.
- Decreased rate of positive resection margins.
- Decreased rate of pancreatic fistula formation.
- Neoadjuvant ↓ LNs metastasis, improves SR.

Disadvantages

- Potential complications from pre-treatment endoscopic procedures (endoscopic ultrasound scan and fine-needle aspiration, and endoscopic retrograde cholangiopancreatography).
- Biliary stent–related morbidity, stent occlusion during neoadjuvant therapy.
- Disease progression obviating resectability, loss of a "window" of resectability may occur (rarely) in the borderline resectable patient.

Palliative Therapy for Pancreatic CA
Palliative Surgery and Endoscopy
- 85%–90% have advanced disease and are not candidates for surgical resection → palliative.
- Pain → oral morphine or invasive retroperitoneal nerve trunk neurolysis, celiac plexus nerve block.
- Jaundice, pruritus, cholangitis, coagulopathy, and hepatocellular failure.
    - → In the past, biliary bypass during laparotomy.
    - → Now most patient has stent, no need for bypass.
    - → If bypass is done → choledochoduodenostomy is unwise as near to tumor.
- Duodenal obstruction: late 20% of patient, routine gastrojejunostomy when exploration is controversial.
- Can do choledochal and gastrojejunostomy in one set and jejunum pass anterior to colon.
- Roux-en-Y lowers risk of cholangitis.
- If laparoscopy → inoperable → ERCP and stent, but not durable like bypass and has high risk of cholangitis, dislodgement, obstruction; it's superior to percutaneous (PBD) but inferior to surgery, with less morbid procedure.
- Metallic is better than plastic.

Palliative Chemotherapy and Radiation
- Advanced and unresectable tumor → systemic chemotherapy (gemcitabine) → improves symptom, weight, ↑ SR in 2 months.
- 5-FU can be used.
- Palliative radiotherapy can be considered.

Ablation for Locally Advanced Unresectable Disease
- Persistent vascular encasement after neoadjuvant contraindication for resection.
- Nanoknife enables treatment of pancreatic tumor, abutting vascular structure.

Variation and Controversies
- Preservation of pylorus → prevents reflux of pancreatic and biliary juices → ↓ marginal ulcer, increases weight.
- Technique: pancreaticojejunostomy → end-to-side, end-to-end, duct mucosa, invagination.
- Some use stent or glue to seal anastomosis.
- Octreotide decreases pancreatic secretion.
- Pancreatic leak is always about 10%.
- Most surgeons place drain around anastomosis.
- Usually pancreatic leak → drain till resolved spontaneously, but if pancreatic and biliary, i.e., activation of pancreatic juice → disruption → necrotizing retroperitoneal infection → erode major artery and vein such as PV or GDA → bleeding.
- Depending on patient situation, either angiography or OR.
- Open packing for diffuse infection and necrosis.
- Some advise for drain after pancreaticoduodenectomy resection, but routine placement is under investigation.
- Routine NJT or gastrostomy becomes less commonly used.
- Complication of NJT → dumping, intestinal obstruction.
- Complication of TPN → line sepsis, ↓ gut mucosa integrity, and hepatic dysfunction.
- Because of high incidence of retroperitoneal LNs metastasis → radical resection.
- Radical resection means:
  o Pancreatic resection to middle body.
  o Segmental resection of portal vein.
  o Resection of retroperitoneal tissue (LNs) + perinephric + region of celiac plexus → ↑ bleeding, but no increase in mortality.
- Total pancreatectomy → in the past, no risk of leak, but complications are brittle DM, exocrine insufficiency.

- Intraoperative radiotherapy (IORTx) to tumor bed, improve local control and palliate symptom → but intraoperative RTx is not superior to standard external beam radiation.

Posto-perative Surveillance
- Recurrence post-resection manifested by liver metastasis.
- Chemoradiation by 5-FU + EB radiation → on weekly basis for 6 months.
- Physical examination and CA 19-9, CT scan every 3 months in the first 2 years or when CA 19-9 is increase or new symptom suggests recurrence.
- Then for the next 3 years, increase interval.
- Surgery for recurrence reserved for patient with symptom such as gastric outlet or bowel obstruction.

Future Therapy
- Gene therapy is under investigation.
- Tumor suppressor gene.
- Cancer cell is forced to express tumor-specific antigen and cytokines → activate immune system → antitumor effect.

Spleen

Embryology and Anatomy

- Encapsulated mass of vascular and lymphoid tissue.
- Largest reticuloendothelial organ in the body.
- Arises from mesoderm by fifth week of GA.
- Spleen has important hematopoietic role till fifth week of GA; after birth, ↓ this role.
- Located in posterosuperior aspect.
- Most common anomaly is accessory spleen → 20% of population and 30% in patient with hematologic disease.
- 80% of accessory spleen found in splenic hilum and vascular pedicle.
  - → Other locations: gastrocolic ligament, pancreatic tail, greater omentum, stomach's greater curvature, splenocolic ligament, small bowels, mesentery, left broad ligament in female, left spermatic cord in male.
- Contains gastric, colic, renal, pancreatic impression.
- The "odd" of spleen: 1-3-5-7-9-11 → the spleen is 1 inch (thickness) by 3 inches (breadth) by 5 inches (length), weighs 7 ounces, and lies between the ninth and eleventh ribs.
- Length is 7–11 cm; weight is 150 g.
- 1–2 notches.
- Suspended by several ligaments:
  1. Splenocolic
  2. Gastrosplenic—contains short gastric vessels
  3. Phrenosplenic
  4. Splenorenal
- All avascular, except gastrosplenic ligament.
- Tail of pancreas lies within 1 cm of splenic hilum.
- Blood supply: splenic artery is the longest and most tortuous of three branches of celiac artery.
- Splenic artery:
  a) Distributed type: short trunk enters 74% of medial surface.
  b) Magistral type: short terminal branch and enters 25%–30% of medial surface.

583

- Spleen also receives blood supply from short gastric branch from left gastroepiploic artery running in gastrosplenic ligament.
- Splenic V + SMV = portal vein.
- Red pulp, 75%, and white pulp, 25%.
- Red pulp: cord lacks endothelial lining but contains macrophage; sinus contains endothelial.
- Red pulp: dynamic filtration system → terminal (periarticular lymph sheath) → T and B lymphocytes.
- White pulp: nodules, when coalesce → as in lymphoproliferative disorder → targeting bacteria and pathogenic.

Physiology and Pathophysiology

- Spleen is rich in collagen and elastic fiber.
- Inflow is 250–300 mL/min.
- Open and close circulation.
- Innate immunity by red pulp → contacts macrophage + removes senile cells.
- Adaptive immunity by white pulp.
- Spleen removes red cells by Heinz body, also removes senile WBCs and platelets.
- 20 mL of RBCs removed daily.
- Extramedullary site for hematopoiesis if required and recycle iron.
- Release Hb bound to haptoglobin.
- B cells → IgM.
- IgM → opsonic antibody from white pulp.
- White pulp = LNs.
- Major source of protein properdin → activation of complement system.
- Splenic reticulendothelial system (RES) clear bacteria that inadequately opsonized from circulation by hepatic RES such as encapsulated bacteria, meningococcal, pneumococcal, haemophilus.
- Spleen is palpable if enlarged at least two times or higher > 15 cm.
- Important to distinguish splenomegaly from hypersplenism.
  - Splenomegaly: abnormal enlargement of the spleen: moderate, massive, hyper splenomegaly $\geq$ 500 g and $\geq$ 15 cm, massive > 1 kg and > 22 cm.

- • Hypersplenism: often associated with splenomegaly but defined as presence of one or more cytopenia in normal functioning bone marrow.
- Diseases causing hypersplenism:
    a) Hemolytic anemia.
    b) Primary disorder of spleen, i.e., high sequestration → infiltrative disorder.
- Half-life of neutrophil is 6 hrs, then spleen clears it.
- Splenomegaly can sequestrate of 80% of the platelet.
- May contribute in immunologic alteration of platelets → thrombocytopenia in the absence of splenomegaly as in ITP.
- Splenic hematopoiesis → abnormal RBCs as in myeloproliferative disorder.

Imaging for Evaluation of Size and Physiology
- All patients should do US and CT.
- Volume (cc) = length (cm) × width (cm) × height (cm).

Plain Radiography
- Splenic calcification can be observed.

US
- In trauma or resuscitation.
- Doppler imaging.
- Splenic artery:
    1. Distributed
    2. Magistral
- US-guided percutaneous aspiration or biopsy is contraindicated because of hemorrhage but can be done with caution.

CT
- Standard for trauma.
- Assesses splenomegaly, solid and cystic lesion.
- Can predict laparoscopic difficulty.
- Without contrast or venous phase → normal splenic tissue.
- In arterial phase = zebra appearance.

MRI
- Ratio of red and white pulps.

Angiography
- Diagnostic and therapeutic (embolization).
- Spleen angioembolization (SAE) → decreases size → limited success as alternative to splenectomy in chronic ITP, ↑ pain, ↑ stay, ↑ pancreatitis.

Nuclear Imaging
- Radioscintigraphy technetium-T99m (sulfer colloid) is helpful to localized accessory spleen after unsuccessful splenectomy, to diagnose splenosis.
- Indium-labeled autologous platelet scan (ILAPS) demonstrates whether platelet sequestration occur in spleen or liver or both.
- Spleen scintigraphy is used for NASH, which can result in nonalcoholic fatty liver disease (NAFLD) → diagnosis of progression from NAFLD to NASH depends on liver Bx.

Indication of Splenectomy
- Most common indication of splenectomy is trauma.
- Most common elective indication for splenectomy is ITP.

a) Benign: RBC disorder, hemoglobinopathy, platelet disorder.
b) Malignant: WBC disorder and bone marrow disorder (myeloproliferative).
c) Others: cyst, tumor infection, abscess, splenic rupture.

a. Benign Disease
1. RBCs disrorders
Congenital
Hereditary Spherocytosis
- Deficiency or dysfunction of one of erythrocytes membrane protein → destabilization of membrane lipid bilayer → release of membrane lipids.
- More spherical, less deformable, and sequestrated in spleen → hemolytic anemia (HA).
- It is the most common HA required splenectomy.
- Autosomal dominant.

- Symptoms: mild jaundice, but patient with mild disease has no anemia.
  - ↓ MCV.
  - ↑ MCHC.
  - ↑ reticulocyte.
  - ↑ lactate dehydrogenase (LDH).
  - ↑ indirect bilirubin.
  - ↓ haptoglobin.
- Indication for splenectomy (main cause) → growth retardation, skeletal changes, leg ulcer, extramedullary hematopoietic tumor.
- Gallbladder should be removed, unless no gallstone.
- Near-total splenectomy is sometimes indicated in children.
- Delaying is appreciated as to prevent OPSI till age of 4–6 years.

Hereditary Elliptocytosis
- Membrane defect (as spherocytosis).
- Hereditary elliptocytosis—the cell is elongated + circular.
- Hereditary elliptocytosis—harmless.
- It affects more than 50% of RBCs to develop symptom.

RBCs Cell Enzyme Deficiency
Pyruvate Kinase Deficiency
- causes congenital chronic hemolytic anemia.
- Varies from well compensated to transfusion dependent.
- Diagnosis: mutation in DNA or genomic level.
- Splenomegaly → splenectomy → alleviate transfusion.
- Should delay splenectomy till 4–6 years.

G6PD
- The most common red blood cells enzyme deficiency overall is G6PD.

- More prevalent than pyruvate kinase.
- 400 million worldwide.
- Mild, moderate hemolytic anemia.
- Avoid drug, fava beans.
- Transfusion according to symptom.
- Splenectomy has many benefits.

Acquired
Warm Antibody Autoimmune Hemolytic Anemia
- Destruction by autoimmune antibody against Ag.
- Classified to primary, secondary.
- Divide to warm, cold.
- In cold, mild symptom, never splenectomy.
- Warm occurs in midlife, more in female, symptom of hemolytic anemia.
    - → ⅓ to ½ presented with splenomegaly.
    - → Symptoms: hemolytic anemia, reticulocytotic, high bilirubin, blood in the urine and stool.
    - → Coombs test distinguishes autoimmune from other hemolytic anemia.
    - → may require splenectomy.
- Treatment: depends on symptom.
- Unstable → steroid.
- Responds to steroid and anti-CD20 antibody.

2. **Hemoglobinopathies**
   Sickle Cell Disease (SCD)
   - Chronic hemolytic anemia.
   - Autosomal dominant.
   - Inherited from one parent (heterozygous) if carriers, if both (homozygous) have SCD.
   - Mutation of adenine to thymine.
   - Microvascular congestion → thrombosis → ischemia → necrosis.
   - Can present with vaso-occlusive crisis (sickle cell crisis).
   - Sequestration in early presentation and subsequent infarction and autosplenectomy.

- Most common indication for splenectomy is recurrent acute sequestration, hypersplenism, and splenic abscess.
- Pre-operative preparation: hydration, prevents hypothermia, and analgesia.
- Splenectomy does not prevent disease rather than palliative.
- If moderately severe → transfusion.
- Acute chest syndrome (new infiltration on CXR, fever, cough, sputum, hypoxia).
- Patient with stroke or severe crisis requires exchange transfusion.
- Cholecystectomy for gallstone disease.
- Hydroxyurea: ↑ HbF, ↓ HbS.

Thalassemia

- α, β, γ.
- Arises from a single gene defect.
    a) Low functioning Hb: microcytic hypochromic.
    b) Insoluble RBC that cannot release oxygen → cells aging.
- Thalassemia major (homozygous).
- Diagnosis on peripheral blood smear, reticulocytosis.
- a thalassemia: a chain needed to form HbA and HbF, so if detected → symptomatic in utero or at birth.
- b thalassemia: presented at 4–6 months, because β involved in adult Hb only.
- Heterozygous (carrier).
- In thalassemia major → pallor, jaundice, growth retardation, hepatosplenomegaly, leg ulcer, large head.
- Treatment: transfuse RBCs to maintain Hb 9 or more + chelating (deferoxamine).
- Splenectomy in patient with excessive transfusion > 200 mL/kg/year.

- After splenectomy → pulmonary hypertension, ↑ infection
  → in children.should be delayed, or to do partial splenectomy

3. **Platelet Disorder**
   ITP
   - Low platelet and mucocutaneous petechial bleeding.
   - Removal of platelet by opsonization by antiplatelet IgG auto-antibody produced in spleen in Fc receptor in spleen and liver.
   - Incidence 100:1,000,000.
   - Symptoms: petechiae and ecchymosis, bleeding epistaxis, menorrhagia, hematuria, melena.
   - Patient with:
     - 30,000 easily bruising
     - 10,000 spontaneous petechiae and ecchymosis
     - < 10,000 spontaneous bleeding
   - Can be acute or chronic.
   - Intracranial hemorrhage (ICH) → 1%, can perform emergent splenectomy.
   - Children: peak at 5 years after URTI.
   - Adult is usually chronic type.
   - Splenomegaly is uncommon.
   - Other diseases resulting in ITP: SLP, antiphospholipid, lymphoproliferative, HIV, HCV.
   - Drugs such as antibiotic, anti-inflammatory, anti-HTN, antidepressant.
   - Treatment:
     - First line: oral prednisolone, 1–1.5 mg/kg/1 day → response for first three weeks, 50%–75%.
     - IVIg 1 g/day for 2–5 days for internal bleeding (impaired IgG in spleen).
     - Rituximab and thrombopoietin receptor agonist.

- Splenectomy when medical treatment fails, i.e., use of steroid, 10–20 mg/ day for 3–6 months to maintain platelet. 30,000, i.e., refractory, 75%–80%.
  - Recurrent thrombosis (lifelong anticoagulation).
  - Recurrent abortion.
- Laparoscopy is the approach of choice.
- Accessory spleen is the main concern.
- In children, ITP is self-limiting and remission is 70%.
- Splenectomy is controversial in patient with ITP, but if ICH, it is a must.

Thrombotic Thrombocytopenic Purpura (TTP)

- Thrombocytopenia + microangiopathy hemolytic anemia + CNS complication.
- Abnormal platelet clumping in arteriole and capillary.
  - → Microvascular thrombosis, decreased lumen size.
  - → RBCs destruction + sequestrated in spleen
- Studies showed large amount of vWF + platelet clumping → produces the disease.
- Incidence 3.7:1,000,000.
- Symptom like ITP, but can be worse: CNS symptoms, renal failure, arrhythmia, petechial hemorrhage in lower limb.
- CNS complication: varies from headache to seizure and coma.
- Diagnosis by peripheral blood smear, schistocyte, nucleated RBCs, basophilic stippling.
- Aortic stenosis.
- TTP distinguishes from autoimmune causes such as Evan syndrome (ITP + autoimmune + hemolytic anemia) by −ve Coombs test.
- Treatment (first line): plasma exchange and replaced by FFP.
- Splenectomy if medical treatment failed.

b. Malignant Disease
1. WBCs
- Role of splenectomy varies.
- Effective in hypersplenism.
- Historically, splenectomy is required for staging of Hodgkin disease, but now replaced by CT and PET scan (FDG-PET).

Hairy Cell Leukemia
- 2% of adult leukemia.
- Splenomegaly, pancytopenia, abnormal lymphocyte.
- Lymphocyte is irregular, hair-like cytoplasm.
- Splenectomy can return cell count to normal by 40%–70%.
- Now new drugs like rituximab.

Hodgkin Disease
- Disorder of lymphoid system characterized by presence of Reed-Sternberg cells.
- 90% of HL has disease lymphadenopathy above diaphragm → LNs is bulky in mediastinum → cough, obstruction, pneumonia.
- LNs below diaphragm is rare.
- Spleen is an occult site of spread.
- Four histologic types.
- Four stages:

  Stage I   Disease limited to one anatomic region

  Stage II   Two sites of disease in diaphragm

  Stage III   Both sides of diaphragm and limited to spleen, LNs, and Waldeyer's ring

  Stage IV   Disease involves bone marrow, lung, liver, skin, GI
- Staging laparoscopy is not done nowadays in the presence of CT and PET.
- Chemotherapy decreases the need for surgery.
- Indication of surgery: clinical suspension of lymphoma without evidence of peripheral disease or restaging after chemotherapy.

Non-Hodgkin's Lymphoma (NHL)

- NHL is all malignancy involved in lymphoid system.
- Proliferation of one of three: NK, T cells, or B cells.
- Classified to nodal and extranodal and indolent, aggressive and very aggressive.
- Symptom (indolent): swollen LNs.
- Symptoms (aggressive): painful swelling and obstruction.
- Staging by history and physical examination, CT CAP + LNS Bx, bone marrow Bx.
- Splenectomy for thrombocytopenia improves 75% of patients.

Chronic Lymphocytic Leukemia

- Currently considered as subtype of NHL.
- It's a progressive accumulation of old and nonfunctioning lymphocyte.
- Symptoms: weakness, fatigue, fever, illness, night sweat, lymphadenopathy, frequent bacterial and viral infection.
- Splenomegaly.
- Splenectomy improves cytopenia by 75%.

Bone Marrow Disorder (Myeloproliferative Disorder)

- Abnormal growth of cells in bone marrow including CML, AML, CMML, essential thrombocythemia, polycythemia, myelofibrosis.
- Splenectomy for symptomatic splenomegaly.
- Can use chemotherapy for splenomegaly.

CML

- Abnormal growth of stem cells in bone marrow.
- Treatment: imatinib or stem cell transplantation.

AML

- Abnormal growth of stem cells in bone marrow, unlike CML, it is rapid and dramatic.
- Treatment: like CML.

Essential Thrombocythemia

- ↑ platelet in bloodstream.
- Diagnosis by exclusion of CML, polycythemia vera.

Polycythemia Vera

- ↑↑ RBCs, WBCs, and platelet.
- Risk of transformation to AML or myelofibrosis.

Myelofibrosis

- Bone marrow fibrosis.

c. **Other Disorders of the Spleen**

Infection and Abscess

- Risk of splenic rupture
- Infectious mononucleosis due to EBV → splenic rupture.
- Also due to malaria, listeria, fungal, and dengue.
- Inflammation → distorted fibrous support → thin capsule.

- **Abscess (Uncommon)**
  - Associated with splenic vesicles, thrombosis, infarction with SCD, and trauma.
  - Mechanism:
    1. Hematogenous infection
    2. Contiguous infection
    3. Hemoglobinopathy
    4. Immunosuppressants (HIV)
    5. Trauma
  - Symptom 16–22 days before diagnosis: fever, LUQ pain, leukocytosis, splenomegaly in ⅓ of patients.

- US or CT is diagnostic, 95%.
- Most common organisms are aerobic (streptococcal, E. coli), mycobacterium TB, salmonella.
- Treatment: IV antibiotic for 14 days.
- Splenectomy is the treatment of choice, but percutaneous drainage can be used.

- **Cyst**
  - Most common caused by parasitic infection (echinococcosis species).
  - Symptom is related to mass.
  - Serology for echinococcosis.
  - If symptomatic → splenectomy (avoid spillage).
  - Resulting from trauma (pseudocyst).
  - Less common: dermoid, epidermoid, and epithelial cysts.
  - Advise patient for intervention to avoid risk of rupture.

Trauma and Metastasis
- Most common primary tumor is sarcoma.
- 0.6% of tumor metastasis, and most is carcinoma.
- The lung is the most common site for tumor that metastasized to spleen.
- Isolated metastasis → laparoscopic splenectomy.

Storage Disease and Infiltrative Disorder
Gaucher Disease
- Inherited lipid storage disease, deposition of glucocerebroside in cells of macrophage and monocyte.
- Due to deficiency of inactivity of lysosomal hydrolase → organomegaly → splenomegaly → hypersplenism.
- Treatment: splenectomy alleviates hematologic abnormality but did not correct underlying process.
- Partial splenectomy can be used in children.

Niemann-Pick Disease
- Inherited disease, abnormal lysosomal storage of sphingomyelin, and cholesterol in cells of macro and mono → splenomegaly
- Four types of disease.

Amyloidosis
- Extracellular protein disposition.
- Ranges from asymptomatic to MOF.
- Primary: plasma cell dyscrasia, 5%.
- Secondary: chronic inflammatory process and splenomegaly.
- Symptom of splenomegaly relieved by splenectomy.

Sarcoidosis
- Noncaseating granulomas, chronic inflammation.
- Symptoms: fatigue, malaise.
- Most affected organ is lung then spleen.
- Splenomegaly, 25%.
- Massive splenomegaly > 1 kg is rare.
- Other affected tissue is LNs, then eye, joint, liver, and heart.
- Splenomegaly can cause hypersplenism → splenectomy.
- Can spontaneously rupture.

Miscellaneous Disorder and Lesion
Splenic Artery Aneurysm
- Most common visceral artery aneurysm.
- Women: men = 4:1.
- Usually arises from middle to distal portion of splenic artery.
- Indications of treatment:
    - → Presence of symptom
    - → Pregnancy
    - → Intention to get pregnant
    - → Presence of pseudoaneurysm with inflammatory process

- Treatment:
    - → If proxicmal or in mid-splenic artery → resection or ligation alone.
    - → If in distal → splenectomy because of proximity to splenic hilum.
    - → Splenic artery embolization is used and produced excellent result, but pain and abscess formation may follow.

Portal HTN

- Splenomegaly from congestion → destructions of cells.
- Splenectomy if hypersplenism.
- Sometimes splenectomy to ↓ esophageal varices → also another option → splenorenal shunt to decompress PHTN.
- If PHTN is secondary to splenic vein thrombosis → splenectomy.
- Patient with isolated gastric varices with normal LFT and no history of pancreatic disease → splenectomy.

Felty Syndrome

- Triad of rheumatoid arthritis (RA), splenomegaly, and neutropenia.
- 3% of all patients with RA.
- Immune complex coats surface of WBCs → sequestration.
- Recurrent infection → splenectomy.
- 5%–10% massive enlargement.
- Treatment: steroid, methotrexate, and splenectomy.
- Response to splenectomy, 80%.

Wandering Spleen

- Congenital anomaly, the spleen floats in abdomen.
- No attachement (ligamenets) to any visceral organ → torsion and infarction.
- Treatment: spleen removal or splenopexy.

Vaccination and Patient Education
- Elective: 2 weeks vaccine prior to splenectomy.
- If emergency situation $\rightarrow$ 2 weeks postoperative to avoid transient immunosuppression in postsurgery.
- Vaccine to encapsulated organism drops risk of OPSI to < 1%.
- Revaccine after 5–10 years due to decline after this period.

Splenectomy Technique
- If thrombocytopenia, do not give platelet before ligation of spleen artery.
  - Open splenectomy
  - Laparoscopic splenectomy
  - Hand-assisted laparoscopic splenectomy
  - Single-incision laparoscopic splenectomy
  - Robotic splenectomy
  - Inadvertent intraoperative splenic injury

Open Splenectomy
- After induction of anesthesia, in supine position, secure the patient to the table with belts.
- Midline of left subcostal incision depends on the size of the spleen and the preference of the surgeon.
- Proper exposure and retraction and inspection for accessory spleens, especially in hematological diseases.
- Medialization of the spleen.
- Move to the splenic inferior attachment to the colon and move upward, using either energy devices or hemostats and ligatures.
- Move upward to the gastrosplenic ligament containing the short gastric vessels, and at this step, the stomach might be very close. Careful dissection must be ensured not to injure the greater curvature.
- Then dissection of the splenocolic ligament.
- Sharp dissection of the lateral attachment of the spleen to the diaphragm and the kidney using blunt dissection, until the spleen is fully mobilized.
- Dissection of splenic hilum to ligation and division of splenic artery then splenic vein, in which artery and vein

should be carefully divided separately, avoiding the potential risk of AV fistula.
- Avoid injuring the tail of the pancreas.

Splenectomy Outcomes
- Appearance of Howell-Jolly bodies and siderocyte and ↑ WBC and continues to rise for several months, ↑ platelet (within 2 days).

- Complication
  o Pulmonary: lower-left lobe atelectasis (most common complication)
  o Risk of DVT is 40% with splenomegaly and myeloproliferative disease.
    ▪ Symptoms: abdominal pain, anorexia, leukocytosis, thrombocytosis.
    ▪ Diagnosis: Doppler US or CT.
    ▪ Start anticoagulant.
    ▪ Before OR evaluation: if patient is obese, of old age, known hypercoagulable state.
    ▪ Should apply compression devise and heparin, 5,000 IU.
  o Intraoperative or post-op hemorrhage, subphrenic hematoma
  o Infectious subphrenic abscess (drain), wound infection
  o Pancreatic pseudocyst and fistula (may be iatrogenic)
  o OPSI
  o Thromboembolic.

- Hematologic Outcome
  o Initial.
  o Long term.
  o ↑ platelet, ↑ Hb in hemolytic anemia.
  o Spherocytosis success rate is 90%–100%.
  o Laparoscopic splenectomy vs. open splenectomy → in laparoscopic, ↑ time, ↑ cost, ↓ stay, ↓ morbidity and mortality, similar blood loss.

Overwhelming post splenectomy infection (OPSI)

- Asplenism → ↑ infection.
- Clinical picture → sepsis.
- Symptom: constitutional manifestation.
- Absent spleen → symptom → fulminant bacteremia → septic shock, low BP, anuria, DIC.
- Patient with hematologic disease or malignancy is in greater risk than trauma patient.
- OPSI is common in pediatric, 4.4% less than 16 years vs. 0.9% and greater risk < 2 years.
- Organisms (50%): streptococcal, H. influenzae B, and N. meningitidis.
- Lifetime risk is < 1%–5%.
- High in hematologic disease more than trauma.
- Risk is < 5 in > 50 age-group.

- Microbiology and Pathogen
    - Loss of splenic macrophage.
    - Loss of RES.
    - Low tufts in production.
    These three → opsonization particularly for encapsulated bacteria.

- Antibiotic and Asplenic Patient
    - Three categories:
        1. For established or presumed infections.
        2. Prophylaxis before invasive procedure
        3. General prophylaxis.
    - Daily dose of antibiotic till age 5 is recommended.
    - Lifelong prophylaxis in patient not responding to vaccines.
    - Asplenic patient is advised to take with him antibiotic if he has symptom.

Endocrine Surgery

Breast

Embryology

- From fifth to sixth gestational age, two ventral band develop, thickened ectoderm (mammary ridges, milk line) from axilla to inguinal region.
- Polymastia: accessory breast.
- Polythelia: accessory nipple.
- Inverted nipple (4%)—failure of the duct to elevate above skin.
- Witch milk → maternal hormone.
- Breast starts to develop at puberty and completes development at the time of pregnancy.
- Amastia → arrest of mammary ridge.
- Poland syndrome: hypoplasia or complete absence of breast + costal and rib defect + hypoplasia of SC tissues in chest and brachysyndactyly.
- Symmastia: webbing between two breasts.
- Polythelia: 1% associated with abnormality in UT, CVS.

Anatomy

- The breast is composed 15–20 ducts, each composed of several lobes.
- Cooper's suspensory ligament: inserted perpendicular into dermis (structural support).
- Boundaries: second to third rib to infra-mammary fold at sixth to seventh rib, lateral border of sternum to anterior axillary line.
- Rest on fascia of pectoralis major, serratus anterior and external oblique, upper rectus sheath.
- Axillary tail extends and crosses anterior axillary line.
- UOQ contains greater volume of tissue and estrogen receptors.
- Contains sebaceous, sweat, accessory glands.
- Smooth muscle circumferential → nipple erection.
- Nipple contains numerous sensory nerve endings, sucking of infant → neurohormonal stimulation.

Inactive and Active Breast
- Each lobe terminates in major duct, 2–4 mm.
- Major duct lined with two layers of cuboidal cells.
- Minor ducts lined by single layer of cuboidal or columnar.
- Lactiferous sinus lined by stratified columnar epithelium.
- In early menstruation, minor ducts is cord like, with estrogen ↑thickness and with pregnancy ↑ proliferation → lymphocyte, plasma cells, eosinophils accumulated in connective tissue.

  NB:

Merocrine	Exocytosis
Apocrine	Loss of cytoplasm
Holocrine	Membrane rupture
Eccrine	Sweat gland

- The milk contains protein component (merocrine) and lipid component (apocrine).
- The first few days, colostrum contains low lipid but is full of antibodies.

Blood Supply
Arterial:
1. Internal mammary artery (perforators)
2. Lateral branch of posterior intercostal artery
3. Axillary artery
   - highest thoracic (superior)
   - lateral thoracic
   - pectoral from thoracoacromial

Venous:
1. Perforator branch of internal thoracic vein
2. Perforator branch of posterior intercostal vein
3. Tributaries of axillary vein

NB: Batson venous plexus (valveless) contributes in metastasis to spine.

Nerves:
- Lateral cutaneous branch (3–6 intercostal nerves): sensory innervation (lateral mammary branch) → exit the intercostal space between slips of serratus anterior.

- Cutaneous branch → cervical plexus → anterior branch of supraclavicular nerve supplies upper breast.
- Lateral cutaneous branch of second intercostal nerve, visualized during axillary dissection, if injured ≥ loss sensation medial aspect of arm.

NB: boundaries of the axilla
- Anterior: pectoralis major and minor
- Posterior: subscapularis muscle
- Medial: serratus anterior
- Lateral: latissimus dorsi

Lymph Nodes
- Axillary LN groups:
  a. Axillary vein group (lateral): 4–6 LNs, lie medial or posteriorly to axillary vein, receive most drainage of upper extremity.
  b. External mammary group (anterior or pectoral): 5–6 LNs, lie along lower border of pectoralis minor, receive most of lateral aspect of breast.
  c. Scapular group (post- or subscapular): 5–7 LNs, lie posteriorly to wall of axilla at the lateral border of scapula, receive lower posterior neck, posterior shoulder.
  d. Central group: 4 LNs, embedded in the fat of axilla, receive from axillary vein, scapula group, breast.
  e. Subclavicular group (apical): 6–12 LNs, lie posterosuperior to upper border of pectoralis minor, receive from all the other groups.
  f. Interpectoral group (Rotter's LNs): 1–4 LNs, between pectoralis major and minor, receive directly from breast. The lymph fluid of this group drains to central and subclavicular.
- LNs assigned in levels according to their anatomical relation of pectoralis minor:

Level I	Located laterally or below pectoralis minor, includes group (a, b, c)
Level II	Deep or beneath pectoralis minor, includes group (d, f)
Level III	Located medially or above pectoralis minor, includes group (e)

- Plexus of lymph nodes arises in interlobular and communicates with subareola.
- Efferent from breast, pass around lateral edge of pectoralis major and pierce clavipectoral fascia and end in extended mammary (pectoral).
- Some LNs drain directly to subscapular.
- From upper breast, few pass directly to subclavicular.
- Axillary receive > 75% of drainage.

Physiology
Breast Development and Function
- Initiated by estrogen, progesterone, prolactin, oxytocin, thyroid hormone, cortisol, GH.
- Estrogen: duct development.
- Progesterone: differentiation of lobular tissue.
- Prolactin: lactogenesis in late pregnancy.
- LH, FSH: regulate release of ER, PR from ovary.
- Size and density: ↑ at the beginning of menstrual cycle followed by engorgement and subsides at the onset of menstruation.

Gynecomastia
- Physiological: neonate, adolescent, senescence because of circulating estrogen.
- Ductal structure increases and elongates.
- During puberty, it's unilateral.
- Dominant mass, firm, irregular.
- Old age → ↑↑ suspicions of malignancy.
- Not premalignant.
- Klinefelter XXY → ↑↑ risk of breast CA.
- Grade

I	Mild increase with no redundancy
IIa	Moderate increase with no redundancy
II b	Moderate increase with redundancy
III	Marked increase, redundancy, ptosis

Causes
- o Estrogen excess
  - ▪ Gonadal origin "tumor"

- - Nontesticular
  - Endocrine
  - Liver disease
  - Nutrition
  o Androgen decreases
    - Senescence
    - Hypogonadism, first/second testicular failure
    - Renal disease
  o Pharmacological: spironolactone, Ranitidine.
  o Systemic disease with idiopathic mechanism

Treatment

- If the cause decreases androgen → give testosterone.
- If medication → D/C.
- If increase is not responding to the therapy → surgical therapy, local excision, liposuction, subcutaneous mastectomy.
- Attempt to reverse gynecomastia with danazol has been successful but with many side effects.

Infectious and Inflammatory Disease

- Lactational is the most common cause while unrelated to lactation is less common.
- Intrinsic (abnormality in the breast).
- Extrinsic (infection of adjacent structure).
- Periductal mastitis, infected sebaceous cyst.

Bacterial Infection

- Causative organism: staph, strep.
- Breast abscess → staph.
- Previously, surgical treatment in terms of incision and drainage.
- Nowadays, antibiotic with repeated aspiration with US-guided; if failed → incision and drainage.
- Pre-operative US is indicated → extension.
- Incision and drainage, antibiotic, warm compresses, wound care.
- If recurrent abscess → wound swab for AFB, anaerobic, fungal, and biopsy at the time of I&D.
- Epidemic puerperal mastitis → rule out MRSA.

- Non-epidemic puerperal mastitis → emptying of milk by pump to shorten the duration.
- If purulent fluid, stop breastfeeding.
- Zuska's disease, recurrent periductal mastitis, recurrent retroareolar infection, abscess, and smoking aggravate the condition → antibiotic + incision and drainage → sometimes wide debridement.

Mycotic Infection
- Rare by infected infant.
- Pus and blood.
- Antifungal.
- Sometimes incision and drainage or partial mastectomy.
- Candida albicans → IV and topical nystatin.

Hidradenitis Suppurativa
- Nipple areola complex (accessory areolar gland) or axilla (sebaceous cyst).
- Chronic acne.
- When located at nipple, areola mimics other chronic inflammatory, Paget's disease, inflammatory breast CA.
- Incision and drainage.
- Excision may be required + skin graft.
- Now immunosuppressant (Humira) is used with impressive result.

Mondor's Disease
- Thrombophlebitis of superficial veins in chest wall and breast.
- Cord-like structure.
- Lateral thoracic vein, superficial epigastric vein, thoracoepigastric vein are most commonly involved.
- Rarely bilateral.
- Self-limiting.
- Uncertain diagnosis of positive mass → biopsy is indicated.
- Treatment: anti-inflammatory, warm compress.
- Resolve within 4 -6 weeks.
- If refractory or persistent → excision of vein.

Benign Disease of the Breast

ANDI Classification of Benign Breast Disease

Age	Normal	Disorder	Disease
Early reproductive 15–25	Lobular development Stromal development Nipple eversion	Fibroadenoma Adolescent hypertrophy Nipple inversion	Giant fibroadenoma Gigantomastia Subareolar abscess Mammary duct fistula
Late reproductive	Cyclic changes of menstruation Epithelial hyperplasia pregnancy	Cyclic mastalgia Nodulation Bloody nipple discharge	Incapacitating mastalgia
Involution 35–55	Lobular involution Duct involution Dilatation Sclerosis Epithelial turnover	Macrocyte Sclerosing lesion Duct ectasia Nipple retraction Epithelial hyperplasia	Periductal mastitis

Early Productive Year
- Fibroadenoma: 15–25 years, usually 1–2 cm, > 5 cm (giant fibroadenoma).
- Massive stromal hyperplasia.
- Nipple inversion → major duct obstruction → subareolar abscess, mammary duct fistula.

Late Reproductive Year
- Cyclic mastalgia and nodularity associated with premenstrual enlargement.
- Painful nodularity that persist > 1 week is considered a disorder.

- Epithelial hyperplasia of pregnancy gives papillary projection → bilateral bloody nipple disease.

Involution
- When stroma is too quick from microcyte → macrocyte.
- 60% of women ≥ 70 years → atypical hyperplasia.
- Duct and lobular atypical hyperplasia, ↑ risk of breast CA by fourfold.

Cancer risk associated with benign breast disorders and in situ carcinoma of the breast	
Abnormality	**Relative risk**
No proliferative lesions of the breast	No increased risk
Sclerosing adenoids	No increased risk
Intraductal papilloma	No increased risk
Florid hyperplasia	1.5- to 2- fold
Atypical lobular hyperplasia	4- fold
Atypical ductal hyperplasia	4- fold
Ductal involvement by cells of atypical ductal hyperplasia	7- fold
Lobular carcinoma in situ	10- fold
Ductal carcinoma in situ	10- fold

Classification of Benign Breast Disease
- Non-proliferative
  - Cyst and apocrine metaplasia
  - Duct ectasia
  - Duct epithelial hyperplasia
  - Calcification
  - Fibroadenoma

- Proliferative without atypia
  - Sclerosing adenosis

- Radial sclerosing lesion
- Duct epithelial hyperplasia
- Intraductal/lobular hyperplasia

• Atypical proliferative lesion
• Atypical ductal and lobular hyperplasia

Pathology of Non-proliferative Disease

- 70% of breast pathology.
- No risk of breast CA.

• Duct ectasia: dilated subareolar ducts, associated with thick nipple discharge (chemical irritation, fatty acid)
→ local inflammatory process with periductal fibrosis → nipple retraction.
Another theory (periductal mastitis) primary pathology → weakening of duct → dilation, calcium deposit, microcalcification—fine.

• Fibroadenoma: abundant stromal tissue with normal cellular elements, Types:

o *Juvenile fibroadenomas (breast mouse).* This is the most common type of breast lump found in girls and adolescents between the ages of 10 and 18. These fibroadenomas can grow large, but most shrink over time, and some disappear. It has **two types:** periductal and intraductal.

o *Complex fibroadenomas.* These can contain changes such as an overgrowth of cells (hyperplasia) that can grow rapidly. A pathologist makes the diagnosis of a complex fibroadenoma after reviewing the tissue from a biopsy.

o *Giant fibroadenomas.* These can grow to larger than 2 inches (5 centimeters). They might need to be removed because they can press on or replace other breast tissue.

- o *Phyllodes tumor.* Although usually benign, some phyllodes tumors can become cancerous (malignant).
- Adenoma: well circumscribed, normal epithelial with spare stroma can be differentiated from fibroadenoma.
- Hamartoma: 2–4 cm, firm, circumscribed.
- Adenolipomas: round nodular of fatty tissue.
- Fibrocystic disease: need biopsy to all cystic diseases, copper disease.

Pathology of Proliferative Disease without Atypia

- Sclerosing adenosis → childbearing age, perimenopausal, no malignant risk. Distorted breast lobules, multiple microcyst, palpable mass, benign calcification managed by observation, image, histopathology.
- Central sclerosis (radial scar)—epithelial proliferative, apocrine metaplasia, papilloma formation, lesion < 1 cm radial scar, larger complex sclerosing lesion originates from terminal branch duct. Difficult to distinguish between radial scar and invasive carcinoma by biopsy (similar to each other) → open surgical biopsy (excisional).
- Mild duct hyperplasia:
  - Mild: presence of 3–4 cell layers above basement membrane.
  - Moderate: more than 5 cell layers.
- Florid ductal hyperplasia:
  - 70% minor ducts, 20% breast tissue.
- Intraductal papilloma (IDP):
  - Affects major duct, premenopause.
  - 0.5–5 cm.
  - Mostly bloody discharge or serous discharge.
  - Grossly pinkish tan, friable, attached to the wall of duct.
  - Rare malignant transformation.
  - Multiple IDPs decrease discharge but increase the risk of malignancy.
  - Ductogram: filling defect.
  - Tx: microductectomy.

Pathology of Atypical Proliferative Disease
- Atypical Ductal Hyperplasia (ADH)
  - Has same of feature of carcinoma in situ but lacks major feature, ADH similar to DCIS.
  - Composed of round, cuboidal, or polygonal enclosed by basement membrane with rare mitosis.
  - If lesion is 2–3 cm → ADH.
  - If lesion > 3 cm → DCIS.
  - Difficult to diagnose with core biopsy → excisional biopsy.
  - 4–7 times ↑ risk of CA.
  - Excision with negative margin is recommended.

- Atypical Lobular Hyperplasia (ALH)
  - Ranging from ALH to LCIS.

Treatment of Selected Benign Breast Disease
- Cyst
  - Prefer to image breast before FNA or core biopsy, i.e., before artifact.
  - Full aspiration → if not blood → discarded.
  - If there is mass → core biopsy with clip to mark it.
  - If it's bloodstained → cytology.
  - A complex cyst is a concern for malignancy; the simple is not.
  - Pneumocystogram → inject air to cyst → mammogram → for any irregularity.

- Fibroadenoma
  - Conservative management.
  - Core needle biopsy with US-guided.
  - If patient is diagnosed with core needle biopsy with US-guided, excision is avoided.
  - Cytoablation and US-guided vacuum-assisted biopsy treatment of fibroadenoma < 3 m.
  - If larger, removed by excision.

- Sclerosing Disorders
    - Elimination of CA risk by physical examination, mammogram, histopathology.
    - Excisional biopsy and histopathology are necessary to exclude CA.
    - Involve via stereotactic biopsy.
    - Not possible to differentiate the lesion from CA by mammogram or FNA or by core biopsy, so vacuum-assisted biopsy or open biopsy is recommended.

- Periductal Mastitis
    - Painful, tender mass behind nipple, areola complex.
    - Aspiration → send for C/S.
    - Empirically, metronidazole + dicloxacin, then according to C/S.
    - Many respond to antibiotic alone.
    - Repeat aspiration using US-guided or incision or drainage.
    - Usually unilocular, not like peripheral abscess.
    - Either incision and drainage or formal surgery.
    - In women of childbearing age → incision and drainage, unless recurrent.

- Fistula
    - Treatment: initially remove fistula tract, allowing to heal by granulation.
    - Definitive: fistulectomy + primary closure + antibiotic and excision of all major ducts.
    - If recurrent → previous site fistulectomy.
    - If diffuse, more than one fistula → total duct excision.
    - Antibiotic for recurrent infection after fistula excision for 2–4 weeks then total ducts excision.

- Nipple Inversion
    - Congenital or after duct ectasia.
    - Inform the patient for complication → ↓ sensation, necrosis.
    - It results from shorted ducts.

- Breast Pain
  - Some diseases that contribute to mastalgia are bone disease costochondritis, fibromyalgia.
  - Aggravating and relieving factor.
  - Unilateral or bilateral.
  - If cyclic bilateral diffuse, improve after menstruation.
  - If noncyclic, not relieved with menses such as cyst, fibroadenoma, and chest wall disease.
  - Medical treatment: reassurance.
    - → Diet modification, warm compress, low fat, decrease caffeine
    - → analgesic: non-steroidal
    - → Vitamin E, fish oil, primrose oil
    - → Topical non-steroidal
  - Meta-analysis: bromocriptine, danazol, evening primrose, tamoxifen.
    - → Tamoxifen is the drug of choice.

Breast Cancer
- Hormonal and non-hormonal risk factors.
- Increase exposure to estrogen has ↑ risk of CA.
- Increase number of menstrual cycle such as early menarche, late menopause, null parity also ↑ risk.
- Obese patient increases risk after menopause as estrogen increases from androstenedione by adipose tissue.
- Non-hormonal like radiation, atomic bomb (Japan), ↑↑ risk because of somatic mutation.
- Alcohol increases risk due to high serum estradiol.
- Exercise, multiparity decrease the risk.

Risk Assessment Modules
- Average lifetime risk is 12%.
- The longer women live without cancer, the lower their risk.
- At 50 years, 11%; 70 years, 7%.
- Gail et al. developed model most commonly used in the USA, which incorporates age, age of menarche, age of first live birth, number of breast biopsy, history of atypical hyperplasia, number of first-degree relative with breast CA.

- It predicts cumulative risk according to decade of life by overall risk score and relative risk from several categories, then risk score compared to general population.
- Model modified for African American.
- Model modified recently to include body weight, mammography density, but exclude age at menarche.
- Claus et al, 2nd models is assume about prevalence of ↑ percentage breast CA gene.
- Compared to Gail, Claus provides more information about family history but excludes other risk factors.
- Neither Gail nor Claus mentioned diet, use of OCP, lactation, radiation, BRCA1 and 2.
- BRCAPRO is a mendelian model that calculates carry mutation of one of the three genes.

Risk Management
- Estrogen before menopause decreases osteoporosis, sleeplessness, lowers coronary heart disease.
- Estrogen + progesterone started with women who did not undergo hysterectomy because estrogen increases uterine CA.
- Evaluate risk vs. benefit of hormone replacement postmenopause.
- Use of hormone is higher by three to four times in breast CA, no prevention against coronary heart disease.

Breast Cancer Screening
- Breast self-exam (BSE) is not recommended because studies showed no decrease in breast CA.
- Clinical breast exam (CBE) increases detection of CA than mammogram alone.
- Mammography uses of BI-RAD system.
- Routine use of mammogram in ≥ 50 years old to reduce mortality by 25%.
- It's controversial because breast density increases, and mammogram is less likely to detect early breast CA.
- High false +ve → unnecessary biopsy.
- Younger women are less likely to have breast CA.

- US can be used in woman with dense breast, i.e., young female.
- Recommendation by ACS → mammogram at 40s + annual clinical breast examination.
- MRI indications: 20%–25% lifetime risk in women with family history, BRCA mutation, radiation between 10–30 years old, recurrent disease, Li-Fraumeni syndrome, Cowden syndrome, LCIS, previous surgery, axillary LNs with no primary, implants.

NCCN Recommendation Regarding Breast Screening Guideline

≥ 25 < 40	CBE Q1–3Y, breast awareness
40–44	Annual CBE, annual mammography
45–50	Annual CBE, annual mammography
50–74	Annual CBE, annual mammography
> 75	no screening as ↓ risk after 75

Chemoprevention

- Tamoxifen selective estrogen blockage, first drug that decreases breast CA.
    - Tamoxifen vs. placebo in random 13,000 patients, decrease 49% of breast CA risk, only in ER +ve with no change in ER −ve.
    - Complications: endometrial CA, thromboembolic events, cataract.
    - Currently recommended if patient has Gail risk of 1.66% or more in 35–59 years old.
    - They compared tamoxifen vs. raloxifene, raloxifene is more effective to decrease breast CA and decrease uterine CA.
    - Raloxifen is 75% more effective than tamoxifen with less side effects.
- Aromatase inhibitors (AI)
    - More effective than tamoxifen.
    - Decreases invasive breast CA by 65%.
    - Side effects: arthritis, hot flashes.

Risk-Reducing Surgery
- Patient with high risk → prophylactic mastectomy ↓ risk by > 90%.
- BRCA1, BRCA2 → mastectomy + bilateral salpingo-oophorectomy.

BRCA Mutation
- BRCA1
    - 5% of breast CA caused by BRCA mutation.
    - Autosomal dominant.
    - Located on chromosome arm 17q.
    - Functions as tumor suppressor gene.
    - Loss of each → initiation of CA.
    - Predisposes 45% of breast CA, 80% of ovarian CA.
    - Risk is 85% of breast CA and 40% of ovarian CA (lifetime).
    - Associated with invasive ductal carcinoma, poorly differentiated, and have triple −ve (ER, PR, HER2), i.e., BCL.
    - Increases bilateral CA.
    - Tenfold higher in Ashkenazi Jewish population.
    - 20% of Ashkenazi women will develop breast CA.

- BRCA2
    - Located on chromosome arm 13q.
    - Risk mutation is 85%.
    - To date, > 250 mutations have been found.
    - 20% of ovarian CA.
    - Autosomal dominant.
    - 50% of children carry risk.
    - Hundredfold increase of breast CA in men, in comparison to general population.
    - Associated with invasive ductal CA, well differentiated.
    - Presented in early age and bilaterally.
    - Associated with prostate, colon, pancreas, gallbladder, stomach CA.
    - Presented in early age in Ashkenazi women.

Identification of BRCA Mutation Carrier

- Obtaining multigenerational family history.
- Assessing appropriate genetic testing.
- Counseling the patient.
- Interpreting the result.
- 50% of BRCA inherited from father.

BRCA Mutation Testing

- BRCA testing and informed consent.
- False −ve, 5%.
- All family members.
- Usually, health insurance does not apply to BRCA testing.

Cancer Prevention in BRCA Carrier

o Risk-reducing mastectomy and reconstruction
o Risk-reducing salpingo-oophorectomy
o Intensive surveillance for breast and ovarian CA
o Chemoprevention

- After mastectomy → there is cancer risk, i.e., because all breast tissues are not removed.
- For BRCA + menopause → advise not to take hormonal replacement.
- Mammogram with high index of suspicion.
- Breast examination every 6 months at 25 years old because of the risk at age of 30s.
- MRI in known BRCA patients can prevent biopsy in benign lesion. Prevents false +ve.
- Recommendation: ACA → annual MRI in women with 20%–25% risk.
- Strong family history.
- Hormonal therapy is not warranted because most BRCA breast CA will have ER −ve.
- 66% of BRCA1 have DCIS, ER −ve.
- Risk of ovarian CA BRCA1, BRCA2 is 20%, 40%, respectively.
- Bilateral salpingo-oophorectomy at age 35–40.
- Recommendation:
  o Yearly transvaginal US, avoid ovulation time.
  o Annual CA 125 at age 25.

- Better treatment is prophylactic surgery.
- Other hereditary syndromes associated with high risk of breast CA:
  - o Cowden disease (PTEN mutation → thyroid CA, gastrointestinal tract CA, benign skin lesion, and SC nodules).
  - o Li-Fraumeni (P53 mutation → sarcomas, lymphomas, adrenal tumor, melanoma).

Epidemiology and Natural History of Breast Cancer
- Most common cancer in women, 29% newly diagnosed CA, 14% CA related to death after lung CA.
- Decreased over years (decrease use of estrogen, women education), 1.4M new cases yearly.
- Increase incidence in African Americans in younger age < 45 with hormonal receptor −ve.
- 250 women left untreated breast CA for 5, 10, 15 years, SR is 18%, 3.6%, 0.8%, respectively.
- 95% died from CA, 5% from other causes.
- 75% developed ulceration.
- The longest-surviving patient lived for 19 years after diagnosis.

Primary Breast CA
- 80% showed productive fibrosis.
- Entrapment shortened suspensory ligament → skin retraction.
- Disruption of lymphoma draining of skin → Peau d'orange.
- Invasion of skin → ulceration.
- Size correlates with disease-free.

Axillary LNs Metastasis
- Size of tumor increases, some cells shed to cellular space → lymph nodes, especially axillary.
- Level I → II → III.
- Women with −ve LNs → 30% recurrence.
- With +ve LNs → 75% risk of recurrence.

Distant Metastasis
- Breast CA has its own blood supply (neovascularization).

- Cells shed into systemic circulation → pulmonary circulation via axillary, intercostal, or vertebra via Batson plexus.
- Metastasis can occur when tumor size > 0.5 cm.
- Patient with −ve ER → increase recurrence within 3–5 years.
- Common sites are bone, lung, pleura, soft tissue, liver. The brain is less common.
- Brain metastasis increases in triple −ve.

Histopathology of Breast CA
Carcinoma In Situ
- There is no invasion to basement membrane
- It was represent 4% of breast CA before mammogram, now increase to 45% after mammogram.
- DCTS is more than LCIS, 2:1.
- Multicentricity: second breast CA outside of breast quadrant of primary CA or at least 4 cm away.
- Multifocality: second breast CA within the same quadrant of primary CA or within 4 cm of it.
- Multicentricity: 60%–90% in LCIS, while 40%–80% in DCIS.
- Bilaterally: 50%–70% in LCIS, while 10%–20% in DCIS.

Lobular Carcinoma In Situ (LCIS)
- LCIS originates from terminal duct lobular unit, only in female.
- Distension and distortion of terminal duct lobular unit.
- Microcalcification occurs in adjacent tissues, neighborhood calcification (unique).
- Average age for disease is 45 years.
- Twelve times more in white than African.
- Not precancerous (not like DCIS), i.e., predict high risk to develop breast CA in the future rather (marker) than precursor.
- Marker to ↑ risk of future breast CA.
- Synchronous invasive CA, 5%.
- In woman with history of LCIS → 65% develop invasive ductal carcinoma.
- Diagnosis of LCIS by cells, distend terminal duct lobular unit, but architecture is maintained.

- Classic LCIS is not treated by excision i.e. patient is not at risk to develop invasive cancer.
- There is variety → pleomorphic LCIS. There will be calcification on suspicious mammogram.
- Difficult to distinguish DCIS from LCIS by histopathology but by IHC staining for E-cadherin.
- In lobular neoplasia such as LCIS, ALH → lack of E-cadherin, while majority of ductal neoplasia → reactivity to E-cadherin.

Ductal Carcinoma In Situ (DCIS)
- Mostly in women, in men it is 5%.
- Intraductal CA = DCIS.
- High risk to progress to invasive CA.
- Histologically, proliferation of epithelial that lining the minor duct → papillary growth pattern, i.e., early, no pleomorphism, mitosis, or atypia.
- Difficult to distinguish from benign disease.
- Papillary coalesces and fills the duct with hyperchromatic and loss of polarity (cribriform growth pattern).
- With pleomorphism of CA cells + high mitotic figures, obliterate lumina and distend the duct (solid growth pattern).
- With continued growth, these cells outstrip their blood supply and become necrotic (comedo growth pattern).
- Calcium deposition occurs in the area of necrosis → feature seen in mammography.
- DCIS classified based on nuclear grade and presence of necrosis.
- Fivefold risk of invasive CA in same breast, same quadrant, i.e., DCIS is precursor of invasive CA.

Invasive CA
- Ductal or lobular.
- LCIS → lobular invasive CA, and all others are invasive ductal CA.
- 10% special type, 90% undefining histology.
- 80% of invasive breast cancer has no special type (NST).

- Foote-Stewart classification:
  o Paget's disease of the nipple
  o IDC adenocarcinoma with productive fibrosis (scirrhous, simplex, NST), 80%
  o Medullary CA, 4%
  o Mucinous CA (colloid), 2%
  o Papillary CA, 2%
  o Tubular CA, 2%
  o Invasive lobular carcinoma, 10%
  o Rare (adenoid cystic, SCC, apocrine)

- Paget's disease—chronic eczematous eruption of the nipple.
  - It may progress to an ulceration.
  - Usually associated with extension of DCIS or IDC.
  - Nipple biopsy → cell identical to DCIS.
  - Pathognomonic → large, pale, vacuolated.
  - Confused with superficial spreading melanoma but can be differentiated by S-100 antigen immunostaining in melanoma and carcinoembryonic antigen (CEA) immunostaining in Paget's disease.
  - Treatment: lumpectomy.
  - Mastectomy (if involved with nipple areola complex).

- IDCA (scirrhous, simplex, NST)
  - 80% of breast CA.
  - 25% LNs +ve.
  - Occurred mostly in peri- or postmenopausal women.
  - Poorly defined margin.
  - 75% ER +ve.

- Medullary CA
  - 4% of breast CA, associated with BRCA1.
  - Grossly soft, hemorrhagic.
  - Rapid increase in size because of necrosis or hemorrhage.
  - 20% bilaterally.
  - Microscopically: Dense lymphoreticular infiltrate (lymphocyte plasma cell).

- Large pleomorphic nuclei + mitosis.
- Sheetlike with minimal or absent ducts.
- 50% associated with DCIS at periphery.
- Women with this tumor have better SR in 5 years than with NST or ILC.

- Mucinous CA (colloid)
  - 2% of breast CA, affects elderly, bulky tumor.
  - Extracellular pools of mucin surrounded by low-grade cancer cells.
  - Cut section of gelatinous fibrosis.
  - 90% +ve hormone receptors.
  - 33% LNs metastasis.
  - 5, 10 years, SR is 75%, 59%.

- Papillary CA
  - 2% of breast CA, affects old age.
  - Small, rarely > 3 cm.
  - Papillae with fibrovascular stalks.
  - 37% ER +ve.
  - Low LNs metastasis.
  - 5–10 years SR similar to mucinous.

- Tubular CA (most favorable tumor)
  - 2% of breast CA, diagnosed by mammogram.
  - Perimenopausal or early post.
  - 94% ER +ve.
  - Long-term SR, 100%.

- ILC (invasive lobular carcinoma)
  - 10%.
  - Small cells, rounded nuclei, scant cytoplasm.
  - Special stain (signet ring cells carcinoma).
  - Poorly defined mass.
  - Multifocal, multicentric, bilaterally.
  - Difficult to detect, 90% ER +ve.

Diagnosis of Breast CA
By triple assessement (Hx and physical examination, image, Biopsy)

History
- 30% discovered by a woman by herself.
- Breast enlargement or asymmetry.
- Nipple retraction or discharge.
- Ulceration or erythema.
- Axillary mass.
- Musculoskeletal discomfort.
- 50% present with no complaint and no physical sign.
- Any women < 45 present with lump → biopsy.

Examination
Inspection
- With arm to her side
- With arm up
- With hand on her hips (with or without pectoralis major contracture)
- Symmetry, size, shape
- Evidence of edema (Peau d'orange)
- Nipple retraction or skin retraction or erythema

Palpation
- Palpate carefully in supine and gently to all quadrants from sternum lateral to latissimus and from clavicle to upper rectus sheath with palm of the hand or tips of fingers (no grasping or pinching), then in LNs, support arm and elbow and stabilize shoulder girdle → all three levels + supraclavicular.
- Use of diagram—location, size, consistency, shape, mobility, fixation.

Imaging Techniques
- Mammogram
  - Deliver 0.1 cGy/study.
  - CXR contains 25% of this dose.
  - No increase of breast CA risk with mammogram.
  - Two views: craniocaudal (CC), mediolateral oblique (MLO)

- MLO shows greatest volume of breast, UOQ + tail.
- CC shows medial aspect.
- Can be used for grid interval procedure, needle localization, and biopsy.
- Mammographic features of breast CA:
  o Irregular speculated solid mass with or without stellate
  o Asymmetric ticking of breast
  o Clustered microcalcification
- It reduces mortality rate by 33%.
- True +ve rate is 90%.
- Only 20% of non-palpable mass → +ve LNs.
- Xeromammogram: same view but lower radiation.
- BI-RAD classification:
  0 Incomplete → need additional image
  1 Normal
  2 Benign
  3 Probably benign
  4 Suspiciously abnormal
  5 Highly suggested to be malignant
  6 Biopsy-proven CA

- Ductogram
  - For nipple discharge especially fluid + blood.
  - Contrast injected into one or more ducts → then mammogram is performed, CC and MLO views.
  - Blunt cannula in supine position.
  - Intraductal papilloma → small filling defect.
  - Cancer → irregular filling defect.

- Ultrasound
  - Second to mammogram.
  - To differentiate between mass and cyst.
  - On ultrasound, benign cyst has smooth contour, rounded or oral shape, weak internal echoes.
  - Breast CA cyst has irregular wall but can have smooth surface with acoustic enhancement.
  - Offer guidance image, FNA biopsy.
  - Not reliable in detecting lesion ≥ 1 cm.

- Regional LNs could be used.
- Sensitivity to LNs is 30%–80%; specificity is 73%–97%.
- Features of involved LNs in CA: cortical thickening change in shape, increase 10 mm, absence of fatty hilum.

- MRI
  - In case of absence finding on mammogram and histopathology, the probability to diagnose CA by MRI is low.
  - Indication: strong family history or carrying known gene mutation at early age.
  - Patient with breast CA has shown a contralateral breast CA in 5.7%.
  - Can detect multifocal, multicentric.
  - No decrease in rate of re-operation in women who underwent MRI perioperatively compared to women with mammography or ultrasound.
  - One study showed MRI increases rate of mastectomy.
  - Useful in patient presented with LNs metastasis without identifiable primary tumor.
  - To assess response to neoadjuvant.
  - Evaluation of recurrence:
    - Previous surgery
    - Previous biopsy
    - Implant
    - Suspicion lesion with +ve histopathology

Breast Biopsy
- Nonpalpable lesion
  - US localization if there is a mass.
  - Stereotactic technique if no mass (microcal) or architectural distortion.
  - Combination of mammogram, US, or stereotactic FNA (100%) accuracy.
  - FNA → cytology.
  - Core needle → does not disturb breast tissue architecture and allows pathologist to determine if invasive component is present.

- Core needle is preferred over open biopsy because single surgery can be obtained.
- Advantages: decrease complication, decrease scar, low cost.

- Palpable lesion
  - FNA or core biopsy, 22 gauges attached to 10 mL syringe.
  - FNA uses syringe holder to control needle, and the other hand positions the mass.
  - After placement → suction.
  - Once cellular material is seen, stop suction → apply it to slides → air-dried 95% ethanol.
  - If breast mass is clinically palpated and radiologically suspicious → FNA is 100% accurate.
  - Core needle by 14 gauges like trucut.
  - Automated devices if available such as vacuum-assisted core biopsy device.
  - 4–12 samples can be taken from different position.
  - Radiopaque marker such as clips should be placed at the site of biopsy to mark the area for future intervention.
  - Specimen placed in formalin → paraffin.
  - If biopsy does not concur with clinical or radiological → multidisciplinary tumor board.

Breast CA Staging and Biomarkers
Staging
- Examine skin, breast tissue, LNs (axillary, supraclavicular, internal mammary).
- Clinical examination for LNs is 33% accurate → US is most accurate (100%).
- FNA or core biopsy for LNs is better than US alone.
- One of the most common predictor for SR in 10–20 years is nodal involvement (axillary).
- Internal mammary drains central and medial breast.
- +ve supraclavicular LNs are no longer stage IV.
- In routine supraclavicular LNs, biopsy is not indicated.

Tx	Cannot be assessed
T0	No tumor

Tis	DCIS, LCIS, Paget's disease
T1	Tumor ≤ 2 cm
T2	2 to ≤ 5 cm
T3	> 5 cm
T4	Any size with invasion to skin or chest wall
T4a	To chest wall (muscle)
T4b	To skin (Peau d'orange), not inflammatory CA
T4c	A + b
T4d	Inflammatory breast CA
Nx	Cannot be assessed, e.g., removed before
N0	No LNs
N1	Metastasis to same-side axillary I, II
N2	Same-side axillary I, II (fixed, matted) or same side internal mammary.
N2a	Metastasis to same-side axillary (I, II), fixed, matted
N2b	Same-side internal mammary but no axillary
N3	Same-side infraclavicular (III), without (I, II) or same side internal mammary + axillary I, II
N3a	Metastasis to same-side infraclavicular
N3b	Metastasis in same side internal mammary + axillary
N3c	Metastasis in supraclavicular LNs.

Pathological Nodal assessement

PNx	Cannot be assessed (removed)
PN0	No LNs metastasis
PN1	1–3 axillary LNs and/or internal mammary
PN2	4–9 axillary or internal mammary
PN3	More than 10 axillary or infraclavicular III

Biomarkers

- Provide tumor outcome irrespective to surgery.
    - Steroid hormone receptor
    - Growth factor and receptor such as HER2/neu EGFR
    - Proliferation such as PCNA, Ki-67
    - Angiogenesis EEGF
    - Mammalian target of rapamycin (mTOR)
    - Tumor suppressor genes P53
    - Cell cycle, cyclin

- Proteasome
- COX-2 enzyme
- PPARS, Apoptosis

- Steroid Hormone Receptors
  - Hormones play an important role in development and progression of breast CA, ER, PR.
  - Hormone therapy, postmenopause, replacement of estrogen and progesterone increase risk by 26%.
  - Patient with hormone +ve has two to three times longer SR with metastatic disease than −ve does.
  - Patient with tumor −ve ER, PR → not a candidate for hormonal therapy.
  - +ve ER, PR 50% response.
  - −ve ER, PR 10% response.
  - One +ve receptor responds to 33% of the therapy.
  - Can be achieved by IHC.
  - Can be obtained by FNA or cure needle.
  - Test should be performed in all invasive CA.

- Growth factor receptor
  - Overexpression of epidermal GFR → increase ER −ve + P53 overexpression.
  - Increase IHC staining for HER2/neu, EGFR associated with highly mutated P53, Ki-67 overexpression, and ER −ve.
  - HER2 is a member of the EGFR family.
  - Homodimerization → thyroxine phosphorylation → change in cell behavior.
  - Overexpression of HER2 → increase proliferation and highly invasive disease and metastasis.
  - Studies showed overexpression of HER2 → proliferation, invasion, metastasis, poor differentiation, +ve LNs, low hormonal expression, increase recurrence.
  - Routine HER2 should be performed by IHC analysis.
  - Patient with HER2 → is candidate for anti-HER2 (Herceptin), recombinant antibody against HER2.

- Herceptin + chemo → decrease risk by 40%–50% and 1/3 of mortality for patient received chemotherapy alone.

• Indices of Proliferation
  - PCNA nuclear protein with DNA polymerase expression increase in GI cells cycle and reach the maximum at G1/S and decrease in G2.
  - IHC staining for PCNA showed proliferation.
  - Good correlation between the following:
    a. Cell cycle, DNA content
    b. Uptake and proliferation in Ki-67 Ag.
  - PGNA, Ki-67 expression, +ve correlated with P53 overexpression, increase S phase, high mitotic index, high histologic grade, and −ve correlated with ER.
  - Ki-67 used with ER, PR, HER (ICH4), or Ki-67 alone = same prediction.

• Indices of Angiogenesis
  - Necessary for growth and invasiveness of breast CA including O_2 and nutrients and secretion of cytokines by endothelial cells (VEGF) → increase recurrence in nodal −ve breast CA.
  - Angiogenesis developed in microvessel density is combined with thrombospondin (−ve modulator for angiogenesis and P53 expression).
  - Both VEGF and angiogenesis have prognostic and predictive value.

• Indices of Apoptosis
  - Alteration of programmed cell death may be triggered by P53.
  - BCI-2 regulates pathway of apoptosis.
  - Overexpression of BCI-2 → increase histological grade and presence of axillary LNs, decrease disease-free.

- Coexpression of Biomarkers

Type	Hormonal status	Her2/neu
Luminal A	ER +and / or PR +	-
Luminal B	ER +and / or PR +	+
BCL	ER - / PR -	-
HER2/neu+	ER - / PR -	+

ER: Estrogen receptor: PR: Progesterone receptor BCL: basal cell like.
- ER, PR, HER2 = most important.
- The website www.adjuvantonline.com is used for calculation and for combination of chemoendocrine.

Overview of Breast CA Therapy
- Type of therapy is determined by stage of the disease, biological subtype, general health (laboratory, image).

In Situ Breast CA (Stage 0)
- Both LCIS and DCIS are difficult to distinguish from atypical hyperplasia or early invasive CA.
- Mammography: to see tumor extension or presence of second CA.

o **Lobular Carcinoma In Situ (LCIS)**
  - Diagnosed by CNBx.
  - Excisional biopsy is warranted to exclusive DCIS or invasive component.
  - 20% of specimen of DCIS or invasive CA to have LCIS.
  - If excisional biopsy reveals LCIS (classic type), no further surgery or radiation needed.
  - Excision with −ve margin is not indicated.
  - If biopsy reveals pleomorphic LCIS (rare) but aggressive (not stained by E-cadherin), it is usually treated as DCIS, i.e., excision with −ve margin.
  - Options include surveillance, chemotherapy prevention (tamoxifen), bilateral prophylactic mastectomy.
  - The goal of treatment is to prevent or detect invasive CA subsequently developed in 35%–35%.

Chemotherapy Prevention

- For high risk of breast CA, chemotherapy prevention should be considered.
- Many trials showed decrease the risk with the use of tamoxifen, raloxifene, aromatase inhibitor.
- 5 years of tamoxifen lowers risk by 50%.
- For menopausal, raloxifene is as effective as tamoxifen.
- Tamoxifen is the only option for premenopausal.
- All causes osteoporosis, osteopenia.
- Patient who underwent hysterectomy, no risk for endometrial CA.

Prophylactic Mastectomy

- Bilateral prophylactic mastectomy provides maximal risk reduction, 90%–95%.
- Not routinely performed, unless with additional risk factor such as strong family history.

Surveillance

- Estimated lifetime risk to develop breast CA, 30%–40%.
- Annual mammography as well as MRI should be considered.
- Ideally, mammography and MRI should be alternated Q6M.
- LCIS is multifocal (50%) and bilateral (30%).

o **Ductal Carcinoma In Situ (DCIS)**
  - 25% of all breast CA.

Diagnosis

- Suspicious with calcification on mammogram → cluster, pleomorphic in size, arranged in linear or segmental distribution.
- Rarely present as palpable mass.
- Can present as Paget's disease of nipple.
- Stereotactic CNBx for diagnosis of suspicious lesion.
- DCIS with microinvasion indicates SLNBx.

- If stereotactic is not amenable → wire localization and excisional biopsy are warranted.
- MRI is controversial.
    - → High in sensitivity for detection of DCIS compared with mammogram but does not decrease rate of +ve margin or the need of re-excision after lumpectomy.
    - → Increases rate of mastectomy and contralateral prophylactic mastectomy and delays surgery.

Treatment

- Prognosis is excellent, SR in 10 years is high, > 95%.
- The goal is to prevent development of invasive CA.
- Different types of DCIS have varied risks associated with local recurrence or progress to invasive CA.
- Surgery then radiation and hormonal (tamoxifen) therapy if ER +ve, showed decrease recurrence and decrease progress to invasive CA.
- Lumpectomy + radiation = mastectomy.
- Lumpectomy + radiation = lumpectomy alone < 5 years, but after 5 years, lumpectomy alone has higher recurrence, 7% vs. 16.4%.
- If lumpectomy has−ve margin more than 1 cm → no benefit from radiation therapy.
- Margin: less than 2 mm has high local recurrence as DCIS grows in skip or branching pattern, so 5 mm or more decreases local recurrence.
- Lesion > 2.5 cm needs −ve margin > 3 mm.
  Lesion < 1 cm needs −ve margin < 3 mm.
- Use of tamoxifen lowers recurrence vs. no tamoxifen, 10% vs. 7%.

Surgery

- Lumpectomy or mastectomy.
- Indication of mastectomy:
    - multicentric
    - extensive DCIS
    - comedo type, +ve margin after lumpectomy.

- recurrence after lumpectomy + radiation.
- Can perform skin-sparing or nipple-sparing mastectomy (but if at proximity of lesion to nipple areola complex, it is not recommended).
- Wire localization: help to do lumpectomy.
- Indication of SLNBx with DCIS:
  - Invasion component defined in final histopathology
  - CNBx revealed microinvasion
  - Comedo type
  - Large tumor > 4 cm

Radiation
- Standard after surgery.
- But can abort radiation therapy if the risk stratification is mild.

Hormonal
- For hormonal +ve → tamoxifen for 5 years decreases recurrence and decreases development of contralateral breast CA, 13% vs. 8%.
- Side effect of tamoxifen: affects quality of life, hot flush, menopausal symptom.
- Increase risk of endometrial CA.
- Increase risk of thromboembolic disease → so you have to see risk stratification.
- aromatase inhibitor used in postmenopause.

Early Invasive Breast CA (Stage I, IIa, IIb)
- Six procpective randomized studies, comparing breast conserving surgery (BCS) to mastectomy = same.
- Majority of studies are about tumor size.
- Lumpectomy + radiation = total mastectomy. However, the recurrence increases without radiation.
- Recurrence with lumpectomy alone is 39% whereas with lumpectomy + radiation, 14%.
- If large tumor, small breast, BRCA mutation, and frozen section came with +ve margin → mastectomy.

- Old patients (multiple comorbidities) with small (T1, N0) low-grade tumor → lumpectomy alone is accepted + tamoxifen if ER +ve.
- BCS to all patients with stage I, II unless relative contraindication.
- Exclusion criteria for BCS is:
  • invasive lobular carcinoma size 2–3 cm
  • ER −ve
  • T3, T4
  • multifocal, multicentric
  • extensive LNs
  • +ve margin
  • +ve margin after re-excision.
  • Prior radiation to the breast or chest wall
  • Scleroderma or SLE.

The optimal management → Mastectomy + axillary staging + radiation.

- Most patients with early-stage, the reconstruction can be performed immediately at the time of mastectomy (skin sparing).
- There is interest for nipple-areola sparing.
  → But if patient is for radiation after mastectomy, not a candidate because of effect of radiation on nipple.
- Immediate reconstruction with implants or autologous tissues, which are transverse rectus abdominis myocutaneous flap (TRAM), deep inferior epigastric perforation falp, latissimus dorsi flap without implant.
- Can delay the implant after radiation using tissue expander.

Lymphadenectomy
- The Standard of Care: If +ve SLNBx → ALND.
- Immediate ALND vs. ALND in delayed fashion once clinically palpable → no difference.
- ALND for axillary staging is not necessary as 75% present with −ve LNs at the time of screening.
- SLNBx identification rate is 97%, and false −ve, 9.7%.
- 26% of −ve clinical LNs have +ve LNs metastasis.
- 60% of +ve SLNBx → no additional +ve LNs identified after ALND.

- The ALMANAC trial, randomized 1,031 patients with primary operable breast cancer to SLN biopsy vs. standard axillary dissection.
  - The incidence of lymphedema and sensory loss for the SLNBx group was significantly lower than with the standard axillary treatment.
  - At 12 months, drain usage, length of hospital stay, and time of resumption of normal day-to-day activities after surgery were also statistically significantly lower in the SLNBx.
- ACOSOG initiated the Z0010 and Z0011.
- Z0010: patient with T2, N0 with +ve 1–2 SLNBx treated with BCS and WBI → 24% have SLNs +ve; in patient with −ve SLNs → 10% have occult metastasis (bone marrow).
- Conclusion: routinely use IHC for SLNBx is not warranted.
- Z0011: the study is about the role of completion ALND on survival of women with positive SLNBx.
- Conclusion: 1–2 +ve SLNBx (Micrometastasis) having BCS with radiation is not require ALND.
- Not eligible for
  - patient who received neoadjuvant chemotherapy or hormonal therapy.
  - Clinically +ve LNs.
  - FNA reveals macrometastasis to LNs.
- Follow-up after 6 years has no difference.
- Old age, higher BMI → ↑ edema.
- ALND increases wound infection, seroma, paresthesia, lymphedema, 13% vs. 2%.
- NCCN guidelines: no different of OS in patient with 1–2 +ve SLNBx treated with BCS → then ALND vs. no additional intervention.
- AMAROS clinical trial: patients with early-stage invasive breast cancer who have no clinical evidence of local spread of disease to axillary lymph nodes, meaning that palpation or ultrasound shows no sign of disease spread, undergo a sentinel lymph node biopsy.
  → Follow-up for 10 years reveals associated with significantly less lymphedema as compared to surgery.

→ In 10 years, 1.82% (11 out 681 patients) of those assigned to axillary radiotherapy had axillary recurrence compared with 0.93% (7 out of 744 patients) of those assigned to axillary lymph node dissection.

→ Patients assigned to axillary radiotherapy went on to develop a second primary cancer compared with patients assigned to axillary lymph node dissection, 11.0% vs. 7.7%.

→ Strongly believe that axillary radiotherapy is a good alternative to axillary lymph node dissection in this group of patients.

Adjuvant Chemotherapy for early breast CA

- Considered in the following:
  - Node +ve
  - Tumor > 1 cm
  - Tumor > 0.5 cm + advance prognostic feature
  - Lymphovascular invasion
  - High nuclear grade
  - HER2 overexpression
  - −ve hormone receptor
- 2 years of tamoxifen, followed by 3 years aromatase inhibitor if ER, PR +ve.
- If HER2 +ve → systemic chemotherapy (Herceptin).

Advanced Local-Regional Breast CA (IIIa–b)

- Aim is surgery + chemoradiation.
- These patients already have distant metastasis by bone scan, PET, CT, even if −ve serum tumor marker.
- 90% are cured.
- Neoadjuvant chemotherapy+ MRM + radiotherapy and endocrine therapy (gold standard)
  - → or endocrine therapy + MRM + radiotherapy + adjuvant chemotherapy → there is no difference.
- Neoadjuvant chemotherapy should be considered in advanced treatment, especially with ER −ve.
- For ER +ve → primary endocrine is considered, especially if multiple comorbidities.
- Surgical (MRM) followed by radiotherapy.

- Chemotherapy for distant metastasis-free.
- Radiotherapy for local-regional metastasis-free.
- Oxford: neoadjuvant + BCS → increases recurrence by 50%.

Distant Metastasis (Stage IV)

- Treatment is not curative, but many prolonge survival.
- Endocrine therapy associated with minimal toxicity is cytotoxic chemotherapy in ER +ve.
- Patient with dyspnea is not a candidate, but pleural effusion can treat with percutaneous drainage.
- If lymphangitis → chemotherapy is the treatment of choice.
- Systemic chemotherapy → ER −ve, visceral crisis, hormone refractory metastasis.

Local-Regional Recurrence

- Underwent mastectomy.
- Underwent lumpectomy.
- Patient who underwent mastectomy should undergo surgical intervention for local-regional recurrence + chemotherapy + antiestrogen are considered and radiation if she or he did not receive it before.
- Patient underwent lumpectomy → mastectomy and reconstruction + chemotherapy + antiestrogen.

Breast CA Prognosis

- OS is 5 years → 89.5% (white, 90%; black, 78%).
- For localized diagnosis: 98.6% (61% of patients).
- For regional diagnosis: 84% (32% of patients).
- For distant metastasis: 24% (5% of patients).

Surgical Technology in Breast CA Therapy
Excisional Biopsy with Needle Localization

- Excisional biopsy: complete removal of breast lesion with margin of normal breast tissue.
- Core needle biopsy is preferred, and excisional biopsy is reserved for normal biopsy discordant with image or physical examination.
- Circumareolar incision for subareolar lesion or near nipple-areola complex.

- Elsewhere → area of tension in skin.
- Lower quadrant lesion → radial incision.
- For upper quadrant → radial incion not recommended → contracture.
- After excision → x-ray to confirm margin, then show the area of pathology with clip, suture, or dye.
- Additional margin if x-ray shows remnant.
- Closure of defect by absorbable 3-0.
- Drain is not recommended.
- Excisional biopsy with needle localization or wire or wire hook.

Sentinel LNs Biopsy

- SLNBx accepted for T1–T2, but it is a must for T3
- For early stage of breast CA with −ve finding on physical examination and imaging.
- Specially (T3, N0) proven that 75% have +ve LNs.
- Sensitivity, 93%.
- False −ve, 7%.
- Accuracy, 95%.
- Not recommended in the following conditions:
  - Inflammatory breast CA
  - Palpable axillary LNs
  - Neo-adjuvant chemotherapy
  - Multicenteric tumor
  - Proven metastasis
  - Prior axillary surgery
  - Prior excisional biopsy
  - Pregnancy (relative)
- Use intra-operative gamma probe.
- Either radioactive colloid or blue dye.
- Should tell the patient → dark urine (green) and allergy → antihistamine or steroid.
- In pregnancy → radioactive colloid is used instead blue dye.
- Four LNs are enough.

Breast Conservation

- Resection of primary breast CA with −ve margin + adjuvant radiotherapy + assessment of LNs status.
- Alternatively called segmental mastectomy, lumpectomy, partial mastectomy, wide local excision.
- Stage I, II → BCT = mastectomy in six studies.
- Three studies showed BCT → increase local recurrence.
- Radiation decreases recurrence by 50%.
- Advantages: increase quality of life, psychological pressure, skin shape.
- Standard for stage 0, I, II.
- If tumor is in upper quadrant → circumareolar (curvilinear).
- If tumor is in lower quadrant → radial incision.
- X-ray to confirm the lesion.
- Request histopathology for ER, PR, HER2.
- Local recurrence by determining adequacy of margins.
- Re-excision if +ve margin reaches 2 mm −ve margin, and if +ve again → mastectomy.
- SLNBx performed before removal of primary tumor.

Mastectomies

- Halsted radical mastectomy (historically) → mastectomy + level I, II, III axillary LNs dissection + pectoralis major and minor resection.
- Modified radical mastectomy (MRM) → mastectomy + level I, II, III axillary LNs dissection + pectoralis minor resection.
- Extended mastectomy → simple + level I.
- Simple mastectomy without skin sparing, no LNs dissection.
- Skin-sparing mastectomy → all breast tissues + nipple-areola complex with skin preservation.
- Nipple-areola sparing mastectomy, criteria for eligibility:
  - Tumor away from areola by 2–3 cm
  - Small breast size
  - Minimal ptosis
  - No prior surgery
  - No tobacco use
  - No prior breast radiation
  - No collagen or vascular disease

Modified Radical Mastectomy

- Modified radical mastectomy + LNs, I, II, III, with preservation of pectoralis major
- Described by David Patey.
- He removes pectoralis minor to access level III but can preserves pectoralis minor and lateral pectoral nerve (neurovascular bundle).
- Boundaries of MRM, anterior margin of latissimus dorsi laterally, midline of sternum medially, subclavius muscle superiorly, and extension of 2–3 cm of inferior mammary line (IMF).
- Axillary vein should be identified with clearance, anterior + interior + subscapular (level I) with care of thoracodorsal nerve.
- Dissection medially, central LNs (level II) with care of long thoracic nerve, if injured → winged scapula + shoulder weakness.
- Divide the pectoralis minor → apical access (level III) → until costoclavicular (Halsted ligament).
- Some divide pectoralis minor, and some preserve it.

Principles

- Review the radiology, lab and histopathology result.
- The standard is lymph node dissection in level II.
- Mark the tumor with permanent marker.
- Plan the skin incision well so it will close without tension.

Preparation

- Tumor board, full staging, consent, NPO, IVF, DVT, prophylaxis, antibiotics (controversial), marking preoperatively, positioning with upper limb abduction.

Procedure

- Supine position with ipsilateral arm 90 degrees abducted under GA.
- Draped from the neck until costal margin.

- Incision: elliptical transverse with 3 cm clearance around the tumor as outlined by marker, and include any biopsy surgical scar.
- Incision from the lateral edge of the sternum to midaxillary line (height below hairline).
- Dissection beyond the subcutaneous tissue is avoided.
- Several clamps applied to the upper half with vertical traction and countertraction on the breast tissue, within 5–8 mm thickness.
- Then start creating the upper flap to the level of the clavicle, then cover with moist lap pad.
- With the same technique, the lower flap is created to the rectus sheath.
- The lateral edge will be the latissimus dorsi, and the lateral edge of the sternum is the medial border.
- Start from the medial aspect by incising the pectoralis fascia from the lateral edge of the sternum and sharply dissected from the pectoralis muscle until the lateral edge of the pectoralis major muscle, and include it with the breast specimen.
- For axillary dissection: retract the pectoralis major with two right-angle retractors.
- Now the interpectoral fat and lymph nodes are in field and should be dissected and retrieved.
- The medial pectoral nerve is identified and preserved.
- To gain access to the axillary vein, the clavipectoral fascia must be incised, tributaries are ligated, and dissection above the vein is avoided.
- Start dissection 5 mm below the vein, then with retracting the pectoralis muscle, the dissection is proceeded to realizing the axillary tissue from the lateral chest wall.
- Serratus anterior facia should not be violated to protect the long thoracic nerve, and search for the long thoracic nerve below it.
- Then identify the thoracodorsal pedicle by identifying the lateral thoracic vein, which is most anterior tributary to the axillary vein.

- The axillary tissue between the two nerves is grasped and removed; with preservation, go to the intercostobrachial nerve if possible.
- Dissection is continued caudally to remove the rest of the axillary content.
- Insert two drains, one in axilla and one under the flaps.

Complications

- Seroma → 30% → so suction drain decreases incidence. Keep it until 30 mL/day.
- Infection, flap necrosis.
- Hemorrhage → if early, need wound exploration (moderate, severe).
- Lymphedema: 20% but increases to 50%–60% with radiation therapy (extensive LNs removal + radiation therapy + obesity), Treatment → physiotherapy, arm elevation, elastic wrap.
  → after 7–10 years → Angiosarcoma.

Reconstruction of Breast + Chest Wall

- Immediate or delayed.
- Usually primary repair with myocutaneous flap from latissimus dorsi, but delay radiation.
- Breast reconstruction after risk-reducing surgery or after mastectomy for early-stage breast CA, allow skin-sparing mastectomy.
- Reconstruction can be expander/implant or autologous tissue (myocutaneous flap), latissimus, or TRAM.
- In advanced CA, reconstruction after complete adjuvant radiotherapy (inferior outcomes).
- TRAM → skin, SC, muscle rectus abdominis + inferior epigastric vessels.
- Free TRAM → microvascular anastomosis.
- If rib-involved CA → resection of two ribs maximum.

Chemotherapy
Neo-adjuvant

- Surgery then chemotherapy *or* neoadjuvant chemotherapy, then surgery which are the same, but neoadjuvant therapy

increases chance of lumpectomies, decreases incidence LNs +ve, i.e., downstaging.
- Neoadjuvant is considered when initial lumpectomy is too large, i.e., big tumor.
- If during neo-adjuvant therapy → increase size of the tumor → poor outcome.
- Current NCCN recommendation, treatments of operable local-regional breast are neoadjuvant chemotherapy with anthracycline or taxane then surgery +/− ALND, followed by adjuvant radiotherapy.
- In HER2 +ve → Herceptin + chemotherapy.
- Advantages:
  - Downstaging to improve eligibility of BCS.
  - High-grade CA, hormonal receptor −ve, triple −ve, or HER2/neu +ve.
  - For systemic, micrometastasis.
  - Give time (3–4 months) to decide mastectomy vs. lumpectomy.
  - Doxorubicin can be given during second, third trimester in pregnancy when radiation is contraindicated, so neoadjuvant chemotherapy → surgery → postpartum radiation.

Adjuvant Chemotherapy for Breast CA
- For patient with −ve LNs, chemotherapy is not recommended.
- Chemotherapy is recommended by NCCN for the following:
  - Blood vessels or lymph node invasion
  - High nuclear grade
  - High histologic grade
  - −ve hormone receptor
  - HER2 overexpression
  - metastasis
- Patient with IIIa → neoadjuvant, anthracycline, or taxane then MRM + ALND and adjuvant radiation.
- Patient with ER +ve responds less to chemotherapy like lobular (chemotherapy-resistant).

Endocrine Therapy

- **Tamoxifen**
  - Meta-analysis: 5 years of tamoxifen decreases 1/3 of mortality in 15 years.
  - 39% decrease in CA risk in contralateral breast.
  - Toxicity: bone pain, hot flashes, nausea, vomiting, fluid retention, thrombotic < 3%, also cataract.
  - Tamoxifen + Aromatse inhibitor increase survival.
  - Considered in DCIS with +ve hormones receptor; the aim is to decrease recurrence after BCT for the contralateral breast.
  - 20 mg PO daily for at least 5 years.
  - ASCO is recommended for 10 years.
  - If the patient becomes menopausal after 5 years of tamoxifen, D/C and start AI for 5 years.

- **Aromatase Inhibitor (AI)**
  - In postmenopausal, AI is considered the first line of therapy.
  - Or after 2-3 years of adjuvant tamoxifen.
  - Decrease recurrence, local and distant metastasis.
  - 2 years of tamoxifen followed by 3 years AI.
  - Less likely than tamoxifen to cause endometrial CA but decreases bone density → osteoporosis can be treated with bisphosphonate.
  - Node −ve or +ve → adjuvant hormonal therapy.
  - Postmenopausal women who had prior exposure to AI → second-line endocrine therapy → pure antiestrogen (fulvestrant) or tamoxifen followed by high dose of androgen.
  - In premenopausal with stage IV, either tamoxifen or oophorectomy (medial surgery or radioablative).

- **Ablative Endocrine Therapy**
  - In the past, oophorectomy, adrenalectomy, and/or hypophysectomy are used to treat metastatic breast CA.
  - Aminoglutethimide block enzymatic conversion of cholesterol of progesterone and inhibit conversion of androstenedione to estrogen in peripheral tissue.

- Aminoglutethimide = adrenalectomy + hypophysectomy.

- **Anti-HER2 Therapy**
  - Tyrosine kinase inhibitor such as Herceptin.
  - Prolonged SR.
  - 20% of breast CA has HER2.
  - DCIS with microinvasive, always ask for HER2/neu as majority of DCIS is overexpressed HER2.
  - Imatinib (oral TKI) can be given as alternative in case of refractory to Herceptin.
  - Patient with HER2 +ve has better outcome with anthracycline.
  - Patient with HER2 +ve tumor benefit from Herceptin + paclitaxel.
  - Cardiotoxicity if Herceptin is given with anthracycline.
  - Herceptin for HER2 +ve and for metastatic disease.
  - Herceptin decreases mortality by 33%.
  - Buzdar report: neoadjuvant with Herceptin + paclitaxel followed by 5 fluorouracil + epirubicin, cyclophosphamide vs. same chemotherapy without Herceptin—first group showed high response by 25%–66%.
  - None of the patients with Herceptin developed CHF.
  - Lapatinib (tyrosine kinase inhibitor) targeting HER2 + EGFR.

Side Effects of Chemotherapy

Class	S/E
Traditional Chemotherapy Anthracycline	
Doxorubicin	Nausea and vomiting, toxic myocarditis, leukemia
Epirubicin	Nausea and vomiting, toxic myocarditis, leukemia

645

Taxanes

Docetaxel	Myelosuppression, neuropathy, hepatic impairment, stomatitis
Paclitaxel	Myelosuppression, neuropathy, stomatitis, renal impairment

Antimetabolite

Cyclophosphamide	Low Na^+, hemorrhagic cystitis, gonadal suppression
Methotrexate	Thrombosis, pancytopenia, RF, pneumonia
Fluorouracil	Angina, arrhythmia, agranulocytosis

Targeted Chemotherapy

Anti-HER2 Neo

Trastuzumab (Herceptin)	↓ EF (LVEF)
Pertuzumab (Perjeta)	Cardiotoxic, birth defect

Endocrine Therapy

Tamoxifen	Endometrial CA, DVT, cataract, headache, emotional disturbance
Anastrozole (AI)	Arthralgia, inhibit androgen to convert to estrogen

Radiation for Breast Cancer

- After breast-conserving therapy (BCS).
- After a mastectomy, especially if the cancer was larger than 5 cm.
- If cancer is found in many lymph nodes or if certain surgical margins have cancer such as the skin or muscle.
- If cancer has spread to other parts of the body, such as bones or brain.
- The main types of radiation therapy that can be used to treat breast cancer are the following:
- External beam radiation therapy (EBRT)
    - This is the most common type of radiation therapy for women with breast cancer.

- A machine outside the body focuses the radiation on the area affected by the cancer.
- If the patient had BCS, you will most likely have radiation to the entire breast (called **whole breast radiation**) and an extra boost of radiation to the area in the breast where the cancer was removed (called the **tumor bed**).
- The standard schedule for getting whole breast radiation is 5 days a week, for about 5–7 weeks.

- **Hypofractionated radiation therapy**
  - The radiation is also given to the whole breast but in larger daily doses (Monday through Friday) using fewer treatments (typically for only 3–4 weeks).

- **Accelerated partial breast irradiation** (APBI)
  - To give larger doses over a shorter time to only one part of the breast.
  - Accelerated partial breast irradiation (APBI) for selected patient DCIS or early stage resulting to tumor bed as most of recurrence happened there, BID × 5 days.
  - ASTRO guidelines for use of APBI:
    - o Women 60 years or older
    - o Unifocal
    - o ER +ve
    - o No LNs
    - o Margin-free at least 2 mm

- Intra-operative breast irradiation (IOBT)
  - In this approach, a single large dose of radiation is given to the area where the tumor was removed (tumor bed) in the operating room right after BCS (before the breast incision is closed).

- **3D conformal radiotherapy (3D-CRT)**
- **Intensity-modulated radiotherapy (IMRT)**
- **Brachytherapy**
- Chest wall radiation
- Lymph node radiation

Special Clinical Situation

- **Nipple Discharge**
  - If unilateral, bloody, spontaneous, localized to single duct, present in 40s → ↑suspecious of malignancy.
  - Mammography, ultrasound, ductogram, cannulation if single discharging duct.
  - Nipple discharge with cancer is either bloody or serous.
  - Presence of Hb can be found in IDP or duct ectasia as well.
  - Excisional biopsy of the duct.
  - Bilateral → suggested benign diagnosis, multiductal ≤ 39 years, milky or blue-green prolactin secretion.
  - Pituitary adenoma (2%) if prolactin high → CT optic nerve to r/o visual compression.

- **Axillary LNs Metastasis with Unknown Metastasis**
  - Women with +ve axillary LNs → may be breast CA for 90%, i.e., occult breast CA.
  - Initial presentation with LNs in 1%.
  - FNA or core biopsy can establish diagnosis.
  - IHC analysis may be classified in melanocytic or lymphoid.
  - Presence of ER or PR suggests breast CA, but not diagnostic.
  - Search for primary includes thyroid, breast, pelvis, rectum.
  - Mammogram, ultrasound, MRI.
  - CXR, LFTs.
  - CT CAP.
  - Upper and lower scope.
  - When breast CA found → ALND + mastectomy + radiation, chemotherapy, endocrine therapy should be considered.

- **Contralateral Prophylactic Mastectomy (CPM)**
  - >5% chance to have a tumor in contralateral breast.
  - Types of patient advised for CPM:
    - History of radiation due to Hodgkin lymphoma

- If she received radiation at 14 years → ↑ risk at 40 years, 50%
- If ER, PR −ve
- Invasive lobular CA
- BRCA1, BRCA2:
    → Cumulative risk is 47% by 25 years.
    → BRCA1 is higher than BRCA2.
    → 3% per year.
- Other gene mutations:
    - PTEN, P53 (Li-Fraumeni syndrome)
    - HER2/neu overexpression
    - Cowden syndrome
- Family history (Caucasian)
- Young age
- Availability of immediate breast reconstruction

Contraindication
- Medical comorbid, distant metastasis, pregnancy, recently treated advanced stage of CA.

Breast CA during Pregnancy
- Occurs in 1:3,000, axillary LNs +ve in 75%.
- 25% of breast nodules developed during pregnancy.
- Ultrasound + core biopsy for diagnosis.
- Mammogram rarely indicated because of low sensitivity during pregnancy and lactation; fetus should be shielded if mammography is needed.
- MRM in first or second trimester.
- During third trimester, lumpectomy + ALND and radiation deferred till delivery.
- Chemotherapy during first-time pregnancy = abortion, 12% birth defect.
- No evidence of teratogenicity when administering chemotherapy during second or third trimester, so chemotherapy in second or third trimester as neoadjuvant can be considered.
- Same staging as nonpregnant.

Male Breast CA

- Less than 1% of all breast CA occurs in men (UK, USA, Jewish, African).
- Preceded by gynecomastia in 20 years.
- Associated with radiation, estrogen therapy, testicular feminizing syndrome, and Klinefelter XXY.
- Rare in young, usually in above 60s.
- Firm, not tender.
- DCIS, 15%; IDC, 85%.
- ILC is rare but reported.
- Same as female breast CA biology, staging and survival.
- Worse in men because more advanced stage at presentation.
- MRM is the treatment of choice.
- SLNBx in LNs −ve.
- Need adjuvant radiation.
- 80% is hormonal +ve.
- Adjuvant tamoxifen is considered.
- Chemotherapy for −ve hormonal receptor and with large tumor, locally advanced.

Phyllodes Tumors

- Includes cystosarcoma phyllodes (10%).
- Classified to benign, borderline, malignant.
- Borderline has high potential for recurrence.
- Difficult to distinguish between benign and malignant and fibroadenoma.
- Sharply demarcated, mixed gelatinous, solid, and cystic.
- Cut section grossly like leaf (phylloid).
- Most malignant contain liposarcoma or rhabdomyosarcoma rather than fibrosarcoma.
- Small tumor needs −ve margin, but when diagnosis confirmed → excision with 1 cm −ve margin.
- Large tumor requires mastectomy.
- ALND is not recommended because rarely involved.

Inflammatory Breast CA

- Stage IIIb, 3% of breast CA.
- Skin changes, induration, edema (Peau d'orange).

- When locally advanced scirrhous → invade dermal lymph → edema.
- 75% present with + LNs.
- PET + CT.
- 25% distant metastasis.
- Surgery alone or surgery + radiation is disappointed.
- Neoadjuvant with anthracycline → dramatic regression by 75%.
- Should know HER2, hormonal receptor.
- Then MRM (local-regional).
- 5 years SR → 30%.

Rare Breast CA

- SCC: metaplasia of ducts, regional metastasis, 25%.
- Adenoid cystic carcinoma.
- Apocrine carcinoma: well differentiated, low mitosis.
- Sarcoma
    - Similar to soft tissue sarcomas.
    - Clinical picture → painless breast mass, large, rapid growth.
    - Diagnosis by core biopsy or open incisional biopsy.
    - Based on cellularity, degree of differentiation, nuclear atypia, mitotic activity.
    - Treatment: wide local excision, i.e., mastectomy. Axillary dissection is not indicated unless +ve.
- Lymphoma
    - Type I ≤ 39, bilateral: Burkitt lymphoma.
    - Type II ≥ 40: B cell type, Hodgkin.
    - It could be occult breast +ve LN.
    - Treatment: mastectomy + ALND for staging.
    - Recurrent or local-regional disease → chemotherapy and radiation.
    - 5–10 years, SR is 74%, 51%.

Thyroid Gland

Embryology
-   Begin to form 24 days after fertilization, the first and the largest endocrine gland in embryo.
-   Its endodermal outpouching on the floor of primordial pharynx becomes thyroid diverticulum.
-   This diverticulum descends from pharynx and passes anterior to the hyoid bone, maintaining a connection at the base of the tongue (thyroglossal duct).
-   Migration is completed at seventh week of GA, and thyroglossal duct is obliterated.
-   Th ventral part of fourth pharyngeal pouch gives ultimobranchial body, which eventually fuses with thyroid to form parafollicular cells that produce calcitonin.
-   It weights 20 g.

Developmental Abnormalities
- **Thyroglossal Duct Cyst and Sinus**
    -   At fifth week, thyroglossal duct starts to obliterate and disappear by eighth week of GA and rarely persists.
    -   Sometimes gets infected.

    ### Diagnosis
    -   Clinically: 1–2 cm, smooth, well defined.
    -   Midline neck mass moves with swallowing and with protrusion of tongue.
    -   No need for image.

    ### Treatment
    -   Sistrunk operation—en bloc resection of cyst excision of central hyoid bone to decrease recurrence.
    -   1% has cancer, 85% is papillary thyroid CA.
    -   Thyroidectomy is debated, but if there are suspicious cells or enlarged LNs, so thyroidectomy is warranted.
    -   MTC never comes with thyroglossal duct cyst.

- **Lingual Thyroid**
  - Failure of median thyroid to descend.
  - Intervention if obstruction such as chocking, dysphagia, hemorrhage.
  - Many will develop hypothyroidism.

  Treatment
  - Exogenous thyroid hormone to suppress TSH, then RAI ablation followed by thyroxin replacement.
  - Surgical intervention is rare.

- **Ectopic Thyroid**
  - Normal thyroid tissue can be found anywhere in the neck and chest, e.g., trachea, esophagus, aorta, heart and often the tongue.

- **Pyramidal Lobe**
  - Projection of Isthmus—50% of population.
  - Distal end of fibrous band of thyroglossal duct is connected with thyroid gland.
  - It could get enlarged and palpable.

Anatomy
- Located posterior to strap muscles (infrahyoid muscles), inferior to cricoid cartilage.
- Extended to midthyroid cartilage superiorly, carotid sheath and sternomastoid laterally, trachea (2nd, 3rd ring) posteriorly and strap muscles anteriorly (sternohyoid, sternothyroid, omohyoid "superior belly," thyrohyoid).
- All innervated by ansa cervicalis C1–C3 except thyrohyoid by hypoglossal nerve (12).
- Need to divide the strap muscle from the upper half to avoid injury of Ansa cervicalis.
- NB: suprahyoid muscles: Digastric (anterior + posterior belly), Geniohyoid, Mylohyoid, Stylohyoid muscles, it is not related to thyroid gland.

Blood Supply

Arterial

- Superior thyroid artery → external carotid
- Inferior thyroid artery → thyrocervical artery → subclavian artery
- Thyroid ima → brachiocephalic

Venous drainage

- Superior thyroid vein → IJV.
- Middle thyroid vein → IJV.
- Inferior thyroid vein → brachiocephalic vein.

Nerves

- Recurrent laryngeal nerve (RLN) arises from vagus nerve.
  - Left RLN crosses aortic arch.
  - Right RLN crosses subclavian artery (more oblique) → non-recurrent, 0.5%–1%.
  - RLN terminates by entering larynx posterior to cricothyroid muscle.
  - RLN innervated all laryngeal muscles except cricothyroid, which is supplied by external superior laryngeal nerve.
- Superior laryngeal nerve arises from vagus, travels along carotid artery, then divided at hyoid bone into two branches:
  - Internal: sensory to supraglottic larynx
  - External: innervate cricothyroid muscle
- Type 2A, the superior laryngeal nerve cross the superior pole, which we should not ligate en bloc (20% injury) → voice fatigue.
- Sympathetic innervation from superior and middle cervical sympathetic ganglion.
- Parasympathetic → vagus nerve.

Lymphatic System

- Lymph nodes in the neck is divided to six levels:
  - I   Submaxillary (rare, 1%)
  - II   Upper jugular
  - III   Middle jugular
  - IV   Lower jugular

V   Posterior triangle

VI   Central

VII   Anterior mediastinal LNs

NB: can skip metastasis occurs to lateral group without invading central group.

Histology

-   Contains 100,000 lobules. Each lobule → 20–40 follicles (3,000,000 follicles in adult).

Physiology

-   **Iodine Metabolism**
    -   Daily requirement is 0.1 mg/day.
    -   In stomach, jejunum, iodine is converted to iodide → transported to thyroid follicular cells by ATP → stores 90% then excreted by kidneys.

-   **Thyroid Hormones**
    -   Iodine + tyrosine + Thyroglobulin (Tg) → T3, T4.
    -   Steps:
        -   Iodide trapping: ATP transports iodide via protein, e.g., thyroglobulin.
        -   Thyroid hormone synthesis
        -   Oxidation of iodide to iodine and iodination of tyrosine.
        -   Monoiodotyrosine (MIT) to Diiodotyrosine (DIT).
        -   Coupling
            MIT + DIT → T3 or two DIT → T4.
        -   Tg hydrolyzed to release free T3, T4
        -   Deiodination of iodine to reuse it.
    -   T4 is 100% released by thyroid, but T3, 20% by thyroid, the other 80% produced by convergen of T4 by liver, muscle, kidney.
    -   In case of Graves' diagnosis → a lot of T3.
    -   Thyroid hormone transported via (bound to) albumin, prealbumin (protein carrier); only 0.02% is free and in active form.
    -   T3 is potent and less tightly bound to protein.
    -   T3 is three to four times more active than T4.
    -   Half-life of T3 is 1 day and T4 is 7 days.

- Secretion controlled by pituitary gland.
- Thyroids have adaptation of less iodine, and it will secrete T3 rather T4.
- If high iodine, high organification → low suppression, Wolff-Chaikoff effect.
- Epinephrine and HCG → stimulate thyroid hormone secretion, thus increase in pregnancy and gynecology malignancy.
- Glucocorticoids inhibit thyroid hormone production.
- In critically ill patient, ↓ thyroid hormone without compensatory increase of TSH → euthyroid sick syndrome.

Thyroid Hormone Function
- Free T3, T4 enter cell membrane by carrier or by diffusion.
- T4 deiodination to T3 and enters the nucleus via active transport.
- T3 receptor is similar to the nuclear receptors of glucocorticoid, estrogen, vitamin D.
- Two types of receptors, α–β in chromosome 3, 17.
- Thyroid hormone affects almost every system:
    - ↑ heart rate.
    - Responsible hypoxia, hypercapnia in respiratory center in the brain.
    - increase motility (gut).
    - Muscle contraction and relaxation.
    - Glycogenolysis, hepatic gluconeogenesis.
    - Absorption (gut), synthesis of cholesterol.

Evaluation of Patient with Thyroid Diagnosis
- We should measure T4 and T3. Some diseases have high T3 (thyrotoxicosis).

- TSH
    - Reflects the ability of anterior pituitary to detect free T4.
    - Small change in T4 → large shift in TSH.
    - To diagnose hypo- and hyperthyroidism and optimize T4 therapy.

- Total T4 (55–150 nmol/L), total T3 (1.5–3.5 nmol/L)
  - Total T4 reflects thyroid gland output.
  - Total T3 is not suitable for screening.
  - Total thyroxine levels are increased not only in hyperthyroid patients but also in those with elevated Tg levels secondary to pregnancy, estrogen/progesterone use, or congenital diseases.
  - Total T4 levels decrease in hypothyroidism and in patients with decreased Tg levels due to anabolic steroid use and protein-losing disorders like nephrotic syndrome.
  - Thyrotoxicosis has normal T4 and high T3.

- Free T4 (12–30) Pmol/L, free T3 (3–9) Pmol/L
  - Early hyperthyroidism has normal total T4 but high free T4.
  - Refetoff syndrome has ↑ T4, but TSH is normal.
  - ↑Free T3 is confirm diagnosis of hyperthyroidism (early) as free T3 and free T4 increase before total T3, T4.

- Thyrotropin-releasing hormone (TRH)
  - Useful to evaluate pituitary TSH.
  - Give 500 ug IV of TRH, and measure TSH after 30–60 min in normal individual. TSH increases by 6 uIU/mL from baseline.

- Thyroid antibody
  - Anti-thyroglobulin (Tg), antithyroid peroxidase (TPO), thyroid stimulating immunoglobulin (TSI).
  - Anti-Tg and anti-TPO = autoimmune thyroiditis, increase in 80% of Hashimoto, also increase in Graves' disease, MNG, neoplasm.
  - Thyroglobuline (Tg) is normally not released in circulation in large amounts but increases dramatically in destructive process Graves' disease, MNG used in DTC for recurrence after thyroidectomy and RAI ablation.

- Calcitonin
  - Secreted by C cells and decreases Ca^{++}.
  - Sensitive marker in MTC.

Thyroid Imaging
- Iodine-123 (diagnostic), I-131 (therapeutic)
  - Small dose = half-life is 12–14 hrs.
  - Large dose = 8–10 days.
  - Isotope → area with less trap = (cold) 20% malignancy, (hot) < 5% malignancy.
- ^{99m}Tc is taken up by thyroid → shorter half-life.
- US distinguishes solid from cystic + size, multicentricity, echotexture, shape calcification, and lymph nodes + guided image.

NB: American College of Radiology - Thyroid Imaging Reporting and Data System (ACR TI-RADS) use a standardized scoring system for reports providing users with recommendations for when to use FNA or ultrasound follow-up of suspicious nodules, and when to safely leave alone nodules that are benign/not suspicious.

TI-RADS 1: Normal thyroid gland, no focal lesion
TI-RADS 2: Benign nodule (0% risk of of malignancy)
TI-RADS 3: probably benign nodules (<5% risk of malignancy)
TI-RADS 4:
> 4a – undetermined nodules (5-10% risk of mailignancy)
> 4b – suspicious nodules (10-50% risk of malignancy)
> 4c – highly suspicious nodule (50-85% risk of malignancy)

TI-RADS 5: probably malignant nodule (>85% risk of malignancy)
TI-RADS 6: Biopsy proven malignancy

- CT, MRI → LNs, extent of large retrosternal extern, relation to airway and vasculature.
- PET (PET-CT) → screen for metastasis, detects 14%–63%.

Benign Thyroid Disorder
Hyperthyroidism
- Result of excess circulating thyroid hormone, should be distinguished between Graves' disease and toxic nodular goiter.

- The former disorder → ↑ radioactive iodine uptake (RAIU), while the latter is low.

High Hormone Synthesis High RAIU	Release of Performed Hormone Low RAIU
Graves' disease	Thyroiditis
Toxic MNG	Acute phase of Hashimoto
Toxic adenoma	Subacute thyroiditis
Drugs (amiodarone, iodine)	Hamburger thyrotoxicosis
Thyroid cancer	
Hydatidiform mole	
TSH-secreting pituitary adenoma	

Diffuse Toxic Goiter (Graves' disease)
- Most common cause of hyperthyroidism, 60%–80%.
- It's an autoimmune disease.
- Positive strong family history.
- Female: male = 5:1
- Peak incidence in 40s–60s.
- Characterized by the following:
  - Thyrotoxicosis
  - Diffuse goiter
  - Extrathyroidal manifestations: ophthalmopathy, dermopathy (pretibial myxedema), acropachy, gynecomastia.

Etiology
- Not known but many hypotheses suggest an autoimmune disease, postpartum, iodine excess, lithium therapy, bacterial and viral infection associated with certain HLA (HLAB8, HLA DR3).
- But HLA-DRB1*0701 is protective.
- Once initiated → sensitized T-helper lymphocytes stimulate B lymphocytes → Antibody against thyroid hormone receptor → TSI thyroid-stimulating antibody → increase thyroid hormone.
- Graves' disease associated with DM-I, Addison's disease, pernicious anemia, myasthenia gravis.

Pathology
- Macro: diffuse, smoothly enlarged.
- Micro: hyperplastic, columnar epithelium with minimal colloid, papillary projection of hyperplastic tissue, high lymphoid and vasculature.

Clinical Feature
- Related to increase thyroid hormone:
  - Heat intolerance, increased sweating, thirst, decreased weight despite higher intake.
  - ↑ adrenergic stimulation, palpitation, fatigue, low emotion, nervousness, tremor.
  - ↑ Gastrointestinal motility → diarrhea.
  - In females: low fertility, amenorrhea, increased abortion.
  - In children: higher growth, early bone maturation
  - CVS → AF, HF.

General Examination
- Weight loss and facial flush.
- Skin is warm and moist (cutaneous VD).
- Tachycardia or AF.
- Wide pulse pressure, fine tremor.
- Proximal muscle group weakness.
- Hyperreflexia.
- 2% dermopathy.
- Deposition of glycosaminoglycan → thickened skin in pretibial region and dorsum of the foot.
- Prominent stare → catecholamine.
- Periorbital edema, conjunctival swelling.
- Gynecomastia.
- Thyroid acropachy (osteal bone formation).
- Onycholysis: separation of fingernails from beds.

Locally
- Diffuse symmetrically enlarged
- +/− palpable pyramidal lobe, +/− <u>Bruit</u> or thrill over thyroid gland
- Also loud venous hum in supraclavicular space.

Ophthalmopathy

- 50% developed ophthalmopathy.
- Eye symptom: lid lag (Von Graefe's sign).
- Spasm of upper eyelid (Dalrymple's sign), i.e., sclera seen between cornea and eyelid.
- Proptosis, limitation of eye movement (involve inferior and medial rectus muscles).
- Keratitis.
- Blindness due to optic nerve involvement.
- All this results from inflammation caused by cytokines released from T-killer lymphocyte.

Diagnostic Test

- Low TSH +/− high T3, T4 (free), usually T3 high in early.
- Technetium scintigraphy.
- Anti-Tg, anti-TPO → increase in 75% but not specific.
- Low TSHR or TSAB are diagnostic, 90%.
- MRI orbit for exophthalmos.

Treatment

- Medical: antithyroid.
- Ablation: I^{131}
- Surgical.

Medical

- Generally administered for preparing for I^{131} therapy or surgery.
- Propylthiouracil, 100–300 mg Q8H (PTU).
- → PTU inhibits the conversion of T4 to T3.
- Methimazole, 10–30 mg Q8H, then OD (long half-life).
- → Decrease thyroid hormone + ↓binding of iodine
- Both pass placenta → ↓ fetal thyroid function and excrete in milk.
- PTU has lower risk to pass placenta.
- Methimazole has congenital aplasia, so PTU is safer in pregnancy.
- Side effects:
  - Reversible granulocytopenia

661

- Skin rash, fever
- Peripheral neuritis
- Polyarteritis, vasculitis, hepatitis
- The dose is titrated as TSH level.
- Improve symptom in two weeks and euthyroid achieved in 6 weeks.
- 40%–80% develop recurrence after 1–2 years, so treatment reserve for small gland < 40 g.
- −ve or low thyroid hormone receptor antibody.
- Rapid ↓ gland size with antithyroid medication.
- For Tachycardia (catecholamines) → β-blocker → decrease pulse + decrease convergen T4 to T3.
  → Propranolol, 20–40 mg PO Q6H.
- If asthmatic patient → use calcium channel blockers.

RAI (I-131)

- Mainstay in USA to avoid surgery, low cost.
- Give antithyroid till euthyroid, then stop to ↑ uptake.
- Oral I-131 consist of 8–12 mCi.
- After treatment with RAI, most patients become euthyroid within 2 months.
- 50% of patients treated with RAI remain euthyroid 6 months after treatment; the remaining have either hyper or hypo.
- After 1 year, 2.5% of patient develop hypothyroid each year.
- It has been documented that RAI leads to progression of ophthalmopathy.
  → Progression of Graves' ophthalmopathy by 33% after RAI compared to 16% after surgery
  → more common in smoker.
- Overall cancer rate is unchanged, nor infertility.
- Small risk of MNG, thyroid cancer, and hyperparathyroidism.
- Unexplained increase in CVS mortality rate.
- Higher initial dose → higher hypothyroidism.

Indication
- Old age.

- Relapse after surgery or medical treatment.
- Small to moderate goiter.
- Failure of medical treatment.
- Medical or surgery is contraindicated.

Contraindication
- Absolute: pregnant patient or breastfeeding or planning to get pregnant.
- Relative: young age, thyroid nodules, ophthalmopathy.

Surgery
- Indication:
    - RAI is contraindicated.
    - Confirmed cancer or suspicion.
    - Young.
    - Desire to conceive.
    - Have severe reaction to antithyroid medication
    - Large goiter causing compressive symptom.
    - Reluctant to RAI.
    - Moderate to severe diagnosis.
    - Smoker.
    - Desire to rapid control of symptoms.
    - Relative → in pregnant patient: (a) rapid control, (b) medication cannot control.
- Surgery is best performed in second trimester.
- Patient should be euthyroid by medical treatment before the surgery.
    - Lugol's iodine or K^+ iodide 7–10 days before surgery.
    - 2–3 drops BID to low vascularity ↓ thyroid storm risk.
    - Iodide inhibits release of thyroid hormone.
    - If urgent surgery → β-Blocker + K^+ iodide.
- Steroid is useful as adjuncts.
- In patient with thyroid cancer, refused RAI, had severe exophthalmos or reaction to antithyroid medication → total thyroidectomy; other than this → subtotal thyroidectomy (7 g remnant).

- Exophthalmos improved after thyroidectomy.
- Subtotal could be bilateral or total lobectomy + subtotal to other side (Hartley Dunhill procedure). → less complication → reentering from one side.
- Recommendation of ATA → total thyroidectomy.
- Recurrent of thyrotoxicosis → RAI.

Toxic Multinodular Goiter

- Occurs in older people who often have nontoxic MNG.
- Clinical picture: insidious, signs of hyperthyroidism.
- Some patients have T3 toxicosis, and some will develop AF, CHF.
- Can be precipitated by iodide-containing drugs, e.g., amiodarone.
- Extrathyroidal symptoms are absent.

Diagnostic Tool

- Low TSH, high free T4, T3.
- RAIU: ↑ uptake in multiple nodules, with suppression of remaining gland.

Treatment

- Thyroidectomy.
- RAI is for old age whos not fit for surgery.
- the uptake is less than Graves' disease→ recurrent hyperthyroidism.

Toxic Adenoma

- Young patient, mutation in TSHR gene, also GSP mutation may occur.
- Must be > 3 cm to produce symptom.
- RAI → hot area with suppression of the remaining gland.
- Rarely malignant.
- Small nodules treatment → medical or RAI.
- Surgery (lobectomy and isthmusectomy) is performed in young patient with large nodules.
- Percutaneous ethanol injection (PEI) has good result but not same as surgery.

Thyroid Storm
- Hyperthyroidism, fever, CNS agitation or depression, CVS, GI dysfunction, including hepatic failure.
- Precipitated by abrupt cessation of antithyroid or infection, surgery, trauma, or result from amiodarone or following RAI.
- Previously, it has high mortality.
- Managed in ICU with β-blocker, O_2, NSAID (not aspirin), PTU, Lugol's iodine, or Na^+ iodine to decrease uptake of iodine.
- Steroid to prevent adrenal exhaustion and block hepatic thyroid hormone conversion.

Hypothyroidism
- Decrease of circulating thyroid hormone → hypothyroidism
- cretinism in neonate → neurological manifestation and mental retardation.
- Pendred syndrome associated with deafness and Turner syndrome.

Causes

Primary	Secondary	Tertiary
Hashimoto thyroiditis	Pituitary tumor	Hypothalamic
RAI therapy for Graves'	Pituitary	insufficiency
Postthyroidectomy	resection	Resistance to
Excessive iodine intake		thyroid hormone
Subacute thyroiditis		
Drugs (lithium)		
Iodine deficiency (rare)		

Clinical Picture
- In utero → cretinism (Down syndrome, dwarfism), failure to thrive, mental retardation, immediate testing and treatment → neurologic and intellectual deficits.
- In childhood and adolescent → delay development + abdomen distension, umbilical hernia, constipation → rectal prolapse.
- In adult → tiredness, weight gain, cold intolerance, constipation and menorrhagia.
- Myxedema: deposition of glycosaminoglycan in SC tissue → facial and periorbital puffiness.

- Skin → dry, rough, yellowish hue (↓ conversion of carotene to vitamin A).
- Hair → dry, brittle, hair loss.
- Loss of outer 2/3 of eyebrows.
- Enlarged tongue.
- ↓ mentality.
- Abdomen: pain and constipation.
- Libido and fertility are impaired.
- CVS → bradycardia, cardiomegaly, low COP.
- If the cause is pituitary → pale waxy skin, loss of body hair, atrophic genitalia.

Laboratory
- Low T3, T4, high TSH.
- In secondary hypothyroidism, decrease TSH and not increased by TSH stimulant.
- Thyroid autoantibody, high in Hashimoto and Graves' disease.
- ECG: bradycardia and low voltage, flattened T wave or inversion.

Treatment
- T4 (thyroxine) 50–200 mcg/day.
- Starting dose of 100 mcg/day.
- Patient with CVS disease → 25–50 mcg, then increase over weeks or months.
- The dose titrated as clinical picture or TSH.
- subclinical hypothyroidism (T3, T4 are normal, but TSH is high)
- controversial: Some evidences showed: patient with subclinical hypothyroidism with high antithyroid antibody → start because eventually they will develop hypothyroid.
- Patient presented with myxedema coma → IV T4, 300–400 mcg with monitor in ICU.

Thyroiditis
- Types: acute, subacute, chronic.

Acute (Suppurative)
- Thyroid gland is usually resist the infection due to increased vascularity, lymphatic, high iodine, and capsulated.

- Mode of infection:
  - Hematogenous or lymphatics
  - Direct spread via thyroglossal duct cyst
  - Penetrating trauma
  - Immunosuppressant usage
- Streptococci and anaerobe, 70%.
- Common in children proceeded by URTI or otitis media.

Clinical Picture
- Severe neck pain radiating to jaw or ear.
- Fever, chills, odynophagia, dysphonia.

Complication
- Systemic sepsis, tracheal or esophageal perforation, jugular vein thrombosis, laryngeal chondritis, sympathetic trunk paralysis.

Diagnosis
- ↑ WBC, FNABx for gram stain, C&S, cytology.
- CT for abscess.
- Persistent Pyriform Sinus
  - Should always be suspected in recurrent thyroiditis in children.
  - Diagnosis → barium esophagography, 50%; CT, 80%; direct endoscopy, 100%.

Treatment
- IV antibiotics + drainage for abscess.
- Thyroidectomy for recurrent abscess, persistent, or failure of open drainage.
- Pyriform sinus → excision (complete).
  - Flexible fiber-optic laryngoscopy is used to identify internal opening and electrocauterization → success rate is similar to open surgery.

Subacute Thyroiditis
- Painful or painless.
- No known etiology, but painful thyroiditis → viral infection.
- Genetic plays role, HLA-B35.

- One model of pathogenesis: viral or thyroid antigens presented by macrophage $\rightarrow$ stimulate cytotoxic T lymphocyte $\rightarrow$ damage thyroid follicular cells.

- **Painful Subacute Thyroiditis**
    - In ages 30–40, sudden or gradual neck pain radiating to mandible or ear proceeded by URTI.
    - The gland increases in size, tender and firm.
    - Hypothyroid then euthyroid, then hypothyroid (20%–30%), and finally, euthyroid (90%).
    - ↑ ESR > 100.
    - Self-limited, symptomatic treatment.
    - Aspirin and NSAID $\rightarrow$ for pain, steroid in severe cases.
    - Short-term thyroxine may be needed.
    - Thyroidectomy for prolonged course or recurrent disease.

- **Painless Subacute Thyroiditis**
    - Considered as autoimmune disease, sporadic or postpartum $\rightarrow$ typically occurs 6 weeks after delivery with ↑ TPO due to ↓ immunity.
    - In ages 30–50s.
    - Normal size or slight enlargement.
    - Laboratory and RAI are same as painful subacute thyroiditis.
    - Normal ESR.
    - Clinical course is same as painful subacute thyroiditis.
    - Patient with symptom $\rightarrow$ β-blocker and thyroid replacement.
    - Thyroidectomy and RAI for recurrent disease.

Chronic (Hashimoto) Thyroiditis
- Transformation of thyroid tissue to lymphoid tissue, most common inflammatory disease leading to hypothyroidism.
- Low iodine intake, infection, interference, lithium, amiodarone.

Etiology, Pathogenesis, Pathology
- Autoimmune disease result of activated T helper lymphocyte → cytotoxic → attack thyroid gland.
- Hypothyroidism results from destruction of thyrocyte by cytotoxic + autoantibody.
- Antibody against Tg, 60%; TPO, 95%; TSHR, 60%; Na$^+$ iodine, 25%.
- Inheritance predisposition: autoantibody.
- Associated with Down and Turner syndromes.
- Grossly mild enlargement, granular, nodular, firm, pale-gray cut.
- Microscopic: infiltrated by small lymphocyte and plasma cells. Thyroid follicles are smaller, decrease colloid, increase connective tissue, and lined by Hürthle cells or Askanazy cells.

Clinical Picture
- Female: male = 10–20:1.
- In ages 30–50.
- Mild enlargement with firm gland, increase the size of pyramidal lobe.
- 20% hypothyroidism, 5% hyper.

Diagnostic Study
- High TSH, high autoantibody.
- US with FNAB for solitary suspension nodules.
- Thyroid lymphoma → eightyfold higher than normal population.

Treatment
- Thyroid replacement for hypo or subclinical hypothyroidism, because hypothyroidism ↑ coronary heart disease by 1.89%.
- Twelve randomized control trials → thyroxine improves lipid profile.
- Surgery for suspicious malignancy or compressive symptom.

Riedel's Thyroiditis
- Known as invasive fibrous thyroiditis.
- Replaces all thyroid tissue by fibrous tissue and also invades adjacent structure.

Etiology
- Autoimmune + lymphoid infiltration.
- response to steroid suggest autoimmune theory.
- Associated with sclerosing syndromes such as mediastinal, retroperitoneal, periorbital, and sclerosing cholangitis.
- It may be the first fibrotic disorder.
- In ages 30–60.
- Painless, hard anterior neck mass.
- Progresses over months to years → dysphagia, dyspnea, choking, hoarseness of voice.
- Hypothyroid + hypoparathyroidism (replaced by fibrous tissue).

Physical Examination
- Need open thyroid biopsy; FNAB is inadequate.

Treatment
- Surgery to decompress trachea by wedge excision of isthmus and to make tissue diagnosis.
- Extensive resection is not advisable, because of obscure landmark by fibrosis.
- Hypothyroidism → thyroxine replacement.
- Steroid and tamoxifen → dramatic response.
- Recently: mycophenolate.

Goiter
- Greek word means any enlargement of the gland.
- Types: diffuse, uninodular, or multinodular.
- Most of nontoxic goiters are results of high TSH, low T3, T4.

Etiology of non-toxic goiter

Classification	Specific Etiology
Endemic	↓ iodine, goitrogens food (cabbage)
Medication	Iodide, amiodarone, lithium
Thyroiditis	Subacute, chromic, Hashimoto
Familial	Impaired, hormone synthesis
Neoplasm	Adenoma, aarcinoma
Resistance to thyroxin	

- High TSH → diffuse thyroid hyperplasia or focal hyperplasia → colloid nodules or microfollicular nodules.
- In the past, the cause was low iodine intake, but now iodinated salt ↓ the incidence.
- Area with decreased iodine → Central Asia, South America, Indonesia (90% has goiter).

Clinical Features
- Asymptomatic for most patients.
- Dyspnea, dysphagia, and rarely dysphonia from RLN injury, but it is common in malignancy.
- Obstruction of venous return in substernal extension → Pemberton's sign.
- Facial flushing from dilation of cervical vein when raising the arms.
- Sudden increase due to hemorrhage.
- Tracheal deviation may be present.

Diagnostic Test
- Patient is usually euthyroid, normal TSH, T3, T4.
- If nodule developed autonomy → high TSH, hypertrophy.
- RAI patchy uptake, hot and cold area.
- FNA is recommended for patient with dominant nodule.
- 5%–10% carcinomas reported of MNG.
- CT when retrosternal and extension or airway compression.

Treatment
- Small diffuse goiter → no treatment.
- Patient with large goiter → thyroxine → ↓ TSH → ↓ size.
- Iodine for endemic goiter.
- Surgery is for the following:
    - Continue to increase despite thyroxine
    - Obstructive symptom
    - Retrosternal extension
    - Suspicion of malignancy in FNA
    - Cosmetically
- Total thyroidectomy, then T4 lifelong.

Solitary Thyroid Nodules
- 4% of individuals, while malignancy, 40:1 million.

History

- Regard nodule onset (change in size) associated with symptoms such as pain, dysphagia/dyspnea, choking.
- Pain is unusual, but if it exists → hemorrhage, thyroiditis, malignancy.
- Patient with MTC → dull, aching pain.
- History of hoarseness → involvement of RLN.
- History of ionizing radiation.
- Family history with thyroid cancer.
- History of external beam radiation:
  Doses of radiation for treatment of the following:
  - o Tinea capitis, 6.5 cGY
  - o Thymic enlargement, 100–400 cGY
  - o Tonsil + adenoid, 750 cGY
  - o Acne vulgaris, 200–1,500 cGY
  - o Hemangioma
  - o Hodgkin lymphoma, 4,000 cGY
- Radiation causes destruction of thyroid.
- Maximum risk after 20–30 years.
- Nuclear bomb → increases benign and malignant thyroid disease.
- Most thyroid cancers after radiation → PTC with presence of RET/PTC translocation.
- 40% chance of thyroid cancer with history of radiation.
- 60% have cancer in the dominant nodule while 40% → another nodule.

Family History

- Increase risk of non-MTC and MTC.
- MTC occurs in isolation or association (i.e., MEN2).
- Nonmedullary occurs with familial cancer syndrome such as Cowden, Werner (FAP), Gardner syndrome (FNMTC).

Physical Examination

- Inspect for swelling, redness, tracheal deviation, dilated veins and previous scar.
- Best palpated behind patient.
- Cricoid cartilage is an important landmark.
- Hard fixed nodules → ↑ suspicious of malignancy.

- Also must palpate anterior and posterior cervical LNs.

Laboratory
- If patient with nodules and hyperthyroidism → 1% to be malignant.
- Tg cannot differentiate between benign or malignant unless increase; it's good for patient who has undergone total thyroidectomy.
- Calcitonin for diagnosis, MTC, MEN2 (not always).
- All patients with MTC → RET oncogene mutation, urine VMA, metanephrine, and catecholamine to rule out pheochromocytoma.

Imaging
- U/S differentiates cystic from solid and for LNs.
- U/S Criteria for malignant feature:
  o Hypoechoic, solid
  o Fine calcification, loss of halo sign
  o taller than width
  o ↑ LNs
- US + FNA biopsy is recommended by ATA for nodule ≥ 1 cm, unless benign feature on US (e.g., cystic, spongiform).
- Twenty-three gauge needles are inserted → several pass with aspiration, then put it on glass, dip it, and let it dry.

Bethesda Classification to Standard Thyroid FNA

Category	Risk of Malignancy (%)	Recommendation
Nondiagnostic	1–4	Repeat FNA
Benign	0–3	Clinical follow-up
FLUS/AUS	5–15	Repeat FNA, clinical F/U, diagnostic lobectomy
Suspicions for Follicular Neoplasm	20–30	Diagnostic lobectomy
Suspicions of Malignancy	60–75	Diagnostic lobectomy with frozen then process
Malignant	97–99	Formal thyroid operation

Management
- Malignant → thyroidectomy.
- Cystic resolves with aspiration by 75% if persist more than three attempts → Lobectomy is recommended.
- if > 4 cm or complex cyst, malignant (15%).
- Colloid → serial US and Tg; if increasing in size, repeat FNA.
- Controversial → levothyroxine to suppress TSH → decreases size of nodule.
- Less than 25% shrink to 50% of size with TSH suppression.
- If patient has previous radiation or +ve family history → thyroidectomy.

Malignant Thyroid Disease
- Presented with neck swelling.
- Molecular genetics of thyroid tumorigenesis has been studied.
- Several oncogene and tumor suppression genes are involved.
- Up to 70% PTC in children → history of radiation.
- RET in chromosome 10 expressed in tissue derived from embryonic CNS and excretory system (Hirschsprung disease) and kidney, known to predisposed MEN2a, b, and MTC.
- Mutation of RAS gene responsible for 20%–40% of adenoma, MNG, PTC, anaplastic.
- BRAF V600E mutation is predispose 40%–44% of PTC and 22% of anaplastic tumor.
  - → BRAF → PTC, anaplastic, studies showed most aggressive tumor → ↑size, invasion.
- PTEN mutation (Cowden's syndrome): intestinal hamartomas, benign and malignant breast tumors, FTC, rarely PTC and Hürthle cell tumor.
- P53 is a tumor suppressor gene that causes cell cycle arrest, allowing DNA repair.
- Mutation is rare in PTC but common in undifferentiated thyroid CA.
- Sometimes Tg decreases because of high anti-Tg.

American Joint Committee on Cancer (AJCC) classification

T0 = No evidence of primary tumor.

T1 = Tumor ≤2 cm in diameter, limited to thyroid.

T2 = Tumor >2 cm but <4 cm in diameter, limited to Thyroid.

T3 = Tumor >4 cm in diameter, limited to thyroid, or any tumor with minimal extrathyroidal invasion

T4a = Any size tumor extending beyond capsule to invade subcutaneous soft tissue, larynx, trachea, esophagus, or recurrent laryngeal nerve, or intrathyroidal anaplastic cancer

T4b = Tumor invading prevertebral fascia, or encasing carotid artery or mediastinal vessels; or extrathyroidal anaplastic cancer

N0 = No regional lymph node metastasis

N1 = Regional lymph node metastasis

N1a = Metastases to level VI (pretracheal, paratracheal, and prelaryn- geal/Delphian lymph nodes)

N1b = Metastases to unilateral, bilateral, or contralateral cervical or su- perior mediastinal lymph nodes

M0 = no distant metastases

M1 = distant metastasis

Papillary and follicular tumors	
Stage	TNM
< 45 Years	
I	Any T, any, N M0
II	Any T, any, N M1
≥ 45 Years	
I	T1, N0, M0
II	T2, N0, M0
III	T3, N0, M0: T1-3, N1 a, M0
IVA	T4a, N0-1a, M0: T1-4a, N1b, M0
IVB	T4b, any N, M0

IVC	Any T, any N, M1
Medullary thyroid cancer	
Stage	TNM
I	T1, N0, M0
II	T2-3, N0, M0
III	T1-3, N1 a, M0
IVA	T4a, N0-1a, M0: T1-4a, N1b, M0
IVB	T4b, any N, M0
IVC	Any T, any N, M1
Anaplastic cancer	
Stage	TNM
IVA	T4b, any N, M0
IVB	T4b, any N, M0
IVC	Any T, any N, M1

Differentiated Thyroid Cancer (DTC)
- 5% is hereditary.
- Surgery is the primary treatment for differentiated thyroid cancer, PTC, FTC
- Aim:
    - Resect primary tumor with LNs.
    - Minimize morbidity.
    - Provide accurate staging.
    - Minimize risk of recurrence.
    - Facilitate adjuvant treatment with RAI.
    - Surveillance.

Papillary Thyroid Cancer (PTC)
- 80% of thyroid CA.
- Predominant thyroid cancer in children and incidence when exposed to external radiation.
- Female: male = 2:1.
- In ages 30–40.
- Symptoms: euthyroid, slow-growing and painless mass, dysphagia, dysphonia, dyspnea with advanced diagnosis.
- LNs are common especially in child and female (young).

- Diagnosis by FNA.
- Ultrasound is recommended to assess gland and central and lateral LNs.
- Sensitivity of US is 90%–100%.
- Distant metastasis is 20%.

Pathology
- Grossly whitish, calcified clump, necrotic or cystic.
- Microscopic:
  - Papillary projection or mixed papilla and follicular structure or pure follicular, crowded nuclei with growing intranuclear cytoplasmic inclusions
  - Orphan annie nuclei
  - Psammoma body
  - Calcification deposition
- Histologic types: pure papillary, follicular, tall cells, columnar, oxyphilic, diffuse sclerosing.
- Multifocality is 85% → high risk of LNs metastasis but rarely invade adjacent structure.
- Poorly different → 1% → worst prognosis.
- Can be presented with minimal or occult disease with LNs enlargement.
- Prognosis is excellent, 95% in 10 years SR.
- Mayo clinic proposed AGES module: Age, histology grade, extrathyroidal invasion, and metastatic size.
- Then AGES modified into MACIS (mostly post-operation): Distant metastasis, age at presentation, completeness of excision, extrathyroidal invasion, size of the tumor.
- De Groot classification:
  - Intrathyroidal extention
  - Cervical LNs
  - Extrathyroidal invasion
  - Distant metastasis

Treatment
- High risk or bilateral disease → total thyroidectomy.
- Low risk or unilateral disease → controversial but proponent of total thyroidectomy because of the following:
  - Enable to use RAI.

- Make serum Tg-sensitive for recurrence.
- 33%–55% die from recurrence.
- Studies showed ↓ recurrence rate and ↑ SR after total thyroidectomy for tumor of 1 cm.
- If patient has tumor of 1–2 cm who was treated with lobectomy → 24% recurrence and 49% increase in mortality.
- ATA guideline: > 1 cm → total thyroidectomy.
- If FNA → PTC → no frozen needed.
- If patient with nodule → ? PTC → lobectomy + isthmusectomy + pyramidal lobe, if +ve for tumor → completion thyroidectomy.
- Thyroid lobectomy is sufficient when tumor < 1 cm in low-risk patient (unifocal), absence of history of prior radiation, and no LNs.
- Intra-operatively: if LNs is enlarged → central VI (6) LNs dissection (CLND).

- Boundaries for central neck LNs group VI (6):
    - Lateral: carotid artery.
    - Inferior: sternal notch and brachiocephalic vessels.
    - Metastasis to central LNs, 20%–90% → only 50% detected by US.

- Argues to use of prophylactic CLND:
    - Micrometastasis can't be detected by US or intra-operative.
    - Improves accuracy in staging such as N1 → RAI indicated.
    - Low post-operative thyroglobulin level → allows utility to detect recurrence.
    - Low recurrence rate.
    - Low rate of re-operation.
    - Same morbidity with thyroidectomy alone.

- Argues against routine CLND
    - ➤ Absence of RCT that shows lower recurrence and mortality.

> Less than ¼ done by endocrine surgeon with high volume.
> RLNs injury and hypoparathyroidism.

- For T1, T2, no need for LNs dissection.
- For T3, T4, prophylactic unilateral or bilateral CLND.
- Dissection of posterior triangle or suprahyoid is usually not necessary unless extensive metastasis in levels II, III, IV.
- Prophylactic modified radical neck dissection (MRND) is never indicated for PTC, even if micrometastasis → RAI.
- MRND is recommended if biopsy proves involvement of lateral neck.
- MRND is to preserve SCM, IJV, spinal accessory nerve.
- Complication: hematoma, seroma, wound infection, chylous ascites, pneumothorax, nerve injury (spinal accessory, hypoglossal nerve, vagus nerve, phrenic nerve, marginal mandibular nerve, sympathetic trunk, brachial plexus, cutaneous cervical plexus).

Follicular Thyroid Cancer (FTC)
- 10%.
- Common with iodine deficiency, long-standing goiter.
- Female: male = 3:1.
- Age 50 years old.

Clinical Presentation
- Solitary nodules, history of rapid increase in size, painless unless → hemorrhage.
- Cervical LNs involvement is uncommon, 5%.
- 1% hyperfunction → thyrotoxicosis.
- FNA is unable to distinguish benign follicular lesion from cancer.
- Pre-operative diagnosis is difficult unless metastasis.
- Large follicular tumor > 4 cm in old man → malignant.
- Because of limitation of FNA → tumor marker and oncogene such as PTEN are most common, then BRAF, RET is considered.
- Peripheral blood TSHR mRNA predicts malignancy.
  → Sensitivity is 90%; specificity is 80%.

Pathology
- Usually solitary lesion, surrounded by capsule, and follicles are present.
- Architecture depends on degree of differentiation.
- Malignancy is defined as capsular or vascular invasion.
- Minimally invasive tumor → encapsulated + microinvasion → outside the capsule (small vessels).
- Wide invasion with large vessels could be encapsulated.

Surgical Treatment
- Patient diagnosed with FNA → follicular lesion → lobectomy → 80% is benign adenoma.
- Total thyroidectomy is recommended in old age, size > 4 cm → 50% cancer.
- ↑ risk: family history, history of radiation.
- Intra-operative frozen is not helpful but should be performed when there's evidence of capsular or vascular invasion.
- Total thyroidectomy when cancer is diagnosed or if angioinvasion.
- I^{-131} can detect and ablate metastatic disease.
- Prophylactic LNs dissection is not recommended because nodal involvement is infrequent, but if +ve → dissection.
- Prophylactic CLND if tumor is large.
- Mortality is 15% in 10 years, 30% in 20 years.

Hürthle Cell Carcinoma
- Found in Hashimoto disease.
- Adenoma (75%), carcinoma (25%).
- Previuosly was a subtype from FTC.
- Behave as FTC, capsular or vascular invasion.
- Cannot be diagnosed by FNA.

Pathology
- Contain abundance of oncocytic or oxyphilic cells.
- Tumor contains sheet of eosinophilia cells.
- Packed with mitochondria.
- Differs from FTC in multifocal and bilaterally by 30%.
- Do not uptake by RAI (5%).

- Nodal metastasis, 25%.
- Increase MR by 20% in 10 years.

Management

- Similar to FTC.
- Lobectomy + isthmusectomy for unilateral adenoma when invasion is found → total thyroidectomy.
- Routine CLND is similar to MTC.
- If lateral LNs is involved → MRND.

Post-operative for DTC

RAI Therapy

- De Groot → RAI reduce recurrence.
- Screening with RAI is more sensitive than CXR or CT for metastasis but less sensitive than Tg for detection of metastasis, except Hürthel cell carcinoma → screening and treatment by removal of all thyroid tissues.
- Metastasis detection and treatment by RAI I-[131], 75%.
- Used in high-risk feature:
  - Subtype of tall cell columnar, insular, poorly different.
  - Intrathyroidal vascular invasion.
  - Gross or micro multifocality.
- ATA guideline in RAI indications:
  - Grossly extrathyroidal extension regardless of size
  - Tumor > 4 cm
  - +ve LNs
  - High-risk feature
  - Poorly differentiated tumor
- Contraindication:
  - Unifocal
  - < 1 cm
  - Multifocal, all < 1 cm
  - No high-risk feature
- Remnant ablation either with thyroid hormone or recombinant TSH.

- If hormonal withdrawal is used, stop T4, 6 weeks before RAI I-[131].
- Patient should receive T3 instead T4 because of short half-life, 1 day vs. 1 week.
- Then stop for 2 weeks to allow TSH elevation before treatment with Low iodine diet during this 2 weeks.
- First, administer initial dose of 1–3 mCi and measure uptake in 24 hrs. Later, volume should be < 1%, represent residual thyroid bed.
- Treatment dose: 30–100 mCi in low risk, 100–200 mCi in high risk.
- If patient has high Tg but −ve RAI → once I-[123] received → repeat image 1–2 weeks.
- 30% will respond properly → ↓ Tg.
- Maximal dose is 200-500 mCi; accumulative dose is → 1,000–1,500.
- Complication: acute and long term:
  - Acute:
    - Neck pain, swelling, and tenderness
    - Thyroiditis (if remnant present)
    - Sialadenitis (50–450 mCi), taste dysfunction
    - Hemorrhage (brain metastases)
    - Cerebral edema (brain metastases, 200 mCi)
    - Vocal cord paralysis Nausea and vomiting (50–450 mCi)
    - Bone marrow suppression
  - Long term:
    - Bone marrow suppression (>500 mCi)
    - Leukemia (>1000 mCi)
    - Ovarian/testicular damage, infertility
    - Increased spontaneous abortion rate
    - Pulmonary fibrosis
    - Chronic sialadenitis, nodules, taste dysfunction
    - Anaplastic thyroid cancer

- o Gastric cancer
- o Hepatocellular cancer
- o Lung cancer
- o Breast cancer (>1000 mCi)
- o Bladder cancer
- o Hypoparathyroidism.

- Sometimes Tg ↓ because anti-Tg is high (Hashimoto).
- External beam radiation and chemotherapy indications:
  - Control unresectable, local invasion
  - Control pain for bony metastasis
  - No role for routine chemotherapy

- Oncogene kinase inhibitor
  - Inhibit mutation V600E BRAF kinase, promising treatment of patient with metastatic PTC.
  - Side effects → nausea and vomiting, skin SCC.

- Thyroid hormone
  - T4 is essential to replace and suppress TSH → ↓ recurrence rate.
  - Guideline: make TSH < 0.1 mu/mL, normal (0.3–2).

- Follow-up of patient with DTC
  - Tg and anti-Tg initial at 6 months interval in low-risk patients who have suppressed Tg.
  - Tg should be measured after T4 or recombinant TSH 12 months after ablation then annually.
  - With clinical exam and Tg level on T4 therapy, single rTSH Tg < 0.5, 98%–99% free of disease.
  - Tg level > 2 following rTSH → high for recurrence.

Surveillance

- After treatment of low-risk patient, −ve TSH stimulant, Tg → no need for whole-body scan.
- Diagnostic whole-body scan 6–12 months after ablation in high-risk patient.
- Ultrasound for thyroid bed and central, lateral LNs 6–12 months after thyroidectomy, then annually for 3–5 years and Tg level.
- Any LNDs 5–6 mm should undergo biopsy.
- PET scan for those with RAI −ve and Tg +ve, poor differentiated or Hürthle cells.

Undifferentiated Thyroid Cancer
Medullary Thyroid CA

- 5% of thyroid CA.
- arise from parafollicular (C-cell) which secrete calcitonin.
- Most of MTC → sporadic but 25% associated with RET proto-oncogene, i.e., MEN2a, b.
- Management is different in heredity vs. sporadic.
- Patient will have LNs +ve in 15%–20%.
- Pain, aching, and local invasion → dysphagia, dyspnea.
- Distant metastasis is common in lung, liver, bone, brain (LLBB).
- Female: male = 1.5:1.
- 50–60 years, but younger with men.
- MTC secretes calcitonin, CEA, PGE_2, and serotonin.
- Increased bowel motility → diarrhea.
- 2%–4% → Cushing → ectopic ACTH.

Pathology

- Unilateral, 80% is sporadic.
- Bilateral, 90% is familial.
- Sheet of neoplastic cells separated by collagen, amyloid.
- IHC of calcitonin (diagnostic marker).

Diagnosis

- History, ↑ calcitonin, ↑ CEA.
- FNA, family history.

- All patients with MTC should screen for RET mutation, primary hyperparathyroidism, pheochromocytoma, serum Ca^{++}, plasma-free metanephrine, or 24-hr urine collection for catecholamine.

Treatment

- Neck ultrasound to evaluate central and lateral LNs.
- Total thyroidectomy → multicentric.
- I^{-131} is not effective.
- If patient with pheochromocytoma → adrenal resection first, because of the effect of massive catecholamine to CVS with anesthesia.
- Central LNDs metastasis is frequently involved → CLND is routine.
- If patient calcitonin > 400 → CT chest, CT liver, or MRI liver, bone scan.
- Indications for bilateral CLND and MRND:
  - Metastatic disease to lateral neck LNs
  - Large tumor
  - MEN2b
- In case of recurrent or advanced disease → debulking to ↓ pain, flushing, diarrhea.
- Radiation is controversial but can be used in T4.
- Liver metastasis → resection; if could not be surgical → ethanol or ablation or RFA.
- Chemothearpy is not effective.
- Direct therapy against RET kinase under investigation for treatment of MTC.
- In patient with ↑ parathyroid gland size during surgery → resection; if normal size → mark it.
- Children with this RET mutation:
- Prophylactic thyroidectomy for MEN2b with/without bilateral CLND at age of 1 year.
- MEN2a → thyroid US and calcitonin at age 3–5.
- If high risk → thyroidectomy and bilateral CLND at age of 5 years.
- I.e., if nodule > 5 mm or high calcitonin.
- If low-risk patient → serial US, calcitonin, and thyroidectomy is delayed.

- Parathyroid gland: leaves normal gland in situ or total parathyroidectomy with auto-TPx.

Follow-Up
- History and physical examination.
- Annual calcitonin, CEA.
- Ultrasound, CT, MRI.
- PET scan.
- 10 years old, SR is 80%, but ↓ 45% with LNs +ve.
- Outcome is better in *non* MEN syndrome.
- Prophylactic thyroidectomy for RET oncogene is strongly advised.

Anaplastic
- 1% of thyroid CA.
- Women > men.
- Incidence at age: 70–80.
- Long-standing neck mass.
- Rapid enlargement with pain.
- Associated symptoms: dysphonia, dysphagia, and dyspnea.
- Enlarged and fixed to adjacent structure.
- Associated with ulceration.
- Mostly presents with metastatic disease.
- FNA: giant and multinucleated cells.
- If spinal cell → sarcoma.
- Core or incisional biopsy if FNA is necrotic.

Pathology
- Gross: firm.
- Microscopic: sheets of cells with marked heterogeneity are seen. The three main histologic growth patterns are spindle cell, squamoid, and pleomorphic giant cell.

Treatment
- Most aggressive type.
  - ➤ SR in 6 months after diagnosis.
  - ➤ Ultrasound, CT, MRI, PET should be performed.
- Lobectomy in VC paralysis.
- If extrathyroidal → en bloc resection.

Lymphoma
- 1% of thyroid CA.
- Most of non-Hodgkin's B cell.
- Developed in lymphocytic thyroiditis.
- Diagnosis by FNA but mostly −ve, especially in low grade.

Treatment
- Rapid response to chemotherapy.
- Radiation and chemotherapy is recommended.
- Thyroidectomy in compression symptoms.
- Prognosis develops on histological type grade.

Metastatic Cancer
- From kidney, breast, lung, melanoma.
- Diagnosis by FNA.
- Treatment: thyroidectomy.

Thyroid Surgery
Pre-operative Preparation
- Tumor board, full staging, consent, NPO, IVF, DVT prophylaxis, antibiotics (controversial), reviewing the ultrasound report, positioning with neck extension (controversial), blood group and save, all labs, specifically bone profile and TFTs, vocal cord, preoperative assessment.

Total thyroidectomy
- Skin incision: a curvilinear incision is placed in a skin crease two fingerbreadths above the sternal notch between the medial borders of the sternocleidomastoid muscles. The width of the incision may need to be extended for large goiters.
- Dividing the platysma and creating the subplatysmal flaps: subplatysmal dissection plane is developed superiorly (platysma is often absent in the midline) in remaining superficial to the anterior jugular veins up to the level of the thyroid cartilage above and the sternal notch below.
- The skin flaps are secured to Jowell's retractor.
- Separating strap muscles and exposing the anterior surface of the thyroid: the fascia between the sternohyoid and

sternothyroid muscles is divided along the midline with diathermy or scissors.

- Medially rotating the thyroid: using gentle digital retraction, the surgeon rotates the thyroid gland medially.
- Dividing the middle thyroid vein.
- Dividing the superior thyroid artery: the retractors are repositioned to allow full visualization of the superior pole of the thyroid and divide the artery as close to the thyroid parenchyma as possible to avoid injury to the external branch of the superior laryngeal nerve.
- Identifying superior parathyroid gland and preserving it: the retractors are again repositioned to expose the lower neck and the inferior thyroid vessels. The vessels are divided and ligated.
- Identifying inferior parathyroid gland.
- Dividing ligament of Berry: the posteromedial aspect of the thyroid gland is attached to the side of the cricoid cartilage and to the first and second tracheal rings by the posterior suspensory ligament / ligament of Berry. In identifying the RLN, avoid any cautery in this area.
- The wound is irrigated, and hemostasis is achieved.
- Wound drainage is not routinely required; if necessary, a suction drain is positioned in the thyroid bed and brought out through a laterally placed skin puncture.
- The strap muscles are approximated for 70% of their length, and the platysma is closed with interrupted absorbable 3-0 sutures.
- Skin closure is achieved, and light dressing is applied.

Complications

- Neck hematoma, temporary or permanent hypocalcemia, and unilateral or bilateral, recurrent or superior laryngeal nerves injury.

Parathyroid Gland

Embryology
- Superior glands from fourth branchial pouch.
- Inferior glands from third branchial pouch, as well as thymus.
- Superior glands located posterior to upper and middle thyroid lobe at cricoid cartilage, 80%.

Anatomy and Histology
- Superior glands dorsal to RLN while the inferior glands ventral to RLN.
- Golden yellow to brown, depending on cellularity and vascularity.
- 7 mm, 40–50 mg.
- Blood supply → inferior thyroid artery for all glands, 20% of superior gland supplied by superior thyroid artery.
- Venous drainage by superior and middle thyroid vein.
- 3% have less than four glands.
- Histology: chief cells, oxyphil cells with stroma of fat tissue.
- Chief cells produce PTH, acidophilic; mitochondria-rich oxyphil cells are derived from chief cells, can be seen around puberty, and increase in numbers in adulthood.
- A third group of cells is known as water-clear cells rich in collagen (unknown function).

Physiology and Ca^{++} Homeostasis
- Extracellular Ca^{++} is ten-thousandfold than intracellular.
- Extracellular Ca^{++}: the majority is in bone, the remaining contributes in muscle contraction, synaptic transmission, CNS, coagulation.
- Intracellular Ca^{++}: cell division, motility.
- Ca^{++} absorbed from bowel in inorganic form.
- 50% is ionized in active form, and the remaining is bounded to albumin and organic ions, phosphate, and citrate.
- Normal is 8.5–10.5 mg/dL; ionized is 4.4 -5.2 mg\dl
- Ca^{++} with relationship to plasma protein (albumin).
- Each gram decrease in albumin → decreases Ca^{++} by 0.8 mg/dL.

Parathyroid Hormone (PTH)
- Parathyroid relies on CASR (Ca^{++}-sensing receptor) to regulate PTH, also stimulated by decrease in vitamin D, catecholamine, Mg^{++}.
    - Half-life is 2–4 min.
    - Increase resorption of bone by osteoclast and release Ca^{++} and phosphate.
    - Inhibit phosphate reabsorption, bicarbonate and Na^+/H^+ exchange $\rightarrow$ metabolic acidosis.
    - Increase PTH, decrease phosphate $\rightarrow$ increase vitamin D $\rightarrow$ increase bowel Ca^{++} absorption.

- Calcitonin from thyroid C cells $\rightarrow$ anti-increase Ca^{++} by inhibiting osteoclast.
    - Control Ca^{++} level, produce pentagastrin $\rightarrow$ PUD and catecholamine.
    - Marker in MTC and treat acute hypercalcemic crisis, decrease phosphate by excretion, and decrease reabsorption.

- Vitamin D
    - Vitamin D3 is produced by skin, metabolized in liver to 25-hydroxyvitamin D, then hydroxylation in kidney $\rightarrow$ 1.25 dihydroxy (active), stimulate and absorb Ca^{++} and phosphate from gut, and resorb Ca^{++} from bone.

Hyperthyroidism
- Primary, secondary, tertiary.
- PHPT $\rightarrow$ high PTH $\rightarrow$ from adenoma, hyperplasia, GI malabsorption, CA.
- SHPT $\rightarrow$ reversed by kidney transplant for CRF.
- THPT $\rightarrow$ after renal transplant.

Primary HPT
- Incidence is 0.1%–0.3%, more in female than male, 4:1.
- Increase PTH $\rightarrow$ increase Ca^{++}, decrease renal excretion, $\uparrow$ vitamin D.

Etiology

- Radiation (low dose), familial predisposition, diet, exposure to sun.
- Renal leak Ca^{++}, i.e., decrease renal function.
- After radiation in 30s–40s, also increase incidence of thyroid neoplasm concomitant.
- Lithium → increase PTH.
- Adenoma, 80%; multiple adenomas/hyperplasias, 15%–20%.

Genetics

- Most of PHPT are sporadic.
- MEN1, MEN2a, isolated familial, jaw tumor syndrome.
- MEN1 by age of 40: parathyroid adenoma, pancreatic neuroendocrine tumor, pituitary adenoma.
  - → 50% of pancreatic NET is gastrinoma, prolactinomas, 10%–15%; insulinoma, 10%–15%.
- MEN2a by germline mutations of RET proto-oncogene.
  - → Parathyroid adenoma, MTC, pheochromocytoma.
- Patient with familial HPT and jaw tumor syndrome → increase risk of parathyroid CA.

Clinical Manifestation

- Kidney stone, painful bone, abdominal groans, psychic moans, fatigue overtones.
- Depression, low appetite, heartburn, constipation.

- Renal disease
  - 80% will have renal dysfunction or symptom.
  - Calculi, calcium phosphate, or oxalate.
  - Nephrocalcitosis, 5%.
  - Hypertension (50%) correlates with renal dysfunction.

- Bone disease
  - Osteopenia, osteoporosis, osteitis fibrosa cystica.
  - ↑ ALP.
  - X-ray hand: subperiosteal resorption in middle phalanx (second, third), bony cyst, tufting of distal phalanx.
  - Skull loss of inner and outer cortices.

- Brown or osteoclastic tumor (hemosiderin).
- Pain and pathological fracture.
- Decrease bone mineral density (BMD).
- If normal ALP → no symptom, almost never have clinically osteitis fibrosa cystica.
- Osteoporosis of lumbar spine will improve after parathyroidectomy.

- Gastrointestinal (GI)
    - ↑ gastrin → because of increase PTH to blood vessels supplying stomach → PUD
    - Pancreatitis because of hypercalcemia.
    - Increase GB stone, increase biliary Ca^{++}.

- Neuropsychic
    - Florid psychosis.
    - Obtundation coma.
    - Depression, fatigue.
    - Because of level of decrease of neurotransmitters.

- Others
    - Muscle weakness.
    - Chondrocalcinosis, gout, pseudogout.
    - Calcification of blood vessels, valves, skin.
    - Palpable mass mimics thyroid nodule.
    - Keratopathy, uveitis, glaucoma.

DDx

- Causes of hypercalcemia.
- HPT and malignancy, 90% of hypercalcemia.
- In the inpatient, malignancy is the most common cause of hypercalcemia, while in outpatient, PHPT.
- Hypercalcemia + malignancy → solid tumor like lung, breast, kidney, neck, and bone metastasis.
- FHH → mutation of CASR.

condition	PTH	Ca^{++}	24 hrs urine Ca^{++}	Phosporus	calcitriol
Primary	↑	↑	↑	↓	↑
Secondary	↑	N or ↑↓	↓	↑	N or ↓
FHH	N	↑	↓	↓	N or ↓
Malignancy	↓	↑	↑	N	N or ↓
Hypopara-thyroidism	↓	↓	↓	↑	↑

N: normal level

Diagnostic Investigations

- **Biochemical Study**
  - PHPT → increase Ca^{++}, normal PTH, or ↑ urine calcium (60%) (PHPT).
  - Decrease phosphate (serum), 50%.
  - Hyperchloremic metabolic acidosis, 80%.
  - Ca^{++} in urine is not routinely done, except for patient with history of FHH.
  - Sometimes normal Ca^{++} with PHPT → due to low vitamin D.
  - FHH has decreased Ca^{++} in urine.

- **Radiological Tests**
  - X-ray hand and skull.
  - Bone marrow density (BMD).
  - Ultrasound → renal stone, ultrasound neck.
  - PT localization is not used to diagnose PHPT rather than localization.

Treatment

- Most authors agree when the patient has symptoms → parathyroidectomy.
- If asymptomatic → controversial.
- National IHCC 1990 suggests if the patient is asymptomatic → follow up with PTH level, serum and urine calcium, vitamin D, ALP.
- Study: even if stable BMD for 8–10 years, after 15 years, it will decrease.

- 40% with follow-up patients need surgery.
- Medical treatment: antiresorptive treatment such as bisphosphonate, selective estrogen receptor modulators (raloxifene).
- Calcimimetics (modify sensitivity of CASR) results in decreased Ca^{++} and PTH.
- Bone density failed to improve with medical treatment.
- Successful parathyroidectomy → increase BMD.
- Decrease risk of pathological fracture.
- 95% success rate with morbidity.
- Currently, surgery is recommended even if slight increase in Ca^{++} level by 1 mg/dL.

Pre-operative Localization Test

- Noninvasive
  - ^{99m}Tc-labeled sestamibi scan, 80% sensitive, concentrated in mitochondria-rich tissue.
  - It was for cardiac workup then showed delayed washout in parathyroid compared to thyroid.
  - Ultrasound identifies adenoma, > 75%.
  - Single-photon emission CT.
  - CT → if adenoma is in mediastinum.
  - 4D CT sensitivity, 88%; sestamibi, 65%; US, 57%.
  - 4D CT + US, 92%.
  - Intra-operative PTH → PTH decrease 50% in 10 min after removal of the diseased gland.

- Invasive
  - Unilateral focused neck exploration.
  - Radio-guided parathyroidectomy (endoscopic or video-assisted approach).
  - Use of localization decreases morbidity (hypoparathyroidism, RLN injury), decreases stay, decreases time, has better cosmesis = traditional bilateral neck dissection.

Operative Approach
- Unilateral neck exploration
    - It was random, but after localization has been enabled → direct approach.
    - Focus on enlarged parathyroid only.
    - Advantages: decreases operative time, stay, RLN injury, and decreases risk of hypoparathyroidism.
    - Disadvantage: missing another adenoma (double adenoma, 0%–10%) such as FHPT, MEN syndrome.
    - Inability to compare either single adenoma or asymmetrical hyperplasia.

- Endoscopic approach
    - Video associated.
    - Total endoscopic technique.
    - Total endoscopic: port placement variable as thyroid, CO_2 insufflation.
    - Disadvantage: increases time, personnel, expensive, not applicable with multiglandular disease, large thyroid mass with previous neck surgery, but can use endoscopic thoracoscopy to remove mediastinal glands.
    - If patient failed localization or intra-operative PTHa adenoma is not detectable or with multiple abnormal glands, family history of PHPT, MEN1, MEN2 → bilateral exploration is recommended.

- Conduct of parathyroidectomy (standard bilateral exploration)
    - General anesthesia, supine position, neck is hyper-extended.
    - 3–4 cm incision just below cricoid cartilage.
    - Same as thyroid, strap muscle separated in midline.
    - Dissection lateral to thyroid.
    - Bloodless field.

- Middle thyroid vein ligated, anterior retraction of thyroid by peanut, or placement of silk 2-0 into thyroid.
- Space between carotid sheath and thyroid opened by gentle blunt dissection.
- Identify RLN.
- 85% found within junction of ITA and RLN by 1 cm.
- The upper glands are usually superior to this junction and posterior to the nerve, whereas lower glands are found inferior to junction and anterior to RLN.
- Parathyroid is surrounded by fat, so any fat should be explored.
- The fascia is incised, often popped out.
- Any suspicious nodule should be aspirated by 1 cc syringe containing NS.
  → very high aspirate of PTH is diagnostic.

- Location of parathyroid gland
  - Majority (80%–85%) of the glands are in their normal position.
  - Abnormal location of upper parathyroid gland → tracheoesophageal groove, 80%; carotid sheath, 12%; retroesophagus, 4%; intrathyroid, 0.2%.
  - Abnormal location of lower parathyroid gland found in thyrothymic ligament (44%) should be mobilized until upper thymus is delivered, intrathymic (26%), intrathyroidal (17%), base of the neck, anterior mediastinum.
  - If failed → intraoperative ultrasound and incision of the thyroid capsule.
  - If failed → thyroid lobectomy.

- Strategies
  - All four should be identified:
    o Single adenoma is presumed if only one gland is identifed and the other is normal, so dissection from surrounding tissue, vascular

pedicle is clamped, divided, and ligated. Do not rupture → parathyromatosis and send it to frozen to be sure.

o If 2 glands are identified, 2 abnormal and 2 normal, patient mostly has double adenoma. → excision for the abnormal glands.

o if triple (3 abnormal and 1 normal), excision of all glands → frozen, could be asymmetrical hyperplasia. This occurs in old age, above 60s.

o If all is enlarged → hyperplasia, 15%, subtotal or total parathyroidectomy with autotransplantation.

- Autotransplantation failure, 5%.
- In case of leaving some parathyroid tissue especially from inferior gland → recurrence.
- If all are removed → autotransplantation → non-dominant forearm, horizontal skin in incision over brachioradialis or in sternocleidomastoid muscle, 1–2 pockets is made, then placed in each pockets a total of 12 pieces.

Indication of Sternotomy

- $Ca^{++} > 13$ mg/dL with normal gland and failed localization.
- Intraoperative PTH assay from large vein still high despite proper exploration, excision of all glands + thyroid lobectomy.
- Inferior glands tends to migrate to anterior mediastinum or thymus, perithymal fat.
- Partial sternotomy down to third intercostal can be to right or left.

Special Situation

- **Normocalcemia with Increased PTH**
  - Should rule out cause of high PTH such as low vitamin D, osteomalacia, renal leak (renal impairment).
  - 19% will become hypercalcemic within 3 years.
  - Limited studies showed → parathyroidectomy is more likely to be unsuccessful.

697

- **Parathyroid Carcinoma**
  - 1% of primary hyperparathyroidism.
  - Suspected if $Ca^{++} > 14$ mg/dL, increases PTH five times, palpable parathyroid gland.
  - 15% LNs metastasis, 33% distant metastasis.
  - Intra-operative → large gray-white adherent to or invasion of muscle, trachea, RLN, increased LNs, so frozen section is unreliable, needs histological examination to rule out vascular or capsular invasion, fibrous stroma, high mitosis.
  - Treatment: neck exploration with en bloc excision with ipsilateral thyroid lobectomy + removal of LNs (tracheoesophageal, paratracheal upper mediastinum).
  - If the strap muscle is involved → resection.
  - MRND if lateral LNs metastasis.
  - Prophylactic MRND is not advisable.
  - Re-operation for local recurrence, metastatic disease.
  - Adjuvant radiation for recurrence, +ve LNs invasion, tumor rupture.
  - Chemotherapy is not effective.
  - Cinacalcet hydrochloride, calcimimetics, CASR to lower Ca^{++} in case of PT carcinoma.
  - Biphosphonate has shown some effectiveness.

- **Familial Hyperparathyroidism**
  - PHPT + syndromes such as MEN1, MEN2a, jaw tumor, etc.
  - 85% diagnosed pre-operative.
  - Patient with hereditary HPT → high multiglandular disease, so they need aggressive approach → bilateral neck exploration + bilateral cervical thymectomy + subtotal or total parathyroidectomy, and autotransplant is appreciated or cryopreserved.
  - If patient with familial HPT and single adenoma with normal, other glands should be resected with ipsilateral gland while the normal contralateral side is biopsied and marked.
    - → So only one side needs exploration in case of recurrence.

- Patient with MEN2a → total thyroidectomy + CLND. Only abnormal parathyroid gland is resected, and the other normal is marked.

- **Neonatal HPT**
  - Increased Ca^{++}, lethargy, hypotonia, mental retardation.
  - Result from mutation of CASR gene.
  - Urgent parathyroidectomy + autotransplant or cryopreservation + thymectomy.
  - Subtotal parathyroidectomy increases recurrence.

- **Parathyromatosis**
  - Multiple nodules of hyperfunctioning area in the neck, mediastinum following previous surgery by ruptured PT gland or subtotal parathyroidectomy.
  - Aggressive local resection of deposit is leading to normocalcemia but still ↑ recurrence.

- **Post-operative Care**
  - Check Ca^{++} every 2 weeks for 6 months then annually.
  - Recurrence, 1%.
  - FHPT → 15% at 2 years, 67% at 8 years with MEN1.

- **Persistent and Recurrent HPT**
  - Persistent: hypercalcemia that fails to resolve after parathyroidectomy.
  - Recurrence refer to HPT after intervention of at least 6 months with documented biochemical normalized Ca^{++}.
  - Persistent is more common than recurrent.
  - Both occur frequently with familial and MEN syndromes.
  - Most common causes:
    - Ectopic parathyroid
    - Unrecognized hyperplasia
    - Supernumerary gland
  - Less frequent: missed adenoma, incomplete resection, parathyromatosis, inexperienced surgeon.

- Most common sites of ectopic are paraesophageal, 28%; mediastinum, 26%; intrathymic, 24%; intrathyroidal, 11%; carotid sheath, 9%; undescended, 2%.
- Once diagnosed if persistent or recurrent → biochemical tests to rule out causes of high PTH, such as renal insufficiency, renal Ca^{++} leak, GI abnormality.
- Detailed family history for familial type, 24-hr urine collection to rule out FHH.
- Redo surgery, decrease cure to 80%–90% compared with 95%–99% on the first surgery as well as ↑ risk of RLN injury, permanent decrease Ca^{++}.
- If patient is symptomatic or with complication → redo surgery.
- Minimal → conservative.
- Pre-operative localization is routinely, like ultrasound, sestamibi, 4D CT if still −ve or equivocal → ultrasound-guided aspiration or high selective venous catheterization for PTH.
- These patients are better approached with focus approach (lateral) via previous incision between sternomastoid and strap muscle.
- Measure intraoperative PTH to ensure and avoid harmful additional exploration.
- Additional techniques → bilateral IJV sampling for PTH, thyroid lobectomy, high ligation of ITA to ensure infarction of parathyroid gland), cervical thymectomy.
- Avoid blind dissection of mediastinum.
- If failed exploration → treat with medical cinacalcet.

- **Hypercalcemic Crisis**
    - High PHPT results in nausea, vomiting, fatigue, decrease of consciousness, which may result from high Ca^{++} level from uncontrolled PTH resulting to polyuria, dehydration, and low renal function.
    - Ca^{++} as high as 16–20 mg/dL.
    - Parathyroid is large, multiple, and could be palpable.
    - Patient with cancer or familial HPT most likely increases Ca^{++}.
    - Treatment → decrease Ca^{++} level followed by surgery.

- IVF NS (0.9%) to keep UOP > 100 cc/hr; once established → furosemide to increase Ca^{++} clearance.
- If life-threatening → dialysis.

Secondary Hyperparathyroidism (Secondary HPT)

- Secondary to renal failure but may occur with low Ca^{++} secondary to low vitamin D or malabsorption.
- Pathophysiology: hyperphosphatemia (resultant low Ca^{++}), low vitamin D, low Ca^{++} intake, malabsorption.
- Generally low Ca^{++} or normal.
- Aluminum hydroxide → phosphate binder increases osteomalacia.
- These patients are usually treated with low-phosphate diet, phosphate binder, and increased vitamin D intake.
- Calcimimetics control HPT in secondary patient.
- Surgical treatments for patient:
  - Ca^{++} increase > 11 mg/dL
  - Calciphylaxis
  - Progressive renal osteodystrophy
  - Bone pain, pruritus
  - Soft tissue calcification, tumoral calcinosis
- If parathyroid > 1 cm by ultrasound → surgery.
- Introduction of calcimimetics → decreases surgery nowadays, but parathyroidectomy increases bone density.
- Parathyroidectomy is considered if PTH remains high of calcimimetics.
  - Calciphylaxis is rare, life-threatening, complication of secondary HPT, skin lesion resulting to necrosis, nonhealing ulcer → sepsis → death.
  - Skin biopsy is helpful to confirm diagnosis.
  - No surgery without documented high PTH.
  - Dialysis → localization → surgery.
- Usually in secondary hyperparathyroidism are asymmetrical hyperplasia.
- Treatment: subtotal resection, leave 50 mg of most normal PT or total parathyroidectomy with autotransplant in brachioradialis in nondominant forearm or cryopreservation; upper thymectomy is usually performed because 15%–20% will have one or more ectopic gland in thymus.

Tertiary Hyperthyroidism (HPT)
- Postrenal transplant with patient with secondary hyperparathyroidism.
- Transplanted kidney at risk of calcification.
- Treatment: wait 1 year after transplantation, then subtotal or total with autotransplant + upper thymectomy.
- Subtotal in these patients → increase recurrence.

Familial hypocalciuric hypercalcemia (FHH)
- FHH is characterized by moderate but significant hypercalcemia associated with ↑ levels of PTH and urinary calcium excretion that appear inappropriate in the presence of the hypercalcemia.

Etiology
- There are 3 genetic types of FHH based on chromosome location.
- FHH type 1 accounts for 65% of cases and is due to inactivating mutations in the *CASR* gene localized to 3q21.1.
- Mutation *GNA11* (19p13.3) seen in FHH type 2 or *AP2S1* (19q13.2-q13.3) seen in FHH type 3 Diagnostic methods

Clinical presentation
- FHH is suspected when mild hypercalcemia is seen along with normal or slightly elevated PTH, relative hypocalciuria, and normal phosphate levels.
- FHH must be suspected in the presence of persistent hypercalcemia despite surgical removal of a parathyroid adenoma.

Management
- The hypercalcemia seen in FHH does not respond to diuretics or bisphosphonates.
- For those with constantly elevated serum calcium concentrations >14mg/dL or in those with NSHPT or relapsing pancreatitis, a total parathyroidectomy can be beneficial.
- FHH does not lower life expectancy and has a benign, stable course.

Complication of Parathyroid Surgery

- Transient or permanent vocal cord palsy, hypoparathyroidism, the latter by inadequate remnant or failure of autotransplant.
- Hypocalcemia developed in patient with increased bone disease (bone hunger).
- Complication: considered permanent if it persists > 6 months.
- Complication rate is 1%.
- In symptomatic, hypocalcemia, 8 mg/dL:
    1. Oral Ca^{++}, 1–2 g Q4H.
    2. Vitamin D.
    3. calcium chloride or gluconate IV is rarely used, only for severe cases.

Hypoparathyroidism

- Congenital abscess of PT gland resulting from DiGeorge syndrome → lack of thymic development.
- Most common cause of low Ca^{++} is thyroid surgery, often developed transient ischemia.
- Usually circumoral and fingertip numbness and tingling. Mutual symptoms: confusions.
- +ve Chvostek sign (contraction of facial muscle), elicited by tapping on facial nerve anterior to ear.
- +ve Trousseau's sign (carpopedal spasm), elicited by blood pressure cuff.

Adrenal Gland

Embryology
- Adrenal gland consists of cortex and medulla.
- At fifth week of gestational, from mesoderm cortex near gonads, adrenogenital ridge is formed; therefore, ectopic tissue can be found in ovary, testes, and spermatic cord.
- Produce steroid at eighth GA week.
- Medulla from ectoderm, neural crest migrates to para-aortic and paravertebra.

Anatomy
- Paired, retroperitoneal, located at superior and medial to kidney at level of eleventh rib.
- Weight: 4–5 g.
- Arterial supply:
  - Superior: inferior phrenic artery.
  - Middle: aorta.
  - Inferior: renal artery.
- Venous.
  - Right: to inferior vena cava (IVC).
  - Left: to left renal vein.
- Accessory veins occur in 5% to 10% of patients—on the right drain into the right hepatic vein or the right renal vein.
- On the left, accessory veins drain directly into the left renal vein.

Physiology
- The gland produces cholesterol, steroid hormone, catecholamines.

Adrenal Cortex
Mineralocorticoids
- From zona granulosa.
- Renin-angiotensin-aldosterone (major) system decreases renal flow; increases Na^+; increases sympathetic tone; increases renin, salt, and water retention; decrease K^+.
- Angiotensinogen + renin $\rightarrow$ angiotensin I + ACE/lung $\rightarrow$ angiotensin II = potent VC.
- Hyperkalemia stimulate to increase aldosterone.

- ACTH, ADH leads to increased aldosterone.
- 50–250 ug/day depends on Na^+ intake.
- 50% bind to globulin, and 50% are free.
- Half-life is 20 min, then cleared by liver and kidney.

Glucocorticoid
- From zona fasciculata.
- Cortisol in complex with plasma, globulin (75%), albumin (25%) (90%), and 10% is free.
- HL is 60–90 min.
- Cortisol is converted to di-tetrahydrocortisone in liver and kidney and conjugated with glucuronic acid in liver to facilitate excretion by kidneys.

Sex Steroid
- Adrenal androgen (zona reticularis).
- Testosterone, estrogen.

Adrenal Medulla
Catecholamine
- Epinephrine, norepinephrine, dopamine.
- Phenylethanolamine N-methyltransferase non-epinephrine is converted to epinephrine only present in adrenal medulla and Zuckerkandl, which is used to distinguish adrenal medulla tumor from extra-adrenal.
- Stored with Ca^{++}, Mg, ATP, chromogranin.
- Metabolism in kidney and liver results to formation of metabolites as metanephrine, normetanephrine.

Pathology
Disorder of Adrenal Cortex

Hyperaldosteronism (mineralocorticoid) (Conn's disease)
- Secondary to high renin-angiotensin system, e.g., renal stenosis, decreases COP, CHF, HF.
- Primary hyperaldosteronism from autonomous aldosterone secretion leads to ↓ renin.
- Between 30–50 of age.
- 1% of hypertension (HTN).

- Persistant hypokalemia.
- 70% solitary adenoma, 30% bilateral hyperplasia.
- Adrenocortical carcinoma and glucocorticoid suppressible hyperaldosteronism (GSH), 1% of the cases.

Symptoms
- Hypertension—difficult to control.
- Muscle weakness, polydipsia, polyuria, nocturia, headache, fatigue resulting from ↓ K⁺.

Laboratory
- Low K⁺, should suspect hyperaldosteronism in patient with hypertension with persistant hypokalemia despite of K⁺ replacement.
- Antihypertensive should be held.
- Plasma aldosterone: renin 1:25 suggested diagnosis.
- The test is performed over 24-hr urine collection for cortisol, Na⁺, aldosterone after 5 days of high-salt diet or 2 L of normal saline in supine position after being on low-salt diet.
- If plasma aldosterone level < 5 mg/dL or 24-hr urinary aldosterone < 14 ug after saline loading, tertiary hyperaldosteronism is ruled out.
- After confirming diagnosis, see results if it's unilateral or bilateral. It's necessary as laboratory is not 100% sensitive.

Radiology
- CT with 0.5 cm cuts, 90% sensitive, usually 0.5–2 cm (unilateral).
- MRI is less sensitive but more specific.
- If adrenal hyperplasia is suspected → selective venous catheterization and adrenal vein sampling (95% sensitive).
- Adrenal vein cannulated, the blood sample obtain for cortisol and aldosterone (both) venous catheterization (IVC) after ACTH administration.
- Complication: venous rupture.
- Scintigraphy: adenoma, bilateral uptake → hyperplasia.

Treatment

- Preoperative control hypertension by spironolactone.
- Unilateral aldosterone-producing tumor is better managed by adrenalectomy.
- If carcinoma → anterior transabdominal approach.
- For other patients, medical treatment (spironolactone, aldosterone agonist, ACE).
- For GSH → dexamethasone, 0.5–1 mg daily.
- Post-operative requiring mineralocorticoid for 3 months.
- 90% improve hypokalemia after adrenalectomy.
- 70% improve hypertension (HTN) after adrenalectomy.
- Some patients get benefit from spironolactone alone.

Cushing Syndrome

- Cushing described patients as having moon face, buffalo hump (fat redistribution), amenorrhea, impotence (in men), hirsutism, purple striae, hypertension, diabetes, etc.
- Cushing syndrome results from cortisol hypersecretion.
- Cushing disease results from pituitary disease (adenoma).
- Found with MEN1 (pituitary tumor).
- Most common cause is exogenous.
- 70% ACTH-producing pituitary tumor (Cushing disease)
- 20% adrenal cause (adenoma, hyperplasia, CA)(Cushing syndrome)
- 10% ectopic ACTH.
- Causes of ↓ cortisol: depression, pregnancy, CRF, stress.

Symptoms

- Classic feature: truncal obesity results from the lipogenic action of excessive corticosteroids centrally and catabolic effects peripherally on 85% of patients.
- Fat deposition also occurs in unusual sites, such as the supraclavicular space and posterior neck region, leading to the so-called buffalo hump.
- Peripheral muscle wasting.
- Purple striae are often visible on the protuberant abdomen.
- Rounding of the face leads to moon faces, and thinning of subcutaneous tissues leads to plethora.

- There is an increase in fine hair growth on the face, upper back, and arms.
- Glucose intolerance, amenorrhea, and decreased libido or impotence.
- HTN.
- Headaches, visual field defects.
- Panhypopituitarism.
- Hyperpigmentation of the skin.
- Excessive action of cortisol centrally and catabolic peripherally.
- Osteoporosis, pathological fracture.

Laboratory

- 1 mg of dexamethasone at 11:00 p.m., then measure level at 8:00 a.m., usually decreases to < 3 ug/dL, but patient with Cushing syndrome does not.
  - False −ve with mild disease, so resulting level < 1.8.
  - False +ve with patient with CRF, depression, phenytoin.
  - In patient with −ve test, 0.5 mg Q6H for 8 doses, i.e., suppression test or measure urinary cortisol resulting to ↑sensitivity of 95%–100% and specificity of 98%.
- Recently: salivary cortisol.
- Usually 24-hr urine collection + overnight dexamethasone confirm diagnosis.
- After diagnosis of high cortisol result, see if ACTH-dependent or not.
  - Normal (100 pg/mL).
  - Adrenal hyperplasia (500 mg/mL).
  - Ectopic source of ACTH (> 1,000).
  - High dose of dexamethasone suppression test to distinguish between ACTH-dependent (pituitary vs. ectopic). Failure to suppress urinary cortisol by 50% confirms ectopic ACTH-producing tumor.
- Patient suspected to have ectopic cause should undergo testing for MTC, pheochromocytoma.
- Bilateral petrosal vein sampling resulted to whether Cushing syndrome or disease, also as well as CRH.
- CRH to determine etiology of syndrome.

- CRH (1 ug/kg) IV serial ACTH every 15 min over 1 hr.
- Primary adrenal hypercortisolism, ACTH < 10.
- Higher in patient who are ACTH-dependent > 30.
- Patient with pituitary tumor will increase more than ectopic.

Radiology

- CT, MRI distinguish adenoma from carcinoma.
- Adrenal adenoma appears darker in T2.
- Radioscintigraphy image using NP-59 distinguishes adenoma from hyperplasia. If cold, mostly cancer.
- In case of ectopic, CT, MRI, chest, and pelvis.

Treatment

- Laparoscopic adrenalectomy for adrenal adenoma.
- Open adrenalectomy for large tumor $\geq$ 6 cm or suspected CA.
- Bilateral adrenalectomy is curative for primary adrenal hyperplasia.
- Treatment of choice of Cushing disease (not syndrome) is trans-sphenoidal excision.
- Irradiation for recurrence after surgery but can lead to hypopituitarism, which can be done by stereotactic radiotherapy or bilateral laparoscopic adrenalectomy.
- If surgical intervention fails → medical treatment: ketoconazole, metyrapone.
- Patient with ectopic → resect ectopic lesion.
- Medical or bilateral laparoscopic adrenalectomy has been used to palliate patients with unresectable disease and those whose ectopic ACTH-secreting tumor cannot be localized.
- Patient for surgery require pre- and post-steroid to suppress the other gland.
- Bilateral adrenalectomy will need cortisone for life + mineralocorticoid.
- Those patients increase risk of infection and thromboembolic complication because ↑ factors VIII, vWF level.
- Replacement after adrenalectomy:
- Hydrocortisone, 10–20 mg in the morning, 5–10 mg at night.
- Fludrocortisone, 0.05 0.1 mg/d.

Adrenocortical CA

- Rare—1:1,000,000.
- Affected age: children and 40–50 years old.
- Majority are sporadia and can be associated with mutation of P53 (Li-Fraumeni syndrome) and MEN I, Loci on 11p (Beckwith-Wiedemann syndrome), 2p (Carney complex).

Symptoms

- 50% are nonfunctioning, and remaining are 30% secrete cortisol, 20% androgen, 10% estrogen, 2% aldosterone, 35% multiple hormones.
- Enlarging abdominal mass, abdominal or back pain, weight loss, anorexia.

Laboratory

- Low electrolyte (K^+).
- Urinary catecholamine to rule out pheochromocytoma.
- 1 mg dexamethasone suppression test.
- 24-hr urine test for cortisol and 17-ketosteroids to rule out Cushing syndrome.
- CT and MRI, 92% have mass > 6 cm.
- CT heterogeneity, irregular margin, hemorrhage, lymphadenopathy, liver metastasis.
- MRI: moderate bright in T2 high enhancement, delayed washout, invasion also to adjacent structure such as liver, inferior vena cava (IVC).
- PET or PET-CT: distinguish benign from malignant.
- Up to 70% present with stage III or IV.

Pathology

- Grossly large, weight is 100–1,000 g, with area of necrosis and hemorrhage.
- On microscopic only: hyperchromatic, large nuclei, difficult to differentiate.
- Capsular or vascular invasion is the most reliable sign.
- Criteria of malignancy on microscopic histology.
- Nuclear grade III–IV, mitosis > 5/150 HPF, atypical mitosis, diffuse architecture, micronecrosis, invasion of venous, sinusoidal and capsular structure.

- Tumor > 4 cm is mostly malignant.
- Marker such as Ki-67 is useful (prolife activity).

Treatment

- Most indicator of survival is complete resection, 5 years, SR is 32%–48%.
- Excision en bloc with LNs and affected organ such (diaphragm, kidney, pancreas, liver, IVC).
- Best accomplished by open approach (thoracoabdominal).
- Prevent spillage.
- Mitotane is adjuvant for irresectable tumor but S/E on GI and CNS.
- Determine blood mitotane to prevent toxicity.
- Surgical debulking for recurrent diagnosis.
- Chemotherapy is also used, but response is rare due to expression of MDR-1 gene.
- Suramin growth factor inhibitor but neurotoxic.
- This CA is reactive, insensitive to radiation.

Sex Steroid Excess

- Adrenal adenoma or carcinoma leads to virilizing syndrome.
- Hirsutism, amenorrhea, infertility, big muscle mass, deepened voice, temporal balding.
- Prematurity in children.
- Feminizing adrenal tumor leads to testicular atrophy, impotence, gynecomastia, vaginal bleeding, increased breast size, and early menarche.

Diagnostic Test

- Excess androgen precursor.
- Measured by plasma or urine 17-ketosteroids + high estrogen level.

Treatment

- Feminizing tumor ⟶ adrenalectomy.
- Malignancy is difficult to diagnose, distinguished by presence of local invasion or metastasis.
- Adrenolytic drug such as mitotane is useful to control symptoms in metastatic disease.

Congenital Adrenal Hyperplasia
- Congenital adrenal hyperplasia (CAH) results from deficiency or absence of enzyme involved in adrenal steroidogenesis (CYP21A2).
- Low glucocorticoid + aldosterone resulting to high ACTH, which leads to overproduction of androgen.
- At birth: diarrhea, hyponatremia, $\uparrow$ K^+, hyperpigmentation.
- Congenital adrenal hyperplasia (lipoid) decreases cholesterol, resulting to disruption of all steroid synthesis, which resulted also to wasting syndrome (most severe form of congenital adrenal hyperplasia).

Diagnostic Test
- Plasma and urinary steroid.
- Dexamethasone suppression test (2–4 mg QID × 7 days) to distinguish congenital adrenal hyperplasia (CAH) from neoplasia.

Treatment
- Medical: cortisol, mineralocorticoid to suppress ACTH.
- Bilateral laparoscopic adrenalectomy (alternative treatment).

Disorder of Adrenal Medulla
Pheochromocytoma
- Rare, 0.3%–0.9% in autopsy and 1.9% in biochemical marker.
- In ages 40–50.
- Extra-adrenal = functional paraganglioma found at the site of sympathetic ganglion.
- 10% tumor, 10% bilateral, 10% malignant, 10% in pediatric, 10% extra-adrenal, 10% familial in MEN2a, MEN2b.
- Autosomal dominant by germinal mutation in RET proto-oncogene.
- Another disease with risk of pheochromocytoma is Von Hippel-Lindau syndrome, which consists of retinal angioma, hemangioblastoma of CNS, renal cyst and carcinoma, pancreatic cyst, epididymal cystadenoma, and pheochromocytoma (14%).

- Also included in neurofibromatosis (NF1) and other neuroectodermal disease (Sturge-Weber syndrome), Carney syndrome (gastric lesion, leiomyosarcoma, pulmonary chondroma, extra-adrenal paraganglioma),

Symptoms

- Headache, palpitation, diaphoresis (triad) and also anxiety, paresthesia, flushing, shortness of breath (SOB), abdominal pain, nausea and vomiting.
- The most common sign is hypertension and ↑ HR.
- Complications: MI, CVA.

    ↑ symptoms by exercise, micturition, defecation.

Diagnostic Tool

- Biochemical
    - 24-hr urine collection for catecholamine and plasma metanephrine → 98%. Sensitivity and specificity, false +ve with caffeine, raw fruit, methyldopa.
    - Fractionated urinary (norepinephrine, epinephrine, dopamine) is sensitive but not specific because extra-adrenal secretes norepinephrine, no epinephrine in extra-adrenal.
    - Chromogranin A is an acidic protein stoned in medulla and other NET.
    - Plasma metanephrine is the first diagnostic tool.

- Radiology
    - CT: 83%–95%, without contrast to decrease hypertension crisis.
    - MRI: 95%–100%, used mostly with pregnant patient.
    - MIBG: taken by medulla as its structure looks like norepinephrine → for localization.

Treatment

- First medical management to control blood pressure and volume by long-acting a-blocker phenoxybenzamine started 1–3 weeks before surgery, 10 mg BID and can increase the dose to 300–400 mg/day + rehydration.

- b-blocker propranolol, 10–40 mg Q6H preoperative to control tachycardia and arrhythmia before surgery in 3–4 days.
- Volume replacement needed to avoid hypotension.
- Ca^{++} channel blocker to inhibit norepinephrine to transported into vascular smooth muscle.
- Some patients need catecholamine inhibitor (metyrosine).
- Adrenalectomy is a treatment of choice.
- Surgery with arterial + venous line, if CHF Swan-Ganz catheter.
- Don't use fentanyl, ketamine, morphine → will stimulate of catecholamines.
- Intra-operative antihypertension is nitroprusside, nitroglycerin.
- Usually via open approach; if < 5 cm → laparoscopy.
- Postoperative will develop VD → need large-volume IV.

Familial Pheochromocytoma
- VHL syndrome, MEN IIa, b, NF1.
- Multiple and bilateral.
- Unilateral adrenalectomy in the absence of contralateral side lesion.
- Bilateral adrenalectomy in the case of Addison's disease + lifelong steroid.
- If bilateral tumor → cortical sparing subtotal adrenalectomy.
- Laparoscopic subtotal is better than total, but recurrence of pheochromocytoma is 20% with VHL and 33% in MEN2.
- Autotransplant of cortex is an option, but it rarely provides full function, so steroid replacement.

Malignant Pheochromocytoma
- 12%–29% of pheochromocytoma is malignant.
- No definitive histological criteria as pleomorphism, atypia, high mitosis, vascular and capsular invasion showed in benign.
- Malignant is diagnosed by invasion to surrounding structure or distant metastasis to bone, liver, LNS, lung, peritoneum, brain, skin, muscle, also in old age and increasing size of the tumor.
- Malignant pheochromocytoma expresses P53, Bcl2, recently Ki-67, metalloproteinase, COX-2.

- When pheochromocytoma + MEN, rarely malignant, but in SDHB mutation, increase risk of malignancy.
- In general:
  - Soft tissue → excision.
  - External beam radiation for irresectable or skeletal muscle metastasis.
  - Therapeutic I-MIBG radiation.
  - If +ve for somatostatin receptor → long-acting octreotide is used.

Adrenal Incidentaloma
- During imaging.
- 0.4%–4%.
- Nonfunctioning cortical adenoma, 36%–94%.
- Subclinical Cushing (8%), resistant to suppression test by dexamethasone, 24-hr urine test for cortisol is normal.
- Adrenal is a common site of metastasis from lung, breast, melanoma, renal CA, lymphoma.
- In unilateral, incidence of metastasis is 32%–73%.
- Investigation:
  - Dexamethasone suppression test.
  - 24-hr urine collection for catecholamine + metanephrine, VMA, and serum metanephrine.
  - Chemistry, aldosterone, plasma renin in hypertension.
  - In patient with subclinical Cushing, three tests:
    o Dexamethasone suppression test
    o Salivary cortisol
    o 24-hr urinary free cortisol
- If lesion

  < 4 cm, 2% malignant.

  4–6 cm, 6% malignant.

  > 6 cm, 25% malignant.
- Benign adenoma: smooth, encapsulated, homogenous.
- On MRI: T2 adenoma has low signal compared to liver while carcinoma increases intensity. Pheochromocytoma is extremely bright.
- Radionuclide NP-59 if uptake is high → benign lesion.

Management
- AAES guidelines.
- Functional or obvious malignant → adrenalectomy.
- Optimal treatment for subclinical Cushing is controversial, but surgery is advisable with suppressed ACTH, high urine cortisol as they are at risk to develop Cushing syndrome, also if hypertension, glucose intolerance, osteoporosis.
- Nonfunctioning, balanced (benefit/risk)—if lesion is suspicious → adrenalectomy.
- Close follow-up if lesion < 4 cm with benign features, but adrenalectomy is advisable for lesion ≥ 4 cm.
- Important points to be considered:
  - Size criteria
  - Size (actual size)
  - Natural history of incidentaloma
- In older patients, usually nonfunctional adenoma; transformation is uncommon.
- Recommendations for intervention:
  - If tumor increases in size by 1 cm over 2 years, follow up.
  - If hormonal abnormality is positive, increase in size.
  - If tumor is high in production, > 3 cm, high NP-59 uptake.
- Surgeon operates on 40 years old with 4 cm lesion while electing 80 years old with same lesion depending on risks and benefits.
- Lesion increasing in size during follow-up → adrenalectomy.
- Myelolipoma → no adrenalectomy unless proven malignant (rare) even if large, which leads to laparotomy removal.
- History of nonadrenal cancer → resection.
- Suspected metastasis → resection for diagnosis.
- Follow up:
  - Dexamethasone suppression test (1 mg) yearly for 5 years.
  - Urinary catecholamine and metabolite for 5 years.
- Adrenalectomy for lesion growth ≥ 1 cm developed during follow-up.

Adrenal Insufficiency (Addison disease)

- Insufficient production of steroid hormones (either glucocorticoids or mineralocorticoids)
- Primary: adrenal disease.
- Secondary: low ACTH.
- Most common causes of primary are autoimmune infection, metastatic disease, adrenal hemorrhage with fulminant meningococcal septicemia, coagulopathy, also trauma, stress, infection.
- Exogenous glucocorticoids are the most common for secondary.

Symptoms

- Should be suspected in stressed patient, MI, sepsis, PE, fever, weakness, confusion, vomiting, lethargy, and abdominal pain.
- Chronic insufficiency: patient with metastatic disease (weight loss).
- Hyperpigmentation, high ACTH.

Laboratory

- Low Na^+, high K^+, eosinophilia, azotemia, hypoglycemia.
- Diagnosed by ACTH test (distinguish primary, secondary).
- ACTH 250 ug IV—cortisol level measured in 0–30, 60 min.

Treatment

- Volume resuscitation, 2–3 L NS 0.9% or D5 in NS.
- Chemistry, low Na^+, high K^+, low glucose, low cortisol.
- ACTH is high in primary, low in secondary.
- Dexamethasone (4 mg IV) or hydrocortisone (100 mg IU) Q8H.
- Once stabilized, it may lead to underlying cause.
- Taper IV to PO.
- Glucocorticoid (PO), 15–20 mg and 10 mg at night.
- Fludrocortisone, 0.05–0.1 mg daily.

Adrenal Surgery

- Laparoscopy vs. open.
- Anterior vs. lateral vs. posterior approach (retroperitoneal).
- The choice depends on size and experience.
- Laparoscopy is the standard for all benign lesions < 6 cm.

- Laparoscopy in CA is controversial, results in recurrence and carcinomatosis, is not appreciated.

Compilation of Adrenal Surgery

- Patient with Cushing syndrome is more prone to be infected.
- Bleeding IVC.
- Injury in liver, pancreas, spleen, stomach.
- Postoperative instability, mostly pheochromocytoma.
- Adrenal insufficiency.
- Treatment of Cushing patient resulting to Nelson disease, from high pituitary tumor resulting to pigmentation, headache, visual field.

Pituitary Gland

Hypothalamus
- Releases TRH, CRH, GnRH, and dopamine.
- Dopamine inhibits prolactin.

Posterior Pituitary
- Secretes two hormones
  - Oxytocin.
  - ADH (vassopressin).

Anterior Pituitary
- ACTH, GH, TSH, FSH, LH, and prolactin.

Prolactinoma
- Most common pituitary tumor.
- Symptoms: amenorrhea, galactorrhea, infertility, poor libido, visual problem.
- Diagnosis: MRI, visual field testing.
- Treatment: if asymptomatic or microadenoma, follow up with MRI.
- If symptomatic or macroadenoma, bromocriptine + transsphenoidal surgery.

Section III

Subspecialty

Pediatric Surgery

Umbilical Hernia

Anatomy
- The umbilicus at birth is surrounded by dense fascial ring. The opening is reinforced by strongly attached remnants of umbilical artery.
- A layer of fascia (Richet fascia) derived from transversalis fascia supplies the base.

Incidence and Natural History
- It's programmed to continuous closure.
- Weeks, months, or years after birth.
- Male = female.
- High incidence in African region.
- Recognized after cord separation and noted well at 6 months.
- Most closed at age of 3 years old.
- Commonly in preterm baby and low birth weight and 75% of infant weighing < 1,500 g.
- Hernia < 1 cm in diameter closed faster than > 1.5 cm.
- Incarceration, strangulation, perforation, evisceration are rare.

Surgical Indication
- Complication is an absolute indication for surgery.
- Persistence and appearance is a relative indication for repair.
- Giant proboscoid hernia is a wide umbilical ring, may consider repair at age of 2 years old.
- Typical umbilical hernia should be observed till age of 2 years old.
- If no improvement in umbilical fascial ring, repair is to be considered.

Surgical Technique, Result, and Complication
- Many techniques: multiple layers of closure after opening the peritoneium, closed technique, i.e., peritoneal inverted or treated like inguinal hernia repair.

- Absorbable and nonabsorbable suture.
- Redundant skin left in place, will improve overtime, and some advocate excision of skin and reconstructions.
- Repair not changed since 1953 (Gross), and closure of fascia in transverse fashion preserves the umbilicus.

Congenital Defect of Abdominal Wall

- Omphalocele
  - Large defect > 4 cm covered by amniotic membrane that contains midgut and others organs such as liver, spleen, gonads.

- Gastroschisis
  - Less than 4 cm defect and has no covering membrane and usually contains midgut, stomach, and gonads.
  - It is almost always in the right side, but exception may occur.
  - Skin bridge may be present between umbilical cord and the defect.
  - At birth, bowel can be perfectly normal, but after 20 min, it will be edematous and thickened.

- Umbilical Cord Hernia
  - Least common.
  - < 4 cm and contains midgut and covered by membrane (confused with omphalocele).

Clinical Feature
Incidence and Associated Condition

- Omphalocele
  - Before, omphalocele was most common; nowadays, second after gastroschisis.
  - 1–25:5,000.
  - Male preponderance.
  - 45% have associated cardiac problem such as VSD, ASD, ectopia cordis, tricuspid atresia, pulmonary hypertension.
  - 20% chromosomal abnormalities such as Down syndrome.

- Large baby (macrosomia) > 4 kg.
- Can be associated with musculoskeletal and neural tube defect.

- Gastroschisis
  - Most common, this is related to high incidence of prematurity and high survival of preterm infant,
    → before 1970, there was no difference between gastroschisis and omphalocele.
  - Incidence is 2–5:10,000.
  - Male more than female.
  - Anomaly with gastroschisis is usually in midgut with intestinal atresia.

Management
- Omphalocele and Gastroschisis
  - Surgical: either primary (immediate), delayed, or staged repair.

- Umbilical Cord Hernia
  - Defect reduced by holding the sac upward and gently massaging the bowel to peritoneum.
  - Fascia is closed primarily, and umbilicoplasty is always feasible.

Inguinal Hernia
Incidence
Inguinal hernia is the most common operation performed by pediatric surgeons.
- Age
  - During first year with peak in first few months.

- Sex
  - Male: female = 3:1 and 10:1.

- Sides
  - 60% are right sides. In male, this possibly results from later descent of right testicle than the left testicle.
  - Bilateral, 10%.

- Family History
  - 11.5% have family history.
  - High incidence in twin, 10% ♂ and 4% ♀.

- Pathogenesis
  - Failure of closure of the processus vaginalis.

Clinical Feature
- Found by parents during bath or during well-child examination by their pediatrician.
- Typical history of intermittent bulge in groin, labia, or scrotum.
- It's most apparent during increase IAP such as crying, straining.
- It's important to sort out inguinal hernia from communicating hydrocele, retractile or undescended testis, and inguinal adenopathy.
- Hernia may be present at birth or after days, weeks, months, or even years later.
- Older children often complain of groin pain during exercises.
- Incarcerated hernia results from entrapment of bowel or other viscera with hernial sac.
- The concern is that the parent may not recognize the symptoms of incarceration. We must intercut parent while waiting for elective surgery.
- Differential diagnosis of a crying baby includes the following:
  1. Need to feed.
  2. Need to change diaper.
  3. Need a nap.
  4. Need an operation.

Radiology Investigation
- Most cases, history and physical examination are enough.
- Previously, contrast herniography; now US (inguinal).

Management
- Inguinal hernia will not resolve spontaneously, so surgical closure is always indicated.
- High risk of incarceration especially young infant.
- 90% of complication is avoided if repair is done within 1 month of diagnosis.
- Exceptions: premature infant, cardiac or respiratory problem.
- Most patients are under general anesthesia with ETT or LMA with some exceptions.

Timing of Surgery
- Most surgeons recommend repair as soon as after diagnosis.
- Less complications.
- Premature infant: most surgeons recommend surgery before discharge after child attained 2 kg.

Technique
- High ligation of hernia sac.

Postoperative Complication
- Scrotal swelling
- Iatrogenic undescended testicle
- Recurrence
- Injury to vas deferens
- Testicular atrophy
- Intestinal injury
- Loss of abdominal doming
- Chronic pain

Undescended Testis
Classification of Undescended Testis
1. Hypoplastic or absent (3%–5%): testis never develops (agenesis) or disappears after intrauterine torsion (vanished).
2. Intra-abdominal testis, i.e., above internal inguinal ring (5%): located within a few centimeters of internal inguinal ring, vessels, and vas, traveling extraperitoneally and entering

testis through short mesorchium, and difficult to find through inguinal approach → use laparoscopy.

3. Canalicular undescended testis:
    o High inguinal: testis at the level or just below internal ring (15%–20%)
    o Low inguinal: testis at the level or above external ring (45%–50%)
4. Retractile (30%): descended testis changing its position, can be brought as far as upper scrotum but retracts immediately once released.
5. The ectopic testis (2%): perineum, femoral, pubic-penile, contralateral hemiscrotum.
6. Secondary cryptorchidism (ascending): testis no longer palpable in scrotum after normal descent or following surgery, e.g., post inguinal hernia repair.

Complication of Undescended Testis

- Temperature effect, if persistent high temperature → progress alteration.
- Normal raise of testosterone in second and third months postnatally failed to develop.
- Germ cell deficiency in cryptorchidism.
- Infertility.
- Malignancy.
- Inguinal hernia.
- Torsion of a cryptorchid testis.
- Trauma.
- Psychological factor.
- Testicular-epididymal fusion abnormalities.

Diagnosis

- Physical examination: palpate and determine the lowest position that it will sit comfortably without tension, which corresponds to caudal limit of tunica vaginalis.
- Examination should be in warm area with child relaxed and in recumbent (supine) position.
- Examination of genitalia and scrotum and inguinal region.

Treatment
- Hormonal treatment
  - Limited use

- Surgical treatment
  - Orchidopexy
  - Laparoscopic exploration if impalpable (1 or 2 stages)

Torsion of the Testis
- Twisting or torsion results in occlusion of gonadal blood supply, which results to necrosis if unrelieved.

Clinical Feature
- Torsion of testis in adolescent, but before puberty, torsion of testicular appendages is more common.
- Clinical picture: sudden onset of pain in the testis, lower abdomen, or groin.
- Previous history with similar pain for incomplete torsion with spontaneous resolution.
- Horizontal lie of testis when patient is standing indicates a long mesorchium.
- Local palpation is painful unless necrotic.
- Hemiscrotum became red, edematous, and if untreated → necrosis and bluish discoloration.

Investigations
- Radioisotope scan and Doppler US.

Treatment
- Treatment of acute scrotum and possible torsion is immediate exploration of scrotum.
- Midline incision is made in scrotum.
- Hemiscrotum is opened with diathermy.
- Edema of scrotum makes tunica vaginalis difficult to identify but can recognize it by efflux of hydrocele fluid.
- Testis is delivered through incision with evidence of torsion.
- If normal → delivered upper pole and look for twist.
- If testis is twisted, untwist and look for viability, then orchidopexy.

Varicocele

- Dilation of the testicular vein in pampiniform venous causes a varicocele.
- The countercurrent heat exchange mechanism in spermatic cord vessels is displaced, resulting to ↑ temperature.
- Progressive dysfunction of testis and epididymis → testicular atrophy and infertility.
- 15% of population.
- 20%–40% of men presenting in infertility clinic.

Clinical Presentation

- Presented as a soft, distensible mass in upper scrotum.
- 80%–90% in left side.
- In supine position, redundant, left hemiscrotum, and horizontal lie of testis.
- On standing fill with blood → bag of worms.
- Grades:
  - Small (I): evident during valsalva maneuver.
  - Medium (II): palpable without valsalva.
  - Large (III): visible as scrotal-occupying lesion.

Etiology

- Lack of valves in left testicular vein.
- Compression of left vein by SMA and aorta.
- Extrinsic pressure on left testicular vein by sigmoid colon.
- Vascular spasm caused by adrenaline coming from left adrenal.

Effect of Varicocele

- Testicular atrophy → infertility (secondary ↑ temperature).
- Serum testosterone is usually normal. Subclinical defect in androgen axis.
- Leydig cell hypoplasia, increased FSH.

Indication for Treatment

- Criteria for treatment are controversial.
- Common indication including symptoms: chronic pain, discomfort, testicular atrophy, infertility in adult, ↑ 10% difference in gonodal volume on orchiopexy.

Operation

- Inguinal exploration is standard procedure with careful ligation of all venous channels.
- Historically, high incidence of hydrocele, accidental ligation of testicular artery → testicular atrophy → recurrent varicocele.
- Alternative procedure: microsurgical dissection of testicular vein.
- Some advocate to use Doppler US and venography intra-operative.
- Some use antegrade sclerotherapy.
- Laparoscopic ligation of testicular vein proximal to internal ring has gained popularity.

Hypertrophic Pyloric Stenosis
History

- Now referred as infantile hypertrophic pyloric stenosis (IHPS).
- Hirschsprung believed this entity was congenital and represents failure of involution of fetal pylorus, and it was (CHPS).
- Most common cause of gastric outlet obstruction.
- Prevalence: 1.5–4 per 1,000 in Caucasian, but it's less in African Americans and Asians.
- Report suggests high incidence.
- Boy > girl, 2:1 to 5:1.
- Associated with variables including both environmental and familial.
- Now thought to be caused by mechanism rather than developmental defect.
- One study on 1,000 births → barium swallow study immediately after birth → no anatomic abnormality of pylorus and not congenital of interest → 5 of them developed pyloric stenosis in these infants.
- Another study with US at birth (1,400) of child after delivery → no abnormalities and 9 developed IHPS.

Anatomy and Histology

- Grossly enlarged pale muscle mass measuring 2–2.5 cm in length and 1–1.5 cm in diameter.
- Histology: muscle hypertrophy and hyperplasia primarily involving circular muscle and hypertrophy of mucosa.
- IHC: high fibroblast, fibronectin, desmin, elastin, collagen.
- Confocal microscopy: abnormal cantoned thicker nerve fiber.

Etiology

- No definitive cause.
- Many genetic and environmental.
- Genetic: races, male predominance, firstborn infant with +ve family history.

Clinical Feature and Differential Diagnosis

- Nonbilious vomiting at 2–8 weeks and peak at 3–5 weeks.
- Initially, not frequent, but after a few days, it will be forceful (projectile) vomiting every feeding.
- Infant remains hungry after vomiting.
- Not ill or febrile.
- If significant delay → dehydration → lethargic infant.
- Some have diarrhea (starvation stool), mimic gastroenteritis.
- Differential diagnosis (DDx) of nonbilious vomiting:
  o Medical causes, gastroenteritis, high ICP, metabolic disorder.
  o Surgical causes, antral web, pyloric atresia, duplicated cyst of antropyloric region, ectopic pancreatic tissue within pylorus (all less common than IHPS).

Diagnosis

- Nonbilious projectile vomiting, visible peristaltic waves in RUQ and hypochondrium, hypokalemic metabolic alkalosis are cardinal features.
- History and physical examination can make diagnosis by 75%.

- Keep child warm, calm to palpate an enlarged pylorus by pacifier or small feeding dextrose (5%).
- If stomach is distended → NGT to decompress and to palpate.
- Infant in supine, legs bent to relax abdominal wall.
- Examining hand should be placed in epigastrium after the edge of liver has been identified with fingertip, gentile pressure deep to liver and progress caudally.
- ⅓ distance between umbilicus and xiphoid (pylorus).
- Should be committing 5–15 min to obtain adequate examination.

Investigation

- U/S is the initial tool and the standard to diagnose IHPS.
- Thickness is 3.5 mm (in premature) to 4 mm. Length is 16 mm or more (some center, 14 mm).
- If U/S is not available or diagnostic → contrast examination (UGI).
- Barium is preferred than gastrografin, then aspirate it to avoid chemical pneumonitis.
- Demonstrate: elongate pyloric channel indentation of antral outline.

Treatment

Preoperative Preparation

- The preparation depends on severity of fluid and electrolyte abnormalities.
- Three levels of severity of serum HCO_3: slight (< 25 mEq/L), moderate (26–35), severe (> 35).
- In addition to high bicarbonate, low K^+, low Cl, dehydration, and malnutrition.
- Should not place NGT routinely, as it removes additional fluid and hydrochloric acid from stomach.
- IVF resuscitation as degree of dehydration, D5 ½ NS + 20 mEq/L of K^+ is optimal resuscitation, and it can increase K^+ to 30 mEq/L if severely low K^+.
- Normalized serum bicarbonate to be below 30 mEq/L.
- Ramstedt pyloromyotomy is the operation of choice.

Postoperative Management
- Most infants can start feeding after 4 hrs.
- Infant with hematemesis from gastritis → delay 6–12 hrs.
- Start feeding as follows:

Pedialyte	30 mL Q3H × 1 day
Full-strength formula	30 mL Q3H × 1 day
	45 mL Q3H × 2 day
	60 mL Q3H × 1 day
	75 mL Q3H × 1 day

Duodenal Atresia, Stenosis, and Annular Pancreas
Overview
- Duodenum is one of the most common sites of neonatal intestinal obstruction.
- 95% SR, the uncommon mortality is related to anomaly of the other organs.
- Historically, duodenal atresia was encountered in association with trisomy 21 (Down syndrome).
- Gradual decrease in incidence because of termination of pregnancy (TOP)

Introduction
- 1:6,000 to 1:10,000.
- Frequently associated with trisomy 21.

Spectrum of Disorder Involved
- Several varieties of intrinsic and extrinsic congenital lesion can cause complete (81%) or partial (19%) obstruction of duodenum.
- Intrinsic: imperforated or perforated web without bowel continuity.
- Extrinsic: annular pancreas, Ladd's band, volvulus.
- Three types of duodenal atresia:
    a) Type I—92%, there's obstruction septum (web) formed from mucosa and SM with no defect on musculosa.
    The mesentery is intact (windsock deformity), a variant of type I (membrane is thin and elongated).

b) Type II—1%, short fibrous cord can't connect two blind ends of duodenum, mesentery is intact.

c) Type III—there's no connection between two blind ends of duodenum with V-shaped mesenteric defect.

Clinical Presentation

- Advances in prenatal care allow majority of duodenal obstruction (complete and incomplete) to be detected at birth.
- Polyhydramnios noted 30%–65% (early clue).
- The classical double bubble identified in fetal US.
- The large bubble is dilated fluid-filled stomach, whereas the other is distended proximal duodenum, and annular pancreas may also be recognized.
- Repeat bilious vomiting is a characteristic clinical feature, because proximal level of intestinal blockage has no distension and upper abdominal fullness may be noted.
- Patient with complete obstruction AXR will confirm diagnosis (double) bubble sign.
- In case diagnosis is suspected but double bubble is not clear, inject 30–60 mL of contrast through NGT and may demonstrate this characteristic sign.
- If partial, it could be delayed when advanced from formula to solid food in infancy, childhood, or even adulthood.
- UGI study is the most useful study for delayed presentation of old infant or children.
- EGD is a useful diagnostic tool and sometimes therapeutic.

Treatment

- Initially NGT or OGT and IVF.
- Replace GI losses.
- PICC for TPN recommended as the finding is commonly delayed for up to several weeks after repair.
- Assume that midgut volvulus is excluded.

- Surgical correction of duodenal obstruction is not emergent and can take place once infant is optimized and associated anomaly have been studied.

Postoperative
- Prolonged feeding intolerance.
- Many prokinetic proposed, but none of them had any benefit.
- If after 3 weeks the normal function is not achieved, then there's a problem, and UGI contrast study will help to search for residual anatomic obstruction, stenosis, and preview unrecognized obstruction, poor peristalsis.

Outcomes
- SR increases from 45% to 95% due to improved diagnosis and postoperative care, and TOP has a role also.
- Mortality is now usually related to associated anomalies.

Jejunoileal Atresia and Stenosis
History
- Jejunoileal atresia and stenosis are the most common congenital anomalies of the small bowel and the major cause of intestinal obstruction in neonates.
- Atresia (complete occlusion of the intestinal lumen) is 95%.
- Stenosis (partial intraluminal occlusion) is 5%.

Etiology
- Intestinal atresia is secondary to late intrauterine mesenteric vascular insult such as volvulus, intussusception, internal hernia, tight anterior abdominal wall defect.

Diagnosis
Clinical Presentation
- Pre- and postnatal clinical sign should elicit suspicion of jejunal atresia.

- These symptoms include polyhydramnios, bilious emesis, abdominal distension, jaundice, failure to pass meconium in the first day.
- Polyhydramnios is observed in 24% of intestinal atresia and 39% with proximal jejunal atresia.
- Bilious vomiting is more common in jejunal atresia (85%), whereas abdominal distension is common with ileal atresia (98%).
- Jaundice with elevation of indirect bilirubin, 32% with jejunal, 20% with ileal.
- Failure to pass meconium.
- Severe distension is associated with respiratory distress because of elevation of diaphragm.
- Intestinal loop and peristalsis may be visible because thin abdominal wall.

Prenatal Image
- U/S: polyhydramnios, small bowel obstruction associated with atresia, volvulus, meconium peritonitis.
- Reliable to detect proximal vs. distal.
- Presence of small bowel atresia is suspected when US reveals multiple distended loops with vigorous peristalsis → distal bowel is collapsed.
- MRI is more accurate than US. In the view of these findings, we recommend any abnormalities of prenatal US should be followed with MRI.

Post-natal Radiographic Finding
- AXR reveals presence of intestinal obstruction (supine and lateral decubitus)
- Proximal jejunum has few air fluid level with no gas beyond the atresia.
- The more distal the atresia, the more apparent the abdominal distension.
- Proximal to atresia → larger loop with significant air fluid level.

DDx
- Other causes of intestinal obstruction include malrotation without volvulus, meconium ileus, intestinal duplication, internal hernia, colonic atresia, adynamic ileus secondary to sepsis, total colonic aganglionosis.
- Contrast enema is valuable to rule out colonic atresia, because coexisting with jejunoileal atresia.

Pathologic Finding
- 1955 classification to different types and recently slight changes:
  1. Type I: mucosal (septal) with intact bowel and mesentery.
  2. Type II: 2 atretic blind ends connected by fibrous cord with intact mesentery.
  3. Type III: 2 separate segments with V-shaped gap in mesentery.
     IIIa: 2 separate segments with V-shaped gap in mesentery.
     IIIb: apple peel appearance (Christmas tree).
  4. Type IV: multiple atresia.

Treatment
- Maintain the newborn in warm environment.
- 10Fr NGT.
- Suction → the color of NGT (green).
- Laboratory workup, CBC, electrolyte, type, and crossmatching.
- Aggressive IVF may be needed.
- Close monitoring, fluid balance (UOP).
- Replace losses of NGT.
- Once resuscitation is completed → OR.

Operative Technique
- Depends on the pathology of atresia.
- I.e., presence of malrotation, volvulus, meconium ileus, or peritonitis.
- Condition of the bowel, patient stability.
- The aim is primary anastomosis to establish bowel continuity.

Meconium Ileus

- Cystic fibrosis (CF) is autosomal recessive among whites in 1 in 29 births; in black, 1 in 17,000; and in Asian, 1 in 190,000.
- Meconium ileus is a sign of CF.
- Characterized by intestinal obstruction secondary to intraluminal accumulation of meconium.
- Meconium ileus is the earliest clinical manifestation of CF.

Pathogenesis

- Then defect of CF is an exocrine, eccrine gland dysfunction, especially mucus secreting and sweat gland.
- Pancreatic achylia was thought to be the mechanism responsible for meconium ileus, but most patients found at age > 1 year.
- Meconium begins to accumulate in utero.
- Abdominal distension, obstruction.
    - → Obstruction in proximal ileum.
    - → Narrow distal bowel.
    - → Colon: beaded (boxcar) meconium.
    - → More distal colon is small, unused (microcolon).

Clinical Feature

Spectrum of Disorder
- Meconium ileus presented as uncomplicated (simple) or complicated.
- Equal distal ileal obstruction in older patient.
- Uncomplicated presented immediately after birth with abdominal distension, feature of inspissated meconium filling, and obstruction of distal small bowel.
- Complicated either in utero or postnatally by perforation and/or necrosis (meconium cyst)

Clinical History
- Family history of CF, 10%–33% with meconium ileus.
- Serial in utero US predicts the infant at risk without complicating meconium cyst.
- Maternal polyhydramnios, 20%.
- High grade of intestinal obstructions.

Physical Examination
- Neonate born with abdominal distension.
- It's the only variety that neonate produce abdominal distension before swallow air.
- Visible peristaltic waves and palpable doughy bowel loops.
- Finger pressure over firm loop of bowel may hold the indentation (Putty sign).
- Simple or uncomplicated meconium ileus has no finding of peritoneal irritation.
- DRE: unremarkable but characteristically on withdrawal of examining finger spontaneously and expulsion of meconium doesn't follow.

Radiological Study
- Distended and echogenic bowel.
- After delivery, uncomplicated, typical obstruction on radiographic series.
- The characteristic findings are as follows:
    1. Great discrepancy in the size of intestinal loop.
    2. No or few air fluid level or erect, because air can't layer above thicker meconium.
    3. Granular (soap bubble) or ground-glass appearance.

Laboratory Testing
- The definitive study to confirm diagnosis of CF is sweat test.
- Use of pilocarpine iontophoresis method.
- Sweat is collected from arm, leg, and back, and the amount of Na, Cl is measured.
- Minimum amount is 100 mg or 15 microliter.
- If exceeding 60 mEq/L (Cl⁻), it is diagnostic of CF.
- Genetic testing for CF is DNA for CFTR.
- If family has known case of CFTR mutation → fetal DNA by amniocentesis.

DDx
- Combination of family history + physical examination + radiology is critical.

- The additional on maternal amniocentesis or sweat test to confirm diagnosis of CF.
- DDx of neonatal intestinal obstruction includes ileal atresia, Hirschsprung's disease, neonatal small left colon, meconium plug syndrome.

Nonoperative Management

- Depends on dissolution of the meconium + patent ileocolon.
- Use of hypertonic solution is 1,900 mOsm/L, such as N-acetylcysteine, gastrografin.
- After admistration → transient osmotic diarrhea and putative osmotic diuresis occur, so importance of fluid resuscitation + radiopaque enables safe fluoroscopy.

Operative Management

- ⅓–½ will undergo operative intervention, represent of simple or uncomplicated meconium ileus who failed contrast enema therapy.
- If complicated, then operative intervention.

➤ Simple Meconium Ileus
- Many operative procedures.
- One of the most common: enterotomy + irrigation.
- Alternative techniques:
  1. Appendectomy with appendicostomy with meconium evacuation or irrigation through this route
  2. Cecostomy
  3. Bishop-Koop procedure

➤ Complicated Meconium Ileus
- Almost always OR.
- Presence of diffuse bacterial peritonitis precludes primary anastomosis.
- Bishop, Mikulicz, Santulli procedures are applicable.

Meckel's Diverticulum

Embryology

- During early embryonic development, the yolk sac nourishes the embryo via vitelline circulation.
- *Vitellus* means "yolk."
- The intracoelomic yolk sac forms the gut and the extracoelomic yolk sac begins to regress and replaced by placenta.
- With growth, the fetal intestine becomes separated from the yolk sac, leaving only a ductal communication (vitelline/ omphalomesenteric duct), which obliterates between fifth to seventh week.
- Variety of anomalies can result from failure of regression → classical Meckel's diverticulum accident, 90%.

Epidemiology

- Most common congenital anomaly of GIT, 1.2%–3% of population.
- Male: female is equal in asymptomatic patient, but in symptomatic, male: female = 2:1.
- The rule of 2:
  - 2 types of heterotopic mucosa
  - 2 ft from ileocecal valve
  - 2 in long
  - 2 cm in diameter
  - 2 years (discovered usually)
  - 2 times common in ♂
  - 2% of population

Pathology

- True diverticulum, containing all bowel layers.
- Always in antimesenteric border.
- 75% not attached to abdominal wall, 25% attached.
- Most diverticula are located within 100 cm from ileocecal valve, 40 cm median.
- At least 5 ft of distal small bowel should be examined to rule out diverticulum.

- Gastric mucosa is the most common type, followed by pancreatic. Others (colonic, endometrial, pancreatic islets) are rare.
- Incidence of gastric mucosa bleeding is 80%.

Clinical presentation

- Most are silent and asymptomatic.
- 50% will present in the first 2 years.
- Most complications will develop before age 10.
- Hemorrhage is the most common in young age whereas obstruction in adult.

Radiology
- ^{99m}Tc (Meckel scan), administer pentagastrin ↑ gastric mucosa uptake and potent stimulation for gastric acid secretion and ↑ gastric motility.
- ^{99m}Tc half-life 6 hrs, maximum concentration in 15–30 min.
- The study is negative in absence of gastric mucosa.
- High false negative in bleeding diverticula.
- Sensitivity is 60%–84% with high false negative.
- Angiography is usually negative unless bleeding rate is high, 0.5 mL/min (rarely indicated).
- CT can diagnose the Meckel diverticulum and reflect the type of complication.
- Wireless capsule endoscopy can diagnose Meckel.

Bleeding
- Meckel is nearly 50% of all GI bleeding in children.
- DDx: intestinal polyp, IBD, intestinal duplication, hemangioma, AVM.
- Color like rectal bleeding: brightened, 35%; maroon or dark red, 40%; tarry, 7%.

Obstruction
- Meckel can cause obstruction by intussusception, volvulus, vitelline band, incarcerated Littre's hernia.

- Intussusception is slightly common in children and volvulus in adult, and it acts as a pathologic lead point.

Inflammation
- Occurs in older children and misdiagnosed as appendicitis.
- 76% of operations are performed for presumed appendicitis.
- Treated by resection anastomosis.
- Rarely exteriorization (stoma) if sick, unstable.

Neoplasia
- Found, 0.5%–4%.
- Malignant is predominant, and benign is reported, but rarely such as lipoma, angioma, neurofibroma.
- Malignant (leiomyosarcoma, carcinoid, adenocarcinoma, villous adenoma, GIST).

Treatment
- Treatment of symptom of Meckel is resection.
- Open or laparoscopy.

Intussusception
Introduction
- Is one of the most frequent causes of acute obstruction in infant and toddler.
- It's probably second most common cause of acute abdominal pain in infant and preschool age after constipation.
- Diagnosis and treatment combined pediatrician, pediatric radiology, and pediatric surgeon.

Incidence and Demographic
- 1–4 in 2,000 infants and children.
- Male: female = 2:1 or 3:2.
- Male after 9 months is 78%.
- 75% within 2 years, 90% within 3 years. More than 40% seen between 3–9 months.

Pathophysiology

Pathologic Anatomy

- Intussusception develops with its prograde bowel peristalsis. The proximal invaginated bowel (intussusceptum) carrries mesentery into distal recipient bowel (intussuscipient).
- The mesenteric vessels are angulated, squeezed, and compressed between layers of intussusceptum → edema of intussusceptum.
- Venous congestion stasis → outpouring mucus and blood from engorged intussusceptum (classic "red currant jelly" stool).
- If this process continues unabated, bowel congestion and pressure high → ischemic changes → bowel necrosis into intussusceptum.

- Permanent
  - Vast majority, 80%.
  - Mostly, symptoms require treatment.

- Transient (Spontaneous Reduction)
  - 20%.
  - During laparotomy, it is a common observation that intussusception of few < 2 cm at different sites that spontaneously reduce and can be seen by CT or US.
  - Also seen with gastroenteritis because of bowel hyperactivity.

Specific

- Idiopathic, no Pathologic Lead Point
  - All intussusceptions have some kind of PLP.
  - Thickened bowel wall lymphoid (Peyer's patch) functions as lead point in so-called idiopathic, 95%.
  - Infant and children have considerable masses of lymphoid tissue.
  - Peyer's patch is usually located in the antimesenteric area of bowel wall.

- Pathologic Lead Point (PLP)
  - Range: 1.5%–12%.
  - ↑ with age, 5% first year, 44% with first 5 years, 60% 5–14 years.
  - PLP is found in 4% of infants who had one recurrence.
  - Most common focal cause is Meckel's diverticulum, followed by intestinal polyp with duplication.
  - Other less common are periappendicitis, stump appendicitis, inversion appendectomy, appendiceal mucocele, local suture line, massive local lymphoid hyperplasia, ectopic pancreas, abdominal trauma.
  - Other diseases cause multifocal bowel wall thickening such as Henoch-Schonlein purpura, CF, celiac disease, hemophilia, neutropenic colitis, Hirschsprung's, enterocolitis, Peutz-Jeghers syndrome, familial polyposis.

Clinical Finding and Physical Examination

- Should be suspected with any two classic symptoms (abdominal pain, vomiting).
- Two colic signs (abdominal mass and rectal bleeding).
- Most cases are diagnosed within 24 hrs.
- In case of recurrence, usually diagnosis is made < 8 hrs.
- High index of suspicion is necessary in any infant or toddler with crampy abdominal pain.
- Sudden onset of severe, colicky, intermittent abdominal pain, which makes infant pull up their legs, is the most classic symptom of intussusception (85%).
- Pain episode lasts for a few minutes, then infant is pale and sweaty and then returns to normal activity for a while.

Diagnosis
Laboratory
- If bowel becomes ischemic, associated with leukocytosis, acidosis, electrolyte imbalance.

Radiologic Diagnosis
- Usually clinically (50%), but diagnosis relies on radiological image.

Plain AXR
- Nonspecific: right-sided soft tissue filled with gas and stool occupies RLQ, mistaken as cecum.
- Can see sign of intestinal obstruction.

US
- In expert hand, US is 100% accurate.
- Portable, noninvasive, no radiation.
- Finding 3–5 cm in diameter mass is typical. Target or doughnut sign on right side.

CT and MRI
- Most institutions don't routinely use CT or MRI.
- Can find intussusception incidentally on image for another reason.
- In pathologic cause can be useful (lymphoma, mass).

Contrast Enema
- Some use it as preferred diagnostic tool.
- Quick, cost-effective, accuracy is 100%.
- If +ve → can become therapeutic.

Treatment
- When history confirms suspicions of intussusception, the surgeon must evaluate for peritonitis or shock to rule out the rare need for emergent surgery.
- If vomiting → NGT.
- IV antibiotic, because vascular supply may be jeopardized + bowel surgery is possible.
- X-match PRBCs.
- Radiological evaluation to confirm diagnosis.
- OR should be notified when non-operative is unsuccessful.

Non-operative Management
Radiological Reduction
- Contraindication: dehydration, shock, peritonitis, evidence of perforation (free air).
- Factors predict unsuccessful reduction:
  o Younger age, < 6 months
  o Rectal bleeding at presentation
  o Picture of intestinal obstruction
  o Long duration of symptoms, > 72 hrs
- Currently the used technique for nonoperative reduction includes pneumatic or hydrostatic pressure enema under fluoroscopy or US.

Post-reduction Care
- After successful reduction, infant and child should be observed.
- If intussusception is recognized early and enema reduction was easy, then patient can be discharged from ER.
- Most patients are admitted.
- If enema reduction succeeded, start clear fluid and progress to diet as tolerated, stop IVF.
- US is important to reevaluate previous partial reduction.

Operative Management
- Seven indications:
  1. Radiological contraindicated
  2. Failed radiological reduction
  3. Incomplete reduction
  4. Peritonitis
  5. Unstable
  6. Pneumoperitoneum
  7. PLP
- Either laparoscopic or open.
- After IVF resuscitation, IV antibiotic.

Disorder of Intestinal Rotation and Fixation

- When the midgut developed, it protrudes out of the abdominal cavity, forming a loop, the SMA forming the axis of the loop.
- The midgut makes a quarter turn of 90° degrees counterclockwise (first), the distal part to the left (cecum) and the proximal part (small bowel) to the right.
- The body is growing, and the abdominal cavity becomes large enough to allow the bowel loops to return.
- The proximal part of the loop returns first; it passes under the distal part and to the left and makes another turn of 90° degrees counterclockwise (second).
- The distal part of the loop returns last; it passes in front of the proximal part and ends up over to the right, completing the (third) quarter turn of 90°degrees.
- The net effect: proximal part of the midgut ends behind the distal part of the midgut, total of 270° degrees.

Classification of Abnormalities of Intestinal Rotation

- Malrotation → Typical
- → Nonrotation
- → Atypical or malrotation variant

Clinical Manifestation

- Ranging from chronic abdominal pain to acute midgut volvulus, ischemic bowel injury.

- Acute Midgut Volvulus
  - The narrow pedicle formed by the base of mesentery in malrotation predisposes the midgut clockwise, twisting from duodenum to transverse colon.
  - Excessive length of mesentery acts like an axis of twist.
  - Greenish vomiting in normal, healthy baby before presentation
  - Crampy abdominal pain.
  - Infant with complete obstructions rapidly develop intestinal ischemia with firm, distended abdominal hypovolemia and shock.
  - Abdominal tenderness varies with degree of vascular compromise.

- Chronic Midgut Volvulus
  - Intermittent or partial midgut volvulus results in lymphatic and venous obstruction with enlargement of mesenteric LNs and most commonly with children more than 2 years old.

Radiologic Diagnosis of Abnormal Rotation and Fixation
- Contrast fluroscopy is essential for diagnosis.
- Normal relation of stomach, duodenum, ligament of Treitz, ileocecal valve shown schematically.
- AXR is often nondiagnostic.
- US, good screening for infant with suspicious midgut to see vascular flow.
- Whirlpool is the flow pattern of SMV and mesentery around SMA in more than 75% of patients with midgut volvulus and best by Doppler.
- CT also demonstrates whirlpool with IV and oral contrast.

Treatment
Preoperative Management
  - Patient suspected with midgut volvulus may be dehydrated → IV resuscitation and prolonged resuscitation is not warranted.
  - Place NGT, IV accesses, and IV antibiotics.

Operative Technique
  - Ladd's Procedure
    1. Evisceration of the bowel and inspection of mesentery root.
    2. Counterclockwise detortion of midgut volvulus.
    3. lysis of Ladd's peritoneal band.
    4. Straightening of duodenum along right abdominal gutter.
    5. Widening of the mesenteric root.
    6. Appendectomy.
    7. Placement of cecum in RLQ and the small bowel to the left.

Necrotizing Enterocolitis (NEC)

- It is an acquired inflammatory disease that affects the gut of newborn
- NEC is a leading cause of infant mortality and morbidity in NICU.
- ↑rate because ↑ preterm birth and advanced NICU care, resulting to ↑ risk of NEC.
- Most common emergency that ↑ mortality and morbidity.
- Pathology remains incompletely understood.

Incidence

- 0.5%–1%, but this number with suspicious case, so it's not accurate.
- It varies according to geographic distribution, i.e., genetic.
- Incidence of NEC in very low birth weight (VLBW) < 1,500 g, varies in the following:
  - Japan, 1%–2%
  - Austria, 7%
  - Greece, 10%
  - Argentina, 14%
  - Hong Kong, 28%.
- NEC account 1%–7% of all NICU admissions or 1–3 per 1,000 live births.

Epidemiology

Age and Maturity

- Predominant in premature LBW infant.
- 7%–13% occur in full term.
- Mean GA is 31 weeks.
- Average weight is 1,460 g.

Feeding

- 90% of NEC develop after feeding initiation.
- After standardization of feeding schedule for infant, 1,250–2,500 g and less than 35 weeks → decrease risk of NEC, 84% in one study.

Pharmacological Agent

- Indomethacin (NSAIDs) uses:
  - ➢ To delay premature labor

> ➤ To decrease polyhydramnios
> ➤ To close PDA.
- It blocks prostaglandin, predisposes spontaneous intestinal perforation (SIP) and NEC.

Cytokines and Growth Factor
- Plays a critical role in meditating interaction among enterocytes, endothelial cells, fibroblasts, and inflammatory cells.

- Growth Factor (GF)
    - EGF is an important factor for developing GI tract and is present in high concentration in human breast milk.

Cytokines
- Overproduction of pro-inflammatory cytokines (IL-1, IL-2, IL-6, IL-8, IL-12, TNF-α, interferon, PAF).
- Overproduction of anti-inflammatory cytokines (IL-4, IL-10, IL-11), excessive supply of immune function.

- TNF-α
    - Inhibition of TNF-α, reduces bowel necrosis.

- NO (Nitric Oxide)
    - Maintains mucosal integrity.

- PAF
    - Plays role in pathophysiology of intestinal injury.

Pathogenesis
- No definite cause.
- Multifactorial etiology involves combinations of mucosal compromise, pathogenic bacteria, and enteral feeding resulting in bowel injury and inflammatory cascade.
- Most important factor is prematurity and enteral feeding of formula.

Pathology
- May involve single (50%) or multiple (discontinues) segments of intestine.
- Most commonly terminal ileum followed by colon.
- Involving of small and large bowels (both), 44%.
- Pan involvement (NEC totalis), 19%; necrosis at least 75% of gut.

Diagnosis

Clinical Features
- Physiologic instability.
- Lethargy, temperature instability, recurrent apnea, bradycardia, hypoglycemia, shock.
- Locals:
  - Abdominal distension, 70%–98%
  - Blood per rectum, 79%–86%
  - High gastric residual after feeding, > 70%
  - Vomiting, > 70%
  - Diarrhea, 4%–26%
  - Gross blood in stool, 25%–63%

- Initially, abdominal distension, mild tenderness.
  - As disease progresses → ↑ tenderness and palpable bowel loops, fixed or mobile mass, abdominal wall crepitus.
  - Edema and erythema of abdominal wall are results of peritonitis, initially 4% but more common later in the cause of disease.
  - In male discoloration of scrotum indicates perforation.

- Disease rapidly progresses and death within 24 hrs.

Laboratory Findings
- Neutropenia, thrombocytopenia.
- Metabolic acidosis.
- Electrolyte derangement.
- Stool sample +ve for occult blood and reducing substance.
- Damaged mucosa leads to carbohydrate malabsorption.

- Bacteria fermentation, ↑ production of lactate.
- CRP serves as an early indicator of NEC when rise is more than 10 within 48 hrs of suspicion.
- Failure of C-RP to return normal → within 10 days, indicator of abscess, stricture, septicemia.

Imaging

- Plain x-ray remains the cornerstone.
- AP and left lateral decubitus or cross table.
- Any or all the following findings:
  - ➢ Ileus pattern (distension)
  - ➢ Pneumatosis intestinalis
  - ➢ PV gas
  - ➢ Pneumoperitoneum
  - ➢ Intraperitoneal fluid
  - ➢ Persistent dilated fixed loop.
- Contrast studies:
  - ➢ May improve diagnostic accuracy in equivocal NEC.
  - ➢ Barium should never be used → peritonitis.

US

- Used to identify necrotic bowel, intraperitoneal fluid, and PV gas.

MRI

- Although MRI is capable of demonstrating cardinal finding of NEC, but utility is limited.

Classification

Modified Bell's criteria:

- Stage 1: suspected NEC—gastric residuals, abdominal distension, occult or gross blood in stool, x-ray normal to mild distension, temperature instability, apnea, bradycardia
- Stage 2: definite NEC—mild to moderate systemic illness, absent bowel sounds, abdominal tenderness, pneumatosis intestinalis or portal venous gas, metabolic acidosis, ↓ platelets

- Stage 3: advanced NEC—severely ill, marked distension, signs of peritonitis, hypotension, metabolic and respiratory acidosis, DIC, pneumoperitoneum if bowel perforation is present

Management
Nonoperative
- In the absence of necrosis or perforation, the mainstay of treatment is supportive.
- NPO, IVF, NGT to decompress.
- CBC, platelet, blood gas, CRP, electrolyte.
- Blood and urine C/S.
- Broad-spectrum antibiotic like penicillin, aminoglycosides + anaerobic coverage for 1–2 weeks.

Indication for Operation
- The principal goal of surgical intervention in NEC is to remove gangrenous bowel and preserve intestinal length.
- Many argue that exploration should not be undertaken until gangrene is present but before perforation.
- No test confirm the intestinal gangrene.
- Thus it remains a controversy regarding indication for operation, most appropriate timing, and optimal surgical treatment.
- The most widely accepted absolute indication is presence of pneumoperitoneum.
- Relative indication:
  o +ve pareacentesis.
  o Abdominal wall erythema
  o Fixed internal loops
  o Palpable abdominal mass
  o PV gas
  o Clinical deterioration despite maximal medical treatment

Hirschsprung's Disease
- Absence of ganglion cell.

Diagnosis
Clinical Presentation
- Neonatal Obstruction
    - 50%–90% present in neonatal period with abdominal distension, bilious vomiting, feeding intolerance.
    - Delayed passage of meconium, 90%.
    - Some cases: cecal or appendiceal perforation may be the initial event.
    - AXR: dilated bowel loops.
    - DDx: intestinal atresia, meconium ileus, meconium plug syndrome.

- Chronic Constipation
    - In childhood or even in adulthood.
    - Typically, in infant while breastfeeding who develops constipation around the time of weaning.
    - Clinical features that lead to diagnosis are failure to pass meconium in first 48 hrs, failure to thrive, and abdominal distension, enema dependency.

- Enterocolitis
    - 10% will present with fever, abdominal distension, diarrhea due to Hirschsprung's associated with enterocolitis (HAEC).

- Associated Conditions
    - Associated with other congenital anomalies:
        - ➢ Malrotation, genitourinary abnormalities
        - ➢ Congenital heart disease
        - ➢ Limb abnormalities
        - ➢ Cleft palate and lip
        - ➢ Hearing Loss, mental retardation
        - ➢ Dysmorphic feature

- Radiological Evaluation
  AXR
  - Bowel obstruction (distal).
  - Water-soluble contrast enema → transition zone between normal and aganglionic bowel.
  - Most important view is lateral view.

  Anorectal Manometry
  - Easier in older patient ↑(false +ve) by contraction of external sphincter and artifact by crying.
  - Normal RAIR to rule out Hirschsprung's and avoid rectal biopsy.

- Rectal Biopsy (Defentive)

Preoperative Management
- Most cases are surgical.
- IVF, IV antibiotic.
- NGT.
- Investigate for other abnormalities.
- Children with enterocolitis, immediate surgery can't be done → decompression by rectal washout (irrigation).
- Patient can be discharged on breastfeeding, elemental formula + rectal irrigation.
- Some need colostomy to decompress.
- Some advocate nonoperative → enemas and laxative.

Surgery: Pull-Through for Hirschsprung's
- The goal is to remove aganglionic bowel and to reconstruct the anus and preserve normal sphincter function.
- Most commonly performed are Swenson, Duhamel, and Soave techniques.
- Can performed by open surgery, laparoscopy, or transanal pull-through.

Anorectal Malformation
Classification

Male	Female
Perineal fistula	Perineal fistula
Rectourethral fistula (bulber and prostatic)	Vestibular fistula
Rectobladder neck fistula	Persistent cloaca ($\leq$ 3 cm, > 3 cm)
Imperforated anus with no fistula	Imperforated anus with no fistula
Rectal atresia	Rectal atresia
Complex defect	Complex defect

Associated Malformation
- 50%–60% had associated anomaly.
- Higher abnormalities associated with higher anomalies.
- Should rule out VACTERL association.

Cardiovascular
- 30%, but only 10% need treatment.
- Most common lesions are ASD, PDA, then TOF, VSD.
- TGA, hypoplastic left heart syndrome (rare).

GIT
- TEF, 10% cases.
- Duodenal obstruction caused by atresia or malrotation, 1–2%.
- Hirschsprung's disease found in 3 of 2,100 patients.

Spinal, Sacral, and Vertebral Anomaly
- Lumbosacral anomalies such as hemivertebrae, scoliosis butterfly vertebrae, hemisacrum are common.
- Most frequent spinal problem is tethered cord.
  - → Also, spinal lipoma, syringomyelia, and myelomeningocele are common cause.
- For spinal anomaly, US or MRI.
- Currarino triad: sacral defect (hemisacrum) and imperforated anus, presacral mass.
- Sacral ratio is a valuable prognostic tool.
  - ➤ Quantity degree of sacral hypodevelopment.

➢ Patient < 0.4 in continue, if ≈ 1.0 good prognosis.

Genitourinary
- ⅓ to ½, vesicoureteral reflux (VUR), then renal agenesis, dysplasia (next most frequent).
- Cryptorchidism up to 20%.
- Hypospadias, 5%.

Gynecologic Anomalies
- In newborn, hydrocolpos → pyocolpos.
- Müllerian anomaly manifests later in teenager having obstruction of menstrual flow.
- Large abdominal collection and peritonitis may develop, and patient may have amenorrhea because of Müllerian structure.
- Can at any level: obstruction of tube, atresia of cervix or blind hemivagina.
- Uterine malfunction (bicornuate uterus and didelphys uterus).
- Vaginal abnormalities (vaginal septum) leading to vaginal atresia.
- During definitive repair at the time of colostomy closure, inspect intra-abdominal gene structure.

Clinical Finding and Initial Management
- You will call to see newborn male with ARM.
- First: perineal inspection.
- It is important to decide about colostomy or primary operation before 20–24 hrs.
- Wait till sigmoid ↑ intramural pressure to force meconium through a fistula → location of distal rectum.
- If meconium is visualized on perineum → rectoperineal fistula.
- If meconium is in urine → rectourinary fistula.
- Radiology before 24 hrs because rectum collapses by muscle tone of surrounding sphincter.
- In female, same as in male, and the most important step is perineal inspection.

PSARP
- Posterior sagittal anorectoplasty.

Colostomy
- Usually performed as first stage in newborn with high anomaly.

Imperforate Anus without Fistula
- Blind end of rectum is located at the same level as in patient with bulbar urethral fistula, because rectum is still attached to posterior urethra, and careful dissection must be observed.

Rectal Atresia and Stenosis
- Usually separated by fibrous tissue.
- Rectum should be mobilized to allow end-to-end anastomosis.
- Anal canal is normal and excellent in bowel control.
- This defect associated with presacral mass often is teratoma, and full evaluation is essential.

Cloaca
- It is considered separately because of its complexity.
- Reconstruction is required to be delicate, with meticulous technique + creativity, imagination, resourcefulness, and expert surgeon.

The Jaundiced Infant—Biliary Atresia
Etiology
- Unknown, multifactorial.
- Theories: genetic, inflammatory, infection is unproven but increase incidence in certain population → genetic.
- 20% associated with other malformation such as developmental delay abnormalities.
- Infectious: reovirus, rotavirus in animal with infection, resulting to biliary atresia.
- Other factors: Bile ducts ischemia, abnormal bile metabolism, pancreaticobiliary maljunction.

Clinical Evaluation

- Combination of progressive jaundice, acholic stool, dark urine, firm hepatomegaly.
- High direct bilirubin rather than indirect.
- Most cases: perinatal course unremarkable and meconium is normal.
- 50% of initial stool is normal then lighter over time.

Diagnosis

- Persistent jaundice, especially with high direct bilirubin.
- No single test to distinguish biliary atresia from other causes of jaundice.
- Combination of examination, blood test, image, and pathology.
- The final diagnosis is almost always with surgical exploration.

US

- Fasting to allow filling of gallbladder.
- Echotexture of liver, presence of ascites, patency of hepatic vasculature.
- Either biliary atresia or choledochal cyst and obstruction.

Hepatobiliary Scintigraphy

- Use of ^{99m}Tc to assess excretion of bile from liver to small bowel = HIDA.

Liver Biopsy

- To differentiate biliary atresia from other cholestatic conditions.
- It's the most accurate nonsurgical diagnostic test.
- Can be performd by pediatrician or by hepatologist.
- Presence of raring degree of inflammation with ductular proliferation resulting to biliary atresia.

Other Tests

- NDT aspiration or prolonged collection, then look for bile.
- ERCP can avoid unnecessary exploration.
- MRI and MRCP have superior accuracy but expensive sedation and not routinely used.

Treatment
- Preoperative care.
- Standard preoperative measures.
- Bowel preparation is not required.
- Preoperative IV antibiotic (broad spectrum).
- Although patient with biliary atresia has normal coagulation, fat-soluble oral suspension KEDA.
  → vitamin K is administered; 1 mg IM should be given.

Surgical Technique
- Roux-en-Y hepatic portoenterostomy procedure (Kasai procedure).
- Excision of entire extrahepatic biliary tree with transection of fibrous plate near the hilum of liver with bilioenteric continuity reestablished with Roux-en-Y.

Congenital Anomaly of Esophagus (esophageal Atresia)
Classification
- Many classifications are used.
- The most useful and simple is Gross and Vogt classification.

Type	Description	Percentage
A(Gross), II(Vogt)	EA with no TEF	6%
B, III	EA with proximal TEF	5%
C, IIIb	EA with distal TEF	84%
D, IIIa	EA with both pouches and fistula	1%
Type E H type	TEF with no EA	4%

Associated Anomalies
- 50%–70% have at least one congenital anomaly.
- Anomalies are most common in EA without TEF and least common in type H.
- 50% are associated with syndromes such as chromosomal, VACTERL, CHARGE, Fanconi anemia.
- The other 50% are nonsyndromic with multiple gene anomalies.

Diagnosis and Clinical Finding
- Not commonly diagnosed prenatally.
- US relies on the finding of small or absent stomach bubble and association with polyhydramnios, with a predictive value of 20%–40%.
- Diagnosis of EA is confirmed by passing catheter through mouth into esophagus and see where the resistance is.
- Sometimes delay diagnosis and history of coughing during feeding → pulmonary infiltrate on CXR.
- Can make diagnosis by barium esophagography in prone position.

Preoperative Treatment
- To prevent pneumonitis from saliva → NGT with continuous aspiration.
- Head up or prone position to lower reflux.
- Broad-spectrum antibiotic.
- IVF D5 ¼ NS should be started.
- Vitamin K before surgery.
- Routine STT intubation → gastric perforation for high distension.

Operative Repair
- Open thoracotomy or thoracoscopic division of fistula with primary anastomosis of esophagus is the operative procedure of choice.

Congenital Diaphragmatic Hernia
Epidemiology and Genetics
- Death due to associated congenital anomaly.
- ⅓ are stillborn (dead).
- Defect on left side is 80% and on right, 20%. Bilaterally rare and higher associated anomaly.
- Usually sporadic.
- Expected recurrent risk in first-degree relative is 2%.
- Structural chromosomal abnormalities, 9%–34%.
- Environmental factors include insecticides, drugs, phenmetrazine, thalidomide, quinine, cadmium, lead.

Associated Anomaly
- Incidence of associated anomaly is 10%–15%.
- 32% skeletal defect includes limb reduction, costovertebral defect.
- 24% cardiac anomaly.

Pathology
- During early development of diaphragm, the midgut is herniated into yolk sac.
- If pleuroperitoneal canal is not closed by the time of midgut return to abdomen during 9–10 weeks → herniation inot the chest.
- Abdominal viscera herniate through lumbocostal triangle into thoracic cavity.

Diagnosis
- Usually, prenatal by US is 40%–90% accurate.
- Detection mean age is 24 weeks, and some report as early as 11 weeks.
- Polyhydramnios (80%) due to kinking of GEJ.
- CXR: loops of bowels in the chest.
- Location of gastric bubbles should be noted, place OGT.
- Contrast study is rarely needed and shift of mediastinum to contralateral side.
- Once diagnosis of CDH is confirmed, then US abdomen, echo, and cranial US.
- Patient presents with recurrent mild respiratory illness, chronic pulmonary disease.
- Occasionally, pneumonia may mask right CDH.

DDx
- Many of chest conditions: congenital cystic disease of lung, primary agenesis of lung, diaphragmatic eventration, anterior diaphragmatic hernia of Morgagni, congenital hiatal hernia.

Treatment
- Should be followed with prenatal US, the time varies of discovering it.

- Should search for another anomaly, CVS, CNS.
- Evaluation of fetal karyotype by amniocentesis, chorionic villus, or fetal blood sample.
- Care support to fetus and mother to achieve full term.
- Prepare parents and inform about treatment and outcome.
- Should refer the mother to tertiary center that has respiratory strategies such as NO, ECMO, oscillating ventilators.

Preoperative Care
Resuscitation
- It's essential to consider that CDH is a physiologic emergency and not a surgical emergency.
- Ventilation.

Pharmacology
- Prostaglandins: PGD_2, PGE, prostacyclin, COX inhibitor indomethacin are disappointing.
- Ca^{++} channel blocker, prostacyclin derivatives, endothelin receptor antagonist, sildenafil.
- Surfactant.
- Nitric oxide.

Surgical Management
- Operative repair: most surgeons prefer subcostal incision or thoracotomy, thoracoscopy.

Cystic Lung Lesion
Congenital Cystic Adenomatoid Malformation (CCAM)
- Also called congenital pulmonary airway malformation (CPAM).
- Prenatal diagnosis is divided into two categories:
  - Macrocystic single or multiple cysts $\geq$ 5 mm.
  - Macrocystic lesion appears as solid mass on US.
- Overall prognosis depends on the size of CCAM.
- Other presentation → pneumothorax, reactive airway disease, and failure to thrive.
- No gender predominance.
- Associated anomaly is very uncommon.
- Tx: excision to prevent recurrent chest infection.

Congenital Lobar Emphysema (CLE)

- Many causes, the main is that affected bronchus allows passage of air on inspiration but limited expulsion of air on expiration, resulting to lobar overexpansion.
- Air trapped in emphysematous lobe may result to the following:
  - Dysplastic bronchial cartilage creates valve-like ball or completes bronchial atresia.
  - Endobronchial obstruction from mucus or extensive mucosal proliferation and infolding.
- Most common sites:
  - LUL   40%–50%
  - RML   30%–40%
  - RUL   20%
  - LLL   1%
- Barotrauma can cause and acquire emphysema → RLL is the commonest site.
- CLE is distinguished from other cystic lesions prenatally by US → echogenicity, high reflectivity compared to CCAM, and absence of systemic arterial supply compared with BPS.
- After birth, CXR → radiopaque of affected lobe because of delayed clearance of fluid.
- Affected lobe pops out through thoracotomy → resection.

Wilms' Tumor (WT) (Nephroblastoma)

- Most common primary malignant renal tumor of children 90%
- Outcomes improve dramatically.
- Long-term survival rate in North America and Europe is 85%.
- SR of low stages is 95%–99%.
- Current treatment is based on multidisciplinary cooperative group by COG, NWTSG, SIOP.

Epidemiology

- In US, there are 500–550 cases of Wilms' tumor per year.
- Second most common malignant abdominal tumor in children after neuroblastoma.
- Risk of developing Wilms' tumor in general population is 1:10,000.

- High in African Americans compared to whites and low in Asians.
- Most presenting age is 12–48 months, more in girls than boys.
- Rare after 10 years and less than 6 months of age.
- Bilateral Wilms' tumor is 4%–13%.
- Children with syndromes such as Beckwith-Wiedemann syndrome have high risk of developing bilateral WT.
- Congenital anomaly either isolated or as a part of congenital anomaly occurs about 10%.
- WAGR syndrome, Beckwith-Wiedemann syndrome, Denys-Drash syndrome (DDS). Other syndromes associated with Wilms' tumor are hemihypertrophy and Perlman syndrome.
- Urological abnormalities such as hypospadias, cryptorchidism, nephromegaly are associated with Wilms' tumor.

Clinical Presentation

- Most presentations with asymptomatic abdominal mass, often discovered by parents or pediatrician.
- Nonpalpable tumor is discovered by US during evaluation of abdominal pain.
- Gross hematuria, 18.2%; microscopic, 24.4%.
- DDx: neuroblastoma, hepatoblastoma, rhabdomyosarcoma, and lymphoma.
- Neuroblastoma is the most common solid tumor in children.
- The difference between neuroblastoma and Wilms' tumor clinically is that patient with neuroblastoma is often ill because of extension of metastatic disease, but in Wilms' tumor, the patient is healthy.

Diagnosis

- US is good for screening examination of a mass to determine its site of origin.
- CT will confirm renal origin and determine if bilateral.
- MRI is currently being evaluated to help distinguish nephrogenic rests from Wilms' tumor and its preferred method to follow children with bilateral Wilms' tumor after resection.
- Most common sites of metastasis spread are lung and liver, so CT chest is indicated.

Screening

- Screening for patient at risk of genetic syndrome such as BWS, IHH, WAGR, DDS, and Perlman syndrome.
- Renal US is a preferred modality for screening available, noninvasive, no radiation, and no sedation, and it's recommended to scan children every 3–4 months.

Staging

- In COG/NWTS protocol, initial surgical resection is recommended in most cases.
- Thus, for unilateral tumor, the pathology is established prior to chemotherapy or radiotherapy.
- SIOP protocol recommends neo-chemotherapy followed by nephrectomy and staging at that time.

COG Stages

Stage I	Criteria: tumor is limited to kidney and completely resected and no Bx and no penetration.
Stage II	Tumor extends beyond capsular but completely resected and penetration of renal capsule.
Stage III	Gross or microscopic residual tumor remains postoperative, spillage −ve LNs, +ve peritoneal cytology, rupture, or Bx before surgery.
Stage IV	LNs or hematogenous metastasis outside the abdomen.
Stage V	Bilaterally.

SIOP Stages

Stage I	Criteria: tumor is limited to kidney and surrounding capsule but no penetration.
Stage II	The tumor is penetrating outside the kidney but completely resected.
Stage III	Incomplete excision of tumor extended beyond resection margin.
Stage IV	LNs or hematogenous metastasis outside the abdomen.
Stage V	Bilaterally.

Treatment
- Success from multidisciplinary studies and cooperative group NWTSG, SIOP, UK CCSG.

Operative Therapy
- Surgical therapy is a primary component in the treatment of Wilms' tumor and other neoplastic renal lesion, either primary or post-neoadjuvant chemotherapy.

Neuroblastoma
- Most common solid tumors in infants and children.
- Originates from neural crest region.
- Arises in adrenal medulla and along the sympathetic ganglion chain from neck to pelvis.
- Incidence is 1 in 7,500 or 10,000.
- Neuroblastoma is responsible for 10% of childhood tumor.
- 15% of children will die.
- 700 cases are diagnosed annually in US.
- 40% are diagnosed by 1 year of age, 75% by 7 years of age, and 98% by 10 years.
- More than ½ are younger than 2 years at the time of diagnosis.
- ♂:♀ = 1–2:1.
- Most common intra-abdominal malignancy in newborn.
- Mother of infant with neuroblastoma experiences flushing HTN during pregnancy, resulting from catecholamines being released from fetal tumor in utero.

Clinical Presentation
- Multiple clinical manifestations related to the site of primary tumor and presence of metastasis.
- 50%–75% presented with abdominal mass.
- Tumor may be hard, nodular, fixed, and painful on palpation.
- Generalized symptoms: weight loss, failure to thrive, abdominal pain, distension, fever, and anemia.
- 25% will have HTN related to catecholamine.
- Hypercalcemia by sudden spontaneous rupture.
- Neoplasm arises from mediastinum, or neck may be involved in stellate ganglion and cause Horner syndrome (ptosis, miosis, anhidrosis, enophthalmos) and heterochromia of iris.

Diagnosis
- 24 hours urine for adrenaline, noradrenaline, dopamin, HVA, VMA.
- AXR (50%) shows fine stippled tumor calcification.
  - ➢ Displaced of the bowel gas by tumor.
- CXR shows posterior mediastinum.
  - ➢ Paraspinal widening.
- US to distinguish cystic from solid, evaluation for IVC obstruction or compression.
- CT: calcification (80%), used to localize lesion and extension.
- MRI for intraspinal tumor extension and also major vascular structure.
- MIBG: for soft tissue and bony disease.

Risk Stratification and Risk-Based Management
- Low risk: surgical resection is curative.
- Intermediate: surgery and chemotherapy.
- High risk: chemotherapy followed by surgery, radiotherapy to achieve local control, myeloablative treatment with bone marrow resource, and biological treatment.

Management
- Initial surgery for extensive stage III and IV should be limited to biopsy and placement of vascular access device.
- After four to five cycles of chemotherapy, second-look surgery is performed.
- Complete surgical resection for primary tumor is an essential component of treatment.
- During resection, there's a need for adequate IV access because the tumor is highly vascular and blood loss is high.
- Blood pressure must be carefully monitored intraoperatively to detect sudden HTN caused by excessive catecholamine released by tumor.
- Surgical approach depends on location of tumor.
- Upper abdominal incision or thoracoabdominal incision.
- Complete dissection of tumor and all regional LNs.
- Neuroblastoma usually adherent to great vessels.

- En bloc contiguous resection of normal surrounding structure such as spleen, stomach, pancreas, and colon almost always can be avoided.
- For locoregional disease that doesn't have MYCN amplification → surgical resection alone is all that's necessary.
- Patient with locoregional disease with poor prognostic biology are high risk and should be treated with chemotherapy.
- Currently: aggressive chemotherapy, followed by surgery and radiotherapy to achieve local control, then followed by myeloablative therapy and autologous stem cell TPx, 13-cis-retinoic acid + immunotherapy.
- Neuroblastoma is radiosensitive, so radiotherapy is an important part of the treatment.

2nd Branchial Anomalies

- Lie between lower anterior border of SCM muscle and tonsillar fossa of pharynx.
- May be is close to Glossopharyngeal nerve, hypoglossal nerve and carotid vessel.
- Cystic lesion common than fistula.
- Cyst present as non-tender soft mass beneath SCM.
- Change in size during URTI in up to 25%.
- The anomalies classified into 4 types.

Type I	Superficial, located deep to platysma along anterior border of SCM.
Type II	Most common and deep to SCM and either anterior or posterior to carotid sheath.
Type III	Pass between carotid bifurcations and lie adjacent to pharynx.
Type IV	Lesions are medial to carotid sheath in close to pharynx.

- Most common presentation:
- Infant and young children with drainage from small cutaneous pit along anterior border of lower SCM.
- Because risk of infection or malignancy → elective excision.
- Treatment with antibiotics ± aspiration or I & D if infection.
- When diagnosis unclear, need Bx to distinguish infected branchial - cleft and lymphadenitis.

- The goal is complete excision without injury to adjacent nerve and vascular structure.
- Transverse cervical skin incision.
- If sinus or fistula, the probe. Can use methylene blue to identify it.
- If tract is long → 2nd incision (stepladder).

1st Branchial Anomalies

- Rare and more common in ♀.
- Should distinguish from preauricular pits and sinuses.
- Remnant may persist anywhere between external auditory canal and submandibular area.
- Often lie in close association to parotid gland and facial nerve.
- Work classified 1st branchial anomaly into:
  → Type I rarer and considered duplication of membranous EAC.
  → Type II contains ectoderm and endoderm which may include cartilage.
- Pass medial to facial nerve and may present in preauricular, infra-auricular and post auricular location.
- Sinus may present with external drainage below the angle of mandible or otorrhea.
- Communication with EAC may be present.
- Complete surgical excision, Take care because proximity to facial nerve.
- Many authors recommended initial exposure of facial nerve and its branches with superficial parotidectomy to ↓ risk of facial nerve injury.
- Necessary to excise involved skin and cartilage of external auditory canal.

3rd and 4th Branchial Anomalies

- Very rare and almost always occur in the in the Lt. side of the neck.
- Mostly presented as sinus or infected cyst rather than fistula.
- Drain into piriform sinus and can combined with piriform sinus tract.
- Superior laryngeal nerve (SLN) represent the nerve of 4th branchial arch.
- 3rd pouch enter piriform sinus above SLN.
- 4th below this nerve.

- 3rd branchial cleft fistula extended from anterior border of SCM, traversing deep to internal carotid artery and glossopharyngeal nerve, piercing thyroid membrane above internal branch of SLN entering pharynx at piriform sinus.
- 4th branchial fistula would course around Rt subclavian artery or aortic arch on the left ascend back up over hypoglossal nerve and enter piriform apex or cervical esophagus.
- History of repeated URTI and sore throat, hoarseness pain and tender over thyroid gland give suspicion of piriform sinus tract.
    Infection may result in thyroiditis (suppurative).
- Any thyroid abscess → branchial remnant.
- Contrast esophagogram after resolution of acute infection can diagnose piriform sinus.
- Other image can visualize air within cyst such U/S, CT and MRI.
- Complete excision is mainstay of management.
- Direct laryngoscopy or rigid laryngoscopy is recommended for accurate diagnosis.
- Standard collar incision is used to identify RLN.
- Partial or ipsilateral thyroid lobectomy with excision of the tract usually required.
- Partial resection of thyroid cartilage may be necessary to remove entire tract.

Thoracic Surgery

Trachea
Anatomy
- The trachea is composed of cartilaginous and membranous portions, beginning with the cricoid cartilage.
- The vocal cords originate from the arytenoid cartilages and then attach to the thyroid cartilage.
- The subglottic space is the narrowest part of the trachea with an internal diameter of approximately 2 cm.
- The remainder of the distal trachea is 10–13 cm long, consists of eighteen to twenty-two rings, and has an internal diameter of 2.3 cm.
- The first tracheal ring is attached directly to the cricoid cartilage; there are approximately two rings for every 1 cm of tracheal length.
- Blood supply includes the inferior thyroid, subclavian, supreme intercostal, internal thoracic, innominate, and superior and middle bronchial arteries.

Tracheal Injury
- Tracheal injury can result from a variety of causes, including inhalation of smoke or toxic fumes, aspiration of liquids or solid objects, endotracheal intubation, blunt and penetrating trauma, and iatrogenic injury during operative procedures.
- Management of smoke or toxic fume inhalation and liquid aspiration is commonly supportive; use of antibiotics, respiratory support, and airway clearance with flexible bronchoscopy are dictated by the patient's condition.
- High cuff pressures can cause ischemia of the contiguous airway wall in as short as 4 hrs. Prolonged overinflation can lead to scarring and stenosis; full-thickness injury can result in fistulae between the innominate artery anteriorly and the esophagus posteriorly. Avoidance requires careful cuff management to keep pressures.

Tracheal Fistulas
Tracheoinnominate Artery Fistula
- Tracheoinnominate artery fistula has two main causes: low placement of a tracheostomy and hyperinflation of the tracheal cuff.
- Tracheostomy placement should be through the second to fourth trachea.
- Tracheal cuff, when hyperinflated, will cause ischemic injury to the anterior airway and subsequent erosion into the artery.
- Present with massive hemoptysis.
- The tracheostomy incision should be immediately opened widely and a finger inserted to compress the artery against the manubrium.
- Emergent surgical resection of the involved segment of artery is performed, usually without reconstruction.

Tracheoesophageal Fistula
- Either congenital or acquired in patients receiving prolonged mechanical ventilatory support concomitant with an indwelling nasogastric tube.
- Airway suctioning reveals saliva and gastric contents.
- Bronchoscopy is diagnostic, alternatively, esophagoscopy.
- Treatment: advance the ETT to ↓ aspiration, gastric decompression. Esophageal diversion can be performed, and once weaned for ventilator → resection and anastomosis.

Tracheal Neoplasms
- Rare. The most common primary tracheal neoplasms are squamous cell carcinomas (related to smoking) and adenoid cystic carcinomas (65%). The remaining 35% is comprised of small cell carcinomas, mucoepidermoid carcinomas, adenocarcinomas, lymphomas.
- The most common radiologic finding of tracheal malignancy is tracheal stenosis but is found in only 50% of cases.
- Stage of presentation is advanced, with approximately 50% of patients presenting with stage IV disease.
- Five-year survival for all tracheal neoplasms is 40% but falls to 15% for those with stage IV disease.

- Squamous cell carcinomas and adenoid cystic carcinomas represent approximately all tracheal neoplasms.
- Neck and chest CT, rigid bronchoscopy.
- If the tumor is judged to be completely resectable, primary resection and anastomosis are the treatments of choice for these tumors.
- Up to 50% of the length of the trachea can be resected with primary anastomosis.

Lungs

Segmental Anatomy

- Right lung is consist of three lobes branched to ten segments.
  - Upper lobe: (1) apical, (2) posterior, (3) anterior.
  - Middle lobe: (4) lateral, (5) medial.
  - Lower lobe: (6) superior, (7) medial basal, (8) anterior basal, (9) lateral basal, (10) posterior basal.
- Left lung is consist of two lobes branched to nine segments.
  - Upper lobe: (1) apical, (2) posterior, (3) anterior, (4) lateral, (5) medial = lingula.
  - Lower lobe: (6) superior, (7) anterior basal, (8) lateral basal, (9) posterior basal.
- Medial basal segment is not present in left lung.

Lymphatic Drainage

- Lymph nodes that drain the lungs are divided into two groups: the pulmonary lymph nodes (N1) and the mediastinal nodes (N2).
- N1: (a) intrapulmonary or segmental node, (b) lobar nodes, (c) interlobar nodes, (d) hilar nodes.
- N2: (a) anterior mediastinal nodes, (b) posterior mediastinal group, (c) tracheobronchial lymph nodes, (d) paratracheal lymph nodes.

Lung Histology

- The lung has two components: the tracheobronchial tree and the alveolar spaces.
- The tracheobronchial tree consists of approximately twenty-three airway divisions to the level of the alveoli.

- The tracheobronchial tree is normally lined by pseudostratified ciliated columnar cells and mucous (or goblet) cells.
- The bronchial submucosal glands can give rise to salivary gland–type tumors, including mucoepidermoid carcinomas and adenoid cystic carcinomas.
- Two cell types:
  - ➢ Type I pneumocytes (gas exchange) comprise 40% of the total number of alveolar epithelial cells but cover 95% of the surface area.
  - ➢ Type II pneumocytes (surfactant production) comprise 60% of the alveolar epithelial cells but cover only 3% of the alveolar surface area.
- In addition, clusters of neuroendocrine cells are seen in the alveolar spaces.

Preinvasive Lesions
1. Squamous dysplasia and carcinoma in situ and cigarette smoke can induce a transformation of the tracheobronchial pseudostratified epithelium to metaplastic squamous mucosa, with subsequent evolution to dysplasia.
2. Atypical adenomatous hyperplasia (AAH), similar to adenocarcinoma in situ, needs thin-section CT. It is possible to detect preinvasive adenocarcinoma lesions. These lesions can be multiple, are typically small (5 mm or less), and have a ground-glass appearance.
3. Diffuse idiopathic pulmonary neuroendocrine cell hyperplasia.

Invasive or Malignant Lesions
- Broadly divided into two main groups: non–small cell lung carcinoma and neuroendocrine tumors.

Non–Small Cell Lung Carcinoma
- Includes large cell, squamous cell, and adenocarcinoma.

- **Adenocarcinoma**
  - The incidence of adenocarcinoma has increased over the last several decades.

- It is now the most common lung cancer, accounting for 30% of lung cancers in male smokers and 40% of lung cancers in female smokers.
- It occurs more frequently in females than in males.
- Needs cytologic and small biopsy specimens and routine molecular testing for known mutations such as EGFR and K-RAS mutations.

Histological Subtypes
- Adenocarcinoma in situ (AIS)
    - Small ($\leq$ 3 cm) solitary adenocarcinomas that have pure lepidic growth.
    - Lepidic growth is characterized by tumor growth within the alveolar spaces.
    - 100% disease-specific survival with complete surgical resection.
    - CT scan, AIS can appear as a pure ground-glass neoplasm.

- Minimally invasive adenocarcinoma (MIA)
    - Less than 5 mm of invasion are noted within a predominantly lepidic growth pattern.
    - Nearly 100% survival when the lesion is completely resected.
    - The invasive component reaches 5 mm or greater in size.
    - The invasive component histologically is acinar, papillary, micropapillary, and/or solid.
    - On CT scan, solid nodule ($\leq$ 5 mm) with a predominant ground-glass component.

- Lepidic predominant adenocarcinoma (LPA)
    - If lymphovascular invasion, pleural invasion, tumor necrosis, or more than 5 mm of invasion, MIA is excluded and the lesion is called lepidic predominant adenocarcinoma.

- Invasive adenocarcinoma
    - Subtypes include the following:

      a. Lepidic predominant
      b. Acinar predominant
      c. Papillary predominant
      d. Micropapillary predominant
      e. Solid predominant

- Often peripherally located and frequently discovered incidentally on CXR.
- Unlike squamous cell cancers, when symptoms occur, they are due to pleural or chest wall invasion (pleuritic or chest wall pain).
- CT scan, a lobar ground-glass opacification may be present.
- Bubble-like or cystic (≤ 2 cm) adenocarcinomas or extensive associated ground-glass components correlate with slow growth and well-differentiated tumors and a more favorable prognosis.
- Pleural retraction is a poor prognostic indicator.
- Additional histologic variants include colloid adenocarcinoma, fetal adenocarcinoma, and enteric adenocarcinoma.

- **Squamous Cell Carcinoma**
  - Representing 30% to 40% of lung cancers, squamous cell carcinoma is the most frequent cancer in men and highly correlated with cigarette smoking.
  - They arise primarily in the main, lobar, or first segmental bronchi referred to as the central airways.
  - Symptoms of airway irritation or obstruction are common and include cough, hemoptysis, wheezing, dyspnea, and pneumonia.
  - Central necrosis is frequent and may lead to the radiographic findings.

- **Large Cell Carcinoma**
  - Large cell carcinoma accounts for 10% to 20% of lung cancers.
  - May be located centrally or peripherally.
  - Can be differentiated by special immunohistochemical stains.

- **Salivary Gland–Type Neoplasms**
  - Histologically identical to those seen in the salivary glands.
  - The two most common are adenoid cystic carcinoma and mucoepidermoid carcinoma.

Neuroendocrine carcinoma (NEC)

- Immunohistochemical staining for neuroendocrine markers (including chromogranins, synaptophysin, CD57, and neuron-specific enolase) is essential to accurately diagnose most tumors.
- Neuroendocrine lung tumors are classified into the following:

- **Grade I NEC (classic or typical carcinoid)**
  - A low-grade NEC; 80% arise in the epithelium of the central airways.
  - It occurs primarily in younger patients.
  - Because of the central location, it classically presents with hemoptysis, with or without airway obstruction and pneumonia.
  - Can lead to life-threatening hemorrhage with even simple bronchoscopic biopsy maneuvers. Regional lymph node metastases, 15%.

- **Grade II NEC**
  - Atypical carcinoid has a much higher malignant potential.
  - Etiologically linked to cigarette smoking.
  - More likely to be peripherally located.
  - Histologic findings may include areas of necrosis, nuclear pleomorphism, and higher mitotic rates.
  - Lymph node metastases are found in 30% to 50% of patients.
  - At diagnosis, 25% of patients already have remote metastases.

- **Grade III NEC**
  - Large cell–type tumors occur primarily in heavy smokers, in the mid to peripheral lung fields. They are often large with central necrosis and a high mitotic rate.

- **Grade IV NEC (small cell lung carcinoma [SCLC])**
  - The most malignant NEC and accounts for 25% of all lung cancers.
  - These NECs often have early widespread metastases.
  - Primarily in the central airways.
  - Symptoms include cough, hemoptysis, wheezing, dyspnea, and pneumonia.
  - Three groups of grade IV NEC are recognized: pure small cell carcinoma (sometimes referred to as oat cell carcinoma), small cell carcinoma with a large cell component, and combined (mixed) tumors.
  - Consists of smaller cells (diameter 10–20 μm) with little cytoplasm and very dark nuclei.
  - These tumors are the leading producer of paraneoplastic syndromes.
  - Pancoast tumor invades apex of chest wall, and patient has Horner syndrome (invasion of sympathetic chain → ptosis, miosis, anhidrosis).

Lung Cancer Management

- Establishing a clear histologic diagnosis early in the evaluation and management of lung cancer is critical to effective treatment.
- Differentiation between adenocarcinoma and squamous cell carcinoma is crucial in patients with advanced stage disease, as treatment with chemotherapy.
- Life-threatening hemorrhage has occurred in patients with squamous cell carcinoma who were treated with bevacizumab.
- EGFR mutation predicts response to EGFR tumor kinase inhibitors and is now recommended as first-line therapy in advanced adenocarcinoma.

Patient Evaluation

- Evaluation prior to treatment encompasses three areas: diagnosis and assessment of the primary tumor, assessment for metastatic disease, and determination of functional status.

Assessment of the Primary Tumor

- Assessment of the primary tumor begins with the history and directed questions regarding the presence or absence of pulmonary, nonpulmonary, thoracic, and paraneoplastic symptoms.
- CXR or CT scan.
- Recommendations for treatment and options for obtaining tissue diagnosis require a thorough understanding and assessment of CT findings.
- Overall, MRI of pulmonary lesions and mediastinal nodes offers no real improvement over CT scanning.

Options for Tissue Acquisition

1. Brushings and washings for cytology
2. Direct forceps biopsy of a visualized lesion
3. Endobronchial ultrasound-guided FNA
4. Transbronchial biopsy
5. Electromagnetic navigation bronchoscopy

Assessment for Metastatic Disease

- Distant metastases are found in approximately 40% of patients with newly diagnosed lung cancer.
- History and physical examination focusing on the presence or absence of new bone pain, neurologic symptoms, new skin lesions, and constitutional symptoms (e.g., anorexia, malaise, and unintentional weight loss of > 5% of body weight).
- The skin should be thoroughly examined.
- Routine laboratory studies include U&E, LFT.
- CT scan, up to 30% of such nodes are enlarged from noncancerous reactive causes such as inflammation due to atelectasis or pneumonia secondary to the tumor.
- No patient should be denied an attempt at curative resection just because of a positive CT.
- Mediastinal lymph node staging by PET scanning appears to have greater accuracy than CT.
- Endoscopic ultrasound (EUS) can accurately visualize mediastinal paratracheal lymph nodes.

- Cervical mediastinoscopy provides tissue sampling of all paratracheal and subcarinal lymph.
- Some surgeons perform mediastinoscopy in all lung cancer patients because of the poor survival associated with surgical resection of N2 disease.
- Pleural effusion associated with a peripheral-based tumor, particularly one that abuts the visceral or parietal pleural surface, does have a higher probability of being malignant, which would alter the pathologic stage of the disease to stage IV (AJCC).
- Bone scans.
- Liver abnormalities that are not clearly simple cysts or hemangiomas and adrenal enlargement, nodules, or masses are further evaluated by MRI scanning and, occasionally, by needle biopsy.

Tumor, Node, and Metastasis—Lung Cancer Staging
- Typically classified into a clinical stage and a pathologic stage.
- Clinical staging information includes the history and physical examination, radiographic test results, and diagnostic biopsy information.
- pTNM is determined, providing further prognostic information.

Assessment of Functional Status
- Patients with potentially resectable tumors require careful assessment of their functional status and ability to tolerate either lobectomy or pneumonectomy.

Lung Cancer Treatment

Grade IV NEC (Small Cell Lung Carcinoma)
- Lobectomy followed by chemotherapy is warranted after surgical mediastinal staging has confirmed the absence of N2 disease.

Early-Stage Non–Small Cell Lung Cancer
- Early-stage disease includes T1 and T2 tumors (with or without N1) and T3 tumors (without N1 nodal involvement).

- Surgical resection depending on tumor size and location, lobectomy, sleeve lobectomy, and occasionally, pneumonectomy, with mediastinal lymph node dissection or sampling, are appropriate for patients with clinical early-stage disease.

Management of Early-Stage Lung Cancer in High-Risk Patient

- Lobectomy may not be an option for some patients with early-stage disease due to poor cardiopulmonary function or other comorbid illnesses.
- Limited resection, defined as segmentectomy or wedge resection, is a viable option for achieving local control in high-risk patients.
- Rationale for chemotherapy in the management of early-stage NSCLC: the role of chemotherapy in early-stage (stage I and II) NSCLC is evolving, with several prospective phase II studies having shown a potential benefit. It is recommended that chemotherapy be considered in high-risk patients (larger tumors, R1).

Evaluation and Management of Locally Advanced NSCL

- Five-year relative survival in patients with locoregional disease is 25%.
- Stage III disease includes patients with small tumors that have metastasized to the mediastinal lymph nodes as well as large tumors invading unresectable structures.
- Patients with clinically evident N2 have a 5-year survival rate of 5% to 10% with surgery alone.
- Number of involved N2 nodal stations in determining whether to proceed with resection following induction therapy.

Surgery in T4 and Stage IV Disease

- Surgery generally does not have a role in the care of patients with any tumor with N3 disease or T4 tumors with N2 disease. Survival rates remain extremely low for these patients.
- The treatment of patients with stage IV disease is chemotherapy.

Neoadjuvant Chemotherapy for NSCLC

- The use of chemotherapy before anatomic surgical resection has a number of potential advantages:
    1. The tumor's blood supply is still intact, allowing better chemotherapy delivery and avoiding tumor cell hypoxia.
    2. The primary tumor may be downstaged, enhancing resectability.
    3. Patients are better able to tolerate chemotherapy before surgery and are more likely to complete the prescribed regimen than after surgery.
    4. Response to chemotherapy can be monitored and used to guide decisions about additional therapy.
    5. Systemic micrometastases are treated.
    6. It identifies patients with progressive disease/ nonresponders and spares them a pulmonary resection.
- The treatment is generally safe, as it does not cause a significant increase in perioperative morbidity.
- Two randomized trials have now compared surgery alone for patients with N2 disease to preoperative chemotherapy followed by surgery.
- Both trials were stopped before complete accrual because of a significant increase in survival for the chemotherapy arm.

Postoperative (Adjuvant) Chemotherapy for NSCLC

- Any patient with nodal metastasis (N1 or N2) or with T3 tumors (defined as tumors > 7 cm, invading chest wall, diaphragm, phrenic nerve, mediastinal pleura, parietal pericardium, or main bronchus tumor < 2 cm distal to the carina, should receive adjuvant chemotherapy.

Options for Thoracic Surgical Approaches

- Video-assisted thoracoscopic surgery (VATS) has become the recommended approach to diagnosis and treatment of pleural effusions, recurrent pneumothoraxes, lung biopsies, lobectomy or segmental resection, resection of bronchogenic and mediastinal cysts, and intrathoracic esophageal mobilization for esophagectomy.
- Open approaches to thoracic surgery. When video-assisted thoracoscopic approach is not possible, an open approach, most

frequently the posterolateral thoracotomy, is used to gain access to the intrathoracic space.

Postoperative Care
- Chest tube management.
- At the conclusion of most thoracic operations, the pleural cavity is drained with a chest tube(s).
- Pain control.

Respiratory Care
- The best respiratory care is achieved when the patient is able to deliver an effective cough to clear secretions.
- Proper pain control.

Pulmonary Infections
Lung Abscess
- Parenchymal necrosis caused by an infectious organism, tissue destruction results in a solitary or dominant cavity measuring at least 2 cm in diameter.
- Lung abscesses are further classified as primary or secondary.
- A primary lung abscess occurs, for example, in immunocompromised patients as a result of highly virulent organisms inciting a necrotizing pulmonary infection or aspirate oropharyngeal or gastrointestinal secretions.
- A secondary lung abscess occurs in patients with underlying conditions such as partial bronchial obstruction, lung infarct, or adjacent suppurative infections.
- Normal oropharyngeal secretions containing many more streptococcus species and more anaerobes than pneumonia, which follows from aspiration, is typically polymicrobial.

Clinical Features and Diagnosis
- The typical presentation may include productive cough, fever (> 38.9°C), chills, leukocytosis, weight loss, fatigue, malaise, pleuritic chest pain, and dyspnea.
- The CXR is the primary tool for diagnosing a lung.
- CT scan of the chest clarifies the diagnosis when CXR is equivocal.

- DDx also includes loculated or interlobar empyema, infected lung cysts or bullae, tuberculosis, bronchiectasis, fungal infections.

Management of Lung Abscess

- Systemic antibiotics directed against the causative organism represent the mainstay of therapy. The duration of antimicrobial therapy varies from 3 to 12 weeks for necrotizing pneumonia and lung abscess.
- Oral therapy can then be used to complete the course of therapy.
- Surgical drainage of lung abscesses is uncommon since drainage usually occurs spontaneously via the tracheobronchial tree.
- External drainage may be accomplished with tube thoracostomy, percutaneous drainage.

Bronchiectasis

- Bronchiectasis is defined as a pathologic and permanent dilation of bronchi with bronchial wall thickening.
- May be localized to certain bronchial segments, or it may be diffused throughout the bronchial tree, affecting the medium-sized airways.

Pathogenesis

- Development of bronchiectasis can be attributed to either congenital or acquired causes.
- Congenital diseases that lead to bronchiectasis include cystic fibrosis, primary ciliary dyskinesia.
- Acquired causes are categorized broadly as infectious and inflammatory.

Clinical Manifestations and Diagnosis

- Typical symptoms are daily persistent cough and purulent sputum production. The quantity of daily sputum production (10 mL to > 150 mL) correlates with disease extent and severity.
- Diagnosis by CXR or CT.

Management of Bronchiectasis
- Standard therapy includes optimizing airway clearance, use of bronchodilators to reverse any airflow limitation, and correction of reversible underlying cause, chest physiotherapy.
- Acute exacerbations should be treated with a 2- to 3-week course of broad-spectrum intravenous antibiotics tailored to culture and sensitivity profiles
- Surgical resection of a localized bronchiectatic segment or lobe, preserving as much functional lung as possible, may benefit patients with refractory symptoms.

Massive Hemoptysis
- Massive hemoptysis is generally defined as expectoration of over 600 mL of blood within a 24-hr period.
- It is a medical emergency associated with a mortality rate of 30% to 50%.
- Anatomy: the lungs have two sources of blood supply—the pulmonary and bronchial arterial systems.
- Most cases of massive hemoptysis involve bleeding from the bronchial artery.
- In many cases of hemoptysis, particularly due to inflammatory disorders.
- Causes: pulmonary, extrapulmonary, and iatrogenic causes.
- Most are secondary to inflammatory processes, aneurysms of the pulmonary artery (referred to as Rasmussen's aneurysm).

Management
- Life-threatening hemoptysis is best managed by a multidisciplinary team of intensive care physicians, interventional radiologists, and thoracic surgeons.
- Treatment priorities begin with respiratory stabilization; intubation with isolation of the bleeding lung may be required to prevent asphyxiation.
- This can be done with mainstem intubation into the nonbleeding lung.
- Surgical intervention: in most patients, bleeding can be stopped, recovery can occur, and plans to definitively treat the underlying cause can be made.

- Surgical treatment is individualized according to the source of bleeding and the patient's medical condition, prognosis, and pulmonary reserve.
- General indications for urgent surgery are in patients with significant cavitary disease or with fungus balls and the walls of the cavities eroded and necrotic; rebreeding will likely ensue.

Chest Wall
Chest Wall Mass
1. Plasmacytoma.
2. Osteosarcoma: alkaline phosphatase levels may be elevated.
3. Ewing's sarcoma: erythrocyte sedimentation rates may be elevated.

- Radiography. CXR may reveal rib destruction, calcification within the lesion.
- CT and MRI provides multiple planes of imaging (coronal, sagittal, and oblique) and better definition of the relationship between tumor and muscle and tumor and contiguous or nearby neurovascular structures.
- Biopsy: the first step in the management of all chest wall tumors is to obtain a tissue diagnosis.
    1. Needle biopsy
    2. Incisional biopsy
    3. Excisional biopsy

Benign Chest Wall Neoplasms
1. Chondroma fibrous dysplasia
2. Osteochondroma
3. Eosinophilic granuloma
4. Desmoid tumors

Other Tumors of the Chest Wall
1. Primitive neuroectodermal tumors (PNETs) and Ewing's sarcoma
2. Plasmacytoma

Mediastinum
- Superior, anterior, middle, and posterior mediastinum.

- Content of superior mediastinum
  - Muscles: origins of the sternohyoid and sternothyroid.
  - Arteries: aortic arch, brachiocephalic artery, left common carotid, and the left subclavian artery.
  - Veins: brachiocephalic veins and upper half of the superior vena cava.
  - Nerves: vagus nerve, phrenic nerve, recurrent laryngeal nerve.
  - Trachea: with paratracheal and tracheobronchial lymph nodes.
  - Esophagus.
  - Thoracic duct.
  - Thymus.
  - From the content, you can predict the DDx of the swelling, e.g., artery → aneurysm, nerve → schwannomas, esophagus → CA, etc.

- Anterior (thymus)
  - Most common site for mediastinal tumor, *T*s:
  - Thymoma (most common anterior mediastinal mass in adults)
  - Thyroid CA and goiters
  - T cell lymphoma
  - Teratoma (and other germ cell tumors)
  - Parathyroid adenomas

- Middle (heart, trachea, ascending aorta)
  - Bronchogenic cysts
  - Pericardial cysts
  - Enteric cysts
  - Lymphoma

- Posterior (esophagus, descending aorta)
  - Enteric cysts
  - Neurogenic tumors
  - Lymphoma thymoma

Thymoma

- All thymomas require resection.
- Thymus is too big or associated with refractory myasthenia gravis → resection.
- 50% of thymomas are malignant.
- 50% of patients with thymomas have symptoms.
- 50% of patients with thymomas have myasthenia gravis.
- 10% of patients with myasthenia gravis have thymomas.

Myasthenia Gravis

- Fatigue, weakness, diplopia, ptosis, antibodies to acetylcholine receptor.
- Tx: anticholinesterase inhibitors (neostigmine), steroids, plasmapheresis.
- 80% get improvement with thymectomy, including patients who do not have thymoma.

Vascular Surgery

Noninvasive Diagnostic Evaluation of the Vascular Patient
- Ankle-Brachial Index
    - ABI is used to evaluate patients at risk for cardiovascular events.
    - ABI less than 0.9 correlates with increased risk of myocardial infarction and indicates significant underlying peripheral vascular disease.
    - Normally, it is more than 1.
    - Patients with claudication typically have an ABI less than 0.5 to 0.7 range.
    - Those with rest pain are in the 0.3 to 0.5 range.
    - Alternative tests include toe-brachial pressures, pulse volume recordings, duplex ultrasound.
- Segmental Limb Pressures
- Pulse Volume Recording
- Radiologic Evaluation of the Vascular Patient
- Ultrasound
    - Requires experienced technicians and may not visualize all arterial segments.
- Computed Tomography Angiography
    - CTA is a noninvasive, contrast-dependent method for imaging the arterial system.
- Magnetic Resonance Angiography
    - MRA has the advantage of not requiring iodinated contrast agents to provide vessel opacification. Gadolinium is used as a contrast agent for MRA studies.
- Diagnostic Angiography
    - Diagnostic angiography is considered the gold standard in vascular imaging.

Basic Principles of Endovascular Therapy
- Needles and Access
    - o Needles are used to achieve percutaneous vascular access.
- Guidewires
    - o Guidewires are used to introduce, position, and exchange catheters.

- Hemostatic Sheaths
  o The hemostatic sheath is a device through which endovascular procedures are performed.
- Catheters
- Angioplasty Balloons
- Stents
  o Vascular stents are commonly used after an inadequate angioplasty with dissection or elastic recoil of an arterial stenosis.
- Stent Grafts
  o The combination of a metal stent covered with fabric gave birth to the first stent grafts. Covered stents have been designed with either a surrounding PTFE or polyester fabric.

Carotid Artery Disease
- Atherosclerotic occlusive plaque is by far the most common pathology seen in the carotid artery bifurcation.
- 30%–60% of all ischemic strokes are related to carotid atherosclerotic bifurcation occlusive disease.

Epidemiology and Etiology of Carotid Occlusive Disease
- TIA is defined as a temporary focal cerebral or retinal hypoperfusion state that resolves spontaneously.
- Longer-lasting neurologic deficits more likely represent a stroke.
- The severity of stenosis is commonly divided into three categories:
  mild (< 50%), moderate (50%–69%), and severe (70%–99%).
- Severe carotid stenosis is a strong predictor for stroke.

Clinical Manifestations of Cerebral Ischemia
- TIA is a focal loss of neurologic function, lasting for less than 24 hrs.

Diagnostic Evaluation
- Duplex ultrasonography is the most widely used screening tool to evaluate for atherosclerotic plaque and stenosis.
- MRA is increasingly being used.

- The advantage of CTA over MRA includes faster grading of carotid stenosis.

Treatment of Carotid Occlusive Disease
- Currently, neurologists prescribe both aspirin and clopidogrel for secondary stroke prevention.
- Medical therapy alone is inferior to surgical endarterectomy in stroke prevention for severe carotid stenosis.
- Carotid endarterectomy.
- Angioplasty and stenting.
- Surgical techniques of carotid endarterectomy.

Nonatherosclerotic Disease of the Carotid Artery
- Carotid coil and kink
- Fibromuscular dysplasia
- Carotid artery dissection
- Carotid artery aneurysms
- Carotid body tumor
- Carotid trauma

Aortoiliac Occlusive Disease
Diagnostic Evaluation
- Have weakened femoral pulses and a reduced ABI.
- Verification of iliac occlusive disease is usually made by color-flow duplex scanning.
- Pulse volume recordings (PVRs) of the lower extremity with estimation of the thigh-brachial pressure index.
- MRA and multidetector CTA are increasingly being used to determine the extent and type of obstruction.

Differential Diagnosis
- Degenerative hip or spine disease, lumbar disk herniation, spinal stenosis, diabetic neuropathy, and other neuromuscular problems.

Collateral Arterial Network
a. SMA to the distal IMA via its superior hemorrhoidal branch to the middle and inferior hemorrhoidal artery to the internal iliac artery (39%)

b. The lumbar arteries to the superior gluteal artery to the internal iliac system (37%)

c. The lumbar arteries to the lateral and deep circumflex arteries to the CFA (12%)

d. Winslow's pathway from the subclavian to the superior epigastric artery to the inferior epigastric artery to the external iliac arteries at the groin

Disease Classification

-   Based on the atherosclerotic disease pattern, aortoiliac occlusive disease can be classified into three types:

Type I

-   Aortoiliac disease, which occurs in 5% to 10% of patients, is confined to the distal abdominal aorta and common iliac vessels.
-   Symptom typically consists of bilateral thigh or buttock claudication and fatigue.
-   Men report diminished penile erection and may have complete loss of erectile function.
-   In the absence of femoral pulses, constitute Leriche syndrome.
-   Rest pain is unusual unless distal disease coexists.
-   Occasionally, patients report a prolonged history of thigh and buttock claudication.

Type II

-   Aortoiliac disease represents a more diffused atherosclerotic progression that involves abdominal aorta with disease extension into the common iliac artery.
-   This disease pattern affects approximately 25% of patients with aortoiliac occlusive disease.

Type III

-   Aortoiliac occlusive disease, which affects approximately 65% of patients.
-   Patients with "multilevel" disease are older, more commonly male, diabetic, and hypertensive, with

associated atherosclerotic disease involving cerebral, coronary, and visceral arteries.

- The most commonly used classification system of iliac lesions has been set forth by the Trans-Atlantic Inter-Society Consensus (TASC) group with recommended treatment options.
- According to this consensus document:
    - Endovascular therapy is the treatment of choice for type A lesions.
    - Surgery is the treatment of choice for type D lesions.
    - Endovascular treatment is the preferred treatment for type B lesions.
    - Surgery is the preferred treatment for good-risk patients with type C lesions.

Surgical Reconstruction of Aortoiliac Occlusive Disease
- Aortobifemoral bypass
- Aortic endarterectomy
- Axillofemoral bypass
- Iliofemoral bypass
- Femorofemoral bypass
- Obturator bypass
- Thoracofemoral Bypass

Complications of Surgical Aortoiliac Reconstruction
- Acute limb ischemia occurring after aortoiliac surgery may be the result of acute thrombosis or distal thromboembolism.
- The surgeon can prevent thromboembolic events by
    a. avoiding excessive manipulation of the aorta,
    b. ensuring adequate systemic heparinization,
    c. judicious placement of vascular clamps,
    d. thorough flushing prior to restoring blood flow.
- Intestinal ischemia following aortic reconstruction occurs in approximately 2% of cases; 0 infection following aortoiliac reconstruction is a devastating complication that occurs in 1% of cases.
- Aortoenteric fistula formation.

Endovascular Treatment for Iliac Artery Disease
Percutaneous Transluminal Angioplasty
- PTA is most useful in the treatment of isolated iliac stenosis of less than 4 cm in length.
- 2-year patency of 86% can be achieved.
- The complication rate is approximately 2%, consisting of distal embolization, medial dissection, and acute thrombosis.

Stenting in Iliac Arteries

Stent Graft Placement for Aortoiliac Interventions

Lower Extremity Arterial Occlusive Disease
- The symptoms of lower extremity occlusive disease are classified into two large categories:
  - Acute limb ischemia (ALI)
  - Chronic limb ischemia (CLI)
- 90% of acute ischemia cases are either thrombotic or embolic.
- Frequently, sudden onset of limb-threatening ischemia may be the result of acute exacerbation of the preexisting atherosclerotic disease.
- Chronic ischemia is largely due to atherosclerotic changes of the lower extremity that manifest from asymptomatic to limb-threatening gangrene.

Diagnostic Evaluation
- Physical examination and confirmed by the imaging studies.
- A well-performed physical examination often reveals the site of lesions by detecting changes in pulses, temperature, and appearances.
- ABI:
  - Noninvasive studies such as Doppler ultrasound, MRA, and CTA.
  - Contrast angiography remains the gold standard for imaging study.

Lower Extremity Occlusive Disease Classification
- Fontaine classification uses four stages:
    - Fontaine I: patients are asymptomatic.
    - Fontaine II: they have mild claudication (IIa), severe claudication (IIb).
    - Fontaine III: they have ischemic rest pain.
    - Fontaine IV: patients suffer tissue loss, such as ulceration or gangrene.
- The TASC taskforce published a guideline separating lower extremity arterial diseases into four types:
    - Type A: lesions are single focal lesions < 3 cm in length.
    - Type B: lesions are single lesions of 3–5 cm in length.
    - Type C: lesions are multiple stenosis or occlusions > 15 cm in length.
    - Type D: lesions are those with complete occlusion of CFA, SFA, or popliteal artery.

Etiology of Acute Limb Ischemia (ALI)
- ALI is defined as sudden loss of limb perfusion.
- The most common etiologies of ALI include embolism, native vessel thrombosis, reconstruction thrombosis, trauma, and complications of peripheral aneurysm.
- Most cases of lower extremity ALI are the result of thrombosis of a prosthetic conduit.
- Symptoms: abrupt pain and loss of sensory or motor function.

Arterial Embolism
- The heart is the most common source of distal emboli; atrial fibrillation is the most common source.

Arterial Thrombosis
- Often has an underlying atherosclerotic lesion at the site of thrombosis or aneurysmal degeneration with mural thrombosis.

Clinical Manifestations of Acute Limb Ischemia
- Five *P*s: pain, pallor, paresthesias, paralysis, and pulselessness, to which some add a sixth *P*, perishing cold.

- Pain is the usual symptom that causes a patient to present to the emergency room.
- Typically, a patient will complain of foot and calf pain. Pulses are absent, and there may be diminution of sensation.
- Inability to move the affected muscle group is a sign of very severe ischemia and necessitates urgent revascularization.
- Arteriography, if it can be performed in a timely fashion, is an excellent modality for localizing obstructions and deciding which type of intervention (endovascular, embolectomy, or bypass).

Treatment Considerations for Acute Limb Ischemia
- Medical treatment (heparin, Plavix, aspirin)
- Endovascular treatment
- Surgical treatment

Embolectomy
- The groin is opened through a vertical incision, exposing the CFA and its bifurcation.
- The artery is clamped and opened transversely over the bifurcation.
- Thrombus is extracted by passing a Fogarty balloon embolectomy catheter.
- Good back-bleeding and antegrade bleeding suggest that the entire clot has been removed.

Bypass Graft Thrombectomy
- Likely to succeed with prosthetic bypasses.

Complications Related to Treatment for Acute Limb Ischemia
- Hemorrhagic stroke from a thrombolysis procedure has been reported to be 1% to 2.3%, with 50% of hemorrhagic complications occurring during the thrombolytic procedure.
- Intracranial hemorrhage.
- Reperfusion injury to the ischemic.
- Compartment syndrome occurs after prolonged ischemia is followed by reperfusion.

Clinical Manifestations of Chronic Limb Ischemia

- Symptoms include claudication or rest pain, tissue and hair loss, ulceration, or gangrene.
- The diagnosis is made with noninvasive diagnostic tests such as the ABI, toe pressures, and transcutaneous oxygen measurements.
- One of the most common site for occlusive disease is in the distal SFA.
- Cramping pain develops in the calf on ambulation, occurs at a reproducible distance, and is relieved by rest weather. It is important to evaluate whether the symptoms are progressive or static. In greater than 70% of patients, the disease is stable, particularly with risk factor modification.
- Progression of the underlying atherosclerotic process is more likely to occur in patients with diabetes, those who continue to smoke, and those who fail to modify their atherosclerotic risk factors.

Treatment Considerations for Chronic Limb Ischemia

- Endovascular treatment
- Percutaneous transluminal balloon angioplasty
- Subintimal angioplasty
- Stent placement
- Stent graft
- Atherectomy
- Laser atherectomy

Surgical Treatment for Chronic Limb Ischemia Due to Femoropopliteal Disease

- Endarterectomy
- Bypass grafting
- Amputation

Nonatherosclerotic Disorders of Blood Vessels
Giant Cell Arteritis (Temporal Arteritis)

- A systemic chronic inflammatory vascular disease.
- Patients tend to be white women over the age of 50 years, with a high incidence in Scandinavia and women of Northern European descent.

- Genetic factors may play a role in disease having been identified.
- Symptoms: headache, fever, malaise, and myalgias.
- Complications may occur, such as visual alterations, including blindness and mural weakness, resulting in acute aortic dissection that may be devastating.
- The diagnostic gold standard is temporal artery biopsy.
- Treatment regimens are centered on corticosteroids.

Takayasu's Arteritis

- Chronic inflammatory arteritis affects large vessels, predominantly the aorta and its main branches.
- Chronic vessel inflammation leads to wall thickening, fibrosis, stenosis, and thrombus formation.
- Symptoms are related to end-organ ischemia, fever, anorexia, weight loss, general malaise, arthralgias, and malnutrition.
- Laboratory: ESR, CRP, WBCs.
- The gold standard for diagnosis remains angiography, showing narrowing or occlusion of the entire aorta or its primary branches.
- Surgical treatment is performed only in advanced stages, and bypass needs to be delayed during active phases of inflammation.
- There is no role for endarterectomy, and synthetic or autogenous bypass grafts need to be placed onto disease-free segments of vessels.
- For focal lesions, there have been reports of success with angioplasty.

Behçet's Disease

- Rare syndrome characterized by oral and genital ulcerations and ocular inflammation, affecting males found, indicating a genetic component to the etiology.
- Vascular involvement is seen in 7% to 38% of patients and is localized to the abdominal aorta, femoral artery, and pulmonary artery.
- Vascular lesions may also include venous complications such as DVT or superficial thrombophlebitis.

- Arterial aneurysmal degeneration can occur; however, this is an uncommon, albeit a potentially devastating complication. Multiple true aneurysms and pseudoaneurysms may develop, and rupture of an aortic aneurysm is the major cause of death.

Raynaud's Syndrome

- A heterogeneous symptom array associated with peripheral vasospasm, more commonly occurring in the upper extremities.
- Intermittent vasospasm classically follows exposure to various stimuli, including cold temperatures, tobacco, or emotional stress.
- Characteristic color changes occur in response to the arteriolar vasospasm, ranging from intense pallor to cyanosis to redness as the vasospasm occurs.
- The digital vessels then relax, eventually leading to reactive hyperemia.
- The majority of patients are young women less than 40 years of age.
- Using vibrating tools may be more predisposed to Raynaud's syndrome.
- Angiography is usually reserved for those who have digital ulceration.
- The majority (90%) of patients will respond to avoidance of cold and other stimuli.
- The remaining 10% of patients with more persistent or severe syndromes can be treated with a variety of vasodilatory drugs.
- Calcium channel–blocking nifedipine is the drug of choice.
- Surgical therapy is limited to debridement of digital ulcerations and amputation of gangrenous digits.

Buerger's Disease (Thromboangiitis Obliterans)

- A progressive nonatherosclerotic segmental inflammatory disease.
- Most often affects small- and medium-sized arteries, veins, and nerves of the upper and lower extremities.
- The typical age range for occurrence is 20 to 50 years.
- More frequently found in males and heavy smokers.

- The cause of thromboangiitis obliterans is unknown; however, use of or exposure to tobacco is essential to both the diagnosis and progression of the disease.
- Pathologically, thrombosis occurs in small- to medium-sized arteries and veins with associated dense PMN aggregation, microabscesses, and multinucleated giant cells.
- Progression of the disease leads to calf claudication and eventually ischemic rest pain and ulcerations on the toes, feet, or fingers. A complete history should exclude diabetes, hyperlipidemia, or autoimmune.
- The occlusions are segmental and show "skip" lesions with extensive collateralization, the so-called corkscrew collaterals.
- Treatment of thromboangiitis obliterans revolves around strict smoking cessation.
- The role of surgical intervention is minimal in Buerger's disease.

Diabetic Foot
- 1:4 develop foot complication in their lifetime.
- Risk factors:
  - ➤ Poor glycemic control
  - ➤ Impaired immune function
  - ➤ Peripheral neuropathy
  - ➤ Vascular insufficiency
- 50% will develop sensory neuropathy → enables detection of traumatic insult because of blunted pain and thermal receptor (proprioception).
- Motor neuropathy is promoted by unrecognized deformities in plantar surface of the foot.
- Autonomic nervous system disruption → natural protecting function of sweat gland → entry of bacteria.
- Hyperglycemia → α neutrophil + poor perfusion of small vessels (endothelial cells dysfunction) → pro-inflammatory cascade.

Microbiology
- Acute: staph, strep.
- Chronic: gram −ve + anerobic.
  - → Initial empiric antibiotic while C/S result.

Clinical Picture
- Minor abrasion to extensive soft tissue destructions underlying muscle and bone.
- Can manifest local and systemic inflammation.
- Sensory neuropathy ↓ pain.
- Charcot arthropathy in which chronic neuropathy leads to joint degeneration.

Diagnosis
1. Determine extent of involvement grossly and by x-ray.
2. Appreciate risk factor.
3. Identify causative organism.

- Debridement of all necrotic tissue.
- Open all sinus.
- ABI to see arterial insufficiency → usually > 1.3.
- Osteomyelitis is suspected when ulcer > 2 cm² or deep > 3 m or sausage toe.
- ESR is high, 70 mL/hr.

Treatment
- Multidisciplinary
    1. Nutritionist: meal with low sugar.
    2. Internist: optimize medication to target HbA1C between 6.5–7.5.
    3. Vascular surgeon: assess vascularity and correct vascular disease.
    4. Physiotherapy.
    5. Occupational therapy for orthotic, cast, boot, protrusion.
    6. Surgeon: debridement of soft tissue ulcer and gangrene of toes merged with amputation with or without extension to head of metatarsal.
    7. If multiple toes → transmetatarsal.
- Restoration of perfusion by revascularization of tibial or pedal artery.
- VAC assists in closure of the open wound.

Thoracic Aortic Aneurysms

- Aortic aneurysms can be either "true" or "false."
- True aneurysms can take two forms: fusiform (common) and saccular.
- False aneurysms, also called pseudoaneurysms, are leaks in the aortic wall that are contained by the outer layer of the aorta.
- Elective resection with graft replacement is indicated in asymptomatic patients with an aortic diameter of at least twice than normal in the involved segment (5–6 cm in most thoracic segments). Elective repair is contraindicated by extreme operative risk due to severe coexisting cardiac or pulmonary disease.
- An emergency operation is performed for any patient in whom a ruptured aneurysm is suspected.
- Staged repair of multiple aortic segments often is necessary.
- An alternative to traditional open repair of a descending thoracic aortic aneurysm is endovascular stent grafting.
- Criteria needs to be satisfied for this treatment option to be considered, including the presence of at least a 2-cm landing zone of healthy aortic tissue proximally and distally to the aneurysm.

Causes

- Nonspecific medial degeneration
- Aortic dissection
- Genetic disorders: Marfan syndrome, Loeys-Dietz syndrome, Ehlers-Danlos syndrome
- Familial aortic aneurysms
- Aneurysms-osteoarthritis syndrome
- Bovine aortic arch
- Poststenotic dilatation
- Infection
- Aortitis
- Takayasu's arteritis, giant cell arteritis, and rheumatoid aortitis
- Trauma

Clinical History

- Normal diameter of ascending aorta is < 2.1 cm.
- Normal diameter of descending aorta is < 1.6 cm.
- Normal diameter of abdominal aorta is 3 cm.

- As expected, aortic diameter is a strong predictor of rupture, dissection, and mortality.
- For thoracic aortic aneurysms > 6 cm in diameter, annual rates of catastrophic complications were 3.6% for rupture, 3.7% for dissection, and 10.8% for death.
- Critical diameters: 6.0 cm for aneurysms of the ascending aorta and 7.0 cm for aneurysms of the descending thoracic aorta. The corresponding risks of rupture after reaching these diameters were 31% and 43%, respectively.

Clinical Manifestation

- Local compression.
- Aneurysmal expansion and impingement on adjacent structures causes mild chronic pain.
- The most common symptom in patients with ascending aortic aneurysms is anterior chest discomfort.
- Aortic valve regurgitation.
- The resulting deformation of the aortic valve leads to progressively worsening aortic valve regurgitation.
- Distal embolization.
- Rupture.

Diagnostic Evaluation

- Plain radiography
- Echocardiography and abdominal ultrasonography
- Computed tomography (CT)
- Magnetic resonance angiography (MRA)
- Invasive aortography and cardiac catheterization

Treatment

Indications for Operation

- Practice guidelines for thoracic aortic disease recommend elective operation in asymptomatic patients when the diameter of an ascending aortic aneurysm is > 5.5 cm, when the diameter of a descending thoracic aortic aneurysm is > 6.0 cm, or when the rate of dilatation is > 0.5 cm/y.
- In patients with connective tissue disorders such as Marfan and Loeys-Dietz syndromes, the threshold for operation

is based on a smaller aortic diameter (4.0–5.0 cm for the ascending aorta and 5.5–6.0 cm for the descending thoracic aorta).

- For women with connective tissue disorders who are considering pregnancy, prophylactic aortic root replacement is considered because the risk of aortic dissection or rupture increases at an aortic diameter of 4.0 cm or greater.

Open Repair vs. Endovascular Repair

- As noted earlier, endovascular repair of thoracic aortic aneurysms has become an accepted treatment option in selected patients, particularly patients with isolated degenerative descending thoracic aortic aneurysms.
- Practice guidelines recommend that endovascular repair be strongly considered for patients with descending thoracic aneurysm at an aortic diameter of 5.5 cm (which is slightly below the 6.0-cm threshold for open repair).
- For endovascular repairs to produce optimal outcomes, several anatomic criteria must be met.
- Anatomic limitation for this therapy relates to vascular access: the femoral and iliac arteries have to be wide enough to accommodate the large sheaths necessary to deploy the stent grafts.
- The patients who theoretically may benefit more from an endovascular approach than from traditional open techniques are those who are of advanced age or have significant comorbidities.
- For example, the open repair of a descending thoracic aortic aneurysm can result in significant pulmonary morbidity.
- Therefore, patients with borderline pulmonary reserve may better tolerate an endovascular procedure than standard open repair.
- In contrast, patients with significant intraluminal atheroma may be better served by an open approach because of the risk of embolization and stroke posed by catheter manipulation.
- Similarly, patients with connective tissue disorders generally are not considered candidates for elective endovascular repair.

Preoperative Assessment and Preparation
- Cardiac evaluation
- Renal evaluation
- Operative repair

Proximal Thoracic Aortic Aneurysms
- Open repair—traditional open operations to repair proximal aortic aneurysms, which involve the ascending aorta, transverse aortic arch, or both, are performed through a midsternal incision and require cardiopulmonary bypass.
- The best choice of aortic replacement technique depends on the extent of the aneurysm and the condition of the aortic valve.
- Distal thoracic aortic aneurysms.
- Open repair.
- Endovascular repair.

Abdominal Aortic Aneurysm (AAA)
Causes and Risk Factors
- A degenerative process in the aortic wall is the most common.
- Atherosclerotic disease, age, male sex, smoking history, family history, hypertension, coronary artery disease, and chronic obstructive pulmonary disease are associated with the development of AAA.
- Other less common causes include inflammation, infection, and connective tissue disease.
- Male sex and smoking are even stronger risk factors in inflammatory AAA.
- Smoking cessation is the first step of medical therapy, followed by surgical repair.
- Infectious or mycotic AAA is rare but is associated with high mortality.
- Patients with connective tissue disorders such as Marfan syndrome and Ehlers-Danlos syndrome tend to have more extensive and larger aneurysms at a younger age.
- Diabetes and black race have negative association with AAA.

Natural History of Aortic Aneurysm
- Exhibits a "staccato" pattern of growth.
- Average aggregate growth is approximately 3–4 mm/year.
- Rupture risk appears to be directly related to aneurysm size as predicted by Laplace's law.
- Women appear to be at higher risk of rupture than men.
- Rapid expansion of > 0.5 cm within 6 months can be considered a relative indication for elective repair.

Risk of Rupture of Abdominal Aortic Aneurysm (AAA) Based on Size

Description	Diameter of Aorta (cm)	Estimated Annual Risk of Rupture (%)	Estimated Five-Year Risk of Rupture (%)
Normal aorta	2–3	0	0
Small AAA	4–5	1	5–10
Moderate AAA	5–6	2–5	30–40
Large AAA	6–7	3–10	> 50
Very large AAA	> 7	> 10	100

Relevant Anatomy
- AAA is defined as a pathologic focal dilation of the aorta that is > 3 cm or 1.5 times the adjacent diameter of the normal aorta.

Clinical Manifestations
- Asymptomatic and are usually found incidentally during workup for chronic back pain or kidney stones.
- 90% of AAAs are infrarenal in location and have a fusiform morphology.
- Thoracoabdominal aneurysms are classified according to the Crawford.

Classification
- Extent I: involves the majority of the descending thoracic aorta as well as the upper abdominal aorta.

- Extent II: involves the majority of the descending thoracic aorta and the majority of the abdominal aorta.
- Extent III: involves the lower descending thoracic aorta and the majority of the abdominal aorta.
- Extent IV: involves most or all the abdominal aorta.
- Extent V: involves the lower descending thoracic aorta and the upper abdominal aorta.

Diagnostic Evaluation

- Ultrasound is safe, widely available, relatively accurate, and inexpensive and thus the screening modality of choice.
- CT scan remains the gold standard for determination of anatomic eligibility for endovascular repair.

Surgical Repair of Abdominal Aortic Aneurysm

- The main advantage of a conventional open repair is that the AAA is permanently eliminated because it is entirely replaced by a prosthetic aortic graft.
- The risk of aneurysm recurrence or delayed rupture no longer exists.
- As a result, long-term imaging surveillance is not needed with these patients.
- Another potential advantage of open repair includes direct assessment of the circulatory integrity of the colon.
- Risks associated with open repair are cardiac complications, myocardial infarction, arrhythmias, or renal insufficiency.

Endovascular Repair of Abdominal Aortic Aneurysm

- For patients who are at increased risk for surgery because of age or comorbidity, endovascular repair is a superior minimally invasive alternative.
- Meta-analyses of published literature have consistently demonstrated significantly decreased operative time, blood loss, hospital length of stay, and overall perioperative morbidity and mortality of endovascular repair compared with open surgical repair.
- Anatomic eligibility for endovascular repair is mainly based on three areas: the proximal aortic neck, common iliac arteries, and external iliac and common femoral arteries.

Classification and Management of Endoleak

- Over half of these endoleaks will resolve spontaneously during the first 6 months, resulting in a 10% incidence of chronic endoleaks in all cases.
- Endoleaks can be detected using conventional angiography, contrast CT, MRA, and color-flow duplex ultrasound.
- Four types of endoleaks:
  o Type I endoleak = attachment site leak (proximal or distal)
  o Type II endoleak = side branch leak caused by lumbar or side branches
  o Type III endoleak = endograft junctional leak due to overlapping device components.
  o Type IV endoleak = endograft fabric or porosity leak

Aortic Dissection

Pathology and Classification

- A progressive separation of the aortic wall layers that usually occurs after a tear forms in the intima and inner media.
- The two channels are called reentry sites.
- Although the separation of layers primarily progresses distally along the length of the aorta, it can also proceed in a proximal direction; this process often is referred to as proximal extension or retrograde dissection.

Classification

- DeBakey classification (types I, II, III):
  o Type I refers to dissections that propagate from the ascending aorta and extend to the aortic arch and, commonly, beyond the arch distally.
  o Type II refers to dissections that are confined to the ascending portion of the aorta.
  o Type IIIa dissections are limited to the descending aorta.
  o Type IIIb dissections that start in the descending aorta that extend proximally to the arch and ascending aorta.

- Stanford classification (types A, B) of aortic dissection:
  - Stanford type A includes dissections that involve the ascending aorta and arch and descending thoracic aorta.
  - Stanford type B refers to dissections that involve only the descending aorta.

Causes
- Smoking, hypertension, atherosclerosis, and hypercholesterolemia are associated with aortic dissection.
- Connective tissue disorders, aortitis, bicuspid aortic valve, or preexisting medial degenerative disease are at risk for dissection, especially if they already have a thoracic aortic aneurysm.
- Aortic injury during cardiac catheterization, surgery, or endovascular aortic repair is a common cause of iatrogenic dissection.
- Other conditions that are associated with aortic dissection include cocaine and amphetamine abuse.

Clinical Manifestations
- The onset of dissection often is associated with severe chest or back pain, classically described as "tearing."
- Most patients with acute aortic dissection (80%–90%) experience severe pain in the chest, back, or abdomen.
- The pain usually occurs suddenly, has a sharp or tearing quality, and often migrates distally as the dissection progresses along the aorta.
- For classification purposes (acute vs. subacute vs. chronic), the onset of pain is generally considered to represent the beginning of the dissection process. Most of the other common symptoms either are nonspecific or are caused by the secondary manifestations of dissection.

Diagnostic Evaluation
- The value of the CXR for detecting aortic dissection is limited, with a sensitivity of 67% and a specificity of 86%.
- Once the diagnosis of dissection is considered, the thoracic aorta should be imaged with CT, MRA, or echocardiography.
- Transesophageal echocardiography (TEE).

Management
Treatment of Ascending Aortic Dissection
Acute Dissection
- Because of the risk of aortic rupture, acute ascending aortic dissection is usually considered an absolute indication for emergency surgical repair.
- Specific patient groups may benefit from nonoperative management or delayed operation.

Treatment of Descending Aortic Dissection
Nonoperative Management
- Nonoperative, pharmacologic management of acute descending aortic dissection results in lower morbidity and mortality rates than traditional surgical treatment does.
- Aggressive imaging follow-up is recommended for all patients with chronic aortic dissection. Both contrast-enhanced CT and MRA scans provide excellent aortic imaging.

Indications for Surgery
- In the acute phase, surgery has been traditionally reserved for patients who experience complications.
- In general terms, such intervention is intended to prevent or repair ruptures and relieve life-threatening ischemic manifestations.
- During the acute phase of a dissection, the specific indications for operative intervention include aortic rupture.

Endovascular Treatment
- Endovascular therapy is routinely used in patients with descending aortic dissection complicated by visceral malperfusion.

Open Repair
- Acute dissection in patients with acute aortic dissection or surgical repair of the descending

thoracic or thoracoabdominal aorta is traditionally associated with high morbidity and mortality.

- Therefore, the primary goals of surgery are to prevent fatal rupture and to restore branch vessel perfusion.

Venous Anatomy

- Lower extremity veins are divided into superficial, deep, and perforating veins.
- The superficial venous system lies above the uppermost fascial layer of the leg and thigh and consists of the great saphenous vein (GSV) and small saphenous vein (SSV) and their tributaries.
- The deep veins follow the course of major arteries in the extremities. In the lower leg, paired veins parallel the course of the anterior tibial, posterior tibial, and peroneal arteries, to join behind the knee, forming the popliteal vein.
- Venous bridges connect the paired veins in the lower leg.
- The popliteal vein continues through the adductor hiatus to become the femoral vein.
- In the proximal thigh, the femoral vein joins with the deep femoral vein to form the common femoral vein, becoming the external iliac vein at the inguinal ligament.
- Cockett's and Boyd's perforators.

Evaluation of the Venous System
Clinical Evaluation

- Evaluation of the venous system begins with a detailed history and physical examination.

Noninvasive Evaluation

- Duplex ultrasonography (DUS) augmented by color-flow imaging is now the most important noninvasive diagnostic method in the evaluation of the venous system.
- Magnetic resonance venography (MRV) and computed tomography (CT) venography are noninvasive techniques for evaluation of pelvic and intra-abdominal veins.

Invasive Evaluation
- Both venography and intravascular ultrasound (IVUS) are used as adjuncts to percutaneous or open surgical treatment of venous disorders.

Venous Thromboembolism
Epidemiology
- DVT and pulmonary embolism (PE), or VTE, remain important preventable sources of morbidity and mortality.

Risk Factors
- The more commonly acquired VTE risk factors include older age (> 40 years), hospitalization and immobilization, OCP, pregnancy and the recently postpartum state, prior VTE, malignancy, major surgery, obesity, nephrotic syndrome, trauma and spinal cord injury, long-haul travel (> 6 hrs), varicose veins, antiphospholipid syndrome, myeloproliferative disorders, and polycythemia.
- Heritable risk factors include male sex, factor V Leiden mutation, prothrombin 20210A gene variant, antithrombin, protein C and protein S deficiencies, and dysfibrinogenemias.

Diagnosis
Clinical Evaluation
- Pain or swelling.
- Clinical symptoms may worsen as DVT propagates and involves the major proximal deep veins.
- Extensive DVT of the major axial deep venous channels of the lower extremity with relative sparing of collateral veins causes a condition called phlegmasia cerulea dolens.
- This condition is characterized by pain and pitting edema with associated cyanosis.
- When the thrombosis extends to the collateral veins, massive fluid sequestration and more significant edema ensue, resulting in a condition known as phlegmasia alba dolens.

- Both phlegmasia cerulean dolens and phlegmasia alba dolens can be complicated by venous gangrene and the need for amputation.

Vascular Radiologic Evaluation
- Duplex ultrasound
- Impedance plethysmography
- Iodine-125 fibrinogen uptake
- Venography

Treatment
- Once the diagnosis of VTE has been made, antithrombotic therapy should be initiated promptly.

Antithrombotic Therapy
- IV or subcutaneous (SC) unfractionated heparin or SC low molecular weight heparin.
- Fondaparinux, a synthetic alternative to heparin to initiate therapy.
- An oral vitamin K antagonist, usually sodium warfarin, is begun shortly after initiation of IV or SC therapy.
- Either SC or IV therapy is continued until effective oral anticoagulation with warfarin is achieved as indicated by an international normalized ratio (INR) ≥ 2 for 24 hrs.
- A minimum of 5 days of heparin or fondaparinux therapy is recommended.
- UFH therapy is most commonly administered with an initial IV bolus of 80 units/kg.

Systemic and Catheter-Directed Thrombolysis
- Patients with extensive proximal, iliofemoral DVT may benefit from systemic thrombolysis or catheter-directed thrombolysis (CDT).
- Several thrombolytic agents are available, including streptokinase, urokinase, alteplase.

IVC Filters
- Placement of an IVC filter is indicated for patients who have manifestations of lower extremity VTE and

absolute contraindications to anticoagulation, those who have a bleeding complication from anticoagulation therapy.

Operative Venous Thrombectomy
-   In patients with acute iliofemoral DVT, surgical therapy is generally reserved for patients who worsen with anticoagulation therapy and those with phlegmasia cerulea dolens and impending venous gangrene.
-   If the patient has phlegmasia cerulea dolens, a fasciotomy of the calf compartments is first performed.

Lymphedema
Pathophysiology
-   Lymphedema is extremity swelling that results from a reduction in lymphatic transport and accumulation of lymph within the interstitial space.
-   It is caused by anatomic and/or physiologic abnormalities such as lymphatic hypoplasia, functional insufficiency, or absence of lymphatic valves.
-   Classification system, described by Allen.
-   Congenital lymphedema, lymphedema praecox, and lymphedema tarda.
-   Secondary lymphedema is far more common than primary lymphedema. Secondary lymphedema develops as a result of lymphatic obstruction or disruption.
-   Axillary node dissection leading to lymphedema of the arm is the most common cause of secondary lymphedema in the United States.
-   Other causes of secondary lymphedema include radiation therapy, trauma, infection, malignancy, and globally, filariasis (an infection).

Clinical Diagnosis
-   Recurrent cellulitis is a common complication of lymphedema.
-   Repeated infection results in further lymphatic damage, worsening existing disease.

Radiologic Diagnosis
- Duplex ultrasound
- Lymphoscintigraphy
- Lymphangiography

Management
- Bed rest and leg elevation
- Intermittent pneumatic compression therapy
- Lymphatic massage
- Compression garments
- Antibiotic therapy
- Surgery (A variety of surgical procedures have been devised for the treatment of lymphedema. Surgical treatment involves either excision of extra tissue or anastomosis of a lymphatic vessel to another lymphatic or vein.)

Surgical management of Obesity

The Disease of Obesity
- Second leading cause of preventable death.
- BMI = weight (kg) / height (m^2).
- WHO classification of obesity:

Classification	BMI
Normal	18–25
Overweight (Preobese)	25–30
Obese (class I)	30–35
Morbid obese (class II)	35–40
Super morbidly obese (class III)	> 40

Prevalence and Contributing Factor
- In the USA, 37% are obese class I and more.
- Children with parent of normal weight, chance of obesity is 10%.
- Children with obese parent, chance is 80%–90%.
- Diet and culture are the most common contributing factors → others are high intake, low activity.
- Weight gain, adipose cell size and number.
- Abdominal wall SC layer or SC in body + vesicle.
- In male, central obesity; in female, peripheral and gluteal → central → DM, HTN, metabolic syndrome.

Medical and Social Problem
- Discrimination.
- Public facilities don't allow participation such as airline seat, bathroom, clothing size option (lazy).
- Medical: degenerative joint disease, low back pain, HTN, obstructive sleep apnea, GERD, GS, DM, increase lipidemic status, high cholesterol, hypoventilation, arrhythmia.
- Right-side hepatic failure, migraine, venous stain, ulcer, DVT, fungal skin rash, stress urinary incontinence, infertility, dysmenorrhea, depression, abdominal wall hernia, and cancer of breast, colon, prostate, and uterus.

Prognosis
- Male will live 12 years less, and female, 9 years less.

Medical Treatment
- ↓ caloric intake, ↑ energy expanded from exercise.
- Diet and exercise, 3% success rate.
- Should be initiated by lifestyle modification, ↓ calorie, ↑ activity → + dietary counseling.
- Decrease daily calories, 500 kcal/day → 3,500/week → loss 1 lb of fat weekly → 8% of weight in 6 months. Diet and exercise, 10% in 6 months.
- Pharmacological: orlistat.
    - → Inhibits gastric and pancreatic lipase → ↓ lipid absorption.
    - → Decrease 6%–10% in 1 year.
    - → If you stop drug → weight gain.
- Liraglutide (Saxenda), SC injection, either daily or weekly.
- FDA → Qsymia and lorcaserin (serotonin I).
- Less than 1% of obese patients undergo surgery annually (including all classes) and 5% of class II and III.

Indication for Bariatric Surgery
- BMI ≥ 40 with or without comorbid disease
- BMI ≥ 35 with comorbid disease

Contraindication
- ASA IV
- Unfit, low IQ to understood operation
- Not willing to change lifestyle post-op
- Drug, alcohol, psycho

Preoperative Preparation
- Patient selection by NIH.
- Screening for hidden disease such as CAD, cardiovascular disease.
- Cardiology consultation.
- ECG, echo, stress test.
- OSA scale indication of sleep apnea in class III (80%) → airway pressure, hypoxia, arrhythmia.

- Pulmonary disease.
- GERD, rule out Barrett's → EGD → better LRY GB.
- Anticoagulant manages preoperative such as the following:
  - Stop warfarin 5 days before surgery and bridge to heparin.
  - If strong history of VTE → IVC before 1 day of OR, then remove 3–6 weeks.
- Some surgeon recommends US for gallstone to perform it as one procedure. But no routine US to detect gallstone.
- Ursodiol, 300 mg PO BID, lowers gallstone by 4% after RYGB.
- Some recommend to decrease calories to decrease weight before surgery, and some data showed increase improvement and outcome.
- Stop smoking.

Bariatric Surgery Procedure
- Laparoscopy vs. open:
  - Laparoscopy: shorter stay, less morbid, less pain, fast recovery. Patient is interested in laparoscopy.
  - Open: upper midline, some left subcostal.
- Pneumoperitoneum pressure, 15–18 mmHg.
- Gold standard is patient safety.
- Indication for conversion to open:
  1. Failure to establish adequate pneumoperitoneum
  2. Hemodynamic adverse reaction of pneumoperitoneum
  3. Intra-abdominal adhesion
  4. Hepatomegaly
  5. Intraoperative complication, e.g., bleeding
  6. Excess thick body
  7. Longitudinal upper abdominal hernia

Postoperative Follow-Up
- Short term up to 2 years.
- Recommendation = 75% of patients follow up 5 years, especially if malabsorption.
- Multidisciplinary nutrition, psychiatry.

Type of Surgery
1. LAGB
2. LRYGB
3. BPD-DS
4. LSG

Outcome of All Bariatric Procedures

Type	Excess WL (%)	Dyslipid (%)	HTN (%)	DM (%)
BPD	70–80	90	80	90
RYGD	60–70	60–70	60	80
SG	50–60	50–60	60	90
LAGB	40–50	60	58	50–60

❖ **Laparoscopic Adjustable Gastric Banding (LAGB)**
- **Background**
  - Place of inflatable silicon band around proximal stomach.
  - Then band attaches with reservoir to allow tightness.
  - Two types of band: original laparoscopy band and Swedish (wider).

- **Technique**
  - Reverse Trendelenburg position, pneumoperitoneum, division of peritoneum at angle of His and division of GH ligament.

- **Patient Selection and Prepreparation**
  - Old patient, medically ill, high risk.
  - Less impressive outcome if BMI > 50.
  - Patient with Nissen fundoplication is a poor candidate for this operation.

- **Postoperative and Follow-up**
  - Diet instruction, pain control.
  - Follow up 2–3 weeks post-op.
  - As no absorption issue → only multivitamin.

- Ursodiol, 300 mg PO BID, as prophylactic for gallstone.
- Adjustment of the band over 2 years.

- **Outcomes**
  - 8 years follow-up.
  - Weight loss, 60%.
  - HTN improvement, 55%.
  - Obstructive sleep apnea, 33%–2%.
  - GERD improvement, 50%.
  - Less morbid and mortality.

- **Complications**
  - Prolapse, slippage, erosion, failure to lose weight.

❖ **Laparoscopic Roux-En-Y Gastric Bypass (LRYGB)**
  - Small gastric pouch, 20 mL.
  - Roux jejunal limb is brought and anastomosis in the pouch.
  - Roux limb can be anterior or posterior to colon.
  - Length from ligament of Treitz to the anastomosis is 20–50 cm, and length of Roux limb is 75–150 cm or 100–150.
  - It's for BMI > 60.
  - Anticolic, less incidence of internal hernia.
  - Needs EGD preoperatively to all patients.
  - The technique by using blue load stapler.

- **Patient Selection**
  - Relative contraindication: previous gastric surgery, previous ARS, iron-deficiency anemia, Barrett's esophagus.

- **Postoperative Care and Follow-Up**
  - It is the best for patient with GERD after confirming rule out of Barrett's esophagus.
  - Postoperative stays 2–3 days in hospital.
  - Postoperative D1 can perform contrast study.
  - Diet advancement after 3 weeks (first clinic visit).
  - Follow up 3, 6 months, 1 year.

- **Outcomes**
    - Lose 60%–70% of weight.
    - Resolution of comorbidity:
        GERD (90%) and venous ulcer
        DM (80%)
        Hyperlipidemia (70%)
        HTN (50%–60%)
    - Achieve < 35 BMI.

- **Complication**
    - Iron-deficiency anemia (66%)
        Vitamin B12 deficiency (50%)
        Vitamin D deficiency (5%)
        Marginal ulcer (15%)
        → PPI, 90% improved, 10% re-op
        Anastomosis stenosis (1%–19% at 6–12 weeks)
    - Requires urgent intervention.
        Small bowel obstruction, vomiting, hematemesis, leak, bleeding.

- ❖ **Biliopancreatic Diversion with Duodenal Switch (BPD-DS)**
    - Resection of the distal ½–⅔ of stomach and creation of an alimentary tract of the distal 200 of ileum, which is anastomosed to stomach.
    - Then biliopancreatic limb anastomosed to alimentary tract either 75–100 cm from iIeocecal valve.
    - Limited because it's difficult.
    - Higher marginal ulcer → DS can solve the problem.

- **Technique**
    - Residual, 200 mL of stomach.
    - For BMI, < 50.
    - Terminal ileum divided at 250 cm from ICV, then anastomosed to stomach and the other end anastomosed to terminal ileum side to side.
    - DS differ from BPD → sleeve gastrectomy on tube calibrated 32-40 French.
    - Duodenum divided in first portion (2 cm from pylorus).

- Prophylactic cholecystectomy as higher incidence of gallstone because malabsorption of bile salt.

- **Patient Selection and Preparation**
    - Frequent and large movement after any large meal.
    - Requires large number of vitamins and mineral replacement.
    - For class II, III.
    - Contraindication: preexisting Ca^{++}, Fe^{++} deficiency.
    - It is complicated and costly.

- **Postoperative and Follow-Up**
    - As Roux-en-Y gastric bypass.

- **Outcomes**
    - Higher weight loss (most), 70% → 58% in 9 months.
    - Increase OR time.
    - Complication rate is 27%–33%.
    - Nutritional complication is 40%–77%.

❖ **Laparoscopic Sleeve Gastrectomy (LSG)**
    - This technique is the easiest.
    - Superior weight loss then LAGB.
    - It passes LRYGB in popularity.
    - More anatomical.
    - Increase 500%.

- **Indication**
    - Patient selection = same with bariatric operation.
    - BMI > 60—super morbidly obese.
    - First and second stage op.
    - Perform to all patients except GERD.

- **Technique**
    - 3–5 cm proximal to pylorus.
    - Green load.

- Pass bougie 32-36, also test for air leak, bleeding, obstruction.
- Important point: not narrow lumen in incisura.
- Some reinforce to stapler line.

- **Postoperative and Follow-Up**
  - 2 days stay in hospital post-op.
  - Routine gastro griffin can be used postoperatively on first day.
  - Follow as LRYGB.
  - Iron, vitamin B12, vitamin D deficiency.
  - Decrease 60–74.8 kg on first year.

- **Outcomes and Complications**
  - Major complication, less than 5%.
  - Weight loss, 5%–85% for 5 years.
  - One study showed LSG superior to LRYGB in weight loss.
  - Most common complication is leak because of high press → angle of His (esophagus) is too tight most commonly.
  - Second → stenosis in incisura.
  - Late leak at week 6.
  - Proximal leak (late) can be possible after 4 months, distal leak (early).

- **Physiology of Weight Loss**
  - Resolution of DM, but not good as RYGB.

Special Issue Relating to the Bariatric Patient in Adolescent and Elderly
- BMI > 30 is 25%.
- 75% of adolescent is above eighty-fifth percentile.
- Recommendation:
  - ➤ 35 BMI with severe comorbid (DM, nonalcoholic fatty liver disease, OSA)
  - ➤ 40 BMI with mild comorbid (HTN, dyslipidemia, insulin resistance)

In Female
- Obesity → high estrogen → low fertility.

Plastic Surgery after Weight Loss
- Abdominoplasty.

Other Techniques
- Gastric plication
- Endoscopic balloon.

Critical Care

Indication of Intubation
- Inability to maintain airway patency
- Inability to protect the airway against aspiration
- Severe tachypnea
- Failure to ventilate
- Failure to oxygenate (low saturation)
- Anticipation of a deteriorating course that will eventually lead to respiratory failure
- ICU basics:
  - $MAP = CO \times SVR.$
  - $CO = SV \times HR.$
  - O_2 consumption $(VO_2) = CO \times (CaO_2 - CvO_2).$
  - Tissue perfusion $= MAP -$ organ pressure.
  - FAST HUGS BID is a mnemonic for ICU patient follow-up.

F	Feeding (enteral, TPN)
A	Analgesia
S	Sedation
T	Thromboprophylaxis
H	Head up
U	Ulcer prophylaxis
G	Glycemic control
S	Spontaneous breathing trial
B	Bowel movement
I	Indwelling catheter
D	Drug de-escalation

- Pulmonary vascular resistance (PVR) can be measured only by using a Swan–Ganz catheter (echo does not measure PVR).
- Wedge pressure measurements should be taken at end-expiration (for both ventilated and nonventilated patients).
- Shock types: see shock chapter.

Receptors:

α-1—vascular smooth muscle constriction

α-2—venous smooth muscle constriction

β-1—myocardial contraction and rate

β-2—relaxes bronchial smooth muscle, relaxes vascular smooth muscle, increases insulin, glucagon, and renin

Dopamine receptors—relax renal and splanchnic smooth muscle

Cardiovascular drugs:

- Dopamine
    - 2–5 µg/kg/min—dopamine receptors (renal)
    - 6–10 µg/kg/min—beta-adrenergic (heart contractility)
    - > 10 µg/kg/min—alpha-adrenergic (vasoconstriction and ↑ BP)
- Dobutamine (3 µg/kg/min initially)
    - Beta-1, ↑ contractility mostly, tachycardia with higher doses
    - Alpha-1, vasoconstriction
- Norepinephrine (5 µg/min initially)
    - Low dose—beta-1 (↑ contractility)
    - High dose—alpha-1 and alpha-2
    - Potent splanchnic vasoconstrictor
- Epinephrine
    - Low dose—beta-1 and beta-2 (↑ contractility and vasodilation)
    - High dose—alpha-1 and alpha-2 (vasoconstriction)
- Nitroglycerin—predominately venodilation with ↓ myocardial wall tension from ↓ preload, moderate coronary vasodilator
- Hydralazine—α-blocker, lowers BP

Ventilation:

- Noninvasive positive pressure volume (NPPV)
- Pressure support ventilation (referred as IPAP)
- CPAP (referred as EPAP)
    1. Assist control ventilation
        Deliver either volume-cycled (volume-assisted control) or time-cycled (pressure-assisted control).

2. Pressure support
    Provide a preset inspiratory pressure-assisted.
    Patient initiates each breath.
3. Controlled mechanical ventilation (CMV)
    Unassisted breath at preset rate; all breath are mandatory.
4. Synchronized intermittent mandatory ventilation (SIMV)
    Deliver either volume-cycled or time-cycled at preset mandatory rate.
    Patient can breath spontaneously between cycles.

Normal Weaning Parameters
- Negative inspiratory force (NIF) > 20
- $FiO_2 \le 40\%$, PEEP 5
- Pressure support 5
- RR < 24/min, HR < 120 beats/min
- $PO_2 > 60$ mmHg
- $PCO_2 < 50$ mmHg
- pH 7.35–7.45
- Saturations > 93%
- Off pressors
- Follow commands
- Can protect airway

Respiratory System
- Total lung capacity (TLC): lung volume after maximal inspiration.
- TLC = FVC + RV.
- Forced vital capacity (FVC): maximal exhalation after maximal inhalation.
- Residual volume (RV): lung volume after maximal expiration (20% TLC).
- Tidal volume (TV): volume of air with normal inspiration and expiration.
- Functional residual capacity (FRC): lung volume after normal exhalation.
- FRC = ERV + RV.

- ↓ FRC in surgery (atelectasis), sepsis (ARDS), and trauma (contusion, atelectasis, ARDS).
- Compliance: (change in volume)/(change in pressure).
    High compliance means lungs ventilates easily.
    Pulmonary compliance decreased in patients with ARDS, fibrotic lung diseases, pulmonary edema, atelectasis.
- Expiratory reserve volume (ERV): volume of air that can be forcefully expired after normal expiration.
- PEEP: improves FRC and compliance by keeping alveoli open → best way to improve oxygenation.
- Excessive PEEP: ↓ RA filling, ↓ CO, ↓ renal blood flow, ↓ urine output, and ↑ pulmonary vascular resistance, risk of barotrauma.
- FEV1: forced expiratory volume in 1 s (after maximal inhalation).
- Minute ventilation = TV × RR.

Anesthesia

American Society of Anesthesiologists (ASA) classification system:
- ASA 1: a normal healthy patient, e.g., fit, nonobese (BMI under 30), a nonsmoking patient with good exercise tolerance.
- ASA 2: a patient with a mild systemic disease, e.g., patient with a well-controlled disease (e.g., treated hypertension, obesity with BMI under 35, frequent social drinker or is a cigarette smoker).
- ASA 3: a patient with a severe systemic disease that is not life-threatening, e.g., patient with some functional limitations as a result of disease (e.g., poorly treated hypertension or diabetes, morbid obesity, chronic renal failure, a bronchospastic disease with intermittent exacerbation, stable angina, implanted pacemaker).
- ASA 4: a patient with a severe systemic disease that is a *constant threat to life*, e.g., patient with functional limitation from severe, life-threatening disease (e.g., unstable angina, poorly controlled COPD, symptomatic CHF, recent myocardial MI, or stroke, less than 3 months).
- ASA 5: a moribund patient who is not expected to survive without the operation, e.g., ruptured abdominal aortic aneurysm, massive trauma, and extensive intracranial hemorrhage with mass effect.
- ASA 6: a brain-dead patient whose organs are being removed with the intention of transplanting them into another patient.
- The addition of E to ASA (e.g., ASA E) denotes an emergency surgical procedure.

Mallampati Classification
- Class 1: soft palate, fauces, uvula, pillars are visible.
- Class 2: soft palate, fauces, portion of uvula are visible.
- Class 3: soft palate, base of uvula are visible.
- Class 4: only hard palate is visible.

There are many forms of anesthesia:
- Topical anesthesia numbs the surface of a tissue, like an ointment or spry, e.g., xylocaine gel, EMLA cream.

- Local anesthesia causes a loss of sensation in a small area, like around an abscess; it can be field block, ring block, nerve block, and infiltration.

Dosage:

Agent	Max Dose without Epi	Max Dose with Epi	Duration of Action	Notes
Lidocaine	5 mg/kg	7 mg/kg	30–90 min	1% = 10 mg/mL
Bupivacaine	2.5 mg/kg	3 mg/kg	6–8 hrs	2% = 20 mg/mL
Mepivacaine	7 mg/kg	8 mg/kg		
Ropivacaine	3 mg/kg			

- Regional anesthesia causes a larger part of the body, like an entire leg, to lose sensation after performing a nerve block.
- Epidural anesthesia is produced when a local anesthetic is injected into the epidural space, the space in between the spinal cord and the bony vertebrae that surround it.
- Spinal anesthesia is produced when a local anesthetic is injected deeper than in an epidural anesthesia, into the spinal subarachnoid space.
- General anesthesia causes the total loss of sensation throughout the body and a loss of consciousness.

Sedative
- It is a substance that produces a state of central nervous system depression, thereby inducing calm while suppressing bodily reactions, but one that does not directly produce sleep. A person who is given a sedative may fall asleep because they are calm and relaxed.

Hypnotic
- It is a substance that depresses the central nervous system and is intended to directly induce sleep.

Anesthesia
- It is defined as a total or partial loss of sensation, with or without an accompanying loss of consciousness.

Pain Management from Weak to Strong Painkiller

-   Paracetamol, either PO, IV, PR (15 mg/kg).
    NB 1 g of IV paracetamol = 4 mg of morphine.
-   NSAIDs.
-   COX-1: aspirin, Ibuprofen.
-   COX-2: Celebrex, meloxicam, Lornoxicam.
-   Combined paracetamol + codeine.
-   Tramadol.
-   Pregabalin (Lyrica): used to treat pain caused by nerve sensitivity or nerve damage, such as shingles, diabetes, nerve pain, and sciatica.
-   Meperidine (pethidine), morphine.
-   Fentanyl: fast-acting, eighty times stronger than morphine (does not cross-react in patients with morphine allergy), no histamine release.

Types of Inductions

Inhalational Induction Agents

-   Cause unconsciousness, amnesia, and some analgesia (pain relief); most have some myocardial depression, ↑ cerebral blood flow, and ↓ renal blood flow.
-   Nitrous oxide: fast, minimal myocardial depression, tremors at induction.
-   Halothane: slow onset/offset, highest degree of cardiac depression and arrhythmias.
-   Sevoflurane.

Intravenous Induction Agents

-   Sodium thiopental (barbiturate)—fast-acting.
    Side effects: ↓ cerebral blood flow and metabolic rate, ↓ blood pressure.
-   Propofol—very rapid distribution and on/off, amnesia, sedative.
    Side effects: hypotension, respiratory depression.
    Do not use in patients with egg allergy.
    Metabolized in liver and by plasma cholinesterase.
-   Ketamine—dissociation of thalamic/limbic systems, places patient in a cataleptic state (amnesia, analgesia), no respiratory depression or hypotension.

Side effects: hallucinations, catecholamine release ($\uparrow CO_2$, tachycardia), $\uparrow$ airway secretions, and $\uparrow$ cerebral blood flow. Contraindicated in patients with head injury. Good for children.

- Etomidate—fewer hemodynamic changes, fast-acting.
  Continuous infusions can lead to adrenocortical suppression.

Muscle Relaxants (Paralytics)

- Diaphragm—last muscle to go down and first muscle to recover from paralytics.
- Neck muscles and face—first to go down and last to recover from paralytics.
- Depolarizing agents—only one is succinylcholine, depolarizes neuromuscular junction, fast, short-acting, causes fasciculations, $\uparrow$ ICP. Side effects $\rightarrow$ malignant hyperthermia.
- Nondepolarizing agents—inhibits neuromuscular junction by competing with acetylcholine, can get prolongation of these agents with myasthenia gravis.
- Histamine release:
  Rocuronium: fast, intermediate duration, hepatic metabolism.
  Pancuronium: slow-acting, long-lasting, renal metabolism.
- Reversing drugs for nondepolarizing agents:
  Neostigmine—blocks acetylcholinesterase, increasing acetylcholine.
  Edrophonium—blocks acetylcholinesterase, increasing acetylcholine.
  Atropine—should be given with neostigmine or edrophonium to counteract effects of generalized acetylcholine overdose.

Benzodiazepines

- Anticonvulsant, amnesic, anxiolytic, respiratory depression, not analgesic, liver metabolism.
- Versed (midazolam)—short-acting, contraindicated in pregnancy, crosses placenta.
- Valium (diazepam)—intermediate-acting.
- Ativan (lorazepam)—long-acting.
- Tx for overdose of these drugs—flumazenil.

Rapid Sequence Intubation

- It can be indicated for recent oral intake, GERD, delayed gastric emptying, pregnancy, bowel obstruction (preoxygenation, etomidate, succinylcholine, then intubation).

Malignant Hyperthermia (MH)

- It is a hereditary, life-threatening, hypermetabolic acute disorder developing during or after receiving general anesthesia.
- Incidence is 1:12,000 in children and 1:40,000 in adults.
- A genetic predisposition (autosomal dominant disorder) and one or more.
- Triggering agents include halothane, enflurane, isoflurane, sevoflurane, and desflurane and the depolarizing muscle relaxant succinylcholine.
- The cause is rise in the myoplasmic calcium concentration in susceptible patients, resulting in persistent muscle contraction.
- ↑ end-tidal CO_2, then fever, tachycardia, rigidity, acidosis, hyperkalemia, arrhythmias, and sudden cardiac arrest.
- A rise in temperature is often a late sign of MH.
- Can be diagnosed with the caffeine halothane contracture test (muscle biopsy).

Treatment

- Call for help.
- Stop all volatile anesthetics and give 100% O_2.
- Hyperventilate the patient up to three times the calculated minute volume.
- Begin infusion of dantrolene sodium, 2.5 mg/kg IV.
- Repeat dantrolene at 1 mg/kg every 6–8 hrs at least twice.
- Give bicarbonate to treat acidosis if dantrolene is ineffective.
- Treat hyperkalemia with insulin, glucose, and calcium.
- Avoid calcium channel blocke

Abbreviation

A

AAA abdominal aortic aneurysm
AB antibody
ABG arterial blood gas
Abx antibiotics
ACBE air contrast barium enema
ACS abdominal compartment syndrome
ADH anti diuretic hormone
AF atrial fibrillation
AFP (a-FP) alpha Fetoprotein
Ag antigen
ALD acute liver disease
ALL acute lymphoblastic leukemia
ALP alkaline phosphatase
ALTEs acute life-threatening events
AMPLE allergies, medications, past history, last meal and events
ANP Atrial natriuretic peptide
ANS autonomic nervous system
APUD amine precursor uptake and decarboxylation
ARDS acute respiratory distress syndrome
ARF acute renal failure
ASAP as soon as possible
ASD atrial septal defect
ASIS anterior superior iliac spine
AVM Arteriovenous malformation

B

BCC basal cell carcinoma
BCS breast conserving surgery
BD bile duct
BMR basal metabolic rate
BP blood pressure
BSE breast self-examination
Bx biopsy

C

CA. cancer
CAD coronary artery disease
CBG capillary blood gas
CBE clinical breast examination
CCK cholecystokinin
CCP common cavity phenomenon
CD Crohn's disease
CF cystic fibrosis
CHD congenital heart disease
CIC clean intermittent catherization
CLD chronic liver disease
CMV cytomegalovirus /control mandatory ventilation
CNBx core needle biopsy
CNS central nervous system
COP cardiac out put
CP cerebral palsy
CPB cardiopulmonary bypass
CPP cerebral perfusion pressure
CRC colorectal Cancer
CRF chronic renal failure
C/S culture & sensitivity
CS cesarean section
CT CAP chest, abdomen and pelvis
CVP central venous pressure
CVS cardiovascular system
CXR chest x-ray
Cx complication

D

DCR damage control resuscitation
DI diabetes insipidus
DIC disseminated intravascular coagulopathy
DL dentate line
DM diabetes mellitus
DRE digital rectal examination
DSD Detrusor sphincteric dyssynergia /disorder of sexual development
DTC differentiated thyroid CA
DVT deep venous thrombosis

Dx diagnosis
DDx differential diagnosis

E
EBV Epstein Barr virus
EBR external beam radiation
ECF extracellular fluid
ECG electrocardiogram
EEG electroencephalogram
EF ejection fraction
EFS event free survival
EGD esophagogastroduodenoscopy
EGG electrogastrogram
ELBW extreme low birth weight
EMG electromyography
EMR endoscopic mucosal resection
ERCP endoscopic retrograde cholangio-pancreatography
ER/ED emergency room
ERUS endorectal U/S
ESD endoscopic submucosal dissection
ESR erythrocyte sedimentation rate
EUA examination under anesthesia

F
FDG-PET fluorodeoxyglucose-positron emission tomography
FEV forced expiratory volume
FFP fresh frozen plasma
FNAB fine needle aspiration cytology biopsy
FOBT fecal occult blood test
FRV functional residual volume
FSR free survival rate

G
GCT germ cell tumors
GCS Glasgow coma scale
GDNF glial cell line–derived neurotrophic factor
GEP gastric emptying procedure
GFN genitofemoral nerve
GIST gastrointestinal stromal tumor

GIT gastrointestinal tract
GSH glucocorticoid suppressible hyperaldosteronism

H
HACE hepatic artery chemo-embolization
Hb hemoglobin
HBV hepatitis B virus
HCV hepatitis C virus
HF heart failure
HGD high grade dysplasia
HIPEC hyper-thermic intra-peritoneal chemotherapy
HIT Heparin induce thrombo-cytopenia
HIV human immunodeficiency virus
HNPCC Hereditary Non-Polyposis Colorectal Cancer
HL Hodgkin lymphoma
HPV human papilloma virus
HR heart rate
HR heart rate
HSV high selective vagotomy

I
IBD inflammatory bowel disease
IBS irritable bowel syndrome
ICC interstitial cell of Cajal
ICF intracellular fluid
ICH intra-cranial hemorrhage
ICP intracranial pressure
ICU intensive care unit
IMA inferior mesenteric artery
IMF inferior mammary line
IMV inferior mesenteric vein
IOC intra-operative cholangiogram
IPMN intra-ductal papillary mucinous neoplasm
ITP Idiopathic thrombocytopenic purpura
IV intra venous
IVC inferior vena cava
IVF intra-venous fluid
IJV internal jugular vein

L

LES lower esophageal sphincter
LFCN lateral femoral cutaneous nerve
LGD low grade dysplasia
LGIB lower gastrointestinal bleeding
LL & BB lung liver, bone, brain
LLQ left lower quadrant
LMWH low molecular weight heparin
LNs lymph nodes
LOH loss of heterozygosity
LRTI lower respiratory tract infection
LUQ left upper quadrant

M

MALT mucosa associated lymphoid tissue
MBP mechanical bowel preparation
MCDK multi-cystic dysplastic kidney
MCUG Micturition Cystourethrography
MIS minimal invasive surgery
MNG multi-nodular goiter
MRCP magnetic resonance cholangiopancreatography
MRI magnetic resonance image
MRND modified radical neck dissection
MRSA Methicillin-resistant Staphylococcus aureus
MTC medullary thyroid CA
MVA motor vehicle accident
MWS Mallory Wiess syndrome

N

NAD nothing abnormally detected
NAIT Neonatal alloimmune thrombocytopenia
NCCN national comprehensive cancer network
NEC necrotizing enterocolitis
NET neuroendocrine tumor
NGT naso-gastric tube
NHL non-Hodgkin lymphoma
NO nitric oxide
NOMI Non-occlusive mesenteric ischemia
NS normal saline
NSAIDs non-steroidal anti-inflammatory drugs

O

OCP oral contraceptive pills
OI oxygen index
OPD outpatient department
OPSI overwhelming post splenectomy infection
OR operative room
OSR overall survival rate

P

PAF platelet activating factor
PBD percutaneous biliary drainage
PCKD polycystic kidney disease
PCO polycystic ovary
PCN percutaneous nephrostomy
PCNL percutaneous nephrostomy lithotripsy
PD pancreatic duct
PDA patent ductus arteriosus
PE pulmonary embolism
PEG percutaneous endoscopic gastrostomy
PEH para esophageal hernia
PEI percutaneous ethanol injection
PET positron emission tomography
PFT pulmonary function test
PHPT primary hyperparathyroidism
PICC peripherally inserted central catheter
PID pelvic inflammatory disease
PKD polycystic kidney disease
PLD polycystic liver disease
PLP pathologic lead point
PNFC peripancreatic fluid collection
PO per-oral
PPI proton pump inhibitor
PR per-rectal
PSARP posterior sagittal anorectoplasty
PTA percutaneous trans-luminal angioplasty
PTC percutaneous transhepatic cholangiography
PTH parathyroid hormone
PUD peptic ulcer disease
PUH para umbilical hernia

PUV posterior urethral valve
PV portal vein / per vaginal
PVL Panton-Valentine-leukocidin

R
RAI radioactive iodine
RBCs red blood cells
RCT randomized control trial
RES reticuloendothelial system
RFA radiofrequency ablation
RL ringer lactate
RLL right lower quadrant
RLN recurrent laryngeal nerve
RPLND retroperitoneal lymph node dissection
RSVG reverse saphenous vein graft
RUQ rtPA recombinant tissue plasminogen activator
right upper quadrant

S
SAH sub-arachnoid hemorrhage
SBP spontaneous bacterial peritonitis/ systolic blood pressure
SC subcutaneous
SCC squamous cell carcinoma
SCM sternocleidomastoid
S\E side effect
SIMV synchronous intermittent mandatory ventilation
SIRS systemic inflammatory response syndrome
SJS Stevens-Johnson syndrome
SLE systemic lupus erythematosus
SLNBx sentinel lymph node biopsy
SMA superior mesenteric artery
SMV superior mesenteric vein
SR survival rate
SSI surgical site infection
SV stroke volume
SVC superior vena cava
SVD Spontaneous vaginal delivery
SVT supra-ventricular tachycardia
SVR systemic vascular resistance
Sx symptoms

T

TAT trans-anastomotic tube
TAH-BSO Total abdominal hysterectomy + bilateral salpingo-oophorectomy
TACE trans-arterial chemoembolization
TB tuberculosis
TBW total body water
TEF tracheoesophageal fistula
Tg thyroglobulin
TGA transposition of great vessels
TIPS transhepatic intrajugular portosystemic shunt
TLESR Transient Lower Esophagus Sphincter Relaxation
TME total mesorectal excision
TNF tumor necrosis factor
TOF tetralogy of Fallot
TPN total parenteral nutrition
TPx transplantation
TRALI Transfusion-related acute lung injury
TTTS Twin-twin transfusion syndrome
Tx treatment

U

UB urinary bladder
UC ulcerative colitis
UDT undescended testis
UES upper esophageal sphincter
UGIB upper gastrointestinal bleeding
UOP urine out put
UPJO Ureteropelvic Junction Obstruction
URTI upper respiratory tract infection
UTI urinary tract infection

V

VAC vacuum assisted closure
VBG venous blood gas
VC vasoconstriction
VD vasodilatation
VR venous return

VSD ventricular septal defect
VUR vesicoureteral reflux
vWF Von Willebrand factor

W

WBCs white blood cells
WLE Wide local excision
WOPN walled off pancreatic necrosis

Index

849

H

Hartmann's procedure, 108, 304, 317, 324, 339, 341
Heineke-Mikulicz, 237
hemangioma, 135, 290, 431, 450, 452–54, 672, 743, 783
    clinical picture, 450
    diagnosis, 451
    etiology, 450
    management, 451
    nonoperative therapy, 452
    prognosis, 452
    surgical approach and technique, 452
hematoma, 84–86, 89, 93, 95–96, 106, 121, 140, 156, 173, 205–6, 398, 679
hemigastrectomy, 263
hemoglobinopathies, 588
hemolysis, 5, 7, 25, 409
Hemolytic Reaction, 28
hemophilia A, 19
hemophilia B, 19
hemoptysis, massive, 86, 775, 788
    management, 788
hemorrhage, 26, 65–66, 71–73, 80, 82, 123, 223, 234, 276, 278, 291–92, 301, 314, 365, 412, 432, 434, 443, 453–55, 526, 532–34, 536, 578, 585, 621, 642, 653, 671–72, 679, 710
    classification of, 71
hemorrhage control, 72–73, 98, 111
hemorrhoid, 320, 384, 386
hemorrhoidectomy
    complication of, 387
    open, 386
    operative, 386
    stapler, 386
    whitehead, 386
hemostasis, ix, 17–18, 20, 22, 24, 26, 28–30, 44, 92, 105, 173, 191, 205, 242, 367, 465, 577, 688
    biology of, 17

tests for, 29
Henley loop, 263
heparin-induced thrombocytopenia and thrombosis (HITT), 21
hepatic encephalopathy, 414–15, 423, 429
hepatic hydrothorax, 421, 424–25
hepatobiliary iminodiacetic acid (HIDA), 233, 478, 481, 491, 761
hepatocellular carcinoma (HCC), 408, 415, 449, 456–57, 504, 511
hepatopulmonary syndrome, 421, 425
hepatorenal syndromes, 421, 425, 427
hereditary elliptocytosis, 587
hereditary spherocytosis, 471, 586
hernia
    congenital diaphragmatic, 763
    diagnosis, 764
    epidemiology and genetics, 763
    pathology, 764
    treatment, 764
    femoral, 145–46, 148, 151
    hiatal, 46, 189–92, 195, 200, 203, 211–12, 232, 245, 248
    approach, 201
    diagnosis, 200
    incidence and etiology, 200
    postoperative consideration and outcome, 202
    result, 202
    surgical indication, 201
    surgical technique, 201
    treatment, 201–2
    inguinal
    anatomy of inguinal anal, 145, 147
    clinical features, 726
    complication, 154–55
    diagnosis, 147
    incidence, 725
    management, 727
    pathophysiology, 147
    physical examination, 147
    postoperative complication, 727
    radiology investigation, 726
    technique, 727